Ultrasound in Obstetrics and Gynecology

A Practitioner's Guide

Ultrasound in Obstetrics and Gynecology

A Practitioner's Guide

Kathryn A. Gill, MS, RT, RDMS, FSDMS

Program Director, Institute of Ultrasound Diagnostics

Spanish Fort, Alabama

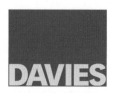

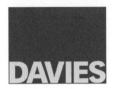

Davies Publishing, Inc.
Specialists in Ultrasound Education,
Test Preparation, and Continuing
Medical Education
32 South Raymond Avenue
Pasadena, California 91105-1961
Phone 626-792-3046
Facsimile 626-792-5308
e-mail info@daviespublishing.com
www.daviespublishing.com

Michael Davies, Publisher
Satori Design Group, Inc., Design
Charlene Locke, Production Manager
Christina J. Moose, Editorial Director
Janet Heard, Manuscript Management
Christian Jones, Production Editing
Daniel Liota, Digital Media
Gina Caprari, Editorial Associate
Stephen Beebe and Jim Baun, Illustration

Notice to Users of This Publication:

In the field of ultrasonography, knowledge, technique, and best practices are continually evolving. With new research and developing technologies, changes in methodologies, professional practices, and medical treatment may become necessary.

Sonography practitioners and other medical professionals and researchers must rely on their experience and knowledge when evaluating and using information, methods, technologies, experiments, and medications described herein, always remaining mindful of their own, their patients', their coworkers', and others' safety and well-being.

Regarding any treatments, procedures, technologies, and/or pharmaceutical products identified, users of this publication are advised to check the most current information provided by product manufacturers and professional societies to verify their latest recommendations regarding methodologies, dosages, timing of administration, practice guidelines, standards of care, and contraindications. It is the responsibility of practitioners, relying on their own experience and knowledge of their patients, to report, make recommendations, and work within these standards, in consultation with other clinicians such as referring and supervisory physicians, to determine to take all appropriate safety procedures and to determine the best treatment of each individual patient.

To the fullest extent of the law, neither Davies Publishing, Inc., nor the authors, contributors, reviewers, or editors assume any liability for any injury and/or damage to persons or property as a matter of products liability, negligence, or otherwise, or from any use or operation of any methods, products, instructions, or ideas contained in the material herein.

Library of Congress Cataloging-in-Publication Data

Gill, Kathryn A., author.
Ultrasound in obstetrics and gynecology : a practitioner's guide / Kathryn A. Gill.
    p. ; cm.
Includes bibliographical references and index.
ISBN 978-0-941022-80-4 (hardcover : alk. paper) — ISBN 0-941022-80-3 (hardcover : alk. paper)
I. Title.
[DNLM: 1. Ultrasonography, Prenatal. 2. Congenital
Abnormalities—ultrasonography. 3. Genital Diseases,
Female—ultrasonography. 4. Pregnancy Complications—ultrasonography. WQ 209]
RG628.3.U58
618.3'07543—dc23

2013019184

Printed and bound in China
ISBN 0-941022-80-3

For
Smitty and Micah Gill,
the two men in my life, for always offering
inspiration, love, and support.
You make my life complete.

Contributors

KATHRYN A. GILL, MS, RT, RDMS, FSDMS
Program Director
Institute of Ultrasound Diagnostics
Spanish Fort, Alabama

JIM BAUN, BS, RDMS, RVT, FSDMS
Clinical Consultant and Educator
Professional Ultrasound Services
San Francisco, California

GEORGE BEGA, MD
Adjunct Assistant Professor of Obstetrics and Gynecology
Department of Obstetrics and Gynecology
Thomas Jefferson University
Philadelphia, Pennsylvania

PAMELA M. FOY, MS, RDMS, FSDMS
Imaging Manager and Clinical Instructor
Department of Obstetrics and Gynecology
Clinical Assistant Professor
School of Health and Rehabilitation Sciences
The Ohio State University
Columbus, Ohio

GEORGE KOULIANOS, MD, FACOG
Director
The Center for Reproductive Medicine
Mobile, Alabama

DANIEL A. MERTON, BS, RDMS, FSDMS, FAIUM
Clinical Instructor and Technical Coordinator
    of Research
The Jefferson Ultrasound Research and Education Institute
Department of Radiology
Thomas Jefferson University Hospital
Philadelphia, Pennsylvania

BRYAN T. OSHIRO, MD
Vice Chairman
Department of Obstetrics and Gynecology
Medical Director
Perinatal Institute
Loma Linda University Medical Center/
    Children's Hospital
Loma Linda, California

JOE RODRIGUEZ, RT, RDMS
Supervisor
Ultrasound Department
Southeast Missouri Hospital
Cape Girardeau, Missouri

MISTY H. SLIMAN, BS, RT(R)(S), RDMS
Adjunct Instructor
American Institute

Reviewers

JIM BAUN, BS, RDMS, RVT, FSDMS
Clinical Consultant and Educator
Professional Ultrasound Services
San Francisco, California

NIRVIKAR DAHIYA, MD
Director—Ultrasound
Assistant Professor—Radiology
Mallinckrodt Institute of Radiology
Washington University Medical School
St. Louis, Missouri

PAMELA M. FOY, MS, RDMS, FSDMS
Imaging Manager and Clinical Instructor
Department of Obstetrics and Gynecology
Clinical Assistant Professor
School of Health and Rehabilitation Sciences
The Ohio State University
Columbus, Ohio

CATHEEJA ISMAIL, RDMS, EdD
Director—Sonography Program
The George Washington University
Washington, DC

DARLA J. MATTHEW, BAS, RT, RDMS
Program Director and Associate Professor
Diagnostic Medical Sonography
Doña Ana Community College
Las Cruces, New Mexico

SUSAN NAGER, BS, RDMS
Diagnostic Medical Ultrasound Instructor
Central Florida Institute
Orlando, Florida

Reviewers *(continued)*

REGINA SWEARENGIN, BS, RDMS
Department Chair, Sonography
Austin Community College
Austin, Texas

JILL D. TROTTER, BS, RT(R), RDMS, RVT
Director, Diagnostic Medical Sonography Program
Vanderbilt University Medical Center
Nashville, Tennessee

ELLEN T. TUCHINSKY, BA, RDMS, RDCS
Director of Clinical Education
Diagnostic Medical Sonography Program
Long Island University
Brooklyn, New York

KERRY E. WEINBERG, MA, MPA, RT(R), RDMS, RDCS, FSDMS
Director and Associate Professor
Diagnostic Medical Sonography Program
Long Island University
Brooklyn, New York

Preface

I ALWAYS KNEW I WANTED TO TEACH. As a little girl, I would line my dolls up at makeshift desks and play teacher for hours. Although my career course did not begin in education, the desire to share my knowledge persisted in the medical environment in which I found myself. At the risk of sounding ancient, I began my sonography career when the technology was so new and schools so few that there were only one or two in the whole country. The technology was foreign and the concepts were challenging, and I knew that, if I ever mastered the techniques myself, I would want to share them with others. So, here I am today writing sonography textbooks with the hope that I can make the educational experience a little less stressful and easier to understand.

There are many excellent sonography reference books related to the Ob/Gyn specialty and I don't claim to have the knowledge base that has already been demonstrated by so many exemplary physician authors. My book is intended to teach the sonography practitioner what to look for, how to document according to published guidelines, and, most important, how to scan. I attempted to organize the material in a way that makes clinical sense and is easy to follow. Each chapter offers scan tips and review questions for self-evaluation as well as the most current protocol guidelines published by the American Institute of Ultrasound in Medicine. The book is intended to provide the basics for the beginner, a good review for the Registry-bound, and a transition for the practitioner entering a more advanced perinatal environment. I use the term *practitioner* to include not only sonographers but also residents, practicing physicians, midwives, physician assistants, and anyone practicing sonography. I believe each can find something of value from this text.

The Ob/Gyn specialty is mostly fun, sometimes heartbreaking, and always challenging. When the patients' hormones are raging and their expectations of the sonography session vary, the sonography practitioner must have an exam system that allows him or her to efficiently perform the study while fielding questions and remaining composed, professional, and genuinely friendly and concerned for the patient's well-being. If this text provides the reader with the confidence required to perform studies related to the Ob/Gyn patient, I will have accomplished my goal.

Kathryn A. Gill, MS, RT, RDMS, FSDMS
Program Director
Institute of Ultrasound Diagnostics

Acknowledgments

I AM VERY PROUD TO HAVE HAD SO MANY TALENTED CONTRIBUTORS and reviewers involved in this project. Teaching can be a challenging profession, and the field of ultrasound is lucky to have so many knowledgeable sonographers willing to share their deep expertise and long experience with us. So I extend my great appreciation to Jim Baun, Dan Merton, Misty Sliman, Pamela Foy, Joe Rodriguez, Dr. George Bega, Dr. Bryan Oshiro, and Dr. George Koulianos for participating in and supporting this ambitious project. In addition, Nirvikar Dahiya, Catheeja Ismail, Darla Matthew, Susan Nager, Regina Swearengin, Jill Trotter, Ellen Tuchinsky, and Kerry Weinberg contributed their significant insights as reviewers.

I would also like to thank the manufacturers for the many images provided for so many of the chapters. The companies from which images were obtained include Siemens, Philips, Hitachi, Medison, and Toshiba. These companies are all staunch supporters of ultrasound education, and we are indebted to them for their never-ending search for the ultimate image.

I have always considered Ob/Gyn sonography to be my specialty since much of my career has involved performing studies in private Ob/Gyn practices. Although the physicians with whom I have worked are too numerous to list, I owe each one a debt of gratitude for tolerating this sonographer's constant barrage of questions regarding cases, treatments, and management options. They taught me so much and played a huge role in making me the sonographer I am today.

Finally, I would like to thank Davies Publishing for taking on this project. Mike Davies, Janet Heard, Christina Moose, Charlene Locke, Christian Jones, Dan Liota, and everyone at Davies Publishing has the patience of Job, which is more than I can say for myself. They graciously and tactfully helped me through all the ups and downs of writing, developing, and perfecting a book, and for that I am very grateful. I know everyone involved is as proud as I am of this new textbook.

Kathryn A. Gill, MS, RT, RDMS, FSDMS
Program Director
Institute of Ultrasound Diagnostics

Contents

Chapter 4 | The Second and Third Trimesters: Basic and Targeted Scans   119

Joe Rodriguez, RT, RDMS, Kathryn A. Gill, MS, RT, RDMS, FSDMS, and Misty H. Sliman, BS, RT(R)(S), RDMS

Chapter 5 | The Placenta and Umbilical Cord   179

Jim Baun, BS, RDMS, RVT, FSDMS, and Kathryn A. Gill, MS, RT, RDMS, FSDMS

Chapter 6 | Ultrasound of the Cervix during Pregnancy   215

Pamela M. Foy, MS, RDMS, FSDMS

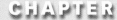

Introduction to Diagnostic Ultrasound

Kathryn A. Gill, MS, RT, RDMS, FSDMS

OBJECTIVES

After completing this chapter you should be able to:

1. Explain the advantages and limitations of B-mode ultrasound imaging.
2. Describe how the body is imaged in two dimensions.
3. List the sonographic criteria necessary to characterize a mass as cystic, solid, or complex.
4. Identify sonographic artifacts and describe their appearance.
5. Explain the relative advantages and disadvantages of the sector, linear, and curved (convex) linear transducers.
6. Demonstrate the various maneuvers used to manipulate the ultrasound transducer.
7. Describe the correct way to hold the transducer while scanning a patient.

B-MODE (BRIGHTNESS MODE) DIAGNOSTIC ULTRASOUND IMAGING provides a dynamic means of evaluating soft-tissue structures of the pelvis and pregnant uterus in cross section. Although the technique of performing diagnostic ultrasound procedures appears effortless, diagnostic ultrasound is one of the most difficult imaging modalities to perform and interpret. Because the inexperienced practitioner can make normal anatomy look abnormal, practitioners must be able to recognize normal patterns before they can appreciate pathology. To help simplify the learning process, this chapter introduces some of the basic concepts and terms used among sonographers, focusing on two-dimensional B-mode imaging. Doppler concepts and applications are addressed elsewhere, including Chapter 12.

THE ADVANTAGES AND DISADVANTAGES OF DIAGNOSTIC ULTRASONOGRAPHY

Advantages

Diagnostic ultrasonography has several advantages over other imaging modalities. In most cases, the sonographic exam is easily tolerated by patients. For evaluating the pelvic area transabdominally, the only required preparation is that the patient has a full urinary bladder. There is usually no need for elaborate bowel preparation, nor is it necessary to introduce contrast agents in order to image soft-tissue organs, as is required for other radiologic procedures. Since the images are produced by using high-frequency sound waves, the patient is not exposed to radiation. To date, no adverse human biologic effects have been demonstrated at the frequency levels used in diagnostic ultrasound. Cross-sectional imaging allows us to easily identify anatomic relationships among organs and other structures and to appreciate depth relationships. Most diagnostic ultrasound systems are portable, and so imaging is not restricted to one department or room. Finally, diagnostic ultrasound procedures are cost- and time-efficient compared to other imaging modalities (Box 1-1).

Box 1-1.	Advantages of B-mode diagnostic ultrasonography.
	Patient tolerates it well
	No bowel preparation is necessary
	Relatively noninvasive
	No radiation to patient
	Anatomic relationships are clearly shown
	Depth relationships are shown
	Time-efficient
	Cost-effective
	Portable

Disadvantages

There are only a few disadvantages to diagnostic ultrasound imaging (Box 1-2). The physics of sound propagation limits the usefulness of ultrasound somewhat in evaluating dense, calcified structures (Figure 1-1) and air-filled organs such as the gastrointestinal tract (Figure 1-2). These structures cause total reflection of the ultrasound and inhibit the sound from penetrating the anterior surface of the structure. In addition, B-mode diagnostic imaging—as distinct from Doppler ultrasonography—does not provide adequate information about function, because the organ, if present, is imaged whether it functions or not. Although efforts are being made through research to improve tissue characterization with ultrasound, the modality is not sensitive enough to distinguish **benign** from **malignant** tissue.

Box 1-2.	Disadvantages of B-mode diagnostic ultrasonography.
	Limited applications
	Inability to determine function
	Inability to distinguish benign from malignant

Nevertheless, sonographic characteristics can suggest that a mass is benign or has a high-risk potential for being malignant.

INFORMATION PROVIDED

Diagnostic ultrasound provides information about the size, shape, echo pattern, and position of organs and other structures. The sonographer knows the normal patterns of all the pelvic organs, including shape, contour,

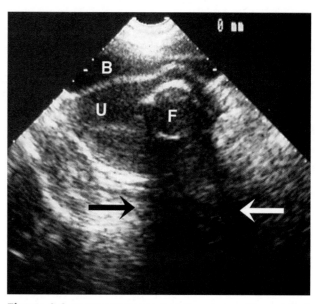

Figure 1-1. *Transverse image through a uterus with a calcified fibroid demonstrating a shadow (arrows) produced from the fibroid. U = uterus, B = bladder, F = fibroid.*

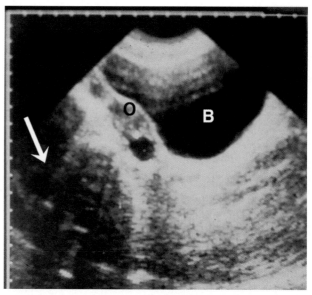

Figure 1-2. *Longitudinal image of an ovary with some shadowing posterior to it from intestinal gas (arrow). B = bladder, O = ovary.*

texture, and internal architecture and relative position. Any disruption of the normal patterns suggests an **anomaly**, or abnormality. When a mass is discovered within or adjacent to an organ, the practitioner should attempt to characterize the mass and determine its origin. To ascertain the size of pelvic organs so they can be compared to normal, measurements are taken in three dimensions. The three measurements include longitudinal, transverse, and anterior/posterior (AP) dimensions (Figure 1-3).

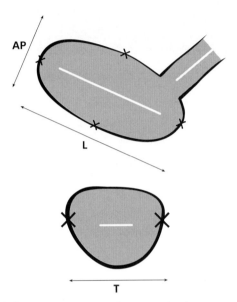

Figure 1-3. *Anatomic drawing demonstrating how to measure an organ or mass in the longitudinal (L), transverse (T), and anterior/posterior (AP) dimensions.*

SCAN PLANES, BODY ORIENTATIONS, AND LABELING

There are two basic scan planes used in diagnostic ultrasound imaging. They are longitudinal (or sagittal) and transverse.

Scan Planes

In **longitudinal** (**sagittal**) imaging, the patient's supine body is divided into right and left sections. An imaginary line down the midline is referred to as **mid-sagittal** (see Box 1-3). The longitudinal (sagittal) image is viewed as though the practitioner were looking at the patient from her right side. On the ultrasound monitor, the patient's head (**cephalic**) is on the left side of the screen and her feet (**caudal**) on the right. The top of the screen is the **anterior** aspect and the bottom of the screen is **posterior** (Figures 1-4 A and B).

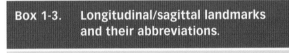

Box 1-3.	Longitudinal/sagittal landmarks and their abbreviations.

M or ML—midline (mid-sagittal)
R—to the right
L—to the left

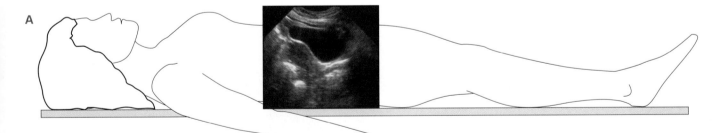

A

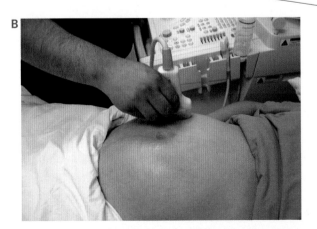

B

Figure 1-4. A *Drawing showing how the body is viewed in the longitudinal plane.* **B** *Image showing transducer placement on abdomen of a pregnant patient for longitudinal imaging. (Figure continues . . .)*

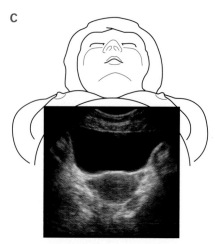

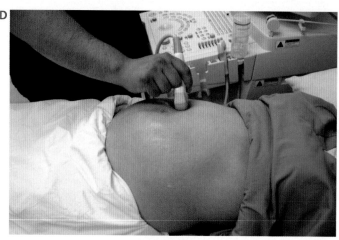

Figure 1-4, continued. C *Drawing showing how the body is viewed from the transverse plane.* **D** *Image showing transducer placement on the abdomen of a pregnant patient demonstrating the transverse orientation. Compression maneuver is also demonstrated.*

Transverse plane imaging visualizes the patient as though she were bisected by an imaginary horizontal line across the waistline into superior and inferior sections (see Box 1-4). The image is viewed as though you were looking at your patient from her feet. On the ultrasound monitor, the patient's right side is on the left side of the screen and her left side on the right. The anterior and posterior aspects are unchanged from that of the longitudinal plane (Figures 1-4 C and D). The **symphysis pubis** describes the line of the union of the bodies of the pelvic bones in the median plane, and the iliac crest or **transcrestal plane** describes the transverse plane at the level of the top of the pelvic bones.

The **coronal plane** divides the patient's body into front and back portions. When scanning in this plane in the long axis, the top of the image would be the lateral aspect, the bottom of the screen would be medial, the right side of the screen would be inferior (caudal), and the left would be superior (cephalic). The sonographer has to indicate whether he or she is scanning from the right lateral approach or the left lateral approach.

Finally, an **oblique** scan plane is any plane that is not longitudinal (sagittal), coronal (A/P), or transverse. Ultrasound has the unique ability to create any type of oblique plane, as the transducer is in the operator's hand. This also makes it imperative to have good knowledge of sonographic anatomy in all planes.

Body Orientations

Other useful terms related to scan planes and body orientations include:

Medial: Toward the center line of the body.

Lateral: Away from the center line of the body.

Proximal: Closer to the point of reference, the origin, etc.

Distal: Farther away from the point of reference, the origin, etc.

Superior: Above; toward the head; generally interchangeable with "cephalad."

Inferior: Below; toward the feet or "caudal."

Superficial: Closer to the surface/skin.

Deep: Farther down from the surface/skin.

Labeling and Documentation

Images should be labeled accurately for documentation purposes. Labeling of scans may vary according to departmental protocols. Some departments choose simply to label images by organ, as demonstrated in Figures 1-5 A and B. Others may label by plane (Figure 1-5C). Guidelines suggested by the American Institute of Ultrasound in Medicine (AIUM) and other laboratory accrediting

Box 1-4.	Transverse landmarks and their abbreviations.

S or SP—symphysis pubis

IC/TCP—iliac crest/transcrestal plane

U—umbilicus

+ = superior movement

− = inferior movement

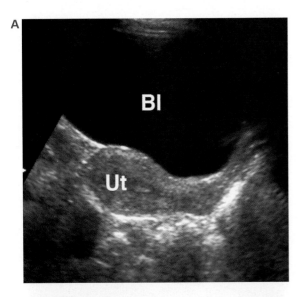

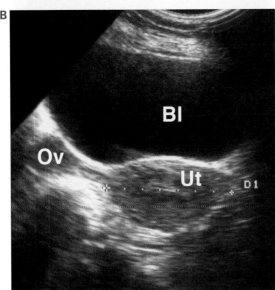

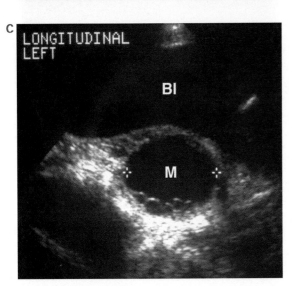

Figure 1-5. A *Longitudinal scan through a normal uterus (Ut = uterus, Bl = bladder).* **B** *Transverse scan through a normal uterus (Ut = uterus, Bl = bladder, Ov = ovary).* **C** *Longitudinal scan through a complex left adnexal mass (calipers; Bl = bladder, M = mass).*

Table 1-1.	Ultrasound labeling guidelines and examples.

Labeling Guideline	Examples
Organ/area of interest	Ovary (ov)
Plane/axis	Longitudinal (lg-long-ln-sag)
Patient position	Left lateral decubitus (LLD)

organizations recommend at the very least that images indicate (1) the organ or area of interest, (2) the plane or axis, and (3) the patient's position if it is other than **supine** (Table 1-1). Whichever labeling protocol you choose, be consistent and as specific as possible.

CHARACTERIZING TISSUE

The descriptive terms used in diagnostic ultrasound help us to characterize the texture and density of tissues. If a structure has many echoes within it, we call it **echogenic**. Echoes that are exaggerated and extremely bright are referred to as being **hyperechoic** (Figure 1-6A), which usually suggests either a very solid, dense structure or the phenomenon of echo enhancement due to the sound beam passing through a fluid component (Figure 1-6B), as described below. **Hypoechoic** describes a structure that is solid but has low-level echoes within it, while **anechoic** denotes a structure without echoes (Figure 1-7). **Echopenic** describes a mass that has a few low-level echoes but is

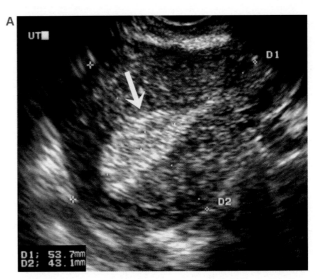

Figure 1-6. A *Longitudinal transvaginal image demonstrating a hyperechoic endometrium (arrow). (Figure continues . . .)*

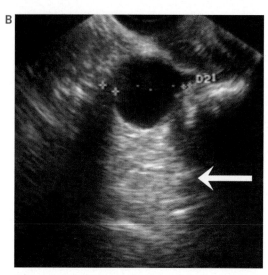

Figure 1-6, continued. B *Coronal transvaginal image of a simple cyst (calipers) showing posterior enhancement (arrow).*

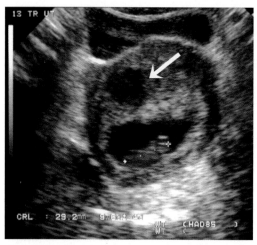

Figure 1-7. *Transverse image of a pregnant uterus. The arrow points to a small hypoechoic or echopenic lesion in the anterior myometrium that is compatible with a small fibroid.*

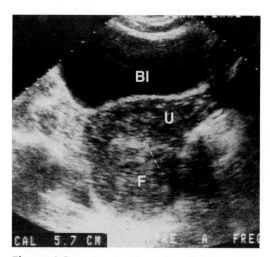

Figure 1-8. *Longitudinal image of the uterus. A fibroid is seen extending off the posterior aspect of the uterus. The fibroid is the same echogenicity (isoechoic) as the uterus. U = uterus, F = fibroid, Bl = bladder.*

less echogenic than its surrounding tissue. When characterizing two structures of equal echogenicity, the sonographer describes them as being **isoechoic** (Figure 1-8). When describing something that is cystic or fluid-filled, we refer to it as being **sonolucent** (see Figure 1-6B).

The terms *homogeneous* and *heterogeneous* are often used in conjunction with these other terms. **Homogeneous** means the echo pattern is smooth and even throughout the defined area (Figure 1-9). **Heterogeneous** indicates an irregular or uneven echo pattern that may even appear to have mixed echogenicities (Figure 1-10).

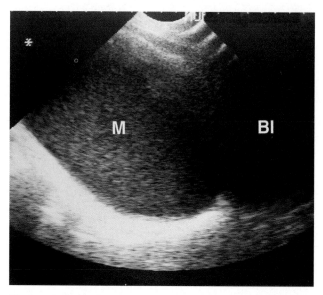

Figure 1-9. *Longitudinal scan through a complex mass containing smooth, homogeneous, low-level echoes. M = mass, Bl = bladder.*

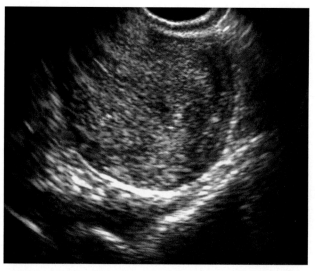

Figure 1-10. *Longitudinal transvaginal image demonstrating a mottled, heterogeneous echo pattern of the uterine myometrium.*

ARTIFACTS

The sonographer must be able to recognize sonographic artifacts, which can mislead one into making a false diagnosis. Conversely, some artifacts are helpful, suggesting the nature of the structure being imaged. For example, posterior enhancement is a characteristic associated with structures containing fluid.

Shadowing

Shadowing is the opposite of posterior enhancement. A shadow is produced when the sound beam is completely reflected or absorbed by the structure being imaged. Posterior shadowing indicates that the tissue producing the shadow is so dense that sound cannot penetrate it or that it completely absorbs sound, inhibiting further penetration (Figure 1-11A). Gas- or air-filled structures also reflect sound and produce shadows (Figure 1-11B). Finally, shadows may result from **refraction** or bending of the sound beam. If an echo is not received by the transducer because of refraction, it will not be displayed on the image. This phenomenon often occurs at the edges of cysts or curved surfaces (see Figure 1-6B).

Posterior Enhancement (Through-Transmission) Artifacts

Posterior enhancement—also known as through-transmission—is a characteristic associated with structures containing fluid. When the sound beam travels through fluid, the echoes posterior to the fluid are brighter than the normal surrounding tissues. Posterior enhancement tells us that there is, indeed, some fluid component within the structure (see Figure 1-6B).

Reverberation Artifacts

Reverberation artifacts are the result of the sound signal bouncing back and forth off of two strong reflective interfaces and can have several different patterns. A reverberation artifact is frequently seen when a fluid-filled structure is in close proximity to the transducer. A good example is the anterior region of the bladder when scanning the pelvis. Soft specular echoes can obliterate details of the anterior bladder wall (Figure 1-12A). Surgical clips, intrauterine devices, or a strong air interface may cause a different type of reverberation artifact called a **ring-down** or **comet-tail artifact**, which appears as multiple parallel lines shaped like a tornado (Figure 1-12B). Comet-tail artifacts are usually smaller versions of ring-down artifacts.

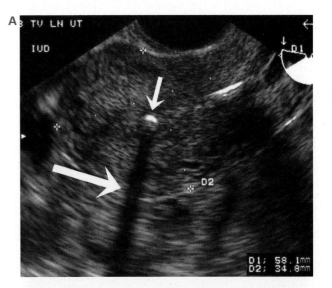

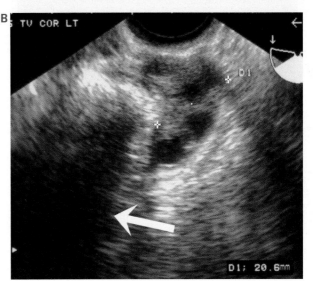

Figure 1-11. A *Longitudinal transvaginal image of a uterus showing shadowing (large arrow) from the endometrial cavity produced by an intrauterine contraceptive device (small arrow).* **B** *Air-filled bowel producing shadowing (arrow) adjacent to the ovary (calipers).*

Side Lobes and Slice-Thickness Artifacts

Side lobe and slice-thickness artifacts interject echoes where they should not be. These are of clinical importance because, for instance, they can make a cyst look like it contains debris and affect the accuracy of measurements (see Figure 1-12A). **Side lobe artifacts** arise from sound beams that lie outside the main beam, which is over the area of interest. The term *side lobe* is used when referring to a single-element transducer, while *grating lobes* is the term associated with the use of a multi-element transducer. With **slice-thickness artifacts**, a simple cyst may fill in with soft echoes, or the wall of the bladder may appear thicker than it actually is.

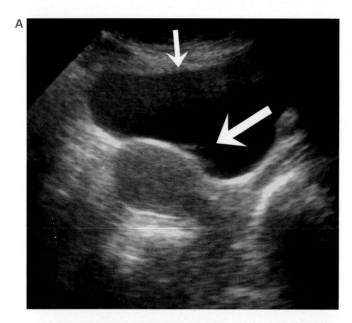

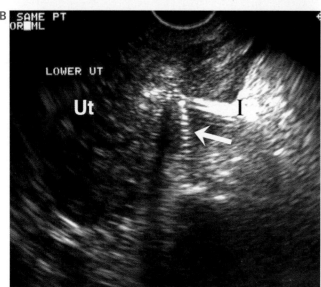

Figure 1-12. A *Longitudinal view of the uterus. Note the soft specular echoes in the anterior aspect of the bladder corresponding to reverberation artifact (small arrow). Slice-thickness artifact is demonstrated by the large arrow.* **B** *Transvaginal image of the uterus. The ring-down artifact (arrow) is produced by an intrauterine contraceptive device (IUCD) that has perforated the lower uterine segment. Ut = uterus, I = IUCD.*

This is because sonography images in two dimensions (height and width), but the anatomic slice actually has three dimensions (height, width, and thickness). When all three dimensions are compressed into two, tissues may be superimposed, creating artifactual echoes that result in diagnostic ambiguity. These artifacts can be eliminated by repositioning the transducer, changing the frequency, and/or adjusting the focal zone.

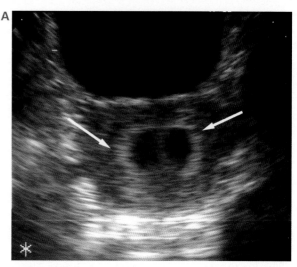

Figure 1-13. *Split-image artifact and corrected view.* **A** *This transverse image shows what appear to be two intrauterine gestational sacs (arrows) that are actually artifactual (split image). Following page:* **B** *and* **C** *With a change in transducer position, only one sac is evident on these longitudinal and transverse images of the same patient.*

Mirror-Image Artifacts

Mirror-image artifacts occur when the sound beam hits a curved structure, focusing and reflecting the sound like a mirror. This most often occurs when scanning pelvic structures through the bladder. A mirror image of the true structure appears immediately posterior to the original reflector.

Split-Image Artifacts

The **split-image artifact** is caused by refraction of the sound as it travels through abdominal muscles. It produces a duplicate image beside the original reflector (Figure 1-13A). Again, a change in transducer placement will verify whether the appearance is artifactual or not (Figures 1-13 B and C).

Propagation Velocity Artifacts

A **propagation velocity artifact** causes a misregistration of information due to the change in sound velocity as it passes through tissues of varying densities and stiffness. If the propagation speed of the ultrasound is slower than expected (i.e., 1540 meters per second), the scanner interprets and displays these delayed echoes as being positioned deeper than the actual structure.

Reverberation and mirror artifacts are also encountered in Doppler ultrasonography.

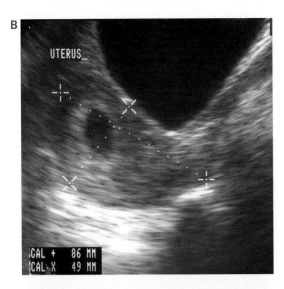

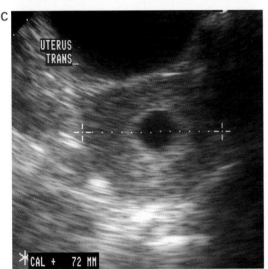

Figure 1-13, continued.

CHARACTERIZING MASSES

Three types of masses can be defined with diagnostic ultrasound: the cyst, solid mass, and mixed or complex mass. Table 1-2 describes the sonographic characteristics specific to these three types of masses. Doppler findings also can be characterized, as described in Chapter 12.

The Cyst

A simple **cyst** is a mass filled with clear, serous fluid. It should have a well-defined border with a strong back wall, no internal echoes, good posterior enhancement, and refractive shadows (Figure 1-14). A mass can be defined as a simple cyst only if it meets *all* the criteria for a cyst—its borders are well-defined, it has no internal echoes, and it exhibits posterior enhancement.

Table 1-2.   Characterizing masses.

Cyst	Solid	Complex
Well-defined borders	Irregular borders	Cystic and solid
No internal echoes	Multiple internal echoes	
Posterior enhancement	No posterior enhancement	

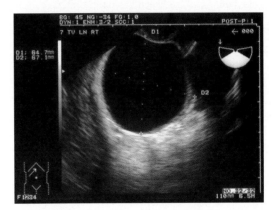

Figure 1-14. *Transvaginal image through a simple cyst.*

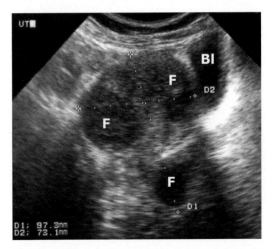

Figure 1-15. *Longitudinal view of uterus. This image demonstrates a uterus containing multiple defined fibroids, solid in echogenicity. Bl = bladder, F = fibroid.*

The Solid Mass

The **solid mass** has ill-defined or irregular borders and contains multiple internal echoes. A solid mass may have variable echogenicity; it may, for instance, be hypoechoic, hyperechoic, and isoechoic to surrounding tissues (Figure 1-15).

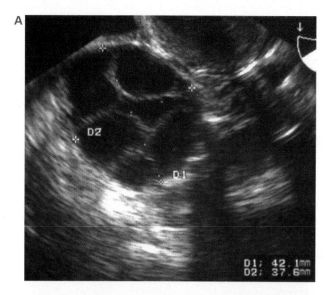

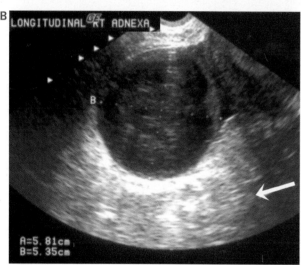

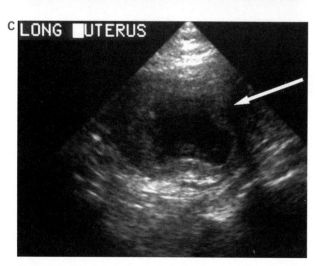

Figure 1-16. A *Transvaginal image demonstrating a multisep-tated, cystic mass (calipers).* **B** *Longitudinal image demonstrating a hemorrhagic cyst in the right adnexa. Although it contains many echoes, note the posterior enhancement (arrow), which indicates fluid components.* **C** *Image of a uterine fibroid undergoing cystic degeneration centrally (arrow).*

The Mixed (or Complex) Mass

The third type of mass is the mixed or complex mass. A **mixed/complex mass** has both cystic and solid characteristics. Three common types of complex masses are regularly seen: those that are predominantly cystic, those that are predominantly solid, and those that contain thick fluid (Box 1-5).

- *Predominantly cystic complex mass*: A complex cyst—a hemorrhagic cyst, for example, or a cystic tumor such as a multiseptated cystadenoma—is a complex mass that is predominantly cystic (Figures 1-16 A and B).

- *Predominantly solid complex mass*: This kind of complex mass includes degenerating tumors. Any solid mass that grows rapidly or outgrows its blood supply will necrose in a process called **cystic degeneration** (Figure 1-16C).

- *Complex masses containing thick fluid*: Blood or pus are examples of thick fluid that complex masses may contain. **Hematomas** and **abscesses** can look very similar sonographically (Figure 1-17). Pus tends to produce more posterior enhancement than blood

Box 1-5.	Types of complex masses.
	Predominantly cystic
	Predominantly solid
	Contain thick fluid

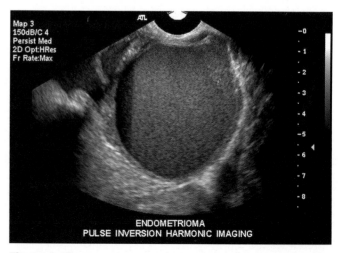

Figure 1-17. *Image of an endometrioma demonstrating very smooth homogeneous internal contents consistent with thick bloody fluid.*

because red blood cells refract sound and the protein content of blood causes more sound absorption. Accompanying clinical information should help to differentiate the two.

CLINICAL DATA

The sonographic examination of an organ consists of four basic evaluations:

1. Shape
2. Echo pattern
3. Position
4. Size

The practitioner must verify that the shape, echo pattern, size, and position of the organ are normal. Any disruption of normal contour, position, size, or echo pattern suggests an abnormality or variant. Knowledge of normal anatomy and normal sonographic patterns is critical in performing diagnostic ultrasound examinations and in making the proper diagnosis.

Another critical element in making a correct diagnosis is the collection of adequate and pertinent clinical information. Different disease processes can have similar sonographic presentations. The combination of clinical information and sonographic findings produces the most correct diagnosis. Many practitioners use clinical data sheets to collect specific information related to the exam, including information about other imaging tests. As illustrated in Appendix C, these forms should address the patient's physical symptoms as well as laboratory tests, past history, and results from other imaging modalities.

TRANSDUCER FORMATS

The format of an ultrasonographic image depends on the type of transducer that is used. There are three primary transducer formats and image shapes (Figure 1-18):

Sector Format

The **sector** image is a triangular pie-shaped wedge. The sector transducer has a smaller face (or "footprint") that allows for scanning in small or tight spaces such as between ribs and under the pubic bone. The main disadvantage of the sector format is that the near field is sacrificed by the apices of the sector image. Images are produced by a single piezoelectric element that sends and receives sound waves.

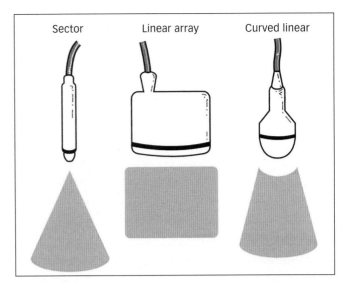

Figure 1-18. *Illustration demonstrating the various shapes of images produced by sector, linear, and curved array transducers. Reprinted with permission from Gill KA: Abdominal Ultrasound: A Practitioner's Guide. Philadelphia, Saunders, 2001.*

Linear Array Format

The **linear array** format is rectangular in shape and allows the practitioner to image a wider field of view. This type of transducer is excellent for scanning second and third trimester pregnancies. Images are produced by multiple piezoelectric elements that are aligned and fired in a sequential, linear fashion.

Convex or Curved Linear Format

The **convex** or **curved linear** format is a good compromise between the sector and the linear array. The footprint or face of the transducer is slightly smaller than that of the linear array, and the curve makes it easier to maintain contact with the skin in small, curved, or depressed areas, as, for instance, with intercostal scanning—scanning between the two costal margins at the xiphoid process—of the liver, spleen, or kidneys. Images are produced in the same manner as with the linear array, except that the elements are aligned in a convex curve.

Phased Array Format

A **phased array** transducer has multiple elements arranged in a circular fashion. Although these elements transmit and receive sound in the same manner as other array transducers, the image shape is that of a sector scan (triangular) because of the circular alignment of the piezoelectric elements.

TRANSDUCER MANIPULATION

Taming the transducer is one of the sonographer's greatest challenges. Good scanning technique requires eyehand coordination and a lot of practice.

Terms used in describing transducer manipulation include *sliding, rocking, tilting* or *angling, rotating,* and *compression*:

- **Sliding** refers to gross movement of the transducer from one location to another and can be done in any direction (Figure 1-19).

- **Rocking** the transducer toward or away from an indicator makes it possible to center the point of interest or actually to extend the field of view in one direction. Another term for this is **in-plane motion**, as it allows for visualization of more anatomy in the original plane slice (Figure 1-20).

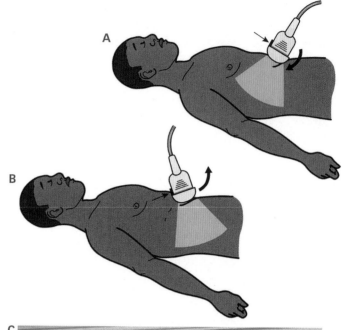

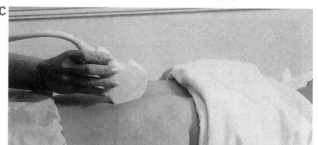

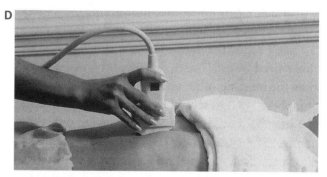

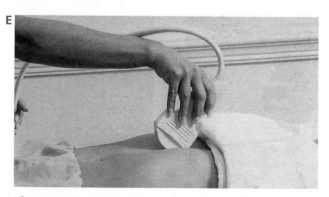

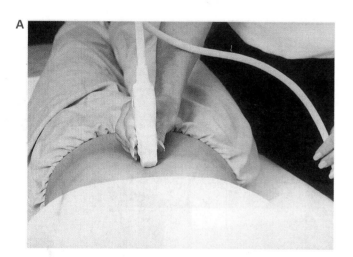

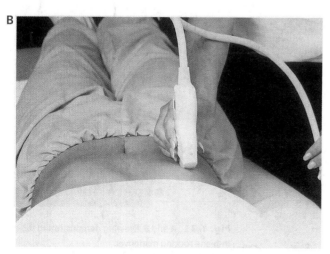

Figure 1-19. A, B *Sliding the transducer from midline to the middle of the right costal. Reprinted with permission from Gill KA:* Abdominal Ultrasound: A Practitioner's Guide. *Philadelphia, Saunders, 2001.*

Figure 1-20. A, B *Rocking the transducer.* **C–E** *Images demonstrating the in-plane rocking motion. Reprinted with permission from Gill KA:* Abdominal Ultrasound: A Practitioner's Guide. *Philadelphia, Saunders, 2001.*

- **Tilting** or **angling** the transducer from side to side (also known as **cross-plane motion**) makes it possible to visualize other planes in the same axis. One can evaluate an entire organ by sweeping through it from side to side and from top to bottom because the sweep is perpendicular to the visualized plane (Figure 1-21).

- **Rotating** the transducer from the 12 o'clock to the 9 o'clock position while holding the transducer in the proper longitudinal plane results in an image of the transverse plane. Rotation of the transducer off of the true longitudinal or transverse plane results in an *oblique view* (Figure 1-22).

- **The compression maneuver**—gently pressing down with the transducer—may be used to displace bowel gas, compress adipose tissue, separate structures, or determine tissue response. When compression is utilized, it should be done gradually and always with consideration of the patient's comfort (Figure 1-23).

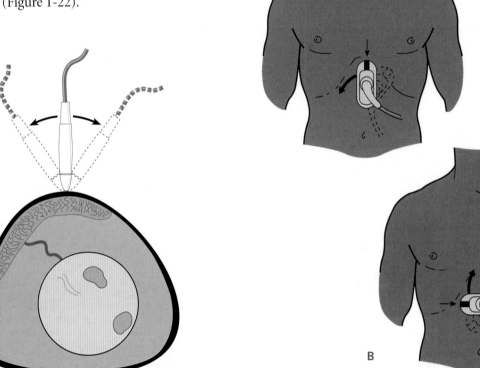

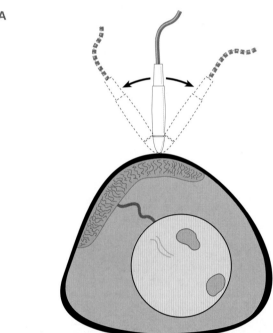

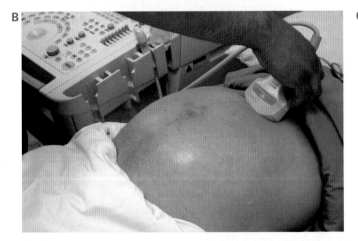

Figure 1-21. A *Tilting the transducer.* **B** *Demonstration of the transducer being tilted cross plane down toward the patient's feet.*

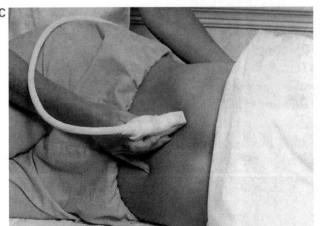

Figure 1-22. A, B *Rotating the transducer.* **C** *Image of a patient in the left lateral decubitus position with the transducer rotated counterclockwise from the longitudinal into the right costal margin. Reprinted with permission from Gill KA: Abdominal Ultrasound: A Practitioner's Guide. Philadelphia, Saunders, 2001.*

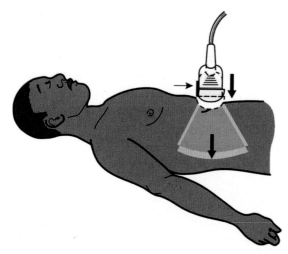

Figure 1-23. *Compression is applied by gently pushing down on the transducer and applying pressure evenly across the entire length of the transducer. Reprinted with permission from Gill KA:* Abdominal Ultrasound: A Practitioner's Guide. *Philadelphia, Saunders, 2001.*

See "Transducer Insertion and Manipulation" in the following introduction to transvaginal technique for additional techniques of probe manipulation used in transvaginal studies.

INTRODUCTION TO TRANSVAGINAL TECHNIQUE

First a note on terminology. The terms ***transvaginal*** and ***endovaginal*** are commonly used interchangeably. So too are the terms ***transabdominal*** (through the abdominal wall) and ***transvesical*** (through the urinary bladder). For instance, one might say, "A transvesical ultrasound examination is performed before an endovaginal examination in order to evaluate the entire pelvis." One might also use the equivalent statement, "A transabdominal ultrasound examination is performed before a transvaginal examination in order to evaluate the entire pelvis." Transabdominal and transvesical examinations both use the anterior approach, while the transvesical examination specifically utilizes the full urinary bladder as an **acoustic window**. Sometimes we do perform transabdominal examinations when the urinary bladder is empty. Nevertheless, it is common for ultrasound practitioners to use these terms interchangeably.

Advantages

Transvaginal sonography is an excellent complement to the transabdominal pelvic evaluation because it can provide additional information that in many cases cannot be obtained with the traditional transvesical approach. Because transvaginal sonography relies on higher-frequency transducers (5–7.5 MHz), tissue resolution is improved. The transducer is placed immediately adjacent to the pelvic structures, and therefore there is no need for great depth penetration to image through abdominal wall, fat, and bowel. Large obese patients and those with thick scarring from previous operations are no longer the challenge they once were. The endometrium and fundal region of the retroflexed uterus can be better imaged as the sound beam can be angled so that it is more perpendicular to the anatomy (Figure 1-24). Products of conception can be

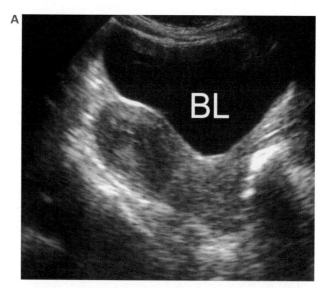

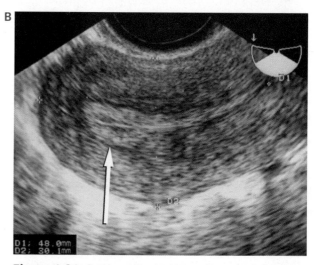

Figure 1-24. A *Transabdominal image through the uterus using the bladder (BL) as an acoustic window. The endometrial stripe cannot be well-defined.* **B** *Transvaginal image showing improved resolution of the endometrium (arrow). Following page:* **C** *Transabdominal image of the right ovary (calipers) revealing little detail of the ovarian architecture (BL = bladder).* **D** *Transvaginal technique allows for visualization of the ovarian parenchyma and individual follicles (arrows).*

imaged 1–2 weeks earlier, and there is no need for bladder filling prior to the examination. The vaginal transducer can also be used to locate areas of tenderness and to help rule out adhesions by checking for organ mobility. See Box 1-6.

Disadvantages

Although transvaginal sonography can provide valuable, additional information, it is not the recommendation of this author to use the technique solely. Due to the lack of penetration provided by higher frequencies, the depth of penetration is only about 6 cm; therefore, anatomy positioned higher in the pelvis will not be imaged. An enlarged uterus filled with fibroids cannot be adequately evaluated, nor can vaginal masses such as Gartner's duct

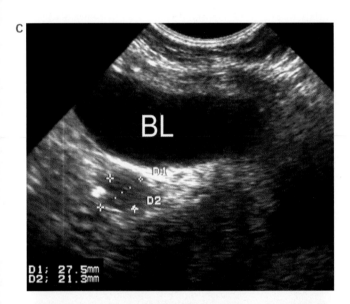

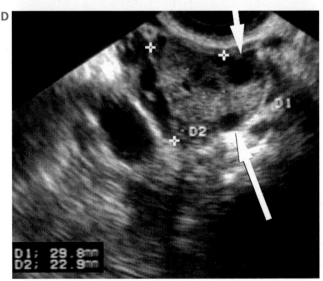

Figure 1-24, continued.

Box 1-6.	Advantages of transvaginal sonography.

Provides information that cannot be obtained transabdominally.

Tissue resolution is improved because of the high-frequency transvaginal transducers.

Large obese patients and those with surgical scarring are more easily imaged.

Endometrium and fundus of a retroflexed uterus are better imaged.

Products of conception can be imaged 1–2 weeks earlier.

Bladder filling is not required.

Areas of tenderness can be localized and evaluated.

Adhesions can be ruled out by confirming organ mobility.

cysts. As the bladder begins to fill, pelvic anatomy is displaced out of the field of view, and artifactual refractive shadows from the bladder edge interfere with imaging. Because the vagina limits transducer movement somewhat, the field of view is also limited. Finally, the transvaginal image gives us a more magnified view of the anatomy, and many times we are not able to appreciate surrounding structures for orientation purposes or to view a mass or structure in its entirety on one image. See Box 1-7.

Box 1-7.	Disadvantages of transvaginal sonography.

Depth of penetration is only about 6 cm, so anatomy higher in the pelvis cannot be imaged.

An enlarged, fibroid-filled uterus cannot be adequately evaluated.

Vaginal masses (e.g., Gartner's duct cysts) cannot be adequately evaluated.

Bladder filling can displace pelvic anatomy from the field of view and can create artifactual refractive shadows.

Field of view is somewhat limited by the limitations of probe manipulation.

The magnified transvaginal image can interfere with orientation and make it difficult to view a mass or structure in its entirety.

One still needs a global view of the pelvis in order to perform a thorough and complete pelvic examination. A transvaginal study without benefit of the transabdominal perspective will eventually result in missed anatomy and pathology. Limited studies performed for embryonic/ fetal viability, follicular monitoring, confirmation of an **intrauterine pregnancy** (**IUP**) (any pregnancy that takes place within the womb), and the like are acceptable but should be documented as limited exams.

Contraindications

Sonographers often make judgment calls concerning images taken during an examination or the technique to be utilized. In some circumstances, transvaginal studies should not be performed, such as in virginal patients, young or old. It is imperative to inquire if the patient is or has been sexually active before performing a vaginal study. This type of questioning should be done in private, away from attending friends or relatives, since the patient may not want them to be privy to this information.

Vaginal atrophy or stenosis is not uncommon among elderly patients and may be seen in patients who have had radiation treatment as well. A transvaginal study would be quite uncomfortable for these patients and may even tear delicate membranes.

Transvaginal studies are also contraindicated in obstetric patients who present with bleeding and a dilated cervix. With cervical dilatation, the risks of introducing infection are increased, as are spontaneous abortion and premature rupture of membranes (PROM).

Others who should not be scanned transvaginally include those with cervical incompetence and a bleeding placenta previa. If the vaginal perspective is needed in these cases, translabial or transperineal scanning can be performed with the transabdominal transducer. See Box 1-8.

Box 1-8.	Contraindications for transvaginal sonography.

Virginal patients

Vaginal atrophy or stenosis

Obstetric patients with bleeding and dilated cervix

Cervical incompetence

Bleeding placenta previa

Instrumentation

As noted above, several types and formats of transducers are commercially available, including sector, linear, curved linear, and phased array. Fields of view range from 85 degree angles to 240 degrees. When evaluating equipment, bear in mind that your choice of transducer may significantly limit your ability to see well if the angle of your field of view is less than 90 degrees. Additional options available include varying the degree of angle, variable focuses, variable frequencies, and a steerable beam.

Transducer housings may have straight handles or bent ("broken") handles (Figures 1-25 A and B). Straight handles are easier to aim, but the bent handles are easier to manipulate if you do not have a gynecologic table. Both are handled similarly in the sagittal plane, but coronal viewing requires more thought with the bent handle because the transducer must be rotated 180 degrees to view the opposite sides of the pelvis. Coronal viewing with the straight handle is accomplished by simply rotating counterclockwise 90 degrees toward you as you would for transverse imaging transabdominally.

Patient Preparation

The vaginal study is a very intimate examination and patients may be somewhat reluctant at first. It is important to take the time to explain the procedure in detail and to answer any questions she may have. Let her know that additional information can be obtained transvaginally, and reassure her that the transducer will be inserted only an inch or two. It might be helpful to use a comparison, such as how far one inserts a tampon or suppository. Additionally, explain that the procedure should not be uncomfortable but, if it becomes so, she should let you know. Once she agrees to have the examination performed, she should be instructed to empty her bladder completely and disrobe from the waist down.

Transducer Preparation

Some recommend preparing the transducer in front of the patient so they can see that the transducer is cleansed, disinfected, and protected by a sheath. Nevertheless, many practitioners prefer to do this while the patient is dressing to save valuable time. The transducer should be cleansed well between patients. Guidelines for cleaning and preparing endocavitary ultrasound transducers published by the American Institute of Ultrasound in Medicine appear in Appendix B.

Once the transducer is cleaned a small dollop of gel is applied to the tip. It is then covered by a protective sheath. If the patient has a known infection, it may be an indication to double sheath the probe. One may choose to use condoms, surgical gloves, or commercially available probe covers. Condoms have been shown to have fewer leakage problems than some commercial probe covers (see Appendix B). Another consideration in choosing probe covers is whether they contain latex or not. Latex allergies are not uncommon, and symptoms can vary from mild welting to severe systemic anaphylaxis. It has been reported that 18%–40% of spina bifida patients are

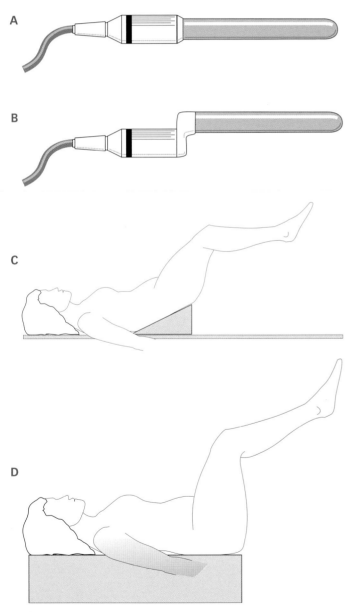

Figure 1-25. A, **B** *The architecture of the straight and bent-handle endovaginal transducers.* **C** *A wedge sponge elevating the patient's hips but not the upper body.* **D** *Elevation of upper and lower body. (Figure continues . . .)*

latex-sensitive. Patients should be questioned about latex sensitivity. Ask them if they have ever experienced a rash, itching, or wheezing after inflating a toy balloon or wearing latex gloves. Latex sensitivities should be reported, and patients should be advised on how to inform others of their allergy. Gloves that are labeled "hypoallergenic" may not always prevent adverse reactions.

Patient Positioning

The patient is positioned on the exam table in the supine lithotomy position. Make sure that she is properly draped and that she is not unnecessarily exposed. A chaperone policy needs to be established when male sonographers are responsible for performing transvaginal studies.

Ideally, a gynecologic table with stirrups and a break-away feature allows for easy performance of the vaginal exam. If such a table is not available, elevate the patient's hips so that the transducer can be manipulated properly for adequate visualization of the uterus and ovaries. This can be accomplished by using sponges or a stack of sheets placed under the hips. Care should be taken to elevate the upper body as well so any free fluid in the pelvis will remain in the pelvis (Figures 1-25 C and D).

Transducer Insertion and Manipulation

The sheathed transducer can be inserted by the sonographer or the patient. Lubricate the end of the transducer with KY jelly or other coupling agent (about 5 cc) for easy insertion. Beware, however, that KY jelly can be spermicidal and should not be used during a fertility-assisted procedure such as ovarian follicular monitoring or artificial insemination. These studies are usually performed during mid-cycle, when the cervical mucus is sufficient for comfortable insertion of the transducer.

Once the transducer is inserted, there are four scanning motions that will be employed. They are angling/tilting, push/pull, rotating, and anterior abdominal pressure (Figures 1-25 E–G). **Angling/tilting** is performed from side to side and up and down in a sweeping motion. **Rotating** the transducer allows you to go from the sagittal to the coronal plane. The transducer should always be rotated in counterclockwise direction so that the orientation of the right and left side of the patient remains consistent. Because you cannot image the entire uterus in one picture, the transducer will have to be pushed in deep for imaging the uterine fundus and must be pulled out slowly for imaging the cervix. Sometimes, anatomy is superiorly located or

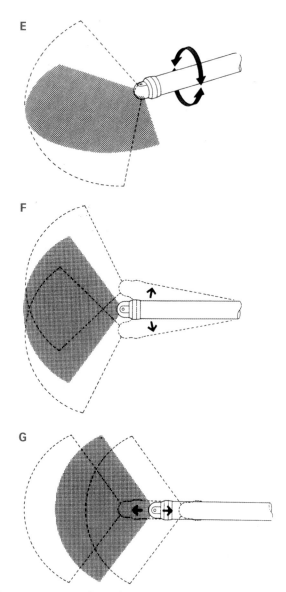

Figure 1-25, continued. E–G *Scanning motions used with transvaginal technique. Reprinted with permission of the Department of Obstetrics and Gynecology, New York University Medical Center.*

just beyond the field of view. In these cases, pressing on the anterior abdomen may help reposition the structure of interest closer to the transducer for better visualization.

Image Orientation

The most difficult part of transvaginal scanning is understanding the image orientation. Organ shapes, echogenicities, and pathologies are the same transvaginally as they are transabdominally. This is true for measurements as well. Other than initial disorientation, nothing about sonographic characteristics is changed. Once you understand how we are looking at the anatomy, image orientation will make sense.

Let's start with what we are most comfortable with, the transabdominal view. Using the full urinary bladder as a window, the practitioner places the transducer on the anterior abdomen and the **long-axis** or longitudinal view of the uterus is demonstrated (Figure 1-26A). A full-bladder technique is required for transabdominal scanning. The filled urinary bladder serves as an acoustic window through which the sound beam can be transmitted. It also displaces the uterus so it lies more perpendicularly to the scan plane, and it helps move the air-filled bowel out of the field of view (Figure 1-26B). Finally, the urinary bladder can serve as an internal cystic reference. (Because vaginal studies are performed with an empty urinary bladder, the patient is instructed to void completely [Figure 1-26C].)

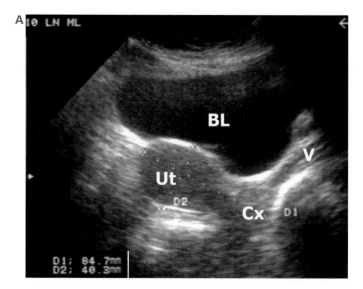

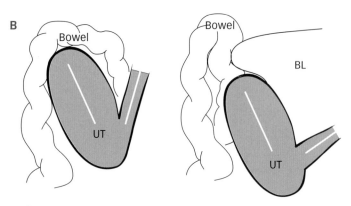

Figure 1-26. A *Longitudinal image of the uterus performed transabdominally through the filled urinary bladder. BL = bladder, Ut = uterus, Cx = cervix, V = vagina.* **B** *Drawing demonstrating how the full bladder affects the pelvic anatomy. UT = uterus, BL = bladder. Following page:* **C** *Transabdominal image through the longitudinal uterus after bladder has been emptied. Bladder residual (arrow). Ut = uterus, Cx = cervix, V = vagina.* **D** *Same Image as C rotated 90 degrees counterclockwise.*

Now rotate this transabdominal image counterclockwise 90 degrees to see the image as if it were performed transvaginally (Figure 1-26D). In the sagittal plane, the bladder will appear in the upper left corner of the image, while the cervix will be seen in the upper right corner (Figure 1-27). As you look at the image, the patient's head would be at the bottom of the image and her feet toward the top of the image. Her anterior abdomen would be toward the left side of the image and her posterior aspect toward the right. We are viewing her anatomy as if she were standing on her head facing the left side of the screen (Figure 1-28). When viewing an **anteflexed**

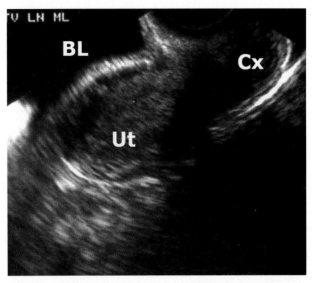

Figure 1-27. *Transvaginal image through the uterus in the longitudinal plane. BL = bladder, Ut = uterus, Cx = cervix.*

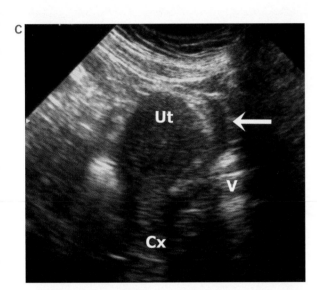

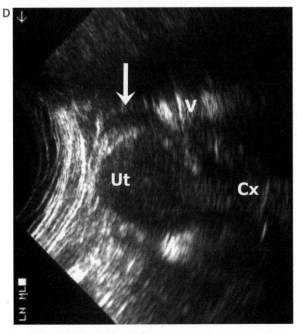

Figure 1-26, continued.

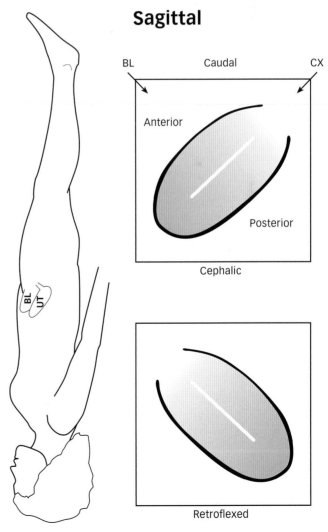

Figure 1-28. *How we view the pelvic anatomy (longitudinally) transvaginally.*

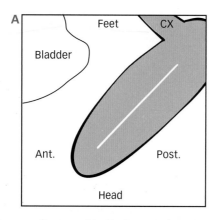

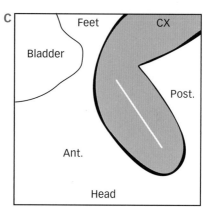

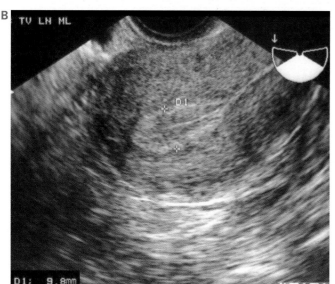

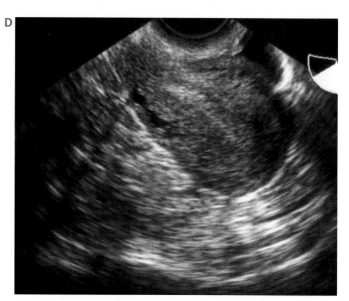

Figure 1-29. A *The longitudinal anteflexed uterus viewed transvaginally.* **B** *Transvaginal image of an anteflexed uterus in the longitudinal plane.* **C** *The longitudinal retroflexed uterus viewed transvaginally.* **D** *Transvaginal image of a retroflexed uterus in the longitudinal plane.*

uterus, the endometrial stripe points toward the left lower corner of the image (Figures 1-29 A and B). If the uterus is **retroflexed**, the endometrial stripe points in the opposite direction, toward the right lower corner of the image (Figures 1-29 C and D).

Coronal imaging maintains the standard right/left orientation used in transabdominal scanning. The only thing different is that the patient's caudal end is toward the top of the image and her cephalic end is at the bottom. We are viewing her as if she were standing on her head with her back side facing us (Figure 1-30).

Pitfalls

The bowel can still be a problem when performing transvaginal studies, especially if the patient has forced fluids in order to fill her bladder for the transabdominal study. Still, active peristalsis should be apparent. Avoid imaging

bowel patterns unless, of course, one sees bowel-related pathology. Static images of bowel can be mistaken for complex adnexal pathology (Figure 1-31).

Engorged pelvic vasculature can be mistaken for dilated fallopian tubes or appear as follicles in an ovary when scanned transversely (Figure 1-32). If one's imaging equipment has color Doppler capability, applying color will provide the answer. Dilated veins caused by pelvic congestion can be identified by slightly increasing the overall gain and watching for the swirling motion of the blood flow within the vessel. This is a helpful technique if color Doppler is not available. Arcuate vessels of the uterus are easily seen with transvaginal technique and should not be mistaken for myometrial cysts (Figure 1-33).

Free pelvic fluid is a common transvaginal finding, especially if a patient is in the middle of her menstrual cycle. One almost always sees a little free fluid in patients during

A

Coronal

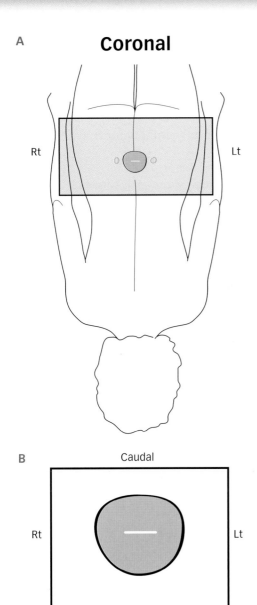

B

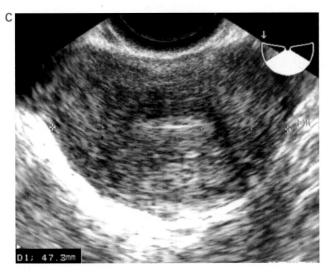

Figure 1-30. A, B *How we view the pelvic anatomy (coronal) transvaginally.* **C** *Coronal transvaginal image through the uterus.*

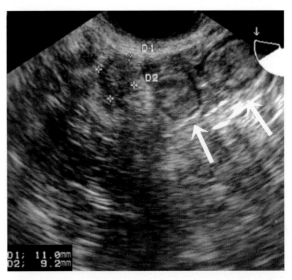

Figure 1-31. *Transvaginal image showing fecal-filled bowel (arrows). A small postmenopausal ovary is being measured between the calipers.*

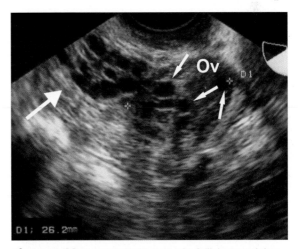

Figure 1-32. *Transvaginal image of a follicle-containing ovary (small arrows) with engorged vessels (large arrow) adjacent to it. Ov = ovary.*

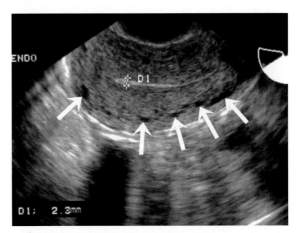

Figure 1-33. *Longitudinal transvaginal image of the uterus showing prominent arcuate vessels (arrows). The endometrium is being measured (calipers).*

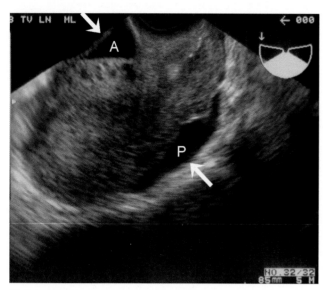

Figure 1-34. *Longitudinal transvaginal image showing free fluid (arrows) in the anterior and posterior cul-de-sacs. A = anterior, P = posterior.*

their reproductive years; it should not be mistaken for pathologic fluid. Moderate free fluid from a ruptured cyst or bleeding will appear, transvaginally, to be quite obvious (Figure 1-34).

STARTING OUT

Now you are ready to begin scanning. Practice makes perfect, and your technique and scan speed will improve over time. In the beginning stages, scan slowly so that you have time to recognize the anatomy as it appears on the display, and how the sonographic image interrelates with the actual anatomy as it is being insonated. If you have to change your transducer position, you should utilize one motion at a time. For example, you should not rock and tilt at the same time. During the learning process, you have to be able to see which motion gives you the desired effects. So tilt or angle first, and then rock to center. Another rule of thumb is to get your patient to help you whenever possible. Give the patient instructions such as changing her position on the table or emptying her bladder. Consider your patient at all times, and tell her to inform you if anything you do becomes uncomfortable.

Establish an exam system and follow it with each and every patient you examine. Following a specific protocol guarantees that each patient receives a complete and thorough examination. Additional images and views may be necessary when pathology or variants are observed. The additional information collected allows for tailoring

exams to each patient's needs. Scanning guidelines recommended by the American Institute of Ultrasound in Medicine can be found in Appendix B. These guidelines provide an excellent basis for establishing your own scanning protocols. Moreover, adherence to the AIUM guidelines represents a minimum standard of care.

REFERENCES

DuBose TJ. *Fetal Sonography.* Philadelphia, Saunders, 1996, pp 37–44.

Gill KA, Tempkin BB: Introduction to ultrasound of human disease. In Curry RA, Tempkin BB: *Sonography: An Introduction to Normal Structure and Function,* 2nd Edition. Philadelphia, Saunders, 2004, pp 497–512.

Hagan-Ansert SL: Introduction to abdominal scanning: techniques and protocols. In Hagan-Ansert SL (ed): *Textbook of Diagnostic Ultrasonography,* 7th Edition. St. Louis, Elsevier Mosby, 2012, pp 132–164.

Hedrick WR, Hykes DL, Starchman DE: *Ultrasound Physics and Instrumentation,* 4th Edition. St. Louis, Elsevier Mosby, 2005.

Hofer M: *Ultrasound Teaching Manual,* 2nd Edition. New York, Thieme, 2005.

Holland CK, Fowlkes JB: Biological effects and safety. In Rumack CM, Wilson SR, Charboneau JW (eds): *Diagnostic Ultrasound,* 4th Edition. St. Louis, Elsevier Mosby, 2011, pp 34–52.

Kawamura DM: Introduction. In Kawamura DM (ed): *Diagnostic Medical Sonography: A Guide to Clinical Practice Abdomen and Superficial Structures,* 2nd Edition. Philadelphia, Lippincott, 1997.

Kawamura DM, Lunsford B: *Diagnostic Medical Sonography: A Guide to Clinical Practice Abdomen and Superficial Structures,* 3rd Edition. Lippincott Williams & Wilkins, 2012.

Kremkau FW: Performance and safety. In Kremkau FW: *Sonography: Principles and Instruments,* 8th Edition. Philadelphia, Elsevier Saunders, 2011, pp 211–237.

Lane A, Tempkin BB: Anatomy layering and sectional anatomy. In Curry RA, Tempkin BB (eds): *Sonography: Introduction to Normal Structure and Function,* 3rd Edition. St. Louis, Elsevier Saunders, 2011, pp 95–128.

Merritt C: Physics of ultrasound. In Rumack CM, Wilson SR, Charboneau JW (eds): *Diagnostic Ultrasound*, 4th Edition. Philadelphia, Elsevier Mosby, 2011, pp 2–33.

Sanders RC, Winter TC: *Clinical Sonography: A Practical Guide*, 4th Edition. Philadelphia, Lippincott Williams & Wilkins, 2006.

Simon BC, Snoey ER: *Ultrasound in Emergency and Ambulatory Medicine*. St. Louis, Mosby–Year Book, 1997.

Strohl L: Ultrasound instrumentation: "knobology," image processing, and storage. In Curry RA, Tempkin BB (eds): *Sonography: Introduction to Normal Structure and Function*, 3rd Edition. St. Louis, Elsevier Saunders, 2011, pp 8–17.

Zweibel WJ: Basic ultrasound physics and instrumentation. In Zweibel WJ, Sohaey R (eds): *Introduction to Ultrasound*. Philadelphia, Saunders, 1998.

SELF-ASSESSMENT EXERCISES

Questions

1. What type of transducer produced this image of an ovarian cyst?

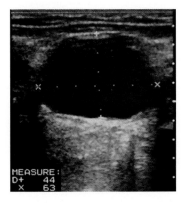

   A. Sector   D. Phased array
   B. Linear   E. Mechanical
   C. Curved linear

2. Which of the following statements about diagnostic ultrasound imaging is correct?

   A. Sonography is an excellent method for imaging the bowel.

   B. Diagnostic ultrasound can differentiate benign from malignant tissue.

   C. Ultrasound imaging can determine organ function and size.

   D. A cystic mass can be readily identified with sonography.

   E. Contrast agents must be used to image soft tissues.

3. Of the following, which is not a criterion for diagnosing a simple cyst?

   A. Well-defined outline
   B. No internal echoes
   C. Poor through-transmission
   D. Refractive edge shadows
   E. Posterior enhancement

4. Why do blood-filled masses show less posterior enhancement than those containing pus?

   A. Red blood cells refract sound.
   B. Blood is thicker than pus.
   C. Blood contains protein and absorbs more sound.
   D. A and B
   E. A and C

5. Which of the following best describes this mass?

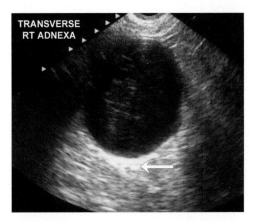

   A. Cystic   D. Complex solid
   B. Solid   E. Homogeneous
   C. Complex cystic

6. In the image from question 5, to what is the arrow pointing?

   A. Reverberation echoes
   B. Posterior enhancement
   C. Refractive shadowing
   D. Slice-thickness artifact
   E. Ring-down artifact

7. As you look at a longitudinal, transabdominal image of a patient, the patient's feet would be toward:

A. The top of the image

B. The bottom of the image

C. The right side of the image

D. The left side of the image

E. Depends on whether patient is supine or prone.

8. As you look at a longitudinal, endovaginal image of a patient, the patient's feet would be toward:

A. The top of the image

B. The bottom of the image

C. The right side of the image

D. The left side of the image

E. Depends on whether the patient is supine or prone.

9. The mass demonstrated by the arrow is:

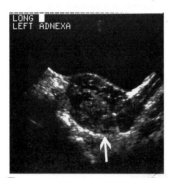

A. Solid   D. Thick fluid

B. Cystic   E. Artifact

C. Complex

10. This image demonstrates, endovaginally, the uterus in the longitudinal plane. What is the uterine position?

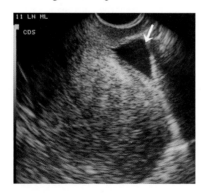

A. Anteflexed   D. Dextroposed

B. Retroflexed   E. Prolapsed

C. Levoposed

11. In the image from question 10, to what is the arrow pointing?

A. Fluid in the bladder

B. Fluid in the anterior cul-de-sac

C. Fluid in the posterior cul-de-sac

D. Fluid in the endometrial cavity

E. Fluid in the space of Retzius

12. When one views a sagittal endovaginal image of an anteflexed uterus, the endometrium will point to:

A. Right upper corner

B. Left upper corner

C. Right lower corner

D. Left lower corner

E. Middle of the image

13. When one views a coronal endovaginal image of the uterus, the patient's left side will be seen at the:

A. Top of the image

B. Bottom of the image

C. Right side of the image

D. Left side of the image

E. Cannot see right and left

14. Of the following statements, which is not true regarding the compression maneuver for scanning?

A. It is used to displace bowel gas.

B. It is used to determine tissue response.

C. It is used to elicit tissue response.

D. It is used to compress fat.

E. It is used to punish the patient.

15. The split-image artifact can be eliminated by:

A. Scanning from a different projection.

B. Having the patient take in a deep breath.

C. Changing the frequency of the transducer.

D. Changing the focus of the transducer.

E. Giving the patient an enema.

Answers

See Appendix F on page 607 for answers and explanations.

Gynecology

Kathryn A. Gill, MS, RT, RDMS, FSDMS

OBJECTIVES

After completing this chapter you should be able to:

1. Discuss the function of the uterus and ovaries.

2. Describe how to determine normal uterine and ovarian measurements for pre- and postmenopausal patients.

3. Explain the menstrual cycle and how it affects the appearance of the endometrium and ovaries sonographically.

4. Identify the normal pelvic structures on a sonogram and describe what potential spaces can harbor pelvic fluid.

5. Identify the locations where fibroids can develop.

6. List the common indications for performing a sonohysterogram.

7. Describe how hormone replacement therapy and certain drugs can affect the postmenopausal endometrium.

8. Explain how to set up for and perform a sonohysterogram.

9. Describe where cysts can be found in the uterus and from where they originate.

10. Describe how endometriosis affects the adnexa and how it appears sonographically.

11. Discuss the causes of pelvic inflammatory disease.

12. Differentiate the benign cystic teratoma from a dermoid and explain their sonographic appearance.

13. Discuss the risk factors for and symptoms of ovarian cancer.

14. Recognize different types of intrauterine contraceptive devices and the complications that can arise from their use.

15. List some normal anatomic structures that can be mistaken for pelvic pathology on clinical exam.

16. Explain how to differentiate a bladder diverticulum from an adnexal cyst.

PELVIC ANATOMY AND PHYSIOLOGY

THE FEMALE PELVIS CAN BE QUITE A CHALLENGE for the sonographer. Different pathologies can look very similar sonographically, and normal structures can simulate abnormalities. When imaging the female pelvis, the examiner naturally concentrates on the uterus and ovaries but also must remain cognizant of the rest of the anatomy and potential spaces contained within the pelvic compartment. The **pelvic girdle** consists of irregular ring-shaped bones that form the pelvic cavity. The **true** or **minor pelvis** is the portion of the pelvic compartment that includes the bladder and pelvic organs (uterus and ovaries). It is the area on which practitioners focus when performing a pelvic sonogram. The **false** or **major pelvis**—which includes the bowel and extends to the **umbilicus**, or naval—also should be evaluated to ensure a complete and thorough examination. Embryologically, the vagina, uterus, and fallopian tubes develop at the same time as the kidneys, and both organ systems develop in the lower abdomen. As embryologic growth continues, the kidneys will rise from their lower lumbar location while the bladder and uterus remain in the pelvic compartment. The ovaries develop in the abdomen and descend into the pelvis, bringing with them the associated vasculature.

Uterus

The uterus is a muscular organ with a central cavity, the sole purpose of which is gestation. The uterus is formed from the fusion of the müllerian ducts. The ovaries, influenced by endocrine sources, produce hormones and **ova** (eggs) for fertilization. Patient age and hormone stimulations influence the sizes and echo patterns of these structures, and they should change accordingly throughout a woman's life. The bladder and uterus are extraperitoneal, as the **peritoneum**, the membrane that lines the abdominal cavity, drapes over them. The ovaries, however, are intraperitoneal, as there is an opening in the peritoneum at the level of the fallopian tube that allows for communication between the abdominal and pelvic compartments.

In the newborn, the uterus may be prominent and have an adult shape due to hormones received from the mother across the placenta. After birth, in the absence of hormone stimulation, the uterus regresses to a size and shape that remain constant until puberty. The infantile uterus has a cylindrical shape; the cervix occupies most of its length, with a small rudimentary body and fundus that occupy only about one-third of the entire uterine length of the uterus (Figure 2-1A). At puberty, as hormone stimulation begins, the body begins to elongate. By adulthood, the **nulliparous uterus** (the uterus of a woman who has not borne children) shows a short cervix constituting only one-third of the length of the uterus (Figure 2-1B). Uterine size may increase slightly with each term pregnancy. At menopause (the end of menstruation and fertility), in the absence of hormone stimulation, the uterus, like the ovaries, will atrophy and may even assume the infantile shape once again (Figure 2-1C). Figure 2-1D illustrates how the uterus changes with age.

Figure 2-1. A *Longitudinal scan showing the appearance of an infantile uterus. The cervix and uterine corpus are indicated by arrows. Notice how prominent the cervix is compared to the nubbinlike corpus. V = vagina, C = cervix, U = uterine corpus.* **B** *Longitudinal image through the normal (nulliparous) adult uterus and a good example of the functional midline. V = vagina, C = cervix, arrows mark cervical length.* **C** *Longitudinal image of a postmenopausal uterus showing an atrophied corpus and fundus. C = cervix, BL = bladder, F = fundus. Following page:* **D** *How uterine size and shape change with age.*

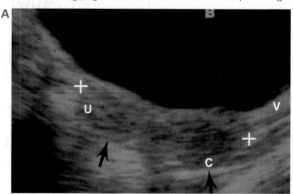

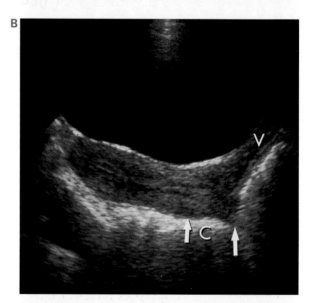

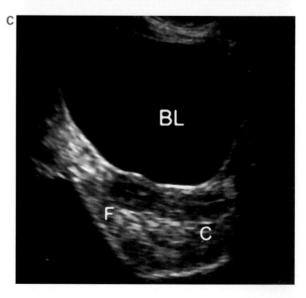

Figure 2-1, continued.

D

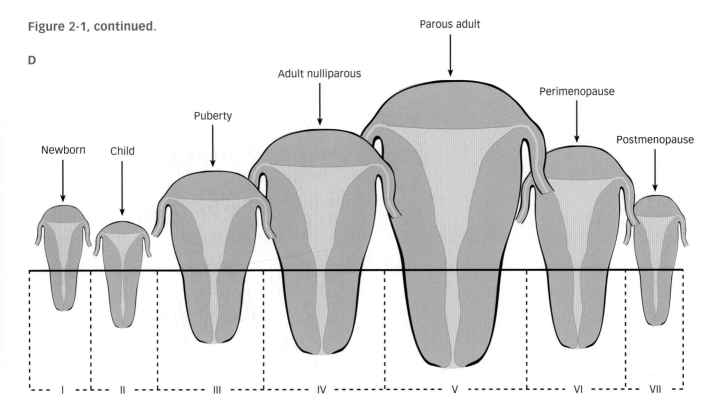

When measuring the uterus, always include the cervix. If a clinician asks for the uterine length excluding the cervix, you must be able to determine where the cervix ends. In a longitudinal scan of the uterus, the cervix ends where you see the uterus bend (Figure 2-2A). As a rule, the nulliparous adult uterus has a longitudinal measurement of 6–9 cm, an anterior/posterior measurement of 3–4 cm, and a transverse measurement of 4–5 cm. One can add 0.5–1 cm to each measurement per term pregnancy. (See Appendix A, Tables 1–4, and Appendix C, "Pelvic Ultrasound Worksheet.")

Although we cannot see all portions of the pelvic anatomy sonographically, we must know them. Figure 2-2B shows a cross-sectional view of the various structures. The uterus has five components—the **vagina** (canal from the vulva to the cervix), **cervix** (the narrow lower end of the uterus between the isthmus and body), **isthmus** (the constricted lower neck of the uterus leading into the body), **corpus** (body), and **fundus** (base)—and three layers consisting of the **endometrium** (inner/mucosal layer), **myometrium** (middle/muscular layer), and **perimetrium** (outer/serosal layer). Note too that the cervix has an opening on the vaginal side, the **external cervical os**, and one on the uterine side, the **internal cervical os**. (See Boxes 2-1 and 2-2.)

A

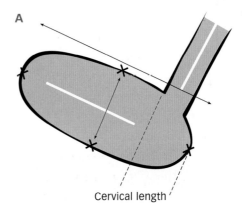

Cervical length

Figure 2-2. A *How to measure the uterus in longitudinal and anterior/posterior dimensions. The long double-headed arrow shows the entire length of the uterus, which includes the cervix. The short double-headed arrow indicates the anterior/posterior measurement of the uterus. The dotted lines indicate where the cervical length should be measured. (Figure continues . . .)*

The sonographic appearance of the endometrium varies according to the age of the patient and the stage of the menstrual cycle. A longitudinal image of the uterus that includes the vagina, cervix, corpus, fundus, and endometrial canal is called the **functional midline**. This view represents the true midline of the uterus, which may or may not be in the midline of the patient. Longitudinal uterine measurements should be obtained from this image (see Figure 2-1B).

B

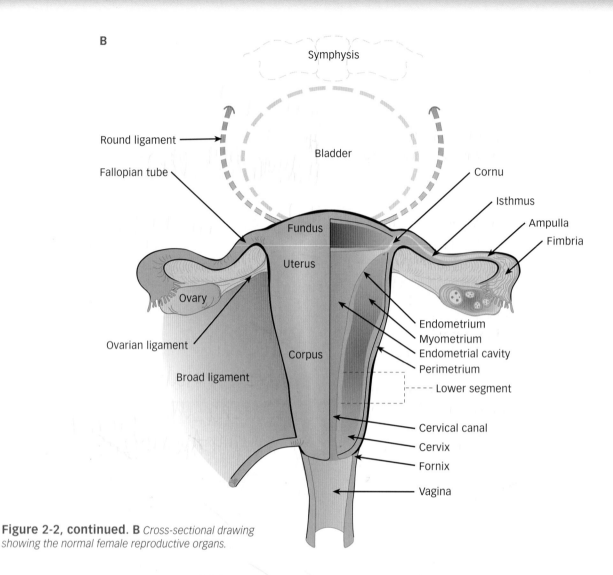

Figure 2-2, continued. B *Cross-sectional drawing showing the normal female reproductive organs.*

Box 2-1.	Components of the uterus.
	Vagina
	Cervix (including internal os and external os)
	Isthmus
	Corpus (body)
	Fundus

Box 2-2.	Layers of the uterus.
	Endometrium (inner/mucosal)
	Myometrium (middle/muscular)
	Perimetrium (outer/serosal)

The ovaries are attached directly to the uterus by the ovarian ligament and indirectly by the broad ligament and **fallopian tubes** (also known as the **oviducts**, **uterine tubes**, or **salpinges**), which lead from the ovaries into the uterus. The fallopian tubes are not routinely imaged sonographically unless they are pathologically dilated. The **uterine cornu** (uterine horn) is the point at which the uterus meets the fallopian tubes. The portion of the tube that inserts into the uterus is called the **interstitial**

portion and is only about 1 cm in length. Medially lies the **isthmus** (the end of the fallopian tube leading into the uterus, not to be confused with the uterine isthmus at the cervical end), and the lateral portion is called the **ampulla**. The ampullary portion is where fertilization usually occurs. The fingerlike projections off the lateral-most end of the tube are called the **fimbria**, and this portion is referred to as the **infundibulum**. The fimbria grab the ovum after ovulation and propel it up into the tube. The broad sheetlike structure to each side of the uterus is the **broad ligament** (Figure 2-2B). Paraovarian cysts can develop within this ligament, and at times the ligament can be seen when there is significant pelvic **ascites** (accumulation of fluid within the peritoneal cavity). The **round ligaments** originate at the uterine horns, pass through the inguinal canal, and end at the labia majoria and mons pubis; they are not visualized, but they may be a source of pain during pregnancy as the uterus enlarges.

Ovaries

The **ovary** is an endocrine organ that influences the menstrual cycle, and its sonographic appearance varies according to the stage of the cycle. A woman has two ovaries, connected to the uterus by the fallopian tubes. Each ovary contains approximately 100,000 eggs or **ova**, more than needed in any one lifetime. The ovaries should be oval or almond-shaped and are recognized by follicular development (Figure 2-3A). Like the size of the uterus, ovarian size depends on the patient's age. As a general rule, the ovaries of women in their reproductive years should not exceed 4 cm in their maximum dimension. For the postmenopausal patient, they should not exceed 2 cm in their greatest dimension. Ovarian volumes may be more helpful to know when you are monitoring ovaries for changes in size or enlargement. (See Tables 5–8 in Appendix A.) In these situations, evaluation and measurements should be obtained using transvaginal technique. Postmenopausal ovaries can be quite difficult to identify because they lack the characteristic follicles and are much smaller. Transvaginal sonography may be more helpful in evaluating the elderly patient as well (Figure 2-3B).

If a patient has elusive ovaries, the internal iliac artery can be used to help localize them, as the ovaries lie just medial and anterior to the internal iliac vessels (Figure 2-3C). The internal iliac artery bifurcates off the common iliac artery to provide oxygenated blood to the pelvic organs, while the external iliac artery sends blood to the lower extremities. The **ureters** (the tubes through which urine passes from kidneys to bladder) are not usually seen unless they are dilated; when dilated, they can be visualized along with the iliac vessels.

Pelvic Muscles

There are five muscle groups in the pelvis that can be identified sonographically (Figure 2-4A). Anatomic drawings can be somewhat difficult to appreciate, and the muscles seem to run together when viewed longitudinally. Therefore, only transverse images are shown in this text.

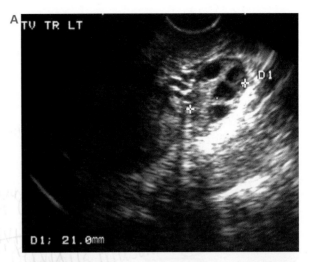

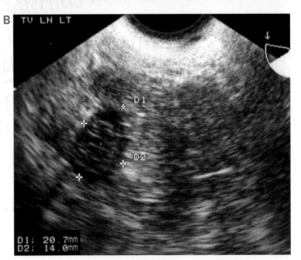

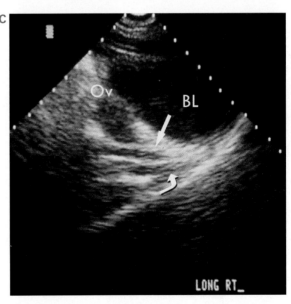

Figure 2-3. A *Transvaginal image of an adult ovary showing multiple follicles.* **B** *Transvaginal image of a postmenopausal ovary seen between the calipers. Follicles have atrophied and are no longer identifiable.* **C** *Longitudinal transvesical scan showing an ovary posterior to the bladder. The internal iliac artery is seen posterior to the ovary (straight arrow) and the internal iliac vein is seen posterior to the artery (curved arrow). BL = bladder, Ov = ovary.*

The five muscle groups include the levator ani, obturator internus, iliopsoas, coccygeus, and piriformis muscles (Box 2-3).

Three of these muscle groups—the levator ani, obturator internus, and iliopsoas—can be routinely imaged at the level of the vagina as one angles the transducer toward the patient's feet (Figure 2-4B). The **levator ani muscles** form the floor of the pelvis, while the **obturator internus** marks the lateral pelvic sidewalls. The **iliopsoas muscles**, a continuation of the abdominal psoas, are large strap

Box 2-3.	Pelvic muscle groups.
	Levator ani
	Obturator internus
	Iliopsoas
	Coccygeus
	Piriformis

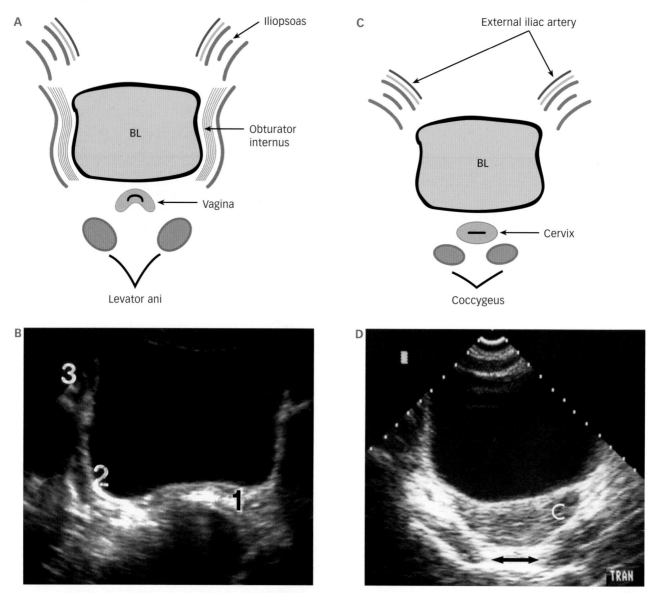

Figure 2-4. A *The level at which the levator ani, obturator internus, and iliopsoas muscles can be identified.* **B** *Transverse image showing the iliopsoas muscle (3) and the obturator internus muscle (2) at the level of the vagina (1). Air in the rectum creates shadowing posterior to the vagina.* **C** *The level at which the coccygeus muscles can be visualized.* **D** *Transverse image at the level of the cervix. The coccygeus muscles can be seen lateral and posterior (arrows). C = cervix. Following page:* **E** *The level at which the piriformis muscles can be imaged.* **F** *Transverse image of the piriformis muscles (curved arrows) seen lateral and posterior to the uterine corpus. Ut = uterus, IP = iliopsoas muscle, BL = bladder.*

muscles that can be seen on most transverse images. Angling toward the patient's head at the level of the cervix, one can see the **coccygeus** (or **pubococcygeus**) **muscles** just lateral to the cervix (Figures 2-4 C and D). Further angulation cephalically reveals the **piriformis muscles** at the level of the uterine corpus (Figures 2-4 E and F). These gray ovoid muscles are commonly mistaken for bilaterally enlarged ovaries because of their close proximity to the uterus.

Pelvic Spaces

As in the upper abdomen, there are several potential spaces within the pelvic compartment, including the posterior cul-de-sac, anterior cul-de-sac, fornices, and space of Retzius. These spaces are not apparent unless fluid is present. Blood, pus, and clear serous fluids can collect within these spaces, indicating certain pathologic processes such as pelvic infection, bleeding from a ruptured ectopic pregnancy, and pelvic ascites. The most commonly imaged space is the **posterior cul-de-sac**, also known as the **pouch of Douglas** or **rectouterine space**. It lies between the posterior uterus and the rectum. The **anterior cul-de-sac** or **uterovesical space** is located between the anterior uterine wall and the posterior bladder. The **fornix** is the space around the cervix, and it has anterior and posterior aspects. Finally, the **space of Retzius** lies between the anterior bladder wall and the pubic bone (Figure 2-5 and Box 2-4).

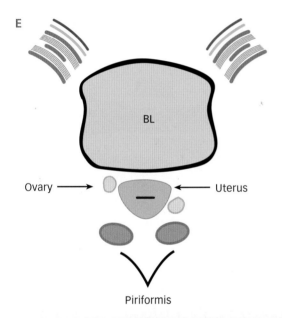

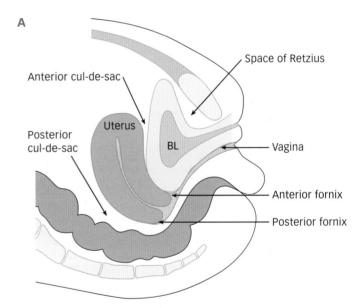

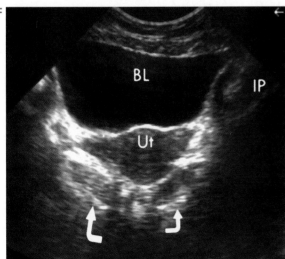

Figure 2-4, continued.

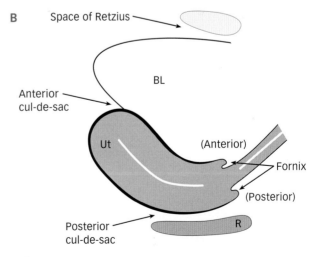

Figure 2-5. A *The various potential pelvic spaces where fluids can collect.* **B** *How these spaces are represented sonographically on a long-axis view of the pelvis. R = rectum. (Figure continues . . .)*

C

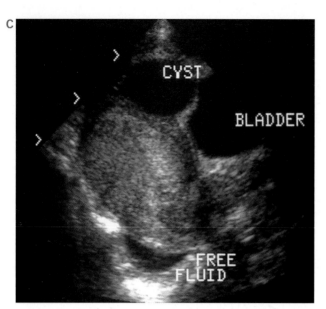

Figure 2-5, continued. C *Longitudinal transvesical image showing a cyst in the anterior cul-de-sac and free fluid in the posterior cul-de-sac.*

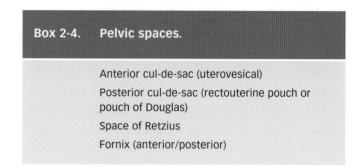

Box 2-4.   Pelvic spaces.

Anterior cul-de-sac (uterovesical)

Posterior cul-de-sac (rectouterine pouch or pouch of Douglas)

Space of Retzius

Fornix (anterior/posterior)

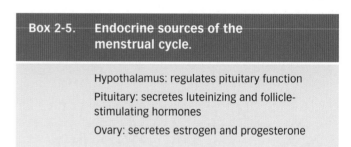

Box 2-5.   Endocrine sources of the menstrual cycle.

Hypothalamus: regulates pituitary function

Pituitary: secretes luteinizing and follicle-stimulating hormones

Ovary: secretes estrogen and progesterone

Menstrual Cycle

In the female patient between the ages of puberty and menopause, normal cyclical changes should occur. This cycle should begin at **menarche** (12–15 years of age) and occur every 28 days. The menstrual cycle is influenced and regulated by three different endocrine sources: the pituitary gland, the hypothalamus, and the ovaries (Figure 2-6). The pituitary gland and hypothalamus, both located in the brain, work together. The **pituitary gland** produces follicle-stimulating hormone (**FSH**) and **luteinizing hormone** (**LH**), while the **hypothalamus** influences the release and inhibition of the pituitary hormones (Box 2-5). At the end of a menstrual cycle when the endometrium has been **sloughed** (shed), estrogen levels are low. At this time, FSH is produced to stimulate **folliculogenesis**. (As a point of interest, FSH in the male stimulates spermatogenesis.) Folliculogenesis results in the development of several follicles (usually between five and eight) within

Figure 2-6. *Diagram and drawing showing how hormonal fluctuations affect the ovaries throughout the menstrual cycle.*

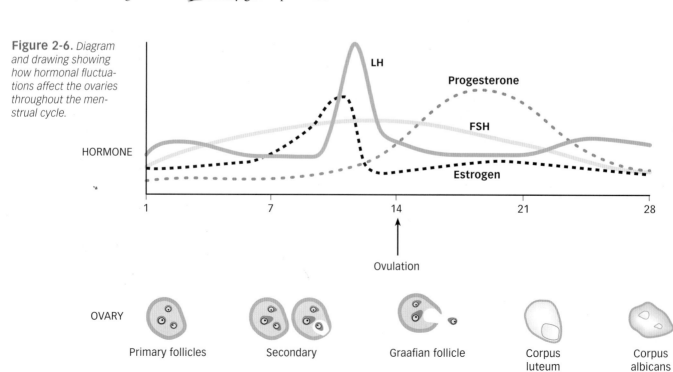

the ovaries (Figure 2-7A). These follicles produce the female hormone **estrogen** and begin the follicular phase of the ovarian cycle (1–14 days). Each follicle contains an egg or **oocyte** surrounded by a layer of cells referred to as the **cumulus oophorus**. Although several follicles develop, only one will usually reach full maturity. This follicle is called the **Graafian** or **dominant follicle**. The follicle measuring more than 11 mm and located closest to the ovarian surface is the follicle that will most likely ovulate (Figures 2-7 B and C). Follicles usually grow at the rate of 2–3 mm per day.

When the dominant follicle grows to approximately 25 mm and the estrogen levels peak, the luteinizing hormone induces **ovulation**. Ovulation typically occurs 14 days after the first day of the **last menstrual period** (**LMP**), at mid-cycle. Some patients claim that they feel a sharp pain or dull cramping when ovulation occurs, called **mittel-schmerz** (German for *middle pain*). Others experience **anovulation**, the failure of the ovary to release an oocyte.

Upon ovulation, the cavity from which the **ovum** or egg emerges becomes filled with a golden, waxy fluid and usually a small bit of blood. This is now referred to as the **corpus luteum cyst**, which produces **progesterone**, the hormone that initiates the **secretory phase** on days 15–28 (Figures 2-7 D and E). Sonographically, one may also appreciate a small amount of fluid in the posterior

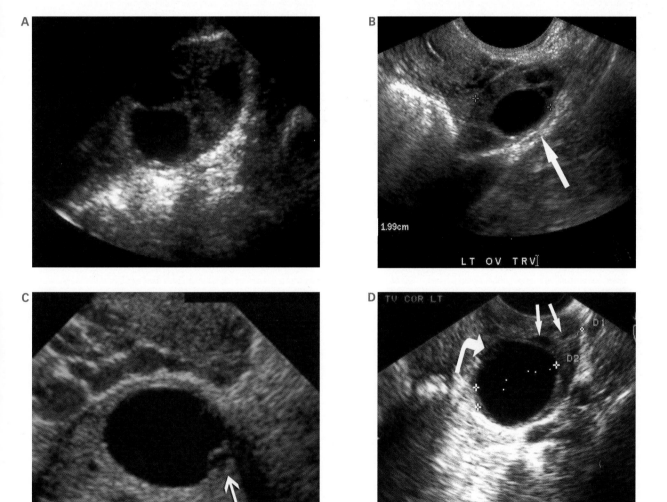

Figure 2-7. A *Transvaginal image of a normal adult ovary showing multiple follicles.* **B** *Transvaginal image showing a normal adult ovary demonstrating a dominant follicle (arrow).* **C** *Transvaginal demonstration of the cumulus oophorus (arrow).* **D** *Transvaginal image of a normal adult ovary demonstrating a corpus luteum cyst with a thickened irregular wall (curved arrow). The other follicles have atrophied and regressed (straight arrows). (Figure continues . . .)*

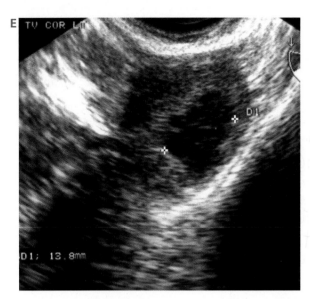

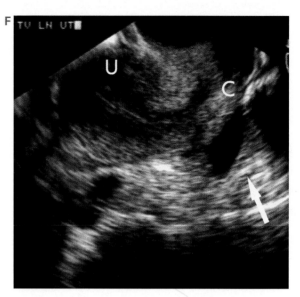

Figure 2-7, continued. E *Transvaginal image of an adult ovary containing a corpus luteum cyst with debris from slight bleeding (calipers).* **F** *Longitudinal image through the uterus showing some free fluid in the posterior cul-de-sac (straight arrow) postovulation. U = uterus, C = cervix.*

cul-de-sac, as fluid will leak out into the peritoneal cavity upon ovulation (Figure 2-7F). By promoting glandular secretions of the endometrium, progesterone causes proliferation of the endometrial lining of the uterus in preparation for receiving the **conceptus**, or blastocyst. In the absence of fertilization, the corpus luteum regresses, causing disintegration of the endometrial lining and subsequent sloughing, an event that transitions to the menstrual phase (days 1–5).

Endometrium

The echogenicity of the endometrium also varies with the menstrual cycle. There are three basic phases: the proliferative, periovulatory, and secretory (Box 2-6). The examiner measures the endometrium across both layers at the widest anterior/posterior diameter (Figure 2-8A). At the end of **menses**, when the endometrium has completely sloughed off, the endometrial stripe is thin, measuring 3–6 mm in diameter. This is the **proliferative phase**, days 6–14 (Figure 2-8B). During mid-cycle, the **periovulatory phase**, the endometrium becomes edematous and begins to thicken, measuring 6–10 mm and presenting a somewhat hypoechoic region around the central echogenic stripe (Figure 2-8C). The **secretory** or **luteal phase** (days 15–28), which begins at ovulation as the onset of menses approaches, is when the endometrium is brightest (most echoic) and thickest, measuring 8–12 mm (Figure 2-8D). During menstrual flow, the endometrial cavity

Box 2-6.	Phases of the menstrual cycle and endometrial thickness.

Proliferative phase, 3–6 mm

Periovulatory phase, 6–10 mm

Secretory phase, 8–12 mm

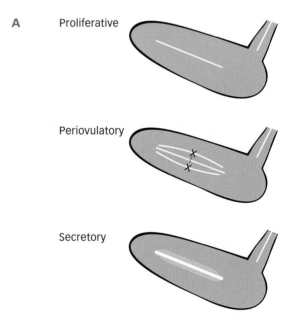

Figure 2-8. A *How the menstrual phases affect the endometrium. Following page:* **B** *Transvaginal image of a proliferative endometrium (calipers).* **C** *Image of a periovulatory endometrium showing multiple layers.* **D** *Transvaginal image of a secretory endometrium (arrow).* **E** *Transvaginal image of an endometrium in a menstruating woman. The endometrium is thick (straight arrow) and the cavity is widened and contains debris and fluid.*

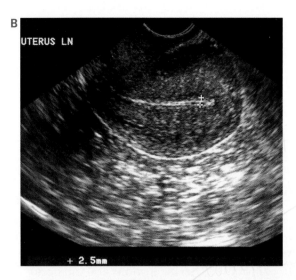

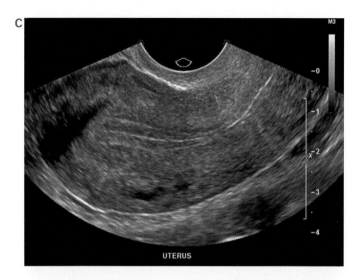

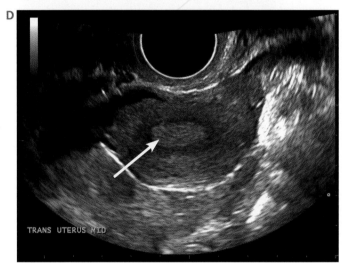

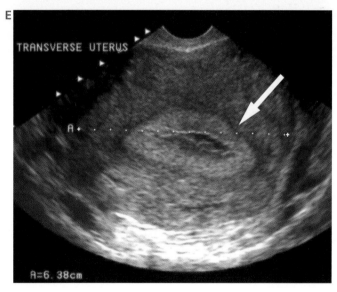

Figure 2-8, continued.

may contain fluid from bleeding, and sometimes clots may give the endometrial stripe a heterogeneous pattern (Figure 2-8E).

Prepubertal and postmenopausal patients present only a faint stripe transabdominally, if one can be seen at all. In the postmenopausal patient, the endometrium should not exceed 5 mm unless the patient is on hormone replacement therapy or other drug therapy, such as tamoxifen (Figure 2-9). Then the endometrium should not exceed 8 mm. If an endometrial measurement is specifically requested by a clinician, it is advised to perform the study transvaginally, since the detail is much better and bladder compression from a transvesical approach will alter the measurement. This is true for ovarian monitoring as well.

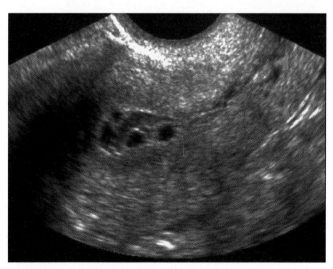

Figure 2-9. *Transvaginal image showing multiple endometrial cysts associated with tamoxifen.*

Uterine Positions

The uterus and ovaries are quite mobile and can assume a variety of positions (Box 2-7). When the urinary bladder is empty, the uterus normally is in the **anteflexed** position, with flexion occurring at the cervix (Figure 2-10A). This causes the fundus of the uterus to point toward the anterior abdominal wall (Figure 2-10B). As the urinary bladder fills, the uterus is pushed downward, displacing surrounding bowel. It remains tilted anteriorly, but the bend at the cervix is unfolded. This position is called **anteverted** (Figures 2-10 C and D). A **retroverted** uterus is one that is tilted posteriorly, while a **retroflexed** uterus bends posteriorly at the cervix, making it appear that there is a septum or interface between the cervix and corpus (Figure 2-11). This usually does not cause the patient to have symptoms, but some women may complain of

Box 2-7.	Uterine positions.
	Anteverted/anteflexed
	Retroverted/retroflexed
	Levoposed
	Dextroposed
	Prolapsed

backaches, **dysmenorrhea** (menstrual pain to the point of interfering with daily activies), or **dyspareunia** (pain during intercourse). Retroflexion may even be associated with fertility difficulties. **Uterine flexions** also can occur at the fundal end of the uterus, although these are less common. Flexions alter the way the examiner measures

A

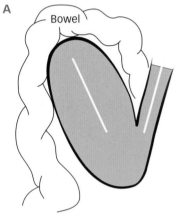

C

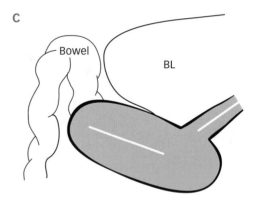

B

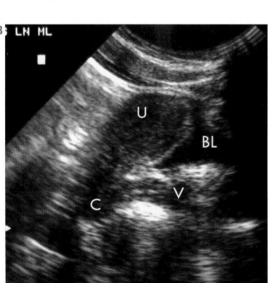

D

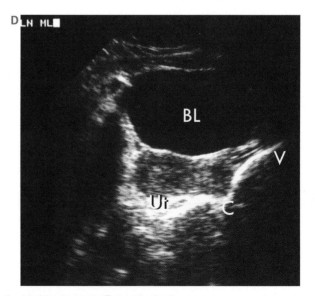

Figure 2-10. A *The position of uterus and surrounding bowel when the bladder is empty.* **B** *Longitudinal transvesical scan showing the anteflexed position of the uterus when the urinary bladder is not adequately filled. BL = bladder, V= vagina, C = cervix, U = uterus.* **C** *The effect a full bladder on the position of bowel and uterus.* **D** *Longitudinal transvesical scan showing an anteverted uterus with the bladder adequately filled. BL = bladder, Ut = uterus, C = cervix, V = vagina.*

A Longitudinal

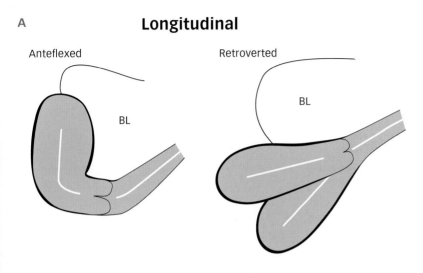

Anteflexed   Retroverted

BL   BL

Figure 2-11. *The difference between version and flexion.* **A** *Anteflexed and retroverted uterus.* **B** *Anteverted and retroflexed uterus.* **C** *Longitudinal transvesical scan through a retroverted uterus. The uterine fundus is indicated by the curved arrow.* **D** *Longitudinal transvesical scan through a retroflexed uterus. The area of flexion is noted by the arrow.* **E** *Longitudinal transvesical image of a retroflexed uterus. Notice the curve of the secretory endometrial stripe (arrows). BL = bladder, OV = ovary.*

B Longitudinal

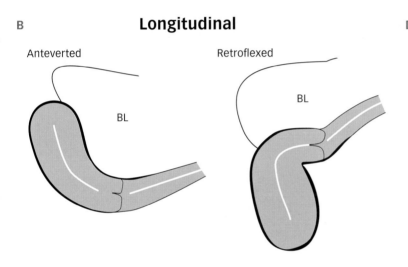

Anteverted   Retroflexed

BL   BL

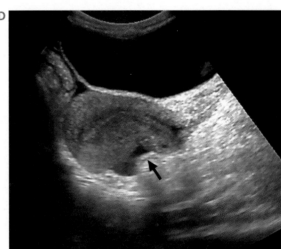

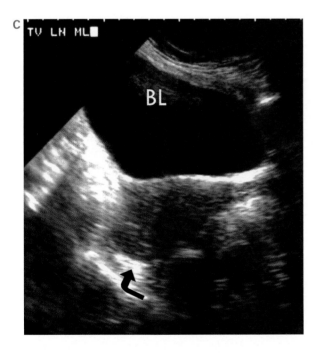

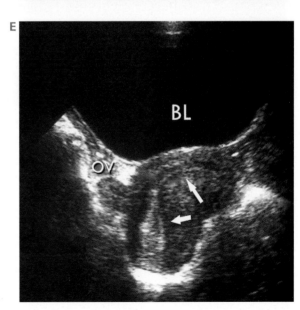

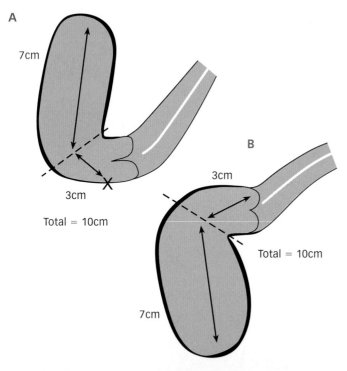

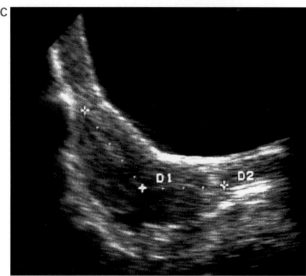

Figure 2-12. *How to measure an **A** anteflexed and **B** retroflexed uterus. **C** Longitudinal transvesical image of an extremely anteverted uterus. Two long-axis measurements are taken and added together to compensate for the flexion.*

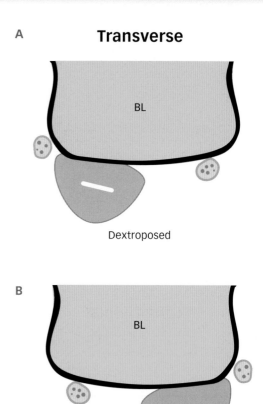

Figure 2-13. A *Dextroposition and* **B** *levoposition of the uterus.*

the uterus in the long axis. One must compensate for the flexion by taking two linear measurements (one of the cervix and one of the uterine body and fundus) and adding them together for the correct long-axis measurement (Figure 2-12). Uterine position can be affected by the degree of bladder filling, fullness of the bowel and rectum, adnexal masses, and poor muscle support. If the uterus is deviated to the right of the midline, it is **dextroposed**. A uterus deviated to the left is **levoposed** (Figure 2-13).

Uterine prolapse occurs when the muscles and ligaments of the pelvis stretch to the point of being ineffective. Prolapse can occur with repeated childbirth, increased abdominal pressure from chronic coughing or heavy lifting, or simply years of having to stand on one's feet. The uterus gradually descends along the axis of the vagina, eventually taking the vaginal wall with it. Symptoms of uterine prolapse depend on the severity of the prolapse and tend to worsen with increased activity. They range from a feeling of pelvic heaviness to dyspareunia, anal pain/pressure, lower back pain, and chronic bladder infections. Uterine prolapse is classified according to three degrees of severity (Figure 2-14):

- *First degree:* cervix is still inside the vagina
- *Second degree:* cervix appears outside the vulva
- *Third degree:* uterus is completely outside the vulva

Uterine prolapse can be temporarily corrected with a **pessary** device or surgically. Pessaries come in a variety of configurations. They expand the proximal vagina and exert pressure on the ligaments, holding the uterus in a forward position (Figure 2-15).

Figure 2-14. *Degrees of uterine prolapse.*

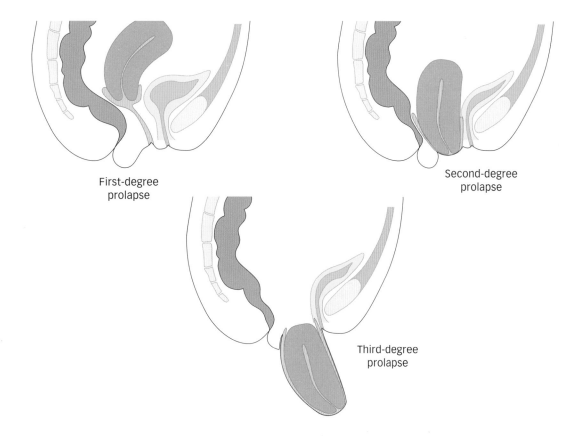

First-degree prolapse

Second-degree prolapse

Third-degree prolapse

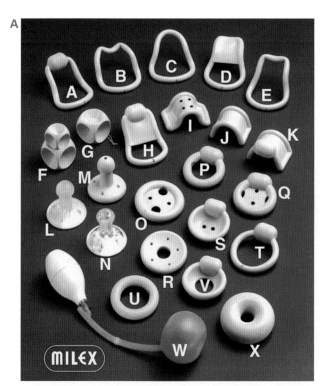

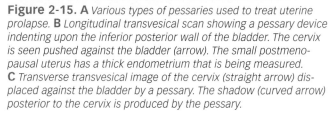

A

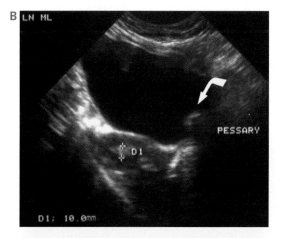

B

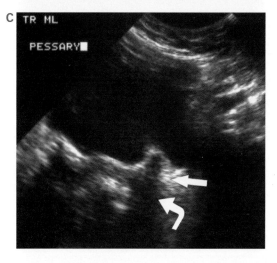

C

Figure 2-15. A *Various types of pessaries used to treat uterine prolapse.* **B** *Longitudinal transvesical scan showing a pessary device indenting upon the inferior posterior wall of the bladder. The cervix is seen pushed against the bladder (arrow). The small postmenopausal uterus has a thick endometrium that is being measured.* **C** *Transverse transvesical image of the cervix (straight arrow) displaced against the bladder by a pessary. The shadow (curved arrow) posterior to the cervix is produced by the pessary.*

Other conditions for which a pessary might be used include vaginal prolapse, enterocele, cystocele, and bladder incontinence. An **enterocele** involves herniation of the sigmoid colon into the upper posterior vaginal vault. A **cystocele** is the result of weak tissues between the vagina and bladder, which allows herniation into the bladder. This causes a bulge along the anterior vaginal wall. Symptoms for these conditions include a heavy or full feeling in the vaginal area and unwanted urine leakage.

Box 2-8.	Pelvic anomalies.
	Uterine agenesis
	Ectopic (accessory/supernumerary) ovaries
	Infantile uterus
	Duplications
	Obstructions

CONGENITAL PELVIC ANOMALIES

Congenital anomalies are present at birth, and those that affect the pelvic organs may also involve other parts of the genitourinary system because the genital and urinary tracts develop embryologically at the same time. Pelvic anomalies that can be identified sonographically include uterine agenesis, ectopic ovaries, malformed uterus, duplications, and gynatresia (Box 2-8).

Uterine Agenesis

Uterine agenesis (absence of the uterus above the vagina) may or may not be associated with vaginal agenesis. When uterine agenesis is discovered, the examiner must determine if ovaries are present (Figure 2-16). Because of the developmental relationship between the genital and

urinary tracts, one should evaluate the kidneys whenever a pelvic anomaly is discovered. Developmental anomalies of the uterus may be encountered as well, including a **unicornuate uterus**, a uterus with only one fully developed müllerian duct.

Ectopic Ovaries

Ectopic (misplaced) **ovaries** are rare and can include accessory and supernumerary ovaries. An ectopic ovary near a normal ovary, attached to it either directly or in the adjacent broad ligament, is an **accessory** ovary, whereas a **supernumerary ovary** is located away from the normal ovary and is not connected to it. Ectopic ovaries may result from the ovary migrating through an inguinal hernia, resulting in a groin or labial location (Figure 2-17).

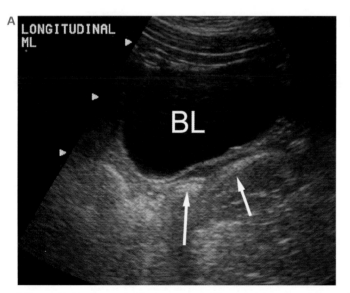
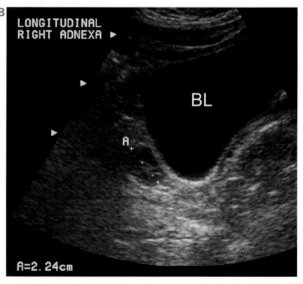

Figure 2-16. A *Longitudinal transvesical image of a patient with uterine agenesis. Note the atretic vagina tapering to a blind end (arrows).* **B** *Longitudinal image of the right ovary in same patient. Only one ovary was identified. BL = bladder.*

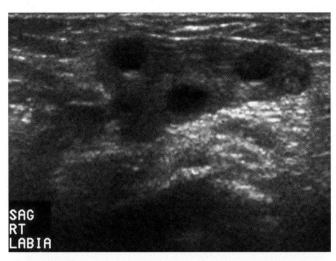

Figure 2-17. *Longitudinal image of an ectopic ovary, labial in location.*

Infantile Uterus

The infantile-shaped uterus may persist in some patients. It is not uncommon for these patients to experience difficulty with fertility, as the endometrium may not develop adequately or there may be associated streak ovaries. The infantile uterus may also be associated with Turner syndrome (see Figure 2-1A).

Duplications

The uterus, fallopian tubes, and superior portion of the vagina develop from the fusion of a pair of tubular structures called the **müllerian ducts**. If normal fusion is disrupted, a variety of presentations may occur (Figure 2-18A). The most common of these is the **bicornuate uterus**, clearly showing two uterine horns and two endometrial canals (Figures 2-18 B and C). This type of anomaly, particularly the T-shaped endometrial cavity, has been associated with in utero exposure to diethylstilbestrol (DES). DES was a drug given to pregnant patients to inhibit spontaneous abortion and preterm delivery from the late 1940s until the early 1970s. It has since been removed from the market, as it was discovered that the offspring of patients who took DES had an increased incidence of gynecologic abnormalities, including cancer. Approximately 1%–5% of patients with uterine duplication experience menstrual disorders and have difficulty with premature delivery, spontaneous abortion, and/or infertility.

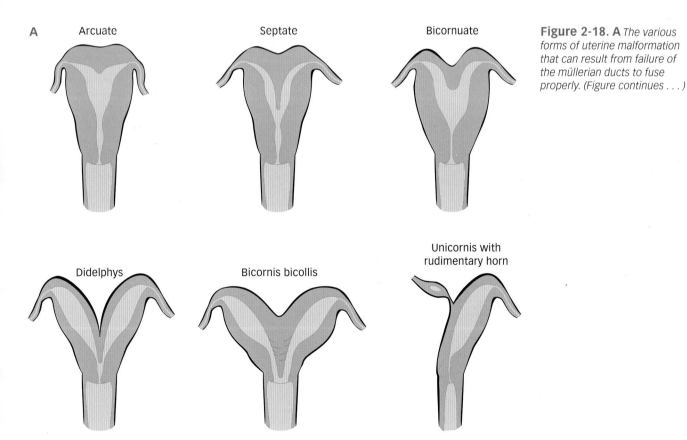

A Arcuate   Septate   Bicornuate

Didelphys   Bicornis bicollis   Unicornis with rudimentary horn

Figure 2-18. A *The various forms of uterine malformation that can result from failure of the müllerian ducts to fuse properly. (Figure continues . . .)*

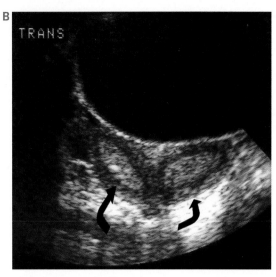

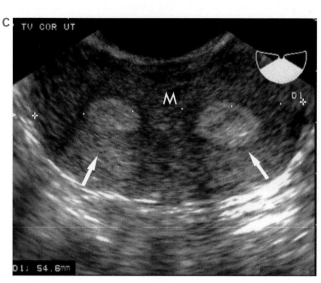

Figure 2-18, continued. B *Transverse transvesical image of a bicornuate uterus. A secretory endometrium is noted in each horn of the uterus (curved arrows).* **C** *Transverse transvaginal image of what upon full examination was confirmed to be a bicornuate uterus, demonstrating myometrium (M) between the two uterine cavities (arrows).*

Gynatresia

Gynatresia is a general term for occlusion of the genital tract and can take several forms. **Cryptomenorrhea** is the congenital or acquired obstruction of menstrual flow. The main symptoms are primary **amenorrhea** (absence or abnormal cessation of the menses) and pelvic pressure or pain. The most common congenital causes include the imperforate hymen, vaginal septum, and vaginal agenesis. Patients are usually in their mid- to late teens. Three degrees are recognized: hematocolpos, hematometra, and hematosalpinx (Figure 2-19A). **Hematocolpos**, generally the result of an imperforate hymen, is a condition in which menstrual blood is retained within a distended vagina (Figure 2-19B). If this condition is untreated, the blood eventually fills the uterine cavity, resulting in **hematometra** (Figures 2-19 C and D). Further progression of the process causes **hematosalpinx**, the accumulation of blood within the uterine tube. Acquired gynatresia may result from cervical malignancy or scarring from radiation treatment.

A

Cryptomenorrhea

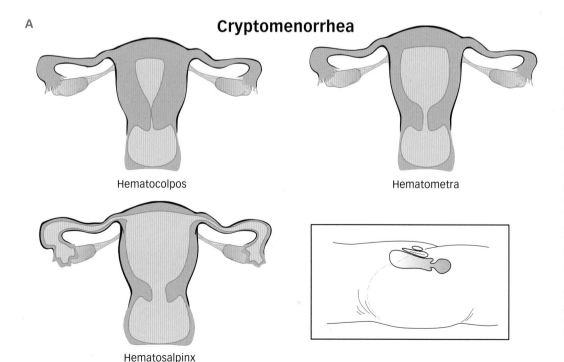

Hematocolpos

Hematometra

Hematosalpinx

Figure 2-19. A *Various degrees to which gynatresia obstructs menstrual flow. Following page:* **B** *Longitudinal transvesical image of a uterus demonstrating hematocolpos. The grossly distended cervix (arrows) shows blood contained within. BL = bladder, Ut = uterus.* **C** *Longitudinal transvesical scan of hematocolpos with hematometra. Hypoechoic blood is seen within the distended endometrial canal and echogenic blood is seen within the distended endocervical and vaginal canals. BL = bladder, Cx = cervix, Ut = uterus.* **D** *Longitudinal transvesical scan of hematometra/hematocolpos. BL = bladder, V = vagina, Cx = cervix, UT = uterus.*

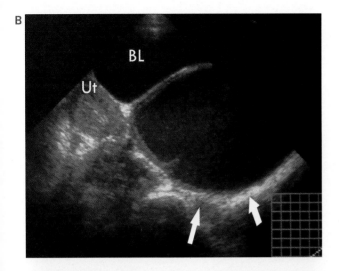

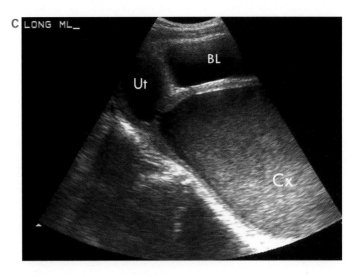

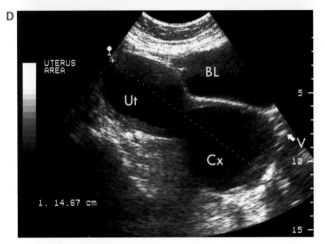

Figure 2-19, continued.

UTERINE PATHOLOGY

Abnormal/Dysfunctional Uterine Bleeding

Three forms of abnormal bleeding may be encountered during the reproductive years. They include mid-cycle bleeding, excessive menstruation (**menorrhagia**), and irregular/excessive bleeding such as bleeding between periods (**metrorrhagia**; see Figure 2-20).

Abnormal uterine bleeding (**AUB**) can be the result of hormonal imbalances, uterine growths, and, less commonly, thyroid/pituitary conditions, bleeding disorders, medications, problems with an intrauterine contraceptive device, or infection/malignancy of the pelvic organs.

Figure 2-20. *Various causes and origins of abnormal and dysfunctional uterine bleeding.*

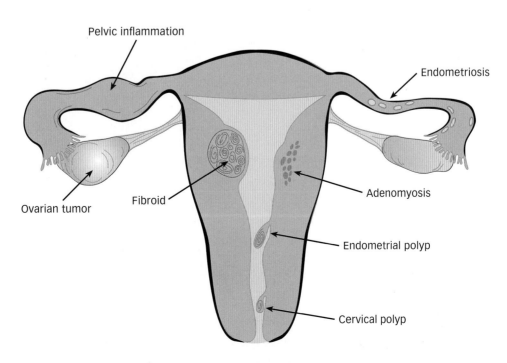

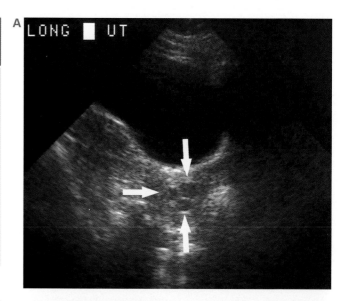

Box 2-9.	Causes of abnormal uterine bleeding (AUB).

Hormonal imbalances

Uterine growths

Thyroid disorders

Pituitary disorders

Bleeding disorders

Medications

Complications from intrauterine contraceptive devices

Pelvic infection

Pelvic malignancy

Box 2-10.	Causes of dysfunctional uterine bleeding (DUB).

Hormonal changes

Diabetes

Thyroid disease

Anorexia

Excessive stress

Obesity

Regular strenuous exercise

Dysfunctional uterine bleeding (DUB) is defined as heavy periods or bleeding between periods caused by a hormonal imbalance and usually occurs when the patient is not ovulating. Causes of DUB include hormonal changes seen in teens and perimenopausal women and in patients with diabetes, thyroid disease, anorexia, excessive stress, or obesity. Women who participate in regular strenuous exercise may also experience hormonal changes that lead to DUB. (See Boxes 2-9 and 2-10.)

Uterine Cysts

The cyst most commonly associated with the uterus is the **nabothian cyst**, found within the cervix. When the lumina of the small glands within the cervical mucosa become obstructed, cystlike structures distend with retained secretions. Nabothian cysts may be singular or multiple, and they vary in size. They are readily identified with transvaginal sonography (Figure 2-21).

Cysts also develop within the vaginal canal. Remnants of the mesonephric duct, these cysts, called **Gartner duct**

Figure 2-21. A *Longitudinal and* **B** *transverse transvesical images showing multiple nabothian cysts indicated by the arrows.* **C** *Trans-vaginal image of large (calipers) and smaller nabothian (arrow) cysts adjacent to each other.*

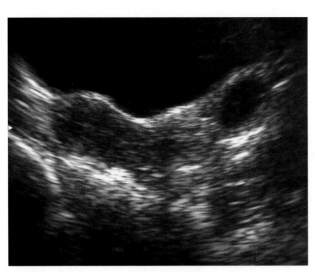

Figure 2-22. *Longitudinal scan showing a rather large Gartner duct cyst in the proximal vaginal canal.*

cysts, are found along the anterolateral wall of the vagina (Figure 2-22). They can be mistaken for cystoceles. Both nabothian and Gartner duct cysts are usually asymptomatic and discovered incidentally during pelvic sonography.

Myometrial cysts have been associated with adenomyosis. They are located between the endometrium and the myometrial border (Figure 2-23A). Care should be taken not to mistake prominent arcuate vessels, which are located around the periphery of the uterus, for myometrial cysts (Figure 2-23B). Small endometrial cysts have been associated with ectopic pregnancy but also are seen during a normal early pregnancy. This finding is therefore usually nonspecific.

Uterine Leiomyomas

Uterine **leiomyomas**, or **myomas**, are benign tumors composed of unstriped (unstriated) muscle and fibrous tissue. When they displace or protrude into the endometrial cavity they are called **submucosal leiomyomas**. These tumors are commonly known as **fibroids** when they appear in the uterus. Although they are not encapsulated, a false capsule from compressed myometrial tissue is formed. Fibroids are the most common tumors found in females, particularly those over age 35. Clinical symptoms include excessive, prolonged periods (**menorrhagia**) with clots, lower back pain, constipation, and urinary frequency. On pelvic examination, the uterus is enlarged and firm (Box 2-11). Fibroids may be associated with infertility or spontaneous abortion. Although there is malignant potential, it is low. Fewer than 5% of fibroids

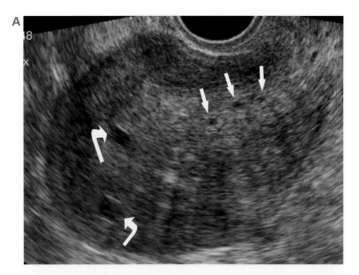

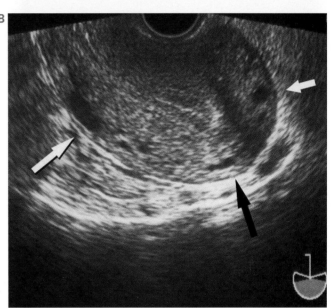

Figure 2-23. A *Longitudinal transvaginal image showing adenomyosis. Multiple small endometrial cysts are indicated by the straight arrows; curved arrows show larger myometrial cysts.* **B** *Longitudinal transvaginal image of a retroflexed uterus with prominent engorged arcuate vessels in a patient who is in the middle of her menstrual cycle. (Figure continues . . .)*

Box 2-11.	Clinical indications of fibroids.
	Menorrhagia
	Lumbar pain
	Constipation
	Urinary frequency
	Enlarged uterus
	African American ethnicity
	More than 35 years of age

C

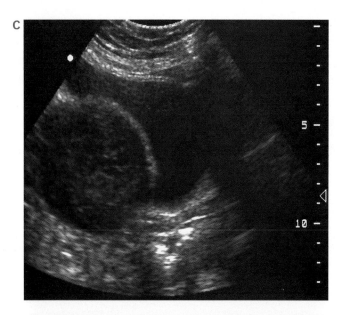

D

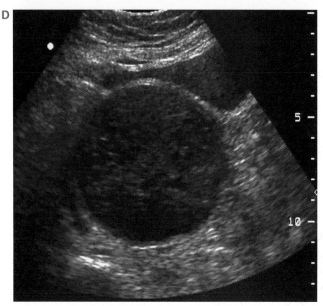

Figure 2-23, continued. C *Longitudinal and* **D** *transverse images of a surgically proven uterine leiomyosarcoma.*

A

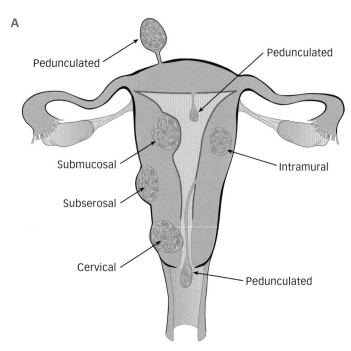

Pedunculated

Pedunculated

Submucosal

Intramural

Subserosal

Cervical

Pedunculated

B

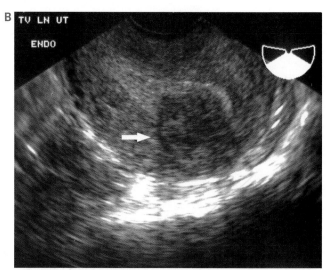

C

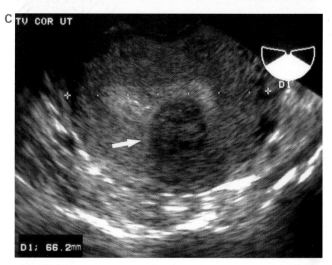

Figure 2-24. A *The various sites of uterine fibroids.* **B** *Longitudinal and* **C** *coronal transvaginal images reveal a submucosal fibroid impinging on the endometrium (arrows).*

are malignant, and of those most occur in the postmenopausal patient as **leiomyosarcoma** (Figures 2-23 C and D). There is a rare pediatric tumor called **sarcoma botryoides**. It is an **embryonal rhabdomyosarcoma** (derived from muscle) usually originating from the upper vagina or cervix.

Fibroids can develop in a variety of locations generally classified as submucosal, intramural, subserous/subserosal, pedunculated, cervical, and tubal (Figure 2-24A and Box 2-12). The **submucosal fibroid** develops underneath the endometrium and may cause endometrial displacement or obliteration (Figures 2-24 B and C). Submucosal

Box 2-12.   Locations of fibroids.

Submucosal (underneath the endometrium)

Intramural (within the muscle layer)

Subserous/subserosal (underneath the outer layer)

Pedunculated (external/internal)

Cervical/tubal

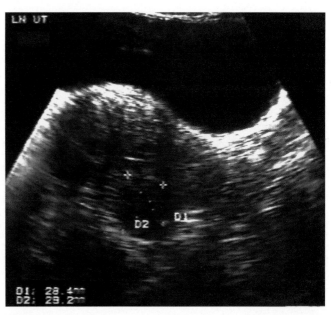

Figure 2-26. *Longitudinal transvesical scan of a posterior subserosal fibroid being measured.*

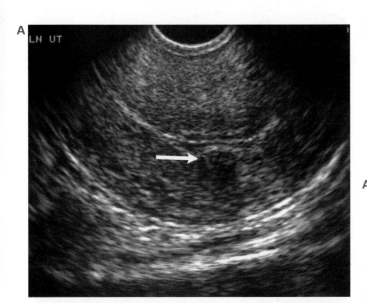

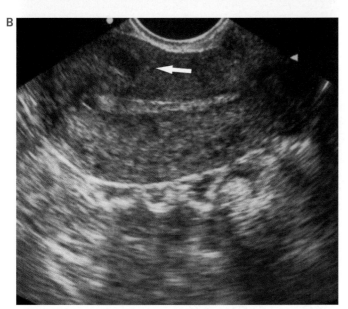

Figure 2-25. A *Longitudinal transvaginal image shows a small hypoechoic fibroid pressing on the endometrial canal (arrow).* **B** *Small fibroid within the anterior myometrium (arrow).*

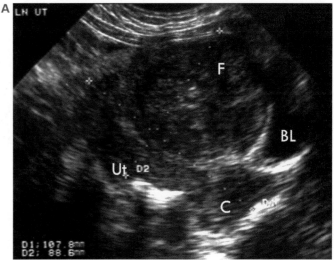

Figure 2-27. A *Longitudinal scan showing a large anterior fibroid. Ut = uterus, F = fibroid, BL = bladder, C = cervix. (Figure continues . . .)*

fibroids tend to be among the most symptomatic, causing abnormal uterine bleeding (Figure 2-25A). **Intramural fibroids** are found within the muscle layer of the uterus. When they are small they may present as incidental findings (Figure 2-25B), but as they grow they cause overall uterine enlargement with or without uterine contour changes (Figure 2-26). **Subserous/subserosal fibroids** are most responsible for producing a very irregular uterine contour (Figure 2-27). The **pedunculated fibroid** can be quite a challenge for the sonographer to identify because it moves on its stalk and simulates, both clinically and

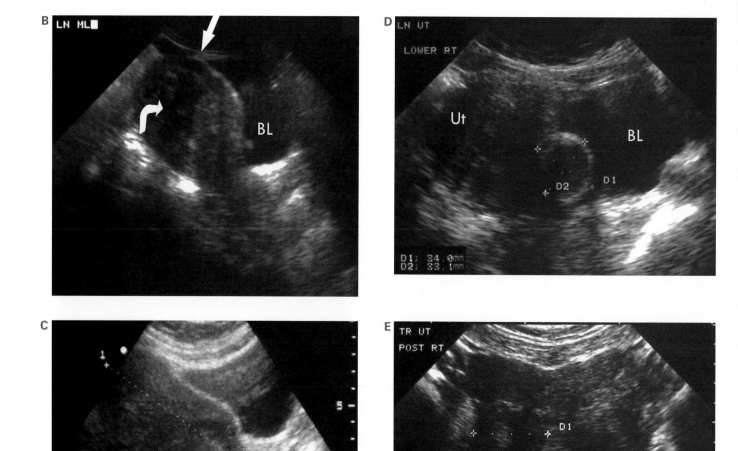

Figure 2-27, continued. B *Longitudinal scan showing a slightly globular uterus with a small hypoechoic fibroid (straight arrow) in the anterior myometrium, which shadows (curved arrow). BL = bladder.* **C** *Longitudinal image of an enlarged uterus containing multiple fibroids, which cause the uterine contour to be irregular.* **D** *Longitudinal image showing a lower uterine segment fibroid (measured) indenting the posterior bladder wall. Ut = uterus, BL = bladder.* **E** *Transverse image through a uterus containing multiple fibroids, one of which is being measured. Note the lobulated contour of the uterus.*

sonographically, an adnexal mass (Figure 2-28). Even a subserous/subserosal fibroid can appear to be an adnexal mass rather than uterine in origin (Figure 2-29). To make the differentiation, the examiner should look at the echo pattern of the mass. Most adnexal masses are cystic or complex. If the mass looks similar to myometrium, it could well be. One must also determine if the mass distorts the endometrial cavity. Larger uterine masses can affect the endometrial position. Although adnexal masses can displace the whole uterus, they do not affect the endometrial cavity. Only 2%–3% of fibroids are located within the cervix or fallopian tube.

Fibroid growth is influenced by estrogen, and after menopause, in the absence of hormone stimulation, fibroids should regress in size. As they grow, fibroids may outgrow their blood supply and necrose or degenerate on the inside (Figure 2-30). When this occurs during pregnancy, it can be a source of pain. Fibroids may calcify (Figure 2-31) or contain scattered calcifications, and

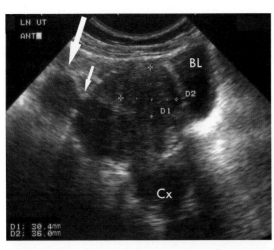

Figure 2-28. *This longitudinal scan shows a uterus containing multiple defined fibroids, one of which is being measured. Superior to the uterine fundus is a pedunculated fibroid (long arrow) and its stalk (short arrow). BL = bladder, Cx = cervix.*

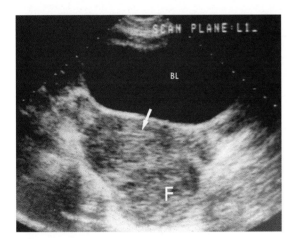

Figure 2-29. *Longitudinal scan through a uterus demonstrating a posterior fibroid. Note how the endometrial stripe is displaced anteriorly by the mass (arrow). F = fibroid, BL = bladder.*

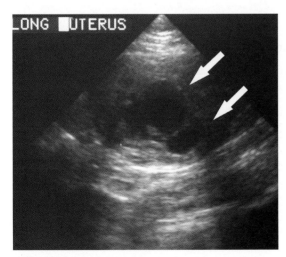

Figure 2-30. *This transverse image through a uterus shows cystic degeneration of fibroids. They appear echo-free and show posterior enhancement indicating a fluid component (arrows).*

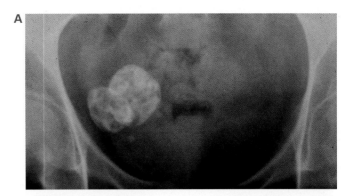

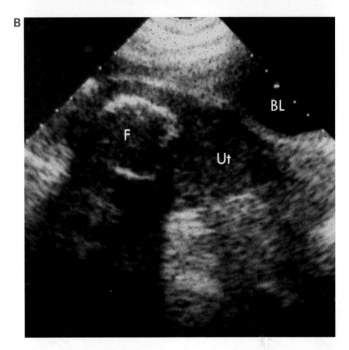

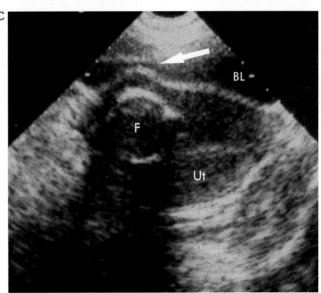

Figure 2-31. A *This flat plate x-ray shows two calcified fibroids in the patient's right adnexa.* **B** *Longitudinal image shows a rounded calcified fibroid in the uterine fundus. F = fibroid, BL = bladder, Ut = uterus.* **C** *Transverse image of same patient. One can appreciate the slight contour irregularity produced by the fibroid (arrow). BL = bladder, Ut = uterus, F = fibroid.*

Calcification

Cystic degeneration

Infertility

Torsion

Malignant potential

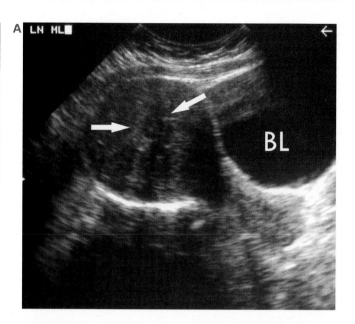

those that are pedunculated may torse and rupture. (See Box 2-13 for the complications associated with fibroids.) Patients with chronic symptoms from fibroids may opt for a hysterectomy. If fertility is an issue, a **myomectomy** can be performed or **gonadotropin-releasing hormone (GnRH)** agonist drugs such as **Lupron (leuprolide)** may be employed to help shrink the tumors.

Endometrial Polyps

Dysfunctional uterine bleeding (DUB) is commonly associated with the **endometrial polyp**, sometimes referred to as an **adenomatous** or **mucous polyp**. These polyps (Figure 2-32) typically are benign pedunculated or sessile projections of the endometrium, and although the menstrual cycles of patients with endometrial polyps are usually normal, menstrual flow is heavier and patients may experience a mild crampy pain. Endometrial polyps can be seen in women of all ages but increase in frequency after age 50 and therefore can sometimes be responsible for postmenopausal spotting/bleeding. Intermenstrual spotting most often is associated with ovulation but may occur when a polyp becomes congested or necrotic. Sonographically, polyps can be difficult to differentiate from a submucosal fibroid unless sonohysterography is performed. The polyps may present as nonspecific focal or diffuse endometrial thickening or as a discrete mass. Color Doppler may assist in demonstrating a vascular stalk, which helps to confirm the presence of a polyp.

Adenomyosis

Adenomyosis, also referred to as **internal endometriosis**, is the result of the endometrium invading the myometrium. It occurs most frequently in women who are **multiparous** (have given birth two or more times). The condition can be localized or diffuse, or it can resemble a fibroid uterus. Patients present with severe dysmenorrhea,

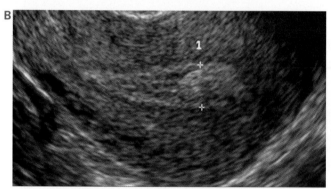

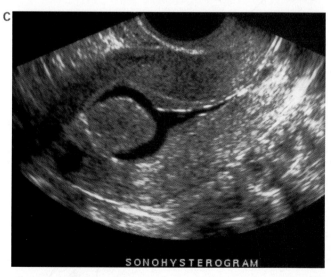

Figure 2-32. A Longitudinal image through a globular uterus with a suspicious hypoechoic nodule seen centrally (arrows). Although originally thought to be a small fibroid, it was later confirmed to be an endometrial polyp. BL = bladder. **B** Longitudinal transvaginal image through a retroflexed uterus showing a hyperechoic nodular region (measured) within the endometrial cavity, typical of a polyp. Notice that it is similar in echogenicity to the endometrium itself. **C** This sonohysterogram shows an endometrial polyp well outlined by the saline.

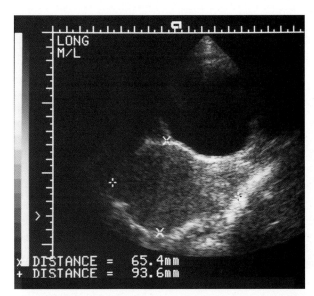

Figure 2-33. *This longitudinal uterine scan shows mild globular enlargement but no defined fibroids. The echo pattern is coarse and somewhat mottled, a presentation associated with adenomyosis.*

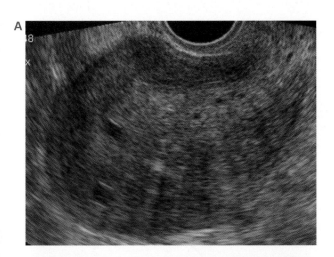

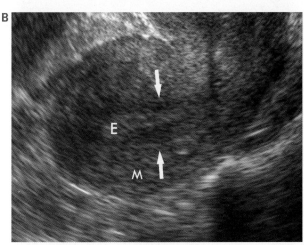

Figure 2-34. A *This transvaginal image shows no junctional zone, streaky shadows, and endometrial/myometrial cysts, all of which are associated with adenomyosis.* **B** *The normal junctional zone (arrows) can be seen quite well on this transvaginal image. E = endometrium, M = myometrium.*

menorrhagia with clots, and dyspareunia. The uterus may be palpably enlarged and tender (Figure 2-33). Adenomyosis is best diagnosed with **magnetic resonance imaging** (**MRI**). Its sonographic characteristics include a coarse and overall mottled appearance of the myometrium, exhibiting streaky shadowing with ill definition or irregular contour of the endometrium (Figure 2-34A). This presentation typically causes a loss of definition of the junctional zone—the hypoechoic area normally seen between the endometrium and myometrium (Figure 2-34B). Small myometrial cysts may be seen in the myometrium extending at least 2 mm beyond the endometrium (Figure 2-34A). Because adenomyosis is hormonally influenced, these cysts may be seen throughout the cycle but are more prominent during the secretory phase. Table 2-1 correlates the clinical and sonographic presentations of adenomyosis.

Endometritis

Box 2-14 lists the causes of **endometritis**, inflammation of the endometrium. This condition is most often the response to infection following abortion, childbirth, insertion of an intrauterine contraceptive device, or acquisition of a sexually transmitted disease. In the postmenopausal patient, senile endometritis may arise from cervicitis or

Table 2-1.	Uterine adenomyosis: correlation of clinical and sonographic presentations.
Clinical	**Sonographic Appearance**
Menorrhagia	Enlarged, tender uterus
Dysmenorrhea	Diffuse streaky shadowing
Dyspareunia	Loss of junctional zone
Multiparous	Endometrial/myometrial cysts

Box 2-14.	Causes of endometritis.
	Abortion/childbirth
	Complications from intrauterine contraceptive devices
	Sexually transmitted disease
	Cervicitis
	Cervical tumor

a cervical tumor. Inflammatory fluid or pus (**pyometra**) may be retained and visualized. Symptoms include pelvic pain, fever, and an elevated white blood cell count. In the postmenopausal patient, it is not uncommon to see endometrial fluid as the endometrium begins to atrophy and degenerate. If the patient is asymptomatic, this fluid is simply an incidental finding and not to be mistaken for endometritis (Figure 2-35).

Endometrial Carcinoma

Endometrial carcinoma is the most common gynecologic malignancy. Although endometrial carcinoma grows much more slowly than cervical cancer, it can grow through the myometrium and into the cervix, adnexa, fallopian tubes, and ovaries. It is associated with excessive estrogen production. Obese, diabetic, hypertensive women and those with estrogen-secreting ovarian tumors are at increased risk, as are postmenopausal patients undergoing hormone replacement therapy. There is a strong predisposition in women with a family history. Hormone replacement therapy causes **atypical hyperplasia** (abnormal overgrowth of tissue) of the endometrium (or **endometrial hyperplasia**), which ultimately undergoes malignant changes (Figure 2-36A). There also seems to be an increased incidence among patients with a history of infertility and DES exposure. (See Box 2-15.) The most common clinical signs of endometrial cancer are postmenopausal bleeding and metrorrhagia.

Endometrial carcinoma is usually diagnosed early because postmenopausal bleeding is a significant symptom. Typically, the most common cause of postmenopausal bleeding is the exogenous administration of estrogen. For postmenopausal women who are not on hormone replacement therapy, endometrial atrophy would be most

Box 2-15. Risk factors for endometrial carcinoma.
Postmenopausal bleeding
Poor fertility history
Obesity
Diabetes/hypertension
Hormone replacement therapy
Estrogen-secreting tumors
Exposure to diethylstilbestrol (DES)

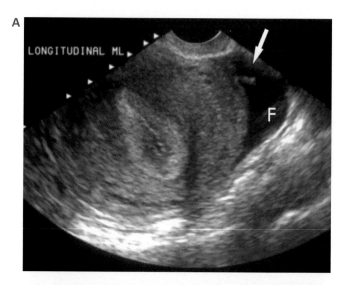

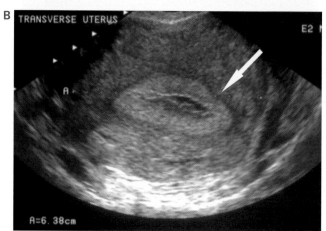

Figure 2-35. A *This transvaginal image shows a retroflexed uterus in a patient presenting with endometritis. There is free fluid in the cul-de-sac and an adhesion seen attached to the uterine fundus (arrow). The endometrium is thickened. F = free fluid.* **B** *Coronal image of endometritis showing the thick endometrium and debris-filled fluid within the endometrial cavity (arrow).*

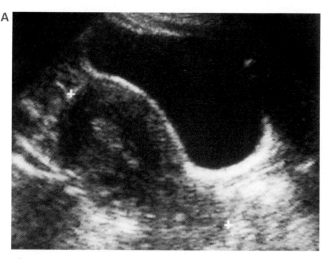

Figure 2-36. A *Longitudinal image of the uterus of an asymptomatic postmenopausal patient not on hormone replacement therapy. The endometrium is too thick. (Figure continues . . .)*

common. Other causes of postmenopausal bleeding include endometritis, cervicitis, benign hyperplasia, polyps, and, rarely, estrogenic ovarian tumors.

Endometrial carcinoma is classified by stage as follows:

- *Stage 0:* suggestive of but not conclusive
- *Stage I:* growth confined to corpus
- *Stage II:* growth extended to cervix
- *Stage III:* growth beyond uterus but not outside pelvis or into bladder/rectum
- *Stage IV:* growth invading rectum/bladder or beyond pelvis

Sonographically, early endometrial carcinoma presents as thickened endometrium. This finding is quite unusual in the postmenopausal patient unless she is receiving hormone replacement therapy. If a patient is on hormone replacement treatment, the postmenopausal endometrium should not measure more than 8 mm (Figures 2-36 B and C). The endometrium of the postmenopausal patient who is not taking hormones should measure no more than 5 mm. Another point to emphasize is the regularity of the endometrium. Normally it is relatively smooth, but it will appear focally thickened and ragged as the cancer spreads into the myometrium (Figure 2-36D). With advanced tumors in Stage III or IV, the entire uterus will be involved, causing significant heterogeneity of the myometrium as well as contour irregularity. Sonographic findings may resemble those for a fibroid uterus, but clinical data should indicate otherwise (Figure 2-36E).

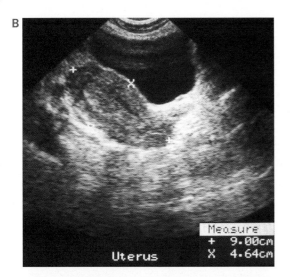

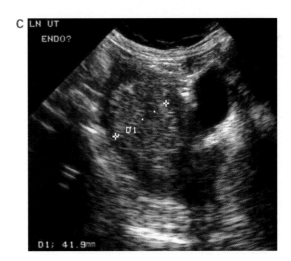

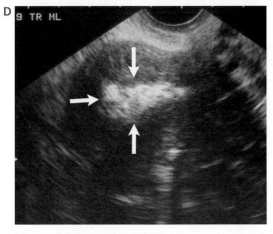

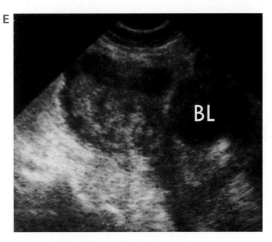

Figure 2-36, continued. B *Postmenopausal patient presenting with bleeding and a grossly thickened endometrium. Note loss of the junctional zone along the posterior wall, indicative of myometrial invasion. Biopsy confirmed endometrial carcinoma.* **C** *This postmenopausal patient shows only a thin rim of myometrium because of endometrial carcinoma.* **D** *Transvaginal image from a postmenopausal patient with bleeding demonstrates a brightly echogenic and very irregular endometrium (arrows).* **E** *This longitudinal image shows an advanced stage of endometrial carcinoma. The uterus is enlarged and irregular in contour. BL = bladder.*

Drug-Induced Conditions

In patients already diagnosed with a condition for which they are undergoing treatment, sonographic findings can reveal drug-related effects on the endometrium. For example, **tamoxifen**, a nonsteroidal antiestrogen drug, is commonly prescribed for therapy in pre- and post-menopausal patients with breast cancer. Premenopausal women may experience an antiestrogen effect, while postmenopausal women usually see a weak estrogenic effect. Because tamoxifen increases the risk of hyperplasia, polyps, and endometrial carcinoma, these patients may be referred for evaluation of endometrial changes, as can others on drug therapies that affect the endometrium. For these patients measurements should always be obtained by transvaginal technique for accuracy and quality of **resolution**, or detail (Figure 2-37).

Uterine Evaluation Using Saline Infusion Sonohysterography

Saline infusion sonohysterography (**SIS**) utilizes endovaginal sonography to evaluate the endometrium and endometrial cavity. This is accomplished by inserting a small catheter into the cervical canal and introducing sterile saline into the endometrial cavity (Figure 2-38). The procedure is very simple, well tolerated, cost-effective, and performed on an outpatient basis. Higher-frequency (5–7.5 MHz) endovaginal transducers provide better visualization and improved resolution in evaluating the female pelvis, and saline infusion sonohysterography can reduce the need for more invasive procedures such as biopsy, hysteroscopy, or dilation and curettage. (See Box 2-16.)

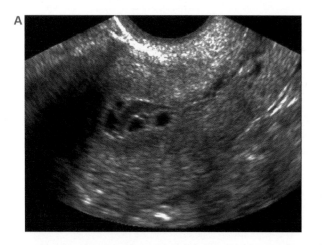

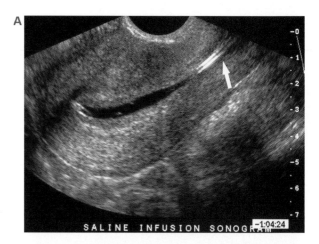

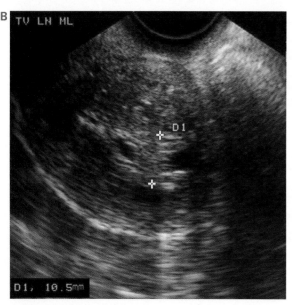

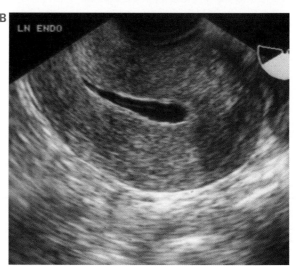

Figure 2-38. A and **B** Longitudinal transvaginal images of a postmenopausal uterus showing saline being introduced into the endometrial cavity by a catheter (A, arrow). The normal endometrium is thin and regular.

Figure 2-37. A and **B** Transvaginal evaluations of a patient on tamoxifen show the classic thickened and cystic endometrium that is a complication of the drug.

Box 2-16. Prime candidates for saline infusion sonohysterography.

History of prior surgery (in symptomatic patients)

Multiple pregnancies (in symptomatic patients)

Previously known fibroids

Patients who are obese

Patients with dysfunctional uterine bleeding

Infertility and patients with recurring miscarriage

Synechiae

Diagnosis of retained products of conception

Monitoring drug therapies

Preoperative evaluation and locating foreign object

Indications for SIS

Synechiae/Asherman Syndrome Patients who have a history of prior uterine operations or multiple pregnancies may have uterine scar tissue and adhesions, or **uterine synechiae** (also called **Asherman syndrome**), which may be associated with abnormal bleeding and/or pain. Synechiae may also lead to the development of polyps within the endometrial cavity. Adhesions within the endometrial cavity appear as bandlike structures bridging and distorting the cavity.

Polyps **Polyps** are fairly common benign lesions in peri- and postmenopausal women. They can have a thin stalk or a broad base and may be multiple. With standard ultrasound technique, either transabdominal or transvaginal, the polyp may appear indistinct or the endometrial echo pattern may have a nonspecific or nodular appearance. It may be difficult to differentiate the presentation from that of a fibroid. Polyps are much easier to identify once they are outlined by fluid, and SIS therefore makes it possible to distinguish a polyp from a submucosal fibroid (Figures 2-39 A and B).

Fibroids Submucosal fibroids are seen clearly with SIS and often have a hypoechoic appearance. SIS enables the sonographer to demonstrate the difference between a polyp extending from the endometrium and a fibroid pressing on the endometrium (Figure 2-39C).

Postmenopausal Patients In a postmenopausal patient presenting with a thickened endometrium greater than 5–8 mm and vaginal bleeding, endometrial carcinoma

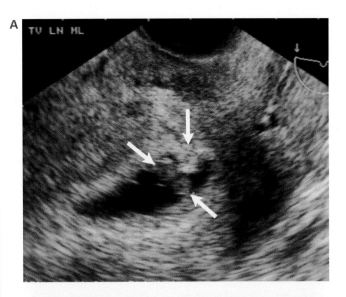

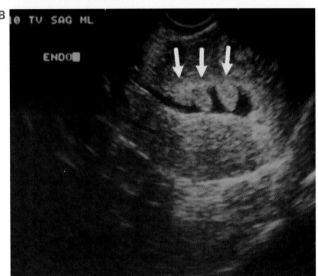

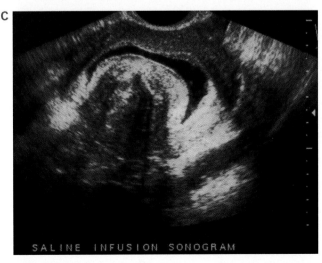

Figure 2-39. A *and* **B** *These sonohysterograms were performed on a 32-year-old patient presenting with irregular bleeding. Multiple polyps are clearly defined (arrows).* **C** *Sonohysterogram shows a submucosal fibroid indenting and displacing the endometrial cavity.*

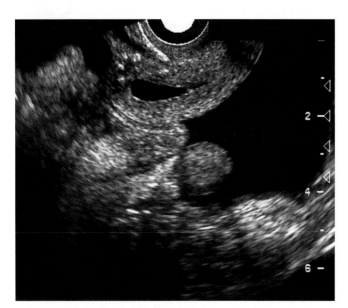

Figure 2-40. *Transvaginal image through the uterus of a post-menopausal patient shows some fluid accumulation within the endometrial cavity. This finding is not uncommon in elderly patients. Note that otherwise the endometrium is thin and regular.*

must be ruled out. These patients are excellent candidates for SIS, as one can more accurately measure the endometrial thickness while better visualizing any irregularities in contour (Figure 2-40).

Infertility When performed with a balloon catheter, SIS can visualize the uterine cavity as well as the patency of the tube. This can be very helpful in evaluating infertility patients as well as those classified as habitual aborters. The endometrium can be monitored during hormone stimulation to help determine the cause of infertility or spontaneous abortion. SIS also helps to identify foreign intrauterine objects, such as an intrauterine contraceptive device that is embedded within the wall of the uterus.

Contraindications for SIS

Pregnancy Patients with a known or suspected intrauterine pregnancy should not undergo SIS. A pregnancy test should be performed prior to scheduling SIS in sexually active patients of childbearing age.

Infection Patients with known or suspected infection should not be considered for SIS, as the procedure could help spread infection throughout the abdominal cavity.

Hemorrhage Patients with uncontrollable uterine hemorrhage should not have SIS, as endometrial tissue could be pushed into the abdominal cavity, leading to endometriosis.

ADNEXAL PATHOLOGY

In addition to becoming familiar with the sonographic signs of intrauterine conditions and pathology, the sonographer must become familiar with those of the **uterine adnexa** or uterine appendages. These include the ovaries, fallopian tubes, and supporting tissues such as the uterine ligaments.

Functional Cysts

Ovarian cysts are the most common pelvic pathology and occur in women of all ages. Cysts can be associated with hormone stimulation from an outside source or simply occur as part of the normal menstrual cycle. The most common physiologic cysts are the follicular and corpus luteum cysts. Theca-lutein cysts are the least common type of functional cyst.

Follicular Cysts

Follicular cysts should be readily identifiable, bilaterally, in patients in their reproductive years. Follicles are only a few millimeters in size at the end of a menstrual cycle and slowly increase in size upon exposure to follicle-stimulating hormone, producing estrogen (Figure 2-41A). Theoretically, the ovaries alternate ovulating, each ovary ovulating every other month. The ovary of the month

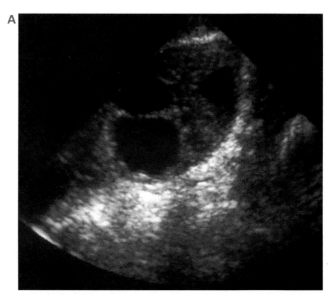

Figure 2-41. A *Transvaginal image of a normal ovary showing several follicles. Ovarian parenchyma can be seen between them. Following page:* **B** *This transvaginal image shows a dominant follicle (arrow). Ut = uterus.* **C** *Transabdominal longitudinal image of a larger dominant follicle that failed to ovulate and involute. It sits in the posterior cul-de-sac, causing anterior displacement of the uterus, which is being measured. BL = bladder, V = vagina, C = cyst.*

should show a dominant follicle around mid-cycle. If a dominant follicle fails to ovulate and involute, it may continue to grow, causing pain. These can grow up to 5 cm or larger and are usually unilocular and thin-walled, meeting all the criteria for a simple cyst (Figures 2-41 B and C). The postmenopausal patient should not show ovarian follicles unless she is on hormone replacement therapy (Figure 2-42). Generally speaking, regardless of the patient's age, simple unilocular cysts measuring less than 3 cm are considered within normal limits and of no real clinical concern.

Corpus Luteum Cyst

Once estrogen levels peak, the luteinizing hormone induces ovulation, producing the **corpus luteum cyst** and progesterone. Most corpus luteum cysts are unilateral and measure 2–4 cm but can grow larger. Upon close examination, these cysts show a more ragged wall than follicular cysts and often contain debris due to a small amount of

hemorrhage that occurs upon ovulation (Figures 2-43 A and B). Some corpus luteum cysts appear quite complex because of the development of fibrinous strands and clotting of blood associated with hemorrhage within the cyst (Figure 2-43C). Hemorrhagic ovarian cysts usually present with a sudden, acute onset of pelvic pain. These findings, when associated with a small amount of fluid within the posterior cul-de-sac, are highly suggestive that ovulation has occurred (Figures 2-43 D and E). Functional cysts usually resolve on their own and follow-up may be indicated after the next cycle to confirm resolution. If the patient is postmenopausal and the diameter of the cyst exceeds 5 cm, follow-up may be indicated in 3–6 months.

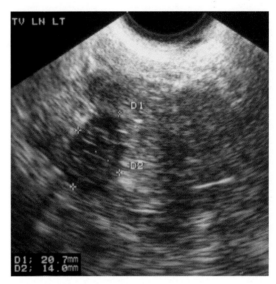

Figure 2-42. *Transvaginal image of a normal postmenopausal ovary (calipers). Note that there are no definable follicles.*

B
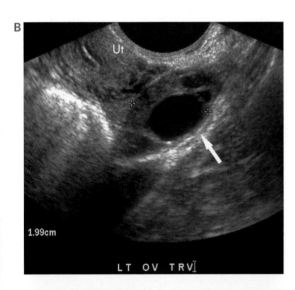

C
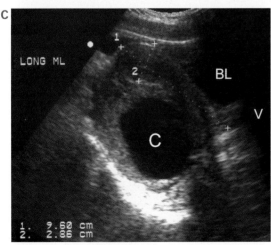

Figure 2-41, continued.

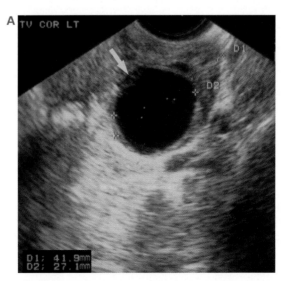

Figure 2-43. A *Transvaginal image of a corpus luteum cyst. Note the thickened irregular wall (arrow). The other follicles have atrophied and regressed. (Figure continues . . .)*

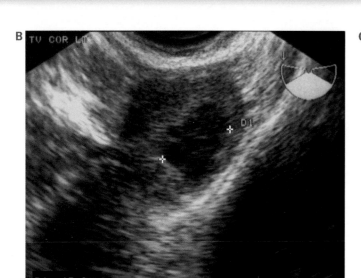

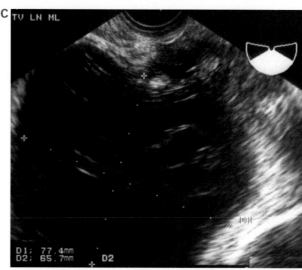

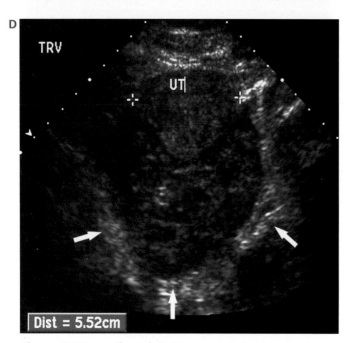

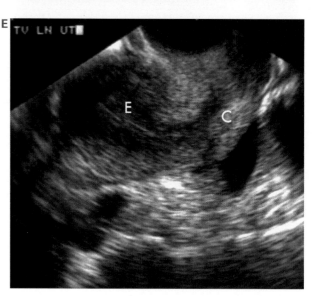

Figure 2-43, continued. B *This transvaginal image of the left ovary shows a corpus luteum cyst filled with debris (calipers). The walls are also quite irregular.* **C** *This image shows a large hemorrhagic ovarian cyst containing multiple fibrinous strands associated with clotting.* **D** *This transverse image shows a large collection of hemorrhagic fluid (arrows) in the posterior cul-de-sac and extending along the lateral margins of the uterus, which is being measured. This patient ruptured a hemorrhagic ovarian cyst. UT = uterus.* **E** *This transvaginal image demonstrates a small amount of free fluid in the posterior cul-de-sac behind the cervix. C = cervix, E = endometrium.*

During early pregnancy, the corpus luteum cyst is critical, as it is responsible for maintaining the pregnancy until the trophoblastic cells are capable of progesterone production. At 6 weeks after the last menstrual period, the corpus luteum can regress without consequence to the pregnancy. The corpus luteum of pregnancy should regress spontaneously by 12 weeks. A cyst that is still present after 16 weeks warrants clinical follow-up.

Theca-Lutein Cysts

Theca-lutein cysts are the result of hyperstimulation of the ovaries and are associated with trophoblastic disease, multiple gestations, ovary-stimulating drugs, and pregnancies complicated by hydrops fetalis. These present as large, bilateral multiseptated cysts and can grow to extend into the upper quadrants of the abdomen (Figure 2-44). Gross enlargement may put the patient at risk for ovarian rupture,

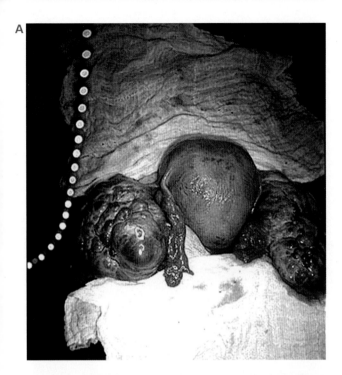

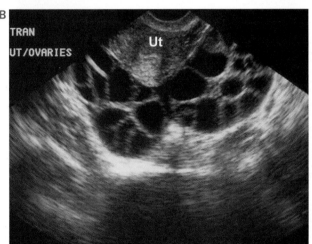

Figure 2-44. A *Surgical specimen of an excised uterus and large theca-lutein cysts.* **B** *Coronal endovaginal image showing bilateral theca-lutein cysts in a patient undergoing fertility assistance. Ut = uterus.*

which can be life-threatening. In the absence of hormone stimulation, the ovaries will eventually regress to normal size. This regression, however, may take 3–4 months.

Nonfunctional Cysts

Polycystic Ovarian Disease

Polycystic ovarian disease (**PCOD**), also known as **Stein-Leventhal syndrome**, is an endocrine disorder whereby excessive **androgen** secretion inhibits maturation of the ovarian follicles. The alteration in feedback to

the hypothalamus results in disturbing the ratio of luteinizing hormone to follicle-stimulating hormone, elevating it as well as increasing serum testosterone and aldosterone levels. The condition is most commonly seen in a younger age group (females in their teens through 20s), and diagnosis is usually performed clinically and serologically. The typical clinical manifestations include obesity, infertility, **hirsutism** (abnormal hairiness), and **oligomenorrhea** (infrequent menstruation). Several reports have suggested an increased incidence of endometrial carcinoma in patients diagnosed with polycystic ovarian disease. Treatment for fertility may include **ovulation induction** with clomiphene citrate or human menopausal gonadotropins or a surgical procedure called the **wedge resection**. Decreasing the amount of ovarian tissue by removing a triangular wedge of tissue causes a reduction in the secretions of androgens, reducing the feedback stimulus to the hypothalamus. Treatment for hirsutism and anovulation is often successful with oral contraceptives.

This condition typically causes enlargement of both ovaries with multiple tiny follicles seen around the periphery of the ovaries. Sonographically, with transabdominal ultrasound, the typical appearance is that of bilaterally enlarged ovaries with the cysts being too small to resolve well (Figure 2-45A). Transvaginally, however, the tiny peripheral cysts can be seen and measure only a few millimeters, giving the classic "string of pearls" appearance (Figure 2-45B). Ovarian enlargement is bilateral and occurs in 70% of cases; however, enlargement may be asymmetric. Although the clinical and sonographic findings described are typical, one must keep in mind that 25%–30% of patients with polycystic ovaries will be relatively asymptomatic and show normal ovaries upon sonographic examination.

Paraovarian Cysts

Paraovarian cysts are located in the broad ligament and are unilocular, thin-walled, and often quite large. When large, these cysts can simulate the urinary bladder. Post-void images can assist in making the diagnosis (Figures 2-46 A and B). Smaller cysts can be found in the **mesosalpinx** (the portion of the uterine broad ligament extending from the ovary to the fallopian tube) and around the terminal portion of the fallopian tube (Figure 2-46C). These are called **hydatids of Morgagni** and **fimbrial cysts**. All of these can simulate an ovarian cyst transabdominally, but one should be able to differentiate with transvaginal technique.

Figure 2-45. A *Image showing the typical appearance of a polycystic ovary. Note the echogenic ovarian parenchyma central to the small peripheral follicles. BL = bladder.* **B** *Transvaginal image of a polycystic ovary exhibiting the classic "string of pearls" sign.*

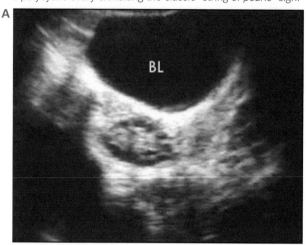

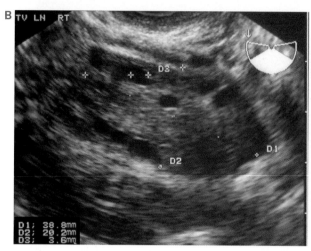

Figure 2-46. A *and* **B** *These transabdominal images show a large paraovarian cyst simulating the urinary bladder.* **A** *Image taken with bladder filled. BL = bladder.* **B** *Image taken postvoid.* **C** *Large paraovarian cyst seen anterior to ovary with the bladder seen inferior to the cyst. OV = ovary.*

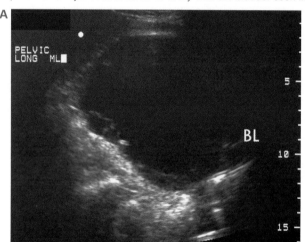

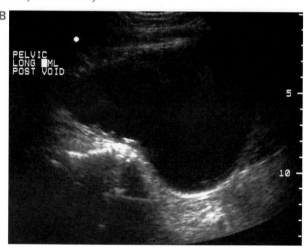

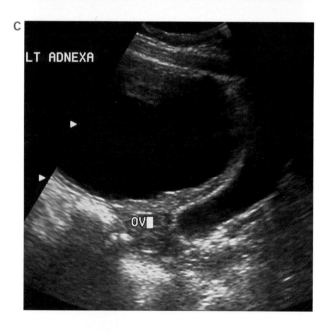

Adnexal Endometriosis

Endometriosis is defined as proliferation of endometrial tissues outside the endometrial cavity and is classified as either internal (adenomyosis, discussed above under "Uterine Pathology") or external (adnexal) in location. This condition appears to have some hereditary predisposition and is seen most frequently among upper-middle-class and professional women who have delayed childbearing. Although the condition is usually considered benign, there is some risk for malignancy. Patients usually present with classic symptoms that occur quite regularly in conjunction with the menstrual cycle. During menses, any ectopic tissues will bleed in response to the hormone stimulation of the cycle. It is not uncommon

Table 2-2. Clinical features for endometriosis.

Location	Clinical Features
Internal/adenomyosis	Intermenstrual pain and menor-rhagia. Palpably enlarged uterus. No pelvic deposit.
Pelvic peritoneum/ligaments	Symptoms indistinguishable from pelvic inflammatory disease. Pain worsens as menses approaches. Uterus may show retroversion from adhesions.
Ovaries	May be enlarged, tender, and fixed by adhesions.
Intestines	May mimic diverticulitis. Marked dyspareunia if rectum is involved. Endometriosis is a differential diagnosis for bowel tumor.
Bladder	Menstrual hematuria.
Umbilicus/scar	Cyclic painful swelling that sometimes bleeds.

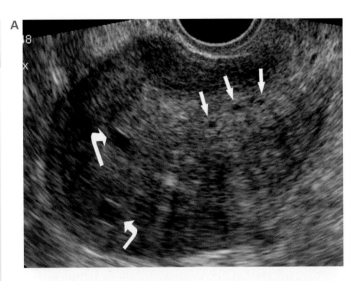

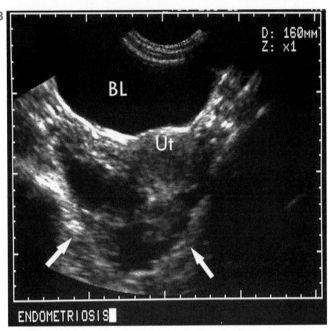

Figure 2-47. A *Transvaginal image of uterine adenomyosis (straight arrows). There is loss of the normal junctional zone. Endometrial as well as myometrial cysts are identified. Note the streaky shadows emanating from the uterus (curved arrows).* **B** *This image shows several ectopic endometrial implants during an active stage of bleeding. The hemorrhagic collection is in the posterior cul-de-sac region and extends into the right adnexa (arrows). BL = bladder, Ut = uterus.*

for adhesions to develop in response to the bleeding tissues, which further complicates the patient's symptoms. Typical symptoms (see Table 2-2) include cyclic pelvic pain (**dysmenorrhea**), lower abdominal and back pain, dyspareunia, dysuria, dyschezia, irregular bleeding, and infertility. If fertility is achieved, the hormones of pregnancy tend to have a therapeutic effect, and after delivery symptoms are not as severe. Other methods of treatment include administration of hormones such as progesterone or danazol, laser surgery, and hysterectomy.

As noted earlier, internal endometriosis, referred to as uterine **adenomyosis**, occurs when the endometrium invades the myometrium. Patients present with an enlarged uterus, dysmenorrhea, and menorrhagia with clots. Sonography is not the best method for evaluating patients with suspected uterine adenomyosis. Nevertheless, studies have suggested that sonographic findings include inhomogeneity of the myometrium with streaky shadowing and the presence of tiny myometrial cysts (Figure 2-47A).

Magnetic resonance imaging is currently the gold standard for diagnosis of both types of endometriosis. Since endometrial cysts are known to be associated with neoplasms such as endometrioid tumors, clear cell carcinomas, and müllerian mucinous borderline tumors, any solid component or nodularity should make one suspicious.

External endometriosis is associated with endometrial tissues found outside the uterus. Several theories exist as to why this occurs, but the most popular theory is that of retrograde spillage of menstrual blood via the fallopian tubes (Figure 2-47B). Retrograde flow of menses can be facilitated by retroversion of the uterus. Mostly retrograde spillage is confined to the pelvic compartment, but migration to remote areas can occur, presumably by a blood route or dissection along retroperitoneal planes.

These deposits are often diffuse and microscopic, making them difficult to evaluate with sonography. Many patients with endometriosis presenting with classic symptoms will show a normal pelvis during ultrasound examination. The structures that are most likely to be affected include the ovary, broad ligament, round ligament, and tubo-ovarian complex. Patients with extensive disease should be evaluated for invasion of other organs and structures, such as the bladder, bowel, and the abdominal wall through a scar. Although these tissues are almost always confined to the pelvic compartment below the umbilicus, rare distant sites have been reported, including the kidney, lung, mediastinum, arm, and nasal cavities.

Bleeding tissues that have been walled off by **lymphocytes** are called **endometriomas** or **chocolate cysts**. These masses are readily identified sonographically but generally cause no symptoms. Endometriomas usually have a thick wall and produce low-level echoes (Figure 2-48), although they can have a variety of sonographic appearances, including that of a cystic, solid, or complex mass. In most cases these masses will show some degree of posterior acoustic enhancement.

Endometriosis can be classified in five stages (Table 2-3), although systems vary (see Appendix C, "American Society for Reproductive Medicine: Revised Classification of Endometriosis"):

- *Stage I*: several small implants on the pelvic peritoneum
- *Stage II*: larger collections of endometrial tissues extending to the uterosacral ligaments, the rectovaginal septum, and/or the ovaries
- *Stage III*: endometriomas (5 mm and larger) on the ovary; possibly superficial implants on the broad ligaments and adjacent structures
- *Stage IV*: endometriomas penetrating the vagina, bowel, or urinary tract that may have migrated to distant sites such as the lymph nodes and umbilicus
- *Stage V*: endometriomas that have become adenocarcinomas

Pelvic Inflammatory Disease

Pelvic inflammatory disease (**PID**) refers to the infection of the fallopian tubes (**salpingitis**), which usually involves the ovaries and surrounding peritoneum. PID can be attributed to a variety of causes, the most common being the ascension of infection due to sexually transmitted diseases. Infection often begins in the vagina and ascends through the cervix and endometrial cavity to

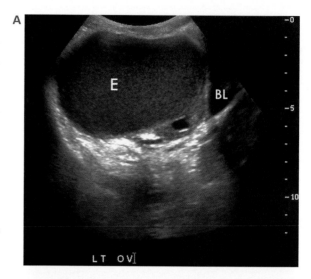

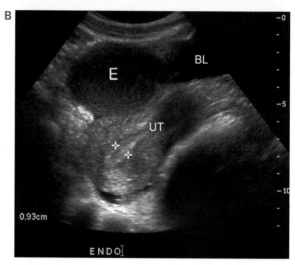

Figure 2-48. A *and* **B** *Longitudinal images of a classic endometrioma. BL = bladder, E = endometrioma, Ut = uterus.*

Table 2-3.	Stages of endometriosis.

Stage	Criteria
I	Small implants on pelvic peritoneum
II	Larger implants extend to: • Uterosacral ligaments • Rectovaginal septum • Ovaries
III	• Endometriomas (5 mm and larger) • Possible implants on broad ligament and adjacent organs
IV	Endometriomas penetrate: • Vagina • Bowel • Urinary tract
V	Endometriomas develop into adenocarcinoma

Box 2-17.	Common causes of pelvic inflammatory disease.

Gonorrhea

Chlamydia

TORCH infections

Intrauterine contraceptive devices

Ruptured appendix

Diverticular disease

Tuberculosis

Surgery

Bacterial infections (e.g., bacteroides, peptostreptococcus)

the tubes and pelvic compartment. Other causes include endometritis from TORCH infections (infections associated with toxoplasmosis, rubella, cytomegalovirus, and herpes), tuberculosis, a ruptured appendix, diverticular disease, intrauterine contraceptive devices, and postsurgical complications (Box 2-17). Symptoms may include pelvic pain that worsens during menses, irregular bleeding, fever, leukocytosis, purulent vaginal discharge, and dyspareunia. On vaginal exam, the cervix and vaginal fornix will be extremely tender, with guarding. Treatment is critical to the preservation of the patient's fertility. Antibiotics are the treatment of choice, followed by aspiration or catheter drainage for those cases that do not respond to oral or intravenous therapy. If untreated, patients may develop right upper quadrant pain due to migration of the infection into the abdomen, causing inflammation around the liver, or **perihepatitis**. When associated with PID, this is called **Fitz-Hugh–Curtis syndrome**.

Uterine findings with PID include mild enlargement of the uterus. Thickening of the endometrium and/or fluid due to endometritis may be seen within the endometrial cavity. Pus may be seen in the posterior cul-de-sac as complex fluid.

The most striking findings with PID are seen in the adnexal regions. Bacteria have a destructive effect on the lining of the fallopian tubes, resulting in the breakdown of tissue and the accumulation of pus within. With acute PID, swollen fallopian tubes filled with pus (**pyosalpinx**) will be seen as sausage-shaped masses lateral and posterior to the uterus. Pus that leaks out of the tube into the surrounding area can lead to further inflammation and the development of a **tubo-ovarian abscess** (**TOA**; see Figures 2-49 A–E). On examination, the abscess usually

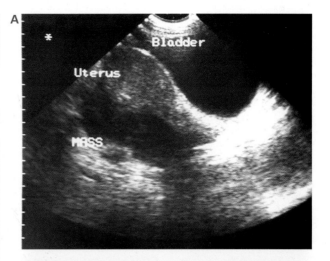

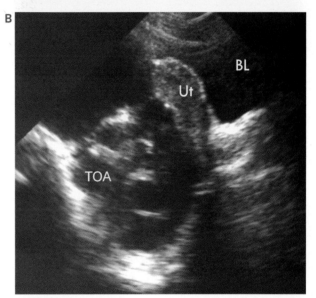

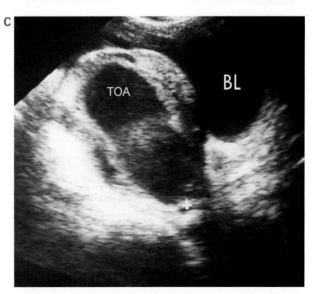

Figure 2-49. A *Image of the uterus with a sausage-shaped mass posterior, typical of a tubo-ovarian complex associated with pelvic inflammatory disease.* **B** *and* **C** *Images of a large tubo-ovarian abscess (TOA). Ut = uterus, BL = bladder. (Figure continues . . .)*

D

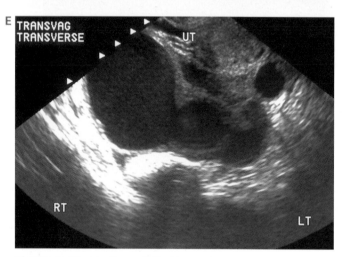

E

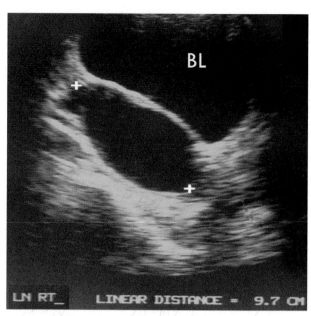

Figure 2-50. *Image of a hydrosalpinx (calipers). BL = bladder.*

Figure 2-49, continued. D *This TOA has a more solid appearance. Ut = uterus, BL = bladder, TOA = tubo-ovarian abscess.* **E** *Complex TOA. UT = uterus.*

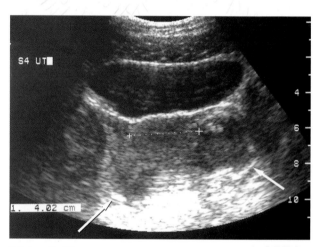

Figure 2-51. *Transverse image of a patient with pelvic inflammatory disease (PID). The uterus is measured (calipers). Bilateral tubo-ovarian abscesses (arrows) create the "indistinct uterus" sign often seen with PID.*

has a thick, shaggy wall and contains low-level echoes. Posterior enhancement should be evident because of the fluid component of pus. Occasionally one might see shadowing emanating from an abscess, as small gas-forming organisms can cause air pockets to develop. Over time, pus confined within a scarred and obstructed tube will liquefy and appear more cystic, turning a pyosalpinx into a **hydrosalpinx** (Figure 2-50). Adhesions frequently develop, fixing the infected mass to the uterus, ligaments, and bowel and resulting in the classic **indistinct uterus sign**, which can also be associated with chronic PID (Figure 2-51).

Ovarian Torsion

The ovaries receive blood from the ovarian arteries as well as branches of the uterine artery. A change in ovarian position could result in **ovarian torsion**, or twisting, causing the arterial supply, lymphatics, and venous drainage to become obstructed. Although this is not considered a common occurrence, ovarian mobility does put these structures at risk for torsion. Anything that causes the ovary to enlarge rapidly or to change position, including pregnancy, can lead to torsion.

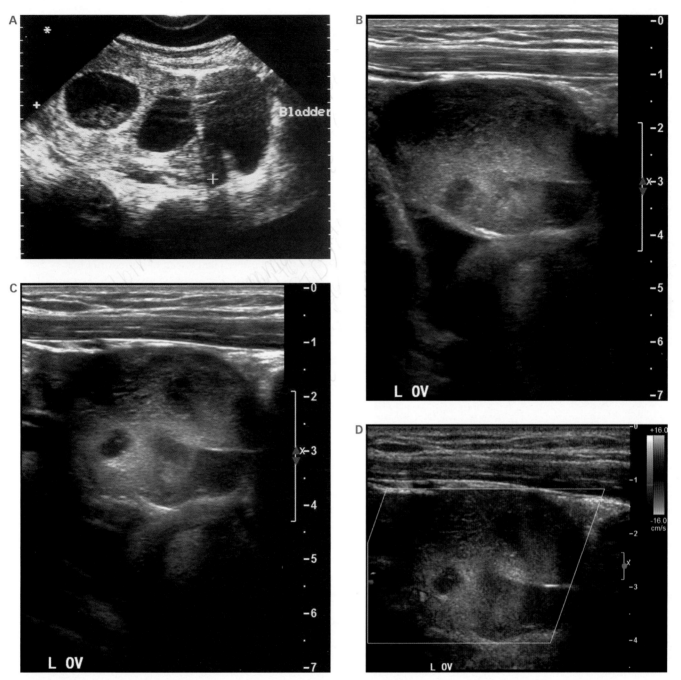

Figure 2-52. A *Longitudinal image shows a grossly swollen ovary with large areas of infarction (calipers) in a patient with ovarian torsion.* **B** *Longitudinal torsed left ovary is enlarged and shows a very hetero- geneous echo pattern with free fluid around it.* **C** *Transverse of the same ovary.* **D** *Color flow application shows no blood flow within the enlarged ovary.*

The most common sonographic appearance of ovarian torsion is one of ovarian enlargement with hypoechoic areas within it corresponding to hemorrhage and/or in- farction (Figures 2-52 A–C). Color Doppler may assist in determining diminished or absent blood flow to the ovary (Figure 2-52D). Typically, patients present with acute lower abdominal pain, nausea, and vomiting. A palpable adnexal mass may be encountered on occasion. Ovar- ian torsion usually occurs on the right side because the sigmoid colon occupies most of the left lower quadrant. Clinical symptoms often mimic other conditions, includ- ing appendicitis and ectopic pregnancy. This condition can occur at any age but is most common in children and women in their reproductive years.

Ovarian Neoplasms

Ovarian neoplasms (tumors) may develop in any age group but are most common in women between the ages of 30 and 60. Many ovarian tumors have malignant potential, even if it is low. Most are asymptomatic and small in the early stages. Many are capable of growing to a large size, at which time they are at risk for torsion or rupture. They can be classified in three categories: epithelial, stromal, and germ cell tumors (Table 2-4). They can also be classified according to whether they are cystic or solid and are so grouped here.

Cystic Neoplasms

Generally speaking, most ovarian tumors are benign and occur in patients who are still in their reproductive years. If an ovarian tumor is discovered in a postmenopausal patient, the finding is a bit more worrisome, as the risk of malignancy increases with age. Although sonography cannot distinguish benign from malignant masses, there are sonographic characteristics that would suggest one over the other. Most unilocular, simple cystic masses measuring less than 6 cm are benign. The more solid the composition of the cystic mass, the higher the risk of malignancy. This includes the thickness of the walls and septae when present, the number of septations, the regularity of the contour, and the overall size of the mass. The association of pelvic ascites with an adnexal tumor is also a high indication for malignancy. Masses that measure more than 10 cm have a malignancy rate higher than those measuring less than 5 cm. If there is a significant decrease in the size of the mass after hormonal treatment, the mass is most likely benign.

Cystadenoma/Cystadenocarcinoma Considered among the most common ovarian neoplasms, the cystadenoma can be classified as serous or mucinous. Both present as multiseptated cystic masses. They are usually unilateral and can grow to become quite large (Figure 2-53). The **serous cystadenoma** contains a clear, watery fluid, while the **mucinous cystadenoma** contains a gelatinous material. Although they look very similar sonographically, the mucinous cystadenoma tends to contain more solid components with papillary projections that grow along the walls and septae (Figure 2-54). Of the two, the serous type is more common; its malignant counterpart, the **serous cystadenocarcinoma**, is the most common ovarian malignancy. The benign cystadenoma has a very high malignant potential; only one in nine remains

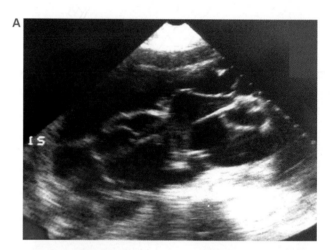
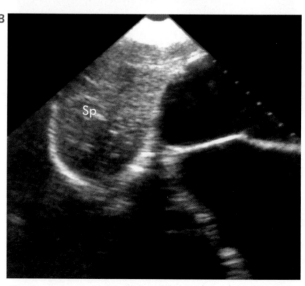

Figure 2-53. A *Transverse transabdominal image through a large serous cystadenoma.* **B** *Longitudinal image through the left upper quadrant of the same patient showing the large mass extending into the abdomen and touching the spleen. Sp = spleen.*

Table 2-4.	Types of ovarian tumor.	
Epithelial	**Stromal Sex Cord**	**Germ Cell**
Serous/mucinous cystadenoma	Fibroma	Teratoma
Cystadenocarcinoma	Sarcoma	Dysgerminoma
Endometrioma/ endometrioid	Thecoma	Gonadoblastoma
Brenner	Granulosa cell	Yolk sac tumor
Clear cell carcinoma	Arrhenoblastoma	

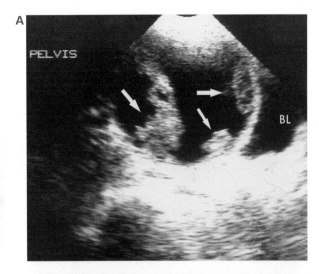

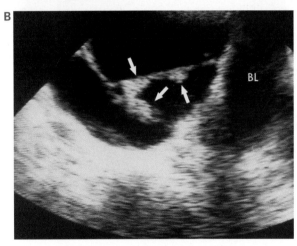

Figure 2-54. A *and* **B** *Longitudinal images of a mucinous cystadenoma. Note the papillary projections growing from the septae (arrows). BL = bladder.*

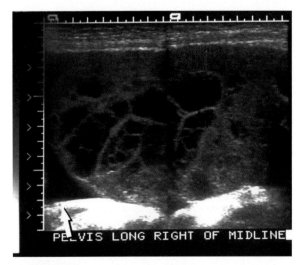

Figure 2-55. *Two linear array images are put together to document this large cystadenocarcinoma. Note the amount of solid component and the thickness of the walls. Ascites can be seen around the superior aspect (arrow).*

benign. Serous tumors tend to grow more rapidly than the very slow-growing mucinous types and are therefore diagnosed earlier (Figure 2-55). Unlike the serous type, the mucinous cystadenoma has a low malignant potential, with only one in seven turning malignant. If a **mucinous cystadenocarcinoma** grows to the point of rupture, it causes **pseudomyxoma peritoni**, a rare condition that involves the gelatinous material spilling out into the abdominal cavity and filling it with the jellylike substance. Mucin-producing cells spread over the parietal and visceral peritoneum, causing a reactive peritonitis with adhesions. Surgery must be performed periodically to remove the exudate, but death eventually results from **cachexia** or obstruction.

Cystic Teratomas **Cystic teratomas** are interesting tumors in that they contain tissues from one, two, or all three fetal layers: endoderm, mesoderm, and/or ectoderm (Box 2-18). They may can contain skin, fat, hair, teeth, fluid, bone, and hormone-producing tissues such as thyroid tissue (Figure 2-56A). A teratoma containing thyroid tissue is referred to as a **struma ovarii**.

Box 2-18.	Tissues found in benign cystic teratomas.
	Endoderm: digestive tract (innermost)
	Mesoderm: connective tissue, bone, blood, and lymph
	Ectoderm: skin, skin glands, hair, nails, nervous system, eyes/ears

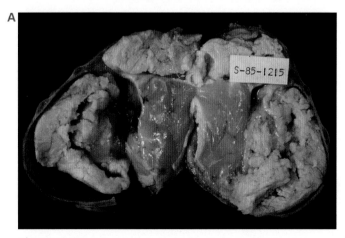

Figure 2-56. A *Surgical specimen of a benign cystic teratoma. (Figure continues . . .)*

Figure 2-56, continued. B *Longitudinal and* **C** *transverse images of a mostly solid teratoma posterior to the uterus. BL = bladder, Ut = uterus, T = teratoma.* **D** *and* **E** *Longitudinal images with solid dermoid seen superior to the retroverted uterus. D = dermoid, Ut = uterus.*

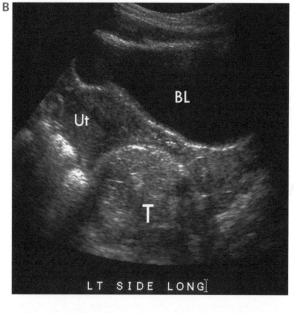

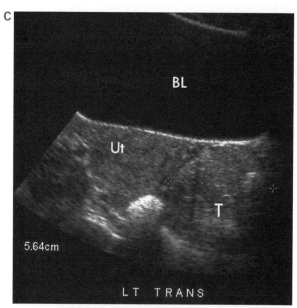

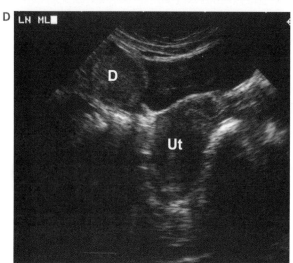

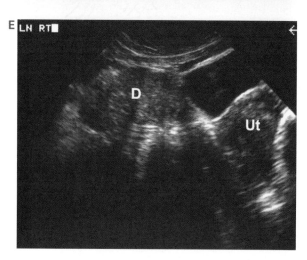

Teratomas are the most common tumor found in patients 20 years of age or younger, and most are benign. They can be categorized as mature (benign), immature (malignant), or **monodermal** (formed of ectoderm only, also known as **dermoid cysts**). In females teratomas are usually associated with the ovaries, and they may be bilateral in up to 20% of patients. Only about 2% of teratomas are malignant, and these are usually seen in young children. Most patients presenting with a teratoma are asymptomatic, but these masses are prone to torse. Torsion will cause pain and, although rupture is uncommon, these symptomatic cystic teratomas are usually surgically resected in order to decrease the risk of torsion and preserve the ovary.

Because teratomas can contain so many different tissue types, they can have a wide variety of echo patterns (Table 2-5). The least common are those that are purely cystic or completely solid (Figures 2-56 B–E). Most will have both cystic and solid components with some region of calcification (Figure 2-57). Dermoid cysts are characterized by a **dermoid plug**, which forms on the cyst's interior surface and can contain bones, teeth, and matted hair extending into the cyst's cavity; on sonography they demonstrate the classic **tip of the iceberg sign**. Lack of sound transmission

Table 2-5. Sonographic categories for dermoids.

Least Common	Most Common
Purely cystic	Complex
Purely solid	Ill-defined

A

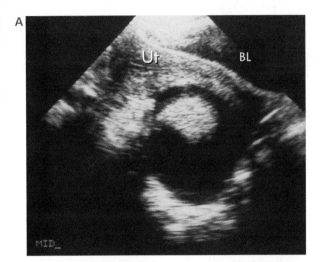

B

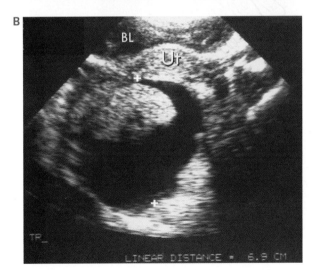

Figure 2-57. A Longitudinal and **B** transverse images showing a complex teratoma in the posterior cul-de-sac displacing the uterus anteriorly. BL = bladder, Ut = uterus.

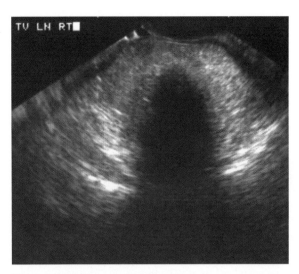

Figure 2-58. Transvaginal image through a teratoma demonstrating the dense shadowing often associated with matted hair and calcification: the "tip of the iceberg" sign.

A

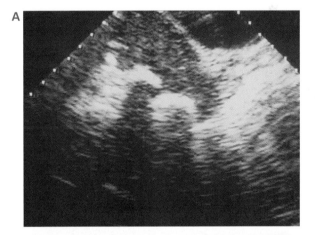

B

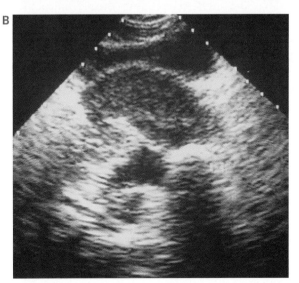

Figure 2-59. A Longitudinal and **B** transverse images demonstrating an area of ill definition where a mass was palpated on physical examination. Note the hyperechoic curvilinear echoes that shadow. At surgery, the patient presented with a benign cystic teratoma behind the uterus.

behind these tissues often inhibits visualization of the entire mass, similar to the way only a small amount an iceberg is visible above the water's surface (Figure 2-58). Teratomas may also present as ill-defined masses with only shadow boundaries, allowing for evidence that a mass that was palpable on physical exam is actually present (Figure 2-59).

Solid Neoplasms

Solid ovarian tumors are rare and can be benign or malignant. Many are hormone-producing, such as the sex cord tumors, which can be either **estrogenic**, producing estrogen, or **androgenic**, producing testosterone. These tumors are mostly hypoechoic and cannot be differentiated sonographically. All solid benign tumors have malignant potential, but it is low.

Granulosa Cell Tumors Granulosa cell tumors, sometimes referred to as **theca cell tumors**, are estrogenic and cause feminizing effects. The postmenopausal patient will present with cyclic vaginal bleeding and develop cystic dysplasia of the breasts. A small percentage of patients will also develop endometrial carcinoma. The young child diagnosed with a granulosa cell tumor presents with precocious puberty. When the tumor is small, it will be solid and hypoechoic, but it tends to undergo cystic degeneration as it enlarges (Figure 2-60A).

Fibromas and Thecomas Seen in the postmenopausal patient, **fibromas** and **thecomas** are sonographically indistinguishable benign tumors that account for about 4%–5% of all ovarian neoplasms. The thecoma, however, is estrogenic, whereas the fibroma is rarely associated with hormone production. The difference lies in the associated symptoms. The thecoma causes postmenopausal bleeding, while the fibroma is relatively asymptomatic. Although the ovarian fibroma has been associated with **Meigs syndrome**, which includes pelvic ascites and pleural effusion, only about 1% actually present with this complication. The fluid can track from the peritoneal to the pleural cavity via the lymphatic system. These findings are seen mostly when the fibroma is more than 5 cm in diameter (Figures 2-60 B and C).

Brenner Tumor The **Brenner tumor** is a solid but benign tumor with estrogenic properties. It constitutes about 2% of ovarian neoplasms. Typically, the Brenner tumor presents sonographically as a highly attenuating mass ranging in size from very small up to 8 cm. It may contain tiny cysts that increase in size upon enlargement of the mass. Although malignant changes are uncommon, the chance for malignancy increases with size (Figure 2-60D).

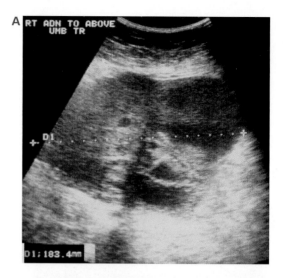

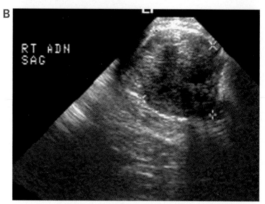

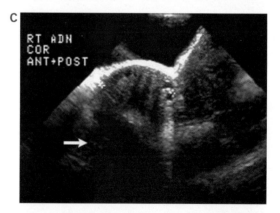

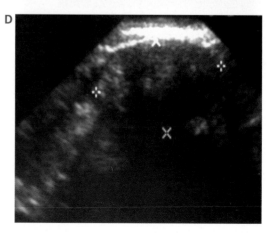

Figure 2-60. A *This image shows a large complex-appearing mass that was proven to be a granulosa cell tumor of the right ovary.* **B** *Endovaginal image of an ovarian fibroma.* **C** *Endovaginal image of a thecoma demonstrating the classic shadowing (arrow).* **D** *Brenner tumor demonstrated on endovaginal exam. B, C, and D are courtesy of Jim Baun, BS, RDMS, RVT, FSDMS, San Francisco, CA.*

Arrhenoblastoma Sometimes referred to as **androblastoma** or **Sertoli-Leydig cell tumor**, the **arrhenoblastoma** is **androgenic**, causing virilism in the patient. Considered rare, these neoplasms are seen mostly in patients in their reproductive years, and 20% are malignant. Upon removal of the tumor, feminine characteristics will return and symptoms regress in the order they appeared, with the exception of vocal changes, which tend to be permanent. Menses should return within two months (Figure 2-61).

Ovarian Malignancy

Ovarian carcinoma (cancer) is a silent killer. Many patients are asymptomatic or present with symptoms so vague—such as fatigue, bloating, and lumbar pain—that they are passed off as trivial complaints. Once symptoms become severe, including abdominal pain and vaginal bleeding, usually only palliative measures can be taken. To complicate the picture, ovarian cancer in general is considered rare. Therefore, patients are not routinely screened unless they meet the high-risk criteria. Patients considered at risk include those with a family history, low **parity** (low number of live-born children), late first pregnancy, infertility, Jewish descent, type A blood, high-fat diet, and the use of feminine hygiene products containing talcum powder. If we can identify those patients at risk and diagnose these tumors when they are still in Stage I, there is a 90%–95% cure rate. Unfortunately, most tumors (70%) are in Stages III and IV at diagnosis (Table 2-6). Some choose to use a scoring system for tumors,

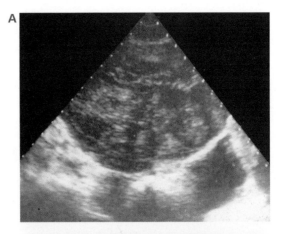

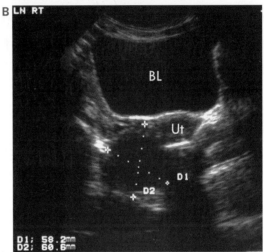

Figure 2-61. A *Image showing a large arrhenoblastoma, heterogeneous but very solid in appearance.* **B** *Transverse image of a small arrhenoblastoma (calipers). It appears quite hypoechoic but shows no posterior enhancement, indicating it is solid. BL = bladder, Ut = uterus.*

Table 2-6.   The staging and treatment of ovarian cancer.

Stage	Treatment
I: Growth limited to the ovary	
Ia: Limited to one ovary; no ascites	Surgery alone
Ib: Limited to both ovaries; no ascites	Surgery alone
Ic: Ascites or (+) peritoneal washings present	Surgery and chemotherapy
II: Pelvic extension	
IIa: Spread to uterus and tubes	
IIb: Spread to other pelvic tissues	Surgery and chemotherapy
IIIc: IIb with ascites	
III: Extrapelvic intraperitoneal spread *and/or* retroperitoneal positive nodes *or* no extrapelvic spread but involvement of intestines/omentum	Extensive surgery and chemotherapy
IV: Distant metastases, pleural effusion	Surgery (as extensive as possible with possible colostomy) followed by chemotherapy and palliative radiation therapy

Table 2-7.   Estimating the likelihood that an ovarian mass is malignant.*

Parameters	0	1	2	3
Wall structure	Smooth or small wall irregularity <3 mm		Solid	Papillary projection
Shadowing	Yes	No		
Septa	None or thin: <3 mm	Thick: >3 mm		
Echogenicity	Sonolucent or low-level echo			Mixed/high

*0 = least likelihood, 3 = greatest likelihood. Based on the scoring system of Lerner et al.

such as the one established by Lerner and colleagues (1994), for assistance in determining the likelihood of malignancy (Table 2-7).

Patients at risk for ovarian cancer are monitored every 6–12 months depending on the number of risk factors they have. Included in the workup is a biannual pelvic examination, pelvic ultrasound, and serum screening such as the **cancer antigen 125 (CA-125)** screening. Sonographic monitoring of the ovaries for ovarian cancer should be performed by transvaginal technique to ensure that ovarian measurements are accurate and consistent. Bladder filling for transabdominal technique can cause displacement and compression of the ovary, making it difficult to image in some cases. If a patient presents with an elevated CA-125, the concern raised is the possibility of malignancy. Practitioners should be aware that the CA-125 is not specific for ovarian cancer and may be elevated with other conditions as well, including endometriosis, pelvic inflammatory disease, degenerating fibroids, cirrhosis of the liver, and early intrauterine pregnancy.

As mentioned previously, the most common ovarian malignancy is the serous cystadenocarcinoma, which is a cystic tumor (Figure 2-62). There are a variety of solid malignant tumors, all of which are relatively rare. The **dysgerminoma** is characteristically ovoid with a smooth capsule. It is usually diagnosed in patients less than 30 years of age, and the younger the patient, the higher the malignancy risk. It is an aggressive tumor that is bilateral in 15% of cases (Figure 2-63). Although a solid tumor, the dysgerminoma may show areas of focal necrosis. (The dysgerminoma is the female counterpart of the seminoma in the male.)

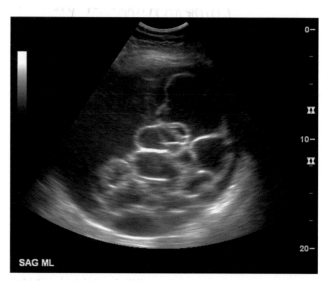

Figure 2-62. *Cystadenocarcinoma.*

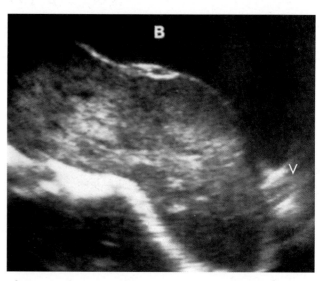

Figure 2-63. *Longitudinal image of a large dysgerminoma in a patient who had a hysterectomy. B = bladder, V = vagina.*

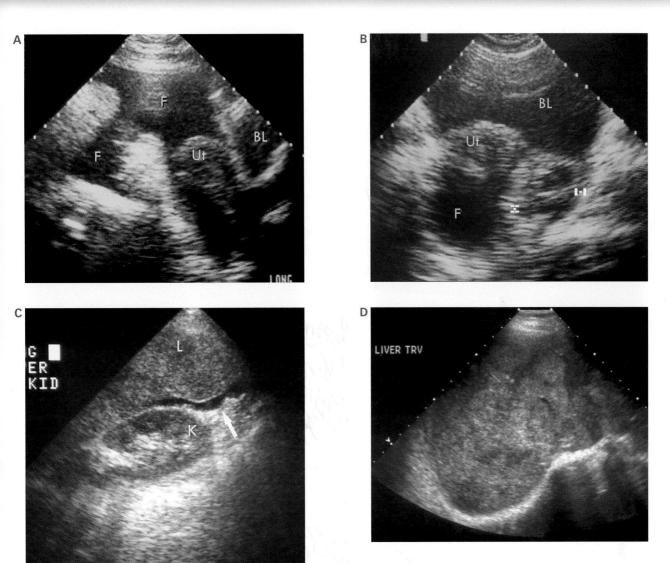

Figure 2-64. A *Longitudinal and* **B** *transverse images of a postmenopausal patient with pelvic ascites (fluid) and a solid left adnexal mass that proved to be malignant. BL = bladder, Ut = uterus, F = fluid.* **C** *Longitudinal image through the right upper quadrant showing extension of ascites in Morison's pouch (arrow). The liver is also enlarged and mottled in appearance. K = kidney, L = liver.* **D** *Transverse image of the liver shows metastatic deposits from the ovarian malignancy.*

The **endodermal sinus/yolk sac tumor** occurs in children and young adults and is highly malignant. These tumors produce alpha-fetoprotein, which can be identified in the blood for diagnostic testing and treatment monitoring.

Krukenberg tumors refer to metastases from primary tumors such as those of the gastrointestinal tract, breast, pancreas, and melanoma. These tumors are bilateral.

Ovarian malignancies can metastasize by four routes. Direct invasion will attack the small and large intestines, fallopian tubes, broad ligament, and uterus. The lymphatic system will allow for spread to pelvic and para-aortic nodes. Peritoneal fluid will carry malignant cells to the pouch of Douglas, paracolic gutters, omentum, right hemidiaphragm, and diffusely into the abdominopelvic compartment. Finally, the bloodborne path spreads the disease to distant sites, including the liver, lung, and skin.

Characteristics that make us suspicious that a pelvic mass is malignant include ascites, irregular walls with a lot of solid component, and metastatic deposits in the liver. Whenever one sees pelvic ascites, the upper abdomen should be evaluated for extension of ascites and possible metastases (Figure 2-64).

INCIDENTAL PATHOLOGY AND MISCELLANEOUS REQUESTS

Sometimes the pelvic sonogram demonstrates structures and pathology that are not necessarily gynecologic in origin. Others may be related but not considered clinically significant. The following include some of those findings.

Intrauterine Contraceptive Device

The sonographer is frequently called upon to look for an **intrauterine contraceptive device (IUCD)** after insertion has been performed and to monitor the position of the device over time. IUCDs should be central in location within the endometrial cavity. They will produce a high reflective echo that casts an acoustic shadow. The echo patterns will vary depending on the material from which the device is made and the type of device. Most will be T-shaped

(Figure 2-65); however, it is still possible to encounter some of the older devices (Figure 2-66). It is important to demonstrate the acoustic shadow, as a normal endometrium will not or should not exhibit shadowing (Figure 2-67).

Several complications can result from IUCDs. Although rare, perforation can occur, usually upon insertion (Figure 2-68). Over time, the device can become embedded into the myometrium, which would cause it to have an eccentric position when evaluated sonographically. If a device perforates all the way through the uterus, it is most difficult to identify sonographically; however, the sonographer can confirm that it is not intrauterine in location. Although relatively effective at preventing pregnancy, the device is not 100% effective: Patients have been known to become pregnant with a device in place. Sonography can assist in locating the device relative to the gestational sac (Figure 2-69). IUCDs, particularly

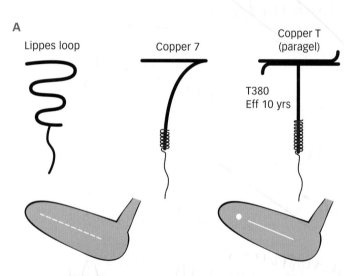

A Lippes loop   Copper 7   Copper T (paragel)

T380 Eff 10 yrs

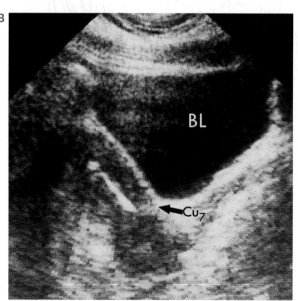

B

BL

Cu₇

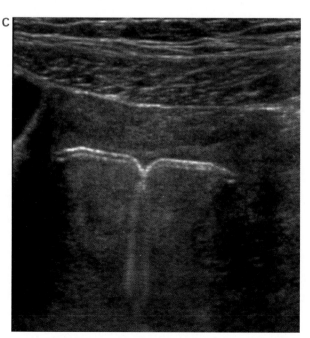

C

Figure 2-65. A *The appearance of the most common intrauterine contraceptive devices and how they are seen sonographically when imaged in long axis.* **B** *Longitudinal image of a Copper-7 intrauterine device in normal position. Cu7 = Copper-7, BL = bladder.* **C** *T-type device shown within the endometrial cavity.*

A

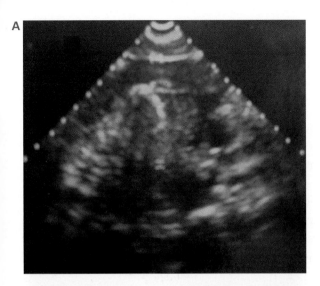

B

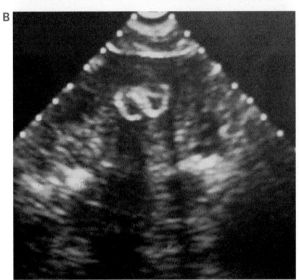

Figure 2-66. A and **B** *Transverse images through the uterus showing the configuration of a Saf-T-Coil intrauterine device.*

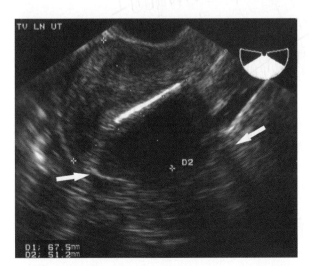

Figure 2-67. *Transvaginal image of a uterus containing an intrauterine contraceptive device. The endometrium can be seen surrounding the device. Posterior shadowing is indicated by the arrows.*

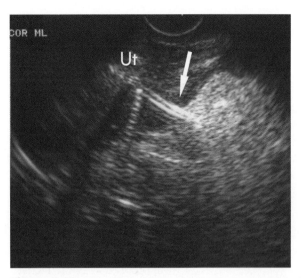

Figure 2-68. *Coronal transvaginal image shows an intrauterine device (arrow) that has perforated the myometrium. Ut = uterus.*

A

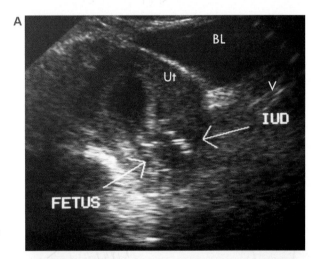

B

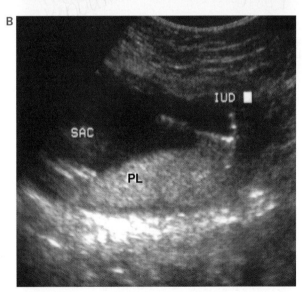

Figure 2-69. A *Longitudinal image of an early intrauterine pregnancy with a Lippes Loop in the lower uterine segment. BL = bladder, Ut = uterus, V = vagina.* **B** *A T-type intrauterine contraceptive device is seen within this second trimester intrauterine pregnancy.*

Figure 2-70. A *and* **B** *Transvaginal images demonstrate a Lippes Loop (arrow) within the uterus of a patient with pelvic inflammatory disease. Ut = uterus, TOA = tubo-ovarian abscess.* **C** *Flat plate x-ray of a female pelvis showing a Lippes Loop intrauterine contraceptive device.* **D** *Longitudinal sonogram demonstrating a Lippes Loop in the uterus.*

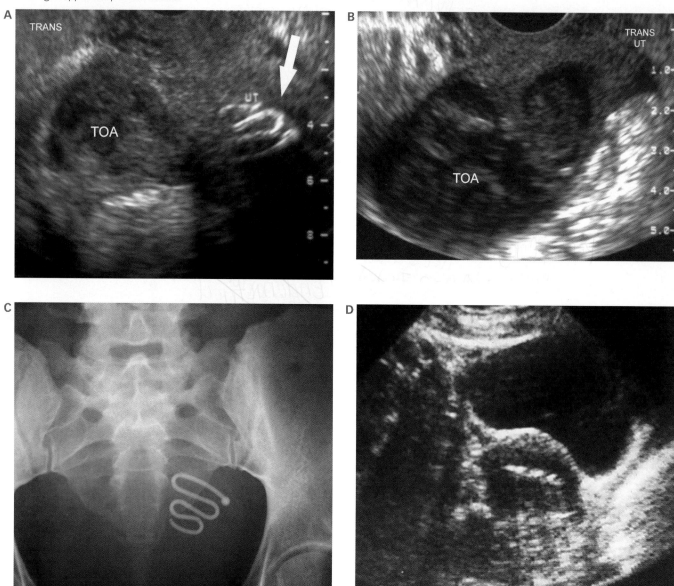

the copper devices, do have some spermicidal properties, but one of the main functions is to inhibit normal implantation of the blastocyst. If a fertilized egg is unable to implant in its normal position, implantation may occur ectopically. Besides being at increased risk for ectopic pregnancy, the patient with an IUCD is also at increased risk for pelvic inflammatory disease, menorrhagia, and dysmenorrhea (Figure 2-70). Finally, menorrhagia with clots may assist with expulsion of the device.

Lymphadenopathy

Sonography is not the best method for evaluating lymph nodes, but if asked to do so the practitioner must remember that they follow the arterial branches. When lymph nodes are grossly enlarged (**lymphadenopathy**), they will be homogeneous, hypoechoic, and lobulated in contour. It is important to pay close attention to the region of the internal and external iliac arteries as well as the iliopsoas margin (Figure 2-71). A good way to

Figure 2-71. A *Transverse and* **B** *longitudinal images through enlarged pelvic lymph nodes located along the iliopsoas margins (calipers).*

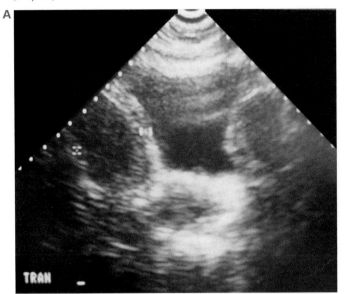

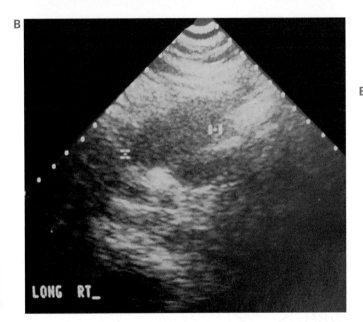

Figure 2-72. A *Longitudinal image of a large hematoma (arrows) that developed following total abdominal hysterectomy. BL = bladder.* **B** *Transverse image taken at the level of the vagina showing a larger hematoma anterior to the bladder posthysterectomy. H = hematoma, BL = bladder. (Figure continues . . .)*

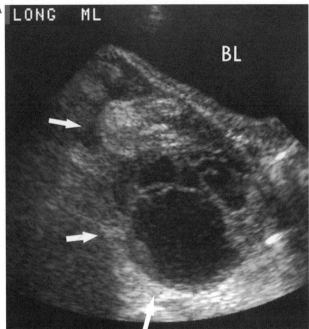

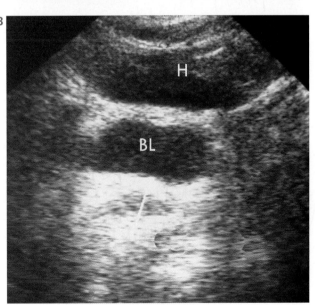

differentiate a node from a lipoma or other solid mass is to identify the hilar vessels for a node; no vascularity is seen in lipomas with color Doppler (CDI) or power **Doppler imaging** (PDI).

Postoperative Complications

Postoperative complications include abscesses and hematomas. These may be found deep in the pelvis (Figure 2-72A) or in surrounding incisions (Figure 2-72B). Abscesses and hematomas can look very similar sono-

graphically; clinical information should help to differentiate the two. Other postoperative complications include the development of **lymphoceles** or **seromas**, which can present as adnexal masses or may occur just under the incision sites. Figure 2-72C shows a posthysterectomy **rectus sheath** hematoma, while Figure 2-72D shows a post–cesarean-section hematoma.

Figure 2-72, continued. C *Transverse image through the abdominal incision posthysterectomy demonstrating a rectus sheath hematoma. BL = bladder, H = hematoma.* **D** *Longitudinal image of a post–cesarean-section hematoma (arrow) in the lower uterine segment. BL = bladder, Ut = uterus.*

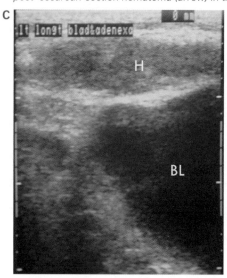

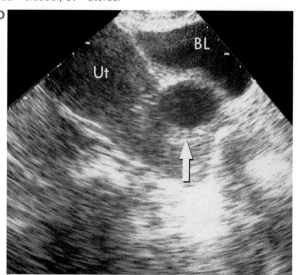

Figure 2-73. A *and* **B** *Longitudinal images showing a tampon (arrow) pushing the cervix against the posterior bladder wall. Ut = uterus, BL = bladder.* **C** *Longitudinal image through the bladder and uterus. A tampon is seen within the vaginal canal (arrow). Ut = uterus, BL = bladder.*

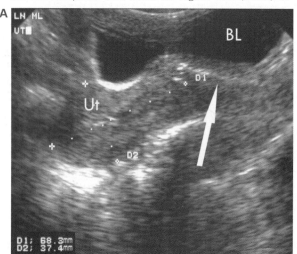

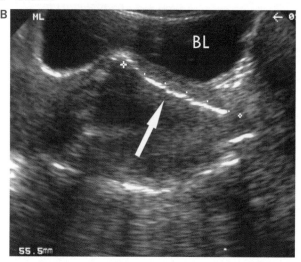

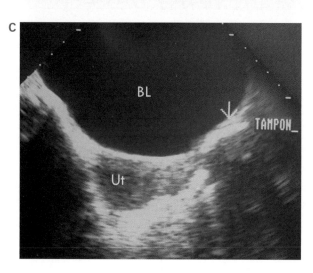

Tampons

Tampons can sometimes cause a mass effect along the posterior bladder wall if they are pushed up into the fornix region. Figures 2-73 A and B demonstrate the effect of a tampon on a retroverted uterus. Shadowing from the tampon might make one suspect a calcified structure. Figure 2-73C shows what appears to be a calcified vagina, but it is only a tampon within the vaginal canal.

Figure 2-74. A *Longitudinal and* **B** *coronal transvaginal images show a hyperechoic area of fibrous scar tissue (arrows) in a patient who had a previous cesarean section.*

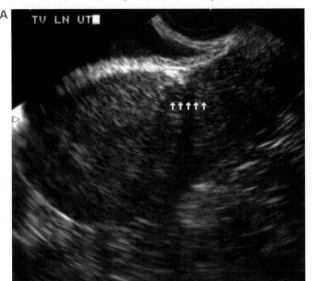
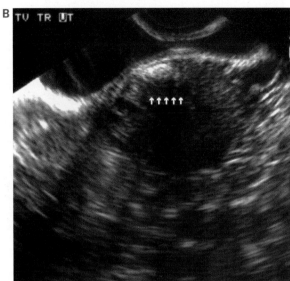

Figure 2-75. A *Longitudinal image showing a kidney displacing the uterus anteriorly. Ut = uterus, BL = bladder, K = kidney.* **B** *Longitudinal image showing the pelvic right kidney just superior to the right ovary. BL = bladder, K = kidney.*

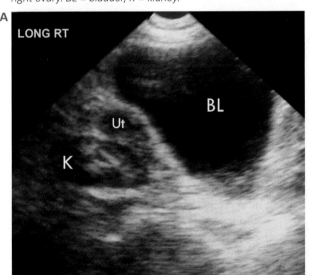
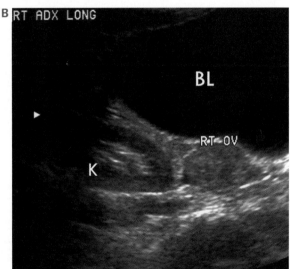

Scarring

Scarring from cesarean sections can cause an indentation into the myometrium, and the fibrous tissue often shadows, as demonstrated in Figure 2-74. Scarring should not be mistaken for a fibroid or adenomyosis.

Pelvic Kidney

The **pelvic kidney** can be a source of confusion for the clinician as well as the ultrasound practitioner. Palpated as an adnexal pelvic mass, the kidney may appear as a solid, heterogeneous mass on ultrasound (Figure 2-75). For this reason, one should always check to make sure both kidneys are in the proper upper abdominal positions when a complex or solid adnexal mass is suspected. A pelvic kidney amid pelvic inflammatory disease may be even more difficult to appreciate than one would expect. Figure 2-76 shows a patient with both kidneys that are pelvic in location and fused. If the practitioner cannot identify kidneys in the normal position, the pelvic mass may be the missing kidney.

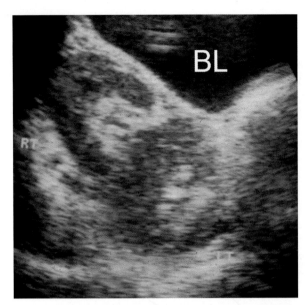

Figure 2-76. *Long-axis image showing fused kidneys posterior to the bladder. BL = bladder.*

Bowel Masses

A bowel mass associated with inflammatory bowel diseases and tumors can mimic an ovarian mass. Care should be taken to identify the ovary separate from the mass. Figure 2-77 demonstrates fluid-filled bowel mimicking a multiseptated cystic mass, which was thought to represent a hyperstimulated ectopic ovary. After a gastrointestinal/small bowel series, which was normal, the patient returned to the ultrasound department for further evaluation of the cystic mass. It was no longer present. Figure 2-78 represents a postmenopausal woman with right lower quadrant fullness and weight loss. Ovaries were not definitely identified, but the large solid mass in the right adnexa was apparent. This adnexal mass was adenocarcinoma of the colon.

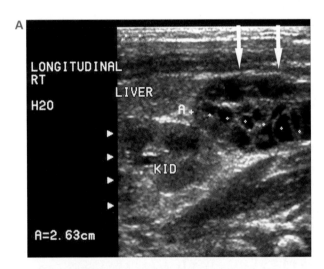

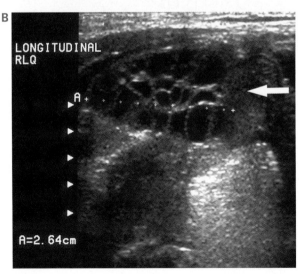

Figure 2-77. A *and* **B** *Longitudinal images through fluid-filled loops of bowel (arrows) simulating a multicystic mass in the pelvis.*

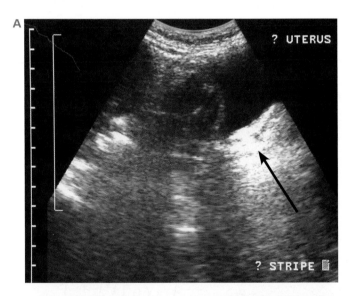

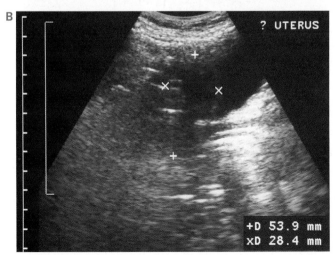

Figure 2-78. A–D *Longitudinal and transverse images through the pelvis of a postmenopausal woman. The mass that was thought to be ovarian in origin proved to be adenocarcinoma of the bowel. (Figure continues . . .)*

Pelvic Congestion

Pelvic congestion is a term often used to describe engorged veins in the adnexal regions. These dilated tortuous tubular structures can provide an interesting sonographic appearance and may be mistaken for a multiseptated or multicystic entity if imaged in cross section (Figure 2-79). Applying color Doppler, when available, will verify that the structure is vascular.

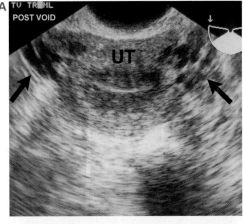

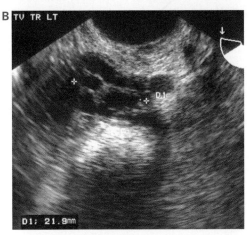

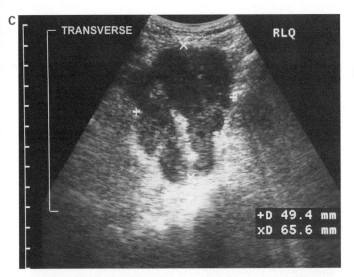

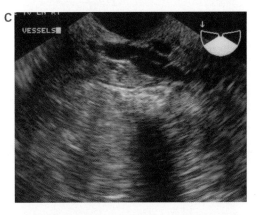

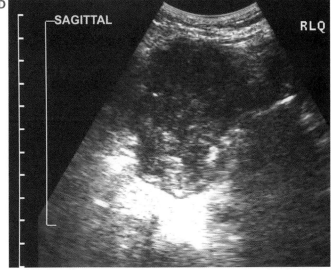

Figure 2-78, continued.

Figure 2-79. A *Transverse image through a postmenopausal uterus showing dilated veins (arrows) in both adnexa. UT = uterus.* **B** *Cluster of dilated veins simulating a multiseptated cystic mass (calipers).* **C** *Longitudinal image through dilated veins showing linear tortuosity.* **D** *Longitudinal image of postmenopausal ovary (calipers) and dilated veins (arrows) surrounding it.*

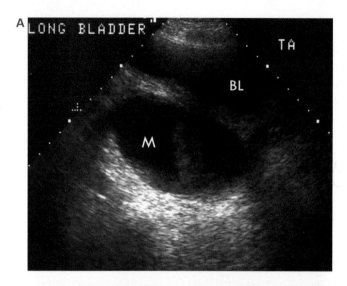

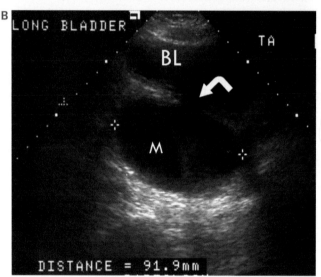

Figure 2-80. A *Longitudinal image showing what looks like a complex cystic mass behind the bladder. BL = bladder, M = mass.* **B** *This longitudinal image shows that the mass communicates (curved arrow) with the bladder, confirming a bladder diverticulum. BL = bladder, M = mass.*

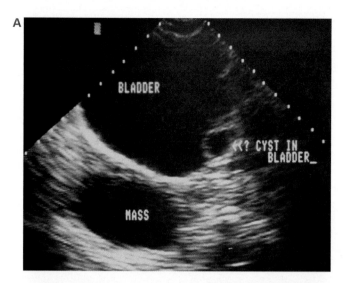

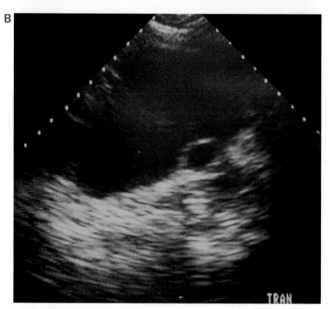

Figure 2-81. A *Longitudinal image shows a cystic mass posterior to the bladder and a ureterocele within the bladder (arrows).* **B** *Transverse imaging proves the ureterocele is from the left side.*

Bladder Diverticuli

A bladder **diverticulum** (outpouching) can easily be mistaken for an adnexal cyst if careful evaluation of the bladder wall is not performed. Unsuspected pathology can be identified if one takes advantage of the patient's full bladder and thoroughly evaluates the continuity and symmetry of the bladder wall. Figure 2-80A shows what appears to be a complex cyst posterior to the bladder. However, further evaluation shows a communication between the bladder and the cyst, indicating a bladder diverticulum (Figure 2-80B). In Figure 2-81A the patient was being evaluated for a possible ovarian cyst. During

the sonographic examination, it was also discovered that she had an **ureterocele** (a ballooning of the lower end of the ureter forming an intravesical pouch) on the left presenting as a cyst on the posterior bladder wall. Transverse imaging shows it is left-sided and located in the region of the **bladder trigone**, the inferior aspect of the urinary bladder where the ureters enter and the urethra exits (Figure 2-81B). Bladder tumors may also be incidental findings of gynecologic scans. Figure 2-82 demonstrate a small polypoid mass on the bladder wall. Figure 2-83 is a sagittal transvaginal image demonstrating a patient with cystitis.

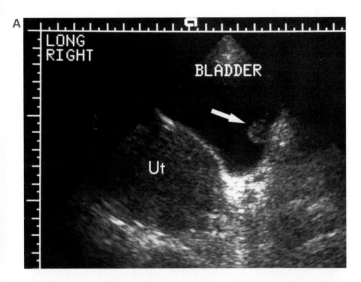

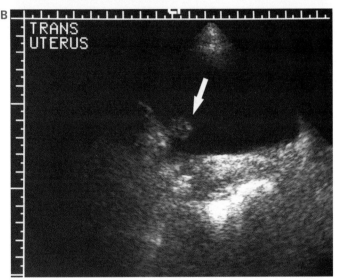

Figure 2-82. A Longitudinal and **B** transverse images of the bladder show a small round, solid lesion on the right inferior aspect of the bladder, consistent with a bladder tumor. Ut = uterus.

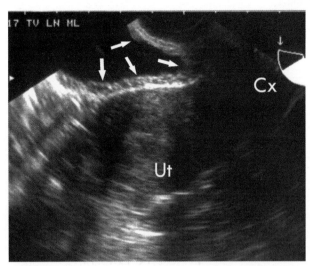

Figure 2-83. Transvaginal image shows some thickening of the bladder wall, which can be indicative of cystitis (arrows). Ut = uterus, Cx = cervix.

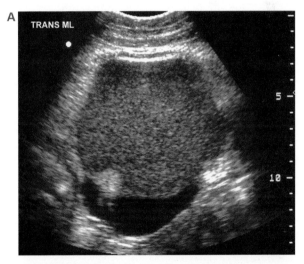

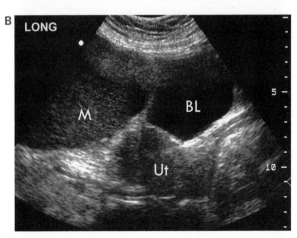

Figure 2-84. A This transverse image shows a well-demarcated complex mass that is pelvic in location gnd thought to represent a benign cystic teratoma. **B** Longitudinal imaging shows it to be superior to the uterine fundus. Surgery reported the mass to be a rare malignancy of the fallopian tube. BL = bladder, Ut = uterus, M = mass.

SCANNING TIPS, GUIDELINES, AND PITFALLS

Sonography is an ever-challenging field. Just when you begin to feel you have seen it all, a case will come along to make you humble again. For example, Figure 2-84 demonstrates a mass discovered in a 48-year-old female who was otherwise asymptomatic. The mass appeared to contain fluid and some brightly echogenic material that shadowed and produced homogeneous low-level echoes. It was thought to be ovarian in nature, probably consistent with a cystic teratoma. Surgery and pathologic resection confirmed it to be a primary papillary adenocarcinoma of the fallopian tube—a very rare tumor and in this case unexpected.

Saline infusion sonohysterography is particularly useful in the examination of the endometrium and endometrial cavity for anomalies. The patient will benefit if the examiner follows proper preparation protocols and is aware of both indications and contraindications for the procedure.

1. Choosing the best time to schedule sonohysterography is important for obtaining the best information. Patients who are on continuous hormone replacement therapy or oral contraceptives can have the examination at any time. Those who are cyclic and who do not take oral contraceptives or those taking a cyclic hormone replacement therapy should have the examination performed just after a cycle, when the endometrium should be the thinnest. Postmenopausal patients who have a transvaginal ultrasound study performed to reveal an endometrial thickness 4–5 mm or less with a hypoechoic junctional zone around it would indicate no further evaluation is necessary. However, postmenopausal patients with an endometrial thickness greater than 4–5 mm are excellent candidates for sonohysterography.

2. If there is no examination table with stirrups, the patient's hips may be elevated for transvaginal scanning using sponge wedges, a stack of sheets, telephone books, or an inverted bedpan. It is important, however, to elevate the patient's upper body as well, so that any free pelvic fluid does not move out of the pelvis.

3. Collect all supplies prior to bringing the patient into the laboratory. Fill the syringe with sterile saline and have it ready.

4. Check the patient's chart or ask about pregnancy. If the patient has not had a pregnancy test, it would be prudent that she have one prior to the procedure.

5. Bring the patient into your laboratory and explain the procedure. Prepare the patient as you normally would for a transvaginal exam. Place a pad under the patient's hips and a paper sheet on the floor for easier cleanup.

6. Perform a regular transvaginal evaluation first:

   A. Insert the **speculum** (open-sided is much easier to remove).

   B. Swab the cervix with a large swab using betadine.

   C. Connect the syringe to the catheter and remove air bubbles completely.

   D. Slide the positioner to mark on the catheter.

   E. Grasping the catheter firmly (ring forceps may be used to hold it), slowly insert the catheter into the external cervical os.

   F. When the catheter is in place, gently remove the speculum.

   G. Insert the transducer anterior to the catheter.

   H. Inform the patient that there may be leakage during the study.

   I. While scanning the endometrial cavity, slowly introduce the saline. Interrogation of all dimensions and measurements of any abnormalities should be taken.

   J. Remove the catheter and document information from the study.

   K. Give the patient a sanitary napkin and explain that it will protect her clothes if all of the fluid has not come out.

7. If there is difficulty entering the cervix due to instability, a **tenaculum** may help to stabilize the cervix for catheter placement.

8. If there is difficulty entering the cervix due to stenosis, a **uterine sound** (an instrument used to measure uterine depth or the distance between the cervix and uterine fundus) might open the way for the catheter to be placed.

9. Difficulty entering the cervix due to pain caused by the procedure is very uncommon but does occur occasionally. If a sound does not open the way for the catheter and the patient is in pain, the procedure may need to be aborted. Slow infusion of saline may deter cramping or pain and minimize discomfort during the examination.

10. Difficulty distending the uterine cavity may call for another syringe to be filled and a second infusion to evaluate the endometrium. (Using a balloon catheter to hold the saline in place for complete evaluation is an option.)

11. For American Institute of Ultrasound in Medicine standards on sonohysterography, see Appendix B.

REFERENCES

Benson CB, Arger PH, Bluth EI: *Ultrasonography in Obstetrics and Gynecology: A Practical Approach to Clinical Problems.* New York, Thieme, 2000, pp 1–67.

Benson CB, Arger PH, Bluth EI: *Ultrasonography in Obstetrics and Gynecology: A Practical Approach to Clinical Problems,* 2nd Edition. New York, Thieme, 2007.

Butani D, Cohen A, Cao S: RCOM Radiological Case of the Month-Pseudomyxoma Peritonei. Appl Radiol 12:36–39, 2005.

Callen PW: *Ultrasonography in Obstetrics and Gynecology,* 5th Edition. Philadelphia, Saunders Elsevier, 2008, pp 887–985.

Chervenak FA, Isaacson GC, Campbell S: *Ultrasound in Obstetrics and Gynecology,* Volume 2, Part 5. New York, Little Brown, 1993, pp 1599–1772.

De Lange M, Rouse GA: *Ob/Gyn Sonography: An Illustrated Review.* Pasadena, CA, Davies Publishing, 2004, pp 227–283.

Fleischer AC: *Sonography in Gynecology & Obstetrics: Just the Facts.* New York, McGraw-Hill, 2004, pp 15–160.

Goldberg BB, McGahan JP: *Atlas of Ultrasound Measurements,* 2nd Edition. Mosby, 2006.

Hassler A, Michael K: The pessary, a method for treating pelvic organ prolapse. J Diagn Med Sonog 21:12–16, 2005.

Hickey J: *Essentials of Obstetrics & Gynecology: A Comprehensive Sonographer's Guide.* Forney, TX, Pegasus Lectures, 2004, pp 3–107.

Hickey J: *Essentials of Obstetrics & Gynecology: A Comprehensive Sonographer's Guide,* 2nd Edition. Forney, TX, Pegasus Lectures, 2008.

Lerner JP, Timor-Tritsch IE, Federman A, et al: Transvaginal ultrasonographic characterization of ovarian masses with an improved, weighted scoring system. Am J Obstet Gynecol 170:81–85, 1994.

Salem S: Gynecology. In Rumack CM, Wilson SR, Charboneau JW: *Diagnostic Ultrasound,* 4th Edition. Philadelphia, Elsevier Mosby, 2011, pp 547–612.

Sanders RC: *Clinical Sonography: A Practical Guide,* 3rd Edition. Philadelphia, Lippincott Williams & Wilkins, 1998, pp 52–75.

Sanders RC, Winter W: *Clinical Sonography: A Practical Guide,* 4th Edition. Philadelphia, Lippincott Williams & Wilkins, 2006.

SELF-ASSESSMENT EXERCISES

Questions

1. Of the following, which is the most common ovarian tumor seen in patients 20 years of age or younger?

    A. Cystadenoma

    B. Cystic teratoma

    C. Fibroma

    D. Dysgerminoma

    E. Brenner tumor

2. This transvaginal image demonstrates a:

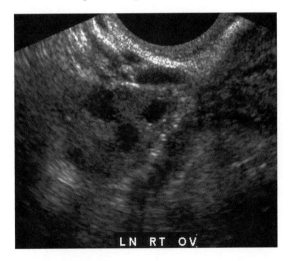

    A. Normal ovary

    B. Multicystic ovary

    C. Polycystic ovary

    D. Hyperstimulated ovary

    E. Postmenopausal ovary

3. A nabothian cyst would be found in the:

A. Broad ligament

B. Ovary

C. Vagina

D. Cervix

E. Endometrium

4. Fitz-Hugh–Curtis syndrome is associated with:

A. Endometriosis

B. Ovarian cancer

C. Ovarian fibroma

D. Intrauterine contraceptive devices

E. Pelvic inflammatory disease

5. Which muscle group forms the floor of the pelvis?

A. Obturator internus

B. Piriformis

C. Coccygeus

D. Levator ani

E. Iliopsoas

6. This 35-year-old infertility patient complains of severe cyclic pain that eases after menses. She has a mass displacing her uterus posteriorly. Her condition most likely is associated with which of the following?

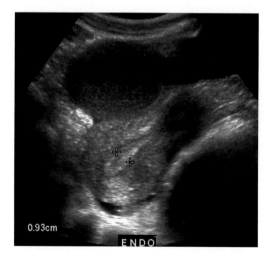

A. Fibroid

B. Endometrioma

C. Dermoid

D. Hemorrhagic cyst

E. Cystadenoma

7. The space located between the posterior bladder wall and the anterior uterus is called the:

A. Anterior cul-de-sac

B. Posterior cul-de-sac

C. Pouch of Douglas

D. Fornix

E. Space of Retzius

8. Of the following ovarian tumors, which is androgenic?

A. Granulosa cell

B. Brenner tumor

C. Fibroma

D. Krukenberg tumor

E. Arrhenoblastoma

9. Androgenic tumors cause:

A. Hirsutism

B. Precocious puberty

C. Fibrocystic breasts

D. Endometrial hyperplasia

E. Postmenopausal bleeding

10. This 47-year-old female complains of menorrhagia and low back pain. She has no history of having any pelvic surgeries. Of the following choices, which is most likely for what is demonstrated on this longitudinal scan through the uterus?

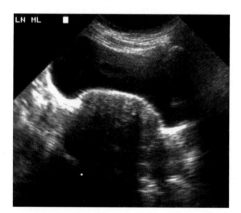

A. Shadowing from bowel overlying the uterus

B. Shadowing from a myomatous uterus

C. Classic example of uterine adenomyosis

D. Poor time gain compensation setting inhibiting visualization of posterior border

E. Classic example of a benign cystic teratoma

11. Of the following positional terms, which is considered normal for most women when the urinary bladder is empty?

   A. Anteverted

   B. Anteflexed

   C. Retroverted

   D. Retroflexed

   E. Levoposed

12. The most common cause of hematocolpos is:

   A. Cervical cancer

   B. Vaginal agenesis

   C. Imperforate hymen

   D. Bladder-vaginal fistula

   E. Acquired gynatresia

13. All of the following can be complications of an intra-uterine contraceptive device *except*:

   A. Ectopic pregnancy

   B. Pelvic inflammatory disease

   C. Menorrhagia

   D. Ovarian hyperstimulation

   E. Uterine perforation

14. Which pelvic mass can be mistaken for the urinary bladder?

   A. Hemorrhagic corpus luteum cyst

   B. Cystadenoma

   C. Benign cystic teratoma

   D. Theca-lutein cyst

   E. Paraovarian cyst

15. Which stage of the menstrual cycle produces a thin endometrium?

   A. Early proliferative

   B. Late proliferative

   C. Periovulatory

   D. Preovulatory

   E. Secretory

16. From this transvaginal longitudinal image, what is the position of the uterus?

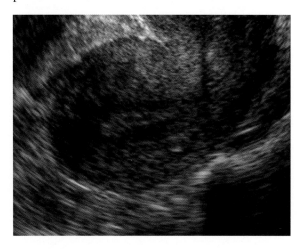

   A. Anteverted

   B. Anteflexed

   C. Retroverted

   D. Retroflexed

   E. Dextroposed

17. What is being measured in this transverse image?

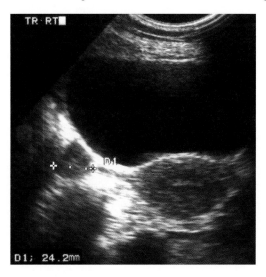

   A. Muscle

   B. Lymph node

   C. Ovary

   D. Cyst

   E. Fibroid

18. Of the following statements which is most true for ovarian tumors?

    A. Most are solid.

    B. Most are benign.

    C. Most are malignant.

    D. Most are androgenic.

    E. Most occur premenopausally.

19. Which statement is *not* true of ovarian teratomas (commonly called dermoids)?

    A. They are monodermal.

    B. They are more common in young adults.

    C. They are often bilateral.

    D. They contain fetal tissues.

    E. They are usually malignant.

20. Which statement is *not* true of the iliac vessels?

    A. The internal iliac artery is also referred to as the *hypogastric artery*.

    B. The pelvic lymph nodes follow the branches of the iliac arteries.

    C. The external iliac artery can be used to localize the ovary.

    D. The internal iliac artery feeds oxygenated blood to the pelvic organs.

    E. In the pelvis, the iliac arteries lie anterior to the veins and the ovaries lie medial to both vessels.

Answers

See Appendix F on page 608 for answers and explanations.

The First Trimester

Misty H. Sliman, BS, RT(R)(S), RDMS, and Kathryn A. Gill, MS, RT, RDMS, FSDMS

OBJECTIVES

After completing this chapter you should be able to:

1. Describe normal prenatal development from conception through the first three months of pregnancy, including fertilization, implantation, and cell division.

2. Explain and describe the anatomy, physiology, and sonographic appearance of the endometrium and gestational sac during the first trimester.

3. List and explain the function and normal sonographic appearance of the key fetal membranes.

4. Distinguish normal from abnormal measurements and sonographic signs.

5. Explain the role of ultrasound in managing patients during the first trimester of pregnancy.

6. Explain the importance of human chorionic gonadotropin (hCG) in pregnancy testing and monitoring.

7. Describe the complications of pregnancy during the first trimester.

8. Recite the key tips for (and explain the pitfalls of) scanning the patient during the first trimester.

IT IS AN AMAZING FACT THAT EVERY HUMAN BEING originates from only two cells. Many changes and a great deal of growth occur in the first few weeks after fertilization. The sonographer must be knowledgeable of developmental changes in order to ascertain that a pregnancy is progressing normally. That is the focus of this chapter.

A few words about the terms used in dating a pregnancy: From a sonographic perspective, the terms **menstrual age** and **gestational age** are interchangeable. Ultrasound calculations and charts used to measure the embryo/fetus are based on menstrual age and calculated from the first day of the last menstrual period (LMP). Embryologic tests, on the other hand, are performed and interpreted in terms of **conceptual** (or **conceptional**) **age**, which is calculated from fertilization and must be considered when reading embryology texts and interpreting actual age. Conceptual age will be two weeks younger than menstrual/gestational age.

Except where noted, this chapter focuses on imaging structures transabdominally. When the practitioner is imaging with transvaginal technique, the products of conception can be identified 1 to 2 weeks earlier than with transvesical imaging.

The three stages of human development include the pre-embryonic, embryonic, and fetal periods. The **pre-embryonic period** begins at the time of fertilization and terminates at the end of the second week. Weeks 2–8 are considered the **embryonic period**. The **fetal period** spans weeks 9–38 (or up to 40; see Figure 3-1).

FERTILIZATION AND PRE-EMBRYONIC DEVELOPMENT

At approximately 14 days after the onset of menses the process of ovulation begins. The **fimbriae**—frondlike appendages at the distal end of the fallopian tube—serve as a mechanical broom, sweeping up the ova as they are expelled from the ovary and whisking them into the fal-

lopian tube. (The fallopian tubes are not routinely imaged unless they are pathologically dilated.) The sperm and the egg (**ovum**) unite, resulting in fertilization. Sperm can live in the female for as long as 24 hours, but the average life span is 4–6 hours. Fertilization usually occurs in the ampullary portion or lateral one-third of the fallopian tube. The fertilized ovum is referred to as the **zygote** (Figure 3-2A). Immediately, the zygote begins to divide into

Figure 3-1. *Progression of pregnancy from conception to term.*

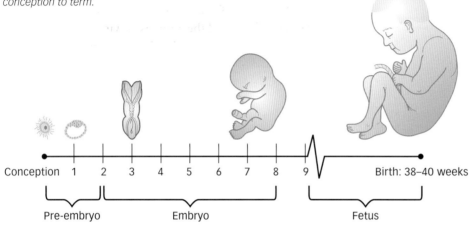

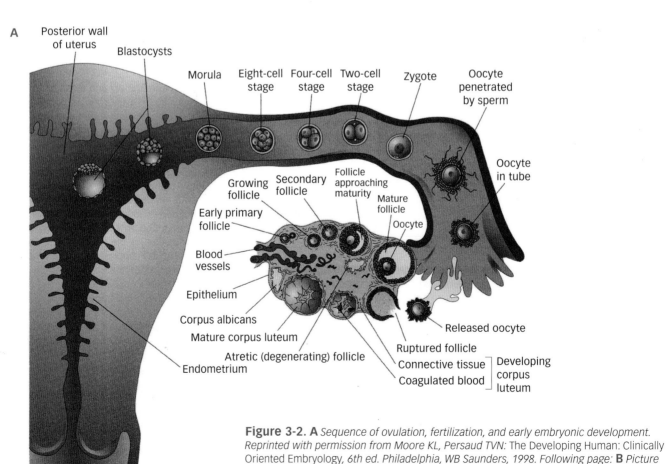

Figure 3-2. A *Sequence of ovulation, fertilization, and early embryonic development. Reprinted with permission from Moore KL, Persaud TVN: The Developing Human: Clinically Oriented Embryology, 6th ed. Philadelphia, WB Saunders, 1998. Following page:* **B** *Picture of a mulberry, which resembles the 12- to 16-cell morula.* **C** *Drawing of progression during pre-embryonic period from fertilization to 2 weeks postfertilization.*

two cells (**blastomeres**). This cell division is referred to as **cleavage**. When cleavage produces a cell mass of 12–16 cells, it is referred to as the **morula**, from the Latin word for mulberry, because that is what the cell mass resembles (Figure 3-2B).

Usually at this point in its development the morula has reached the cornual or interstitial portion of the fallopian tube and tumbles into the endometrial cavity of the uterus. By now, 6–7 days have elapsed since fertilization, and cell division has continued. Now the product of conception is referred to as the **blastocyst**, consisting of an outer cell mass (**trophoblast**), an inner cell mass (**embryoblast**), and fluid from the uterus that forms a cavity pushing the inner cell mass to one side (Figure 3-2C). The trophoblast consists of a single spherical layer that sur-

rounds the inner cell mass and the fluid-filled cavity. The blastocyst wanders within the uterine cavity for 2–3 more days before it finds just the right spot for implantation. It will embed itself in the secretory endometrium in much the same way a sand crab burrows into the sand.

During the second week after fertilization, the **bilaminar** (**embryonic**) **disc** (Figure 3-3A) forms within the blastocyst from two primary germ layers, the endoderm and the ectoderm, and further develops into the **trilaminar disc** (endoderm, ectoderm, and mesoderm; Figure 3-3B). From the inner cell mass, two cavities develop—the primary yolk sac and the amniotic cavity. Finally, two layers of trophoblast differentiate into cytotrophoblast and syncytiotrophoblast. These changes occur between days 7 and 12 postfertilization.

B

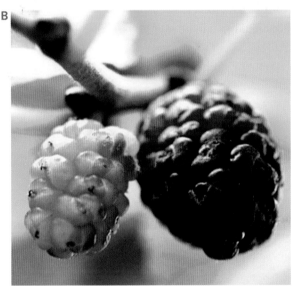

Bilaminar Disc

A

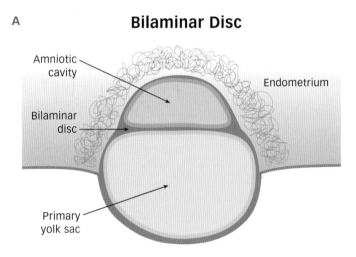

Amniotic cavity

Endometrium

Bilaminar disc

Primary yolk sac

C

Pre-embryonic

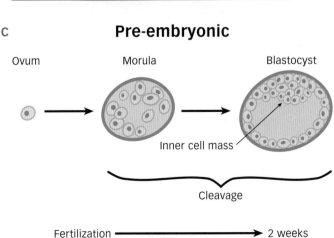

Ovum   Morula   Blastocyst

Inner cell mass

Cleavage

Fertilization ⟶ 2 weeks

Figure 3-2, continued.

B

Trilaminar Disc

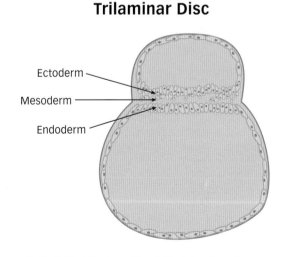

Ectoderm

Mesoderm

Endoderm

Figure 3-3. A *The bilaminar disc.* **B** *The trilaminar disc.*

THE ENDOMETRIUM AND GESTATIONAL SAC

Anatomy

The lining of the uterine cavity into which the blastocyst implants itself consists of three areas that usually can be imaged sonographically early in the pregnancy:

- Decidua basalis
- Decidua vera/parietalis
- Decidua capsularis

The **decidua basalis** is that portion of endometrium where the blastocyst attaches and the placenta develops (**syncytiotrophoblast**), the decidua basalis thereby becoming the maternal surface of the placenta. The syncytiotrophoblast is actively erosive and has been described as being invasive, ingestive, and digestive. It invades the endometrial stroma and contains capillaries, glands, and the blastocyst. Implantation usually begins around day 21, menstrual age. By 28 days' menstrual age, the blastocyst is completely covered by that part of the endometrium called the **decidua capsularis**. The endometrium lining the rest of the uterine cavity is the **decidua vera**, also called the **decidua parietalis** (Figure 3-4). The syncytiotrophoblast will continue to proliferate into two layers called the **cytotrophoblast** and the syncytiotrophoblast at the embryonic pole. During this trophoblastic development, small spaces appear between the invading trophoblast and the inner cell mass. These spaces coalesce and form the slitlike **amniotic cavity**. As the amniotic cavity grows, a thin epithelial roof called the **amnion** develops. Other cells arise from the cytotrophoblast to form the **exocoelomic membrane**, which lines a large cavity called the **exocoelomic cavity**, or **primary yolk sac**.

Fetal Membranes

Amnion

Early in the pregnancy the amnion is smaller than the yolk sac, but as the embryo grows the amnion stretches and surrounds the embryo, secreting and filling with amniotic fluid. Occasionally it can be seen as early as 5–6 weeks as the **double bleb sign** (Figure 3-5). At this time the amnion is only 2 mm in diameter and appears as a small circular structure adjacent to the yolk sac. The embryonic disc lies between the larger yolk sac and amnion and is

Figure 3-4. *The fetal membranes and intrauterine relationships.*

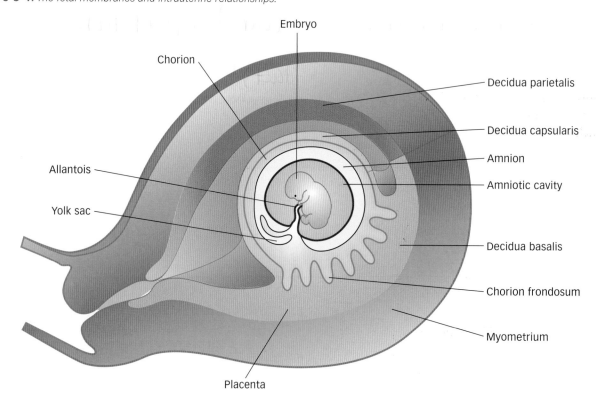

Embryo

Chorion

Decidua parietalis

Decidua capsularis

Amnion

Amniotic cavity

Allantois

Yolk sac

Decidua basalis

Chorion frondosum

Myometrium

Placenta

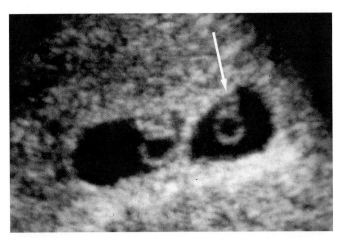

Figure 3-5. *Twin intrauterine gestational sacs showing the double bleb sign (arrow) in the sac to the left in this transverse image. The yolk sac is the larger rounded structure with the embryonic disc situated between the amnion (arrow) and the yolk sac.*

connected to the trophoblast by a stalk that will become the **umbilical cord**. You may actually see cardiac motion in the region of the embryonic disc before a defined embryo is identified (Figure 3-6A). As the amniotic sac enlarges, the amnion appears as a thin, free-floating membrane (Figure 3-6B). The amniotic sac continues to grow and expand until it fuses with the chorion at about 12–16 weeks (Figure 3-6C). Chorioamniotic separation that persists after 16 weeks is worrisome and may be related to malformations such as limb deformities, cleft defects, and amputations.

Allantois
The **allantois** is part of the connecting stalk of the embryo. It gives rise to part of the umbilical cord and bladder (**urachus**). The **vitelline** (**omphalomesenteric**) **duct**, often mistaken for the umbilical cord, can occasionally be seen as a cord connecting the embryo to the yolk sac (Figure 3-7). See Chapter 5 for additional information on the vitelline/omphalomesenteric duct.

Chorion
Cytotrophoblastic cells of the blastocyst surround the embryo and eventually become the **placenta**. The extraembryonic mesoderm and trophoblast make up the **chorion**. Because the **chorion** develops first, we see it as the thickened, echogenic ring (decidual ring) of the **gestational sac**, also referred to as the **extraembryonic coelom**. The chorion secretes **human chorionic gonadotropin** (hCG), a protein hormone secreted by the placenta and present in the blood and urine of a pregnant woman.

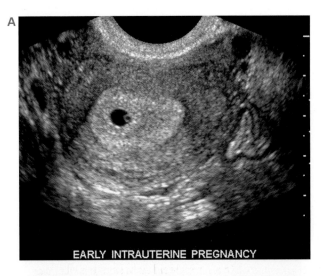

EARLY INTRAUTERINE PREGNANCY

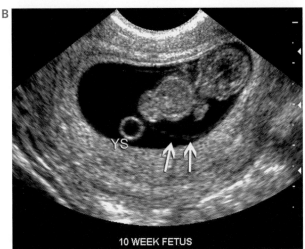

10 WEEK FETUS

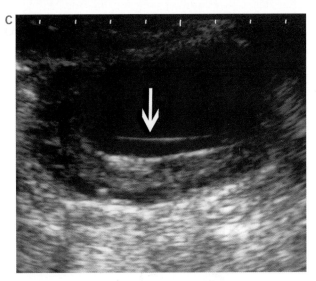

Figure 3-6. A *Transvaginal scan showing an early intrauterine gestational sac containing a yolk sac. An embryo is not identifiable at this time.* **B** *An embryo surrounded by the amnion (arrows). The yolk sac is outside the amnion. YS = yolk sac.* **C** *Amnion (arrow) is still separated from the chorion at 14 weeks.*

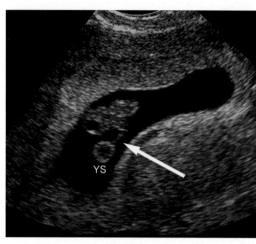

Figure 3-7. *Transvaginal image demonstrating a normal intrauterine pregnancy. The vitelline duct (arrow) is situated between the rounded yolk sac and the echogenic embryonic pole. YS = yolk sac.*

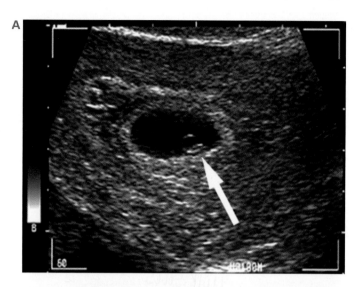

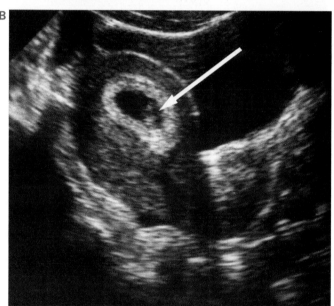

Figure 3-8. A *Transvaginal image showing a well-defined yolk sac with the slitlike embryonic disc adjacent to it (arrow).* **B** *Transabdominally the yolk sac is visualized (arrow) but not as clearly defined.*

Yolk Sac

The **primary yolk sac** gives rise to the intestines and germ cells and degenerates before we are able to see sonographic evidence of pregnancy. As the embryo grows, the yolk sac gets smaller and will become partly incorporated into the embryonic gut (Figure 3-8A). If the yolk sac persists, it will develop into an outpouching of the ileum in the adult known as Meckel diverticulum, the most common congenital defect of the gastrointestinal tract. As the primary yolk sac regresses and is pinched off by the extraembryonic coelom, it gives rise to the secondary yolk sac. It is actually the **secondary yolk sac** that is identified sonographically. By 5–6 weeks we begin to appreciate the secondary yolk sac as a small, echo-free circular structure within the gestational/chorionic sac. It is an essential structure of a normally progressing pregnancy, responsible for **hematopoiesis** (the production of all blood cell types) and transfer of nutrients. Transabdominally, the secondary yolk sac should be seen when the mean sac diameter is 20 mm; transvaginally, it can be imaged at a mean sac diameter of 8–10 mm (Figure 3-8B). Visualization of the yolk sac will distinguish a true gestational sac from a pseudosac. The yolk sac will grow away from the embryo and eventually be seen between the amnion and chorion.

Sonographic signs of a normal yolk sac include these key features:

- *Shape:* perfectly round
- *Size:* at 5–10 weeks neither smaller than 2 mm nor larger than 6 mm
- *Sonographic appearance:* anechoic

Sonographic signs of an abnormal yolk sac include these hallmarks:

- Misshapen (oval, elongated, hourglass; Figure 3-9A)
- Solid (Figure 3-9B)
- Calcified
- Enlarged or too small (Figure 3-9C)
- Absent (Figure 3-9D)

Visualization of an abnormal yolk sac may indicate an abnormal pregnancy and impending demise.

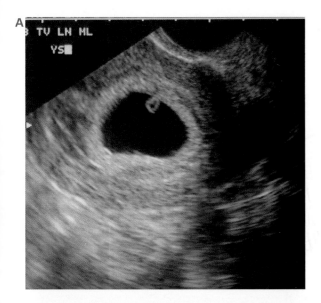

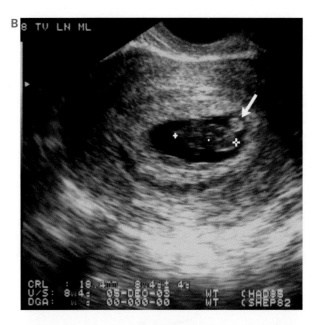

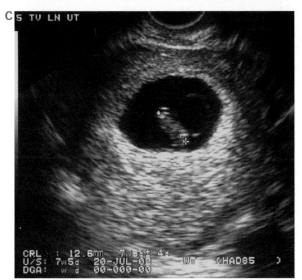

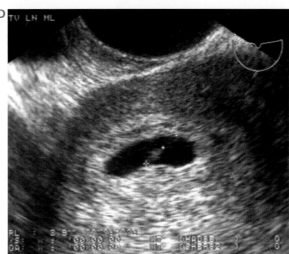

Figure 3-9. A *This transvaginal image shows a rather large gestational sac containing an irregularly shaped yolk sac but no embryo.* **B** *In this image of an early pregnancy measuring 8½ weeks in size, the yolk sac (arrow) was seen as a solid nodular structure next to the fetal pole, which showed no cardiac activity.* **C** *This image shows a large yolk sac measuring approximately 11 mm next to a fetal pole measuring almost 8 weeks in size. No cardiac activity was demonstrated, indicating a failed pregnancy.* **D** *This intrauterine sac shows an embryonic pole being measured, but no yolk sac was definable.*

Sonographic Appearance

The sonographic appearance of the intrauterine gestational sac in relation to the deciduae capsularis and parietalis, the two layers of endometrium it lies between, is that of a double ring—hence the term **double decidual ring** (Figure 3-10A). It is the deciduae capsularis and parietalis with the hypoechoic cavity sandwiched between them (Figure 3-10B).

Very early in pregnancy, before one can appreciate the gestational sac, the **decidualized endometrium** is thick and brightly echogenic. The arcuate vessels of the uterus are engorged and prominent (Figure 3-11A). Occasionally, small (2–5 mm) decidual cysts are imaged in the junctional zone before the intrauterine sac itself can be visualized (Figure 3-11B). Unlike gestational sacs, these cysts do not have echogenic rings around them. Decidual cysts have been associated with ectopic pregnancy and with adenomyosis as well as with normal intrauterine pregnancies and are not specific to either one (Figure 3-11C).

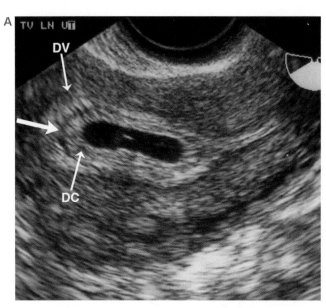

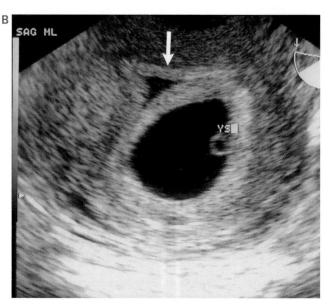

Figure 3-10. A *The double decidual ring can be clearly demonstrated transvaginally. Notice the hypoechoic uterine cavity indicated by the bold arrow. DC = decidua capsularis, DV = decidua vera.* **B** *Transvaginal image clearly showing a gestational sac within the endometrial cavity (arrow).*

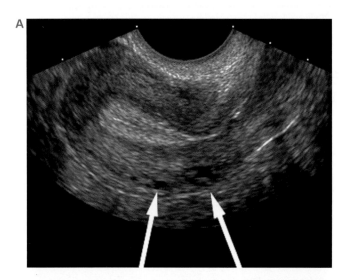

Figure 3-11. A *Transvaginal image of the uterus with a decidual-ized endometrium and engorged arcuate vessels seen peripherally (arrows).* **B** *A decidual cyst (arrow) is seen in this patient who had an ectopic pregnancy. There is no double decidual ring. The arrowheads define the uterine border in long axis.* **C** *A decidual cyst (arrow) can be associated with ectopic pregnancy, early normal pregnancy, or adenomyosis.*

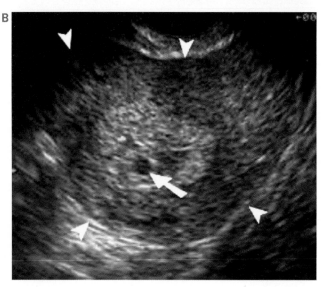

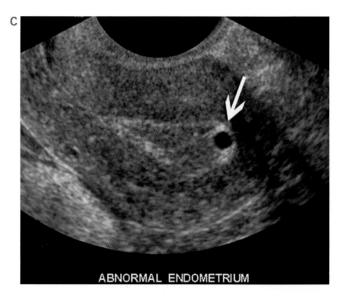

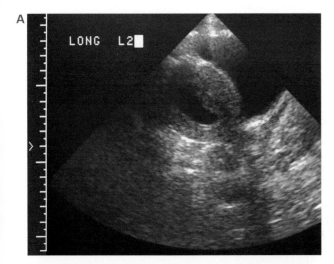

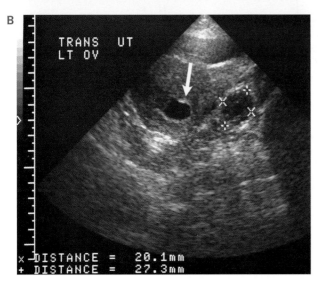

Figure 3-12. A *A collection of fluid is shown within the endometrial cavity of this uterus with a decidualized endometrium. Known as a pseudosac, this finding can be associated with an ectopic pregnancy.* **B** *Transverse image shows the pseudosac (arrow) within the endometrial cavity and an ectopic pregnancy in the left adnexa (calipers).*

Identification of a double decidual ring makes it possible to differentiate a normal intrauterine gestational sac from intracavitary fluid within a decidualized endometrium (**pseudosac**) usually around 5 weeks, transabdominally, when the sac is approximately 1 cm in diameter (Figure 3-12). The practitioner should keep in mind that transvaginal technique allows us to see evidence of an intrauterine pregnancy 1–2 weeks earlier, at 4–4½ weeks' LMP.

Mean Sac Diameter

A normal gestational sac should grow 1–2 mm per day up to 10 weeks. Prior to the imaging of an embryo, sac measurements can be taken to estimate gestational age.

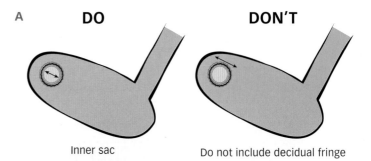

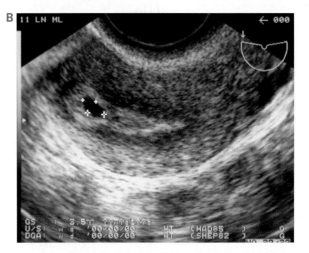

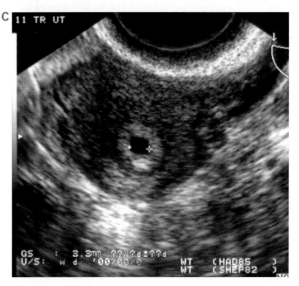

Figure 3-13. A *The correct way to measure a gestational sac.* **B** *Longitudinal image showing long-axis and anterior/posterior sac measurements.* **C** *Correct transverse measurement of the gestational sac.*

When measuring the sac (Figure 3-13), do not include the decidual fringe around it. Measure from one inner sac wall to the other inner sac wall. The **mean sac diameter** (**MSD**) can be calculated using the following formula:

$$(\text{sac length} + \text{height} + \text{width}) \div 3 = \text{MSD (mm)}$$
$$\text{MSD (mm)} + 30 = \text{gestational days}$$

EMBRYONIC DEVELOPMENT

Weeks 3–8 are the embryonic period during which major morpho-/organogenetic events occur and when the conceptus (developing embryo) is most vulnerable to teratogenic agents. During the third week the three germ layers (endoderm, mesoderm, and ectoderm) develop as well as three very important structures: the primitive streak, notochord, and neural tube. The **primitive streak** gives rise to mesenchymal cells, which form connective tissues. The primitive streak forms near the caudal end of the embryonic disc, and as it lengthens the cranial portion becomes more bulbous. By the end of the fourth week it diminishes in size and regresses to become an insignificant structure near the sacrococcygeal region. The **notochord** forms the origin of the axial skeleton, and the **neural tube** forms the central nervous system. All the major organ systems have developed by 8 weeks.

FETAL DEVELOPMENT

Embryonic/Fetal Pole

An embryo can be imaged transabdominally at 6–7 weeks. Transvaginally it can be imaged 1–2 weeks earlier. Once an embryonic pole is identified, the **crown-rump length** (**CRL**) should be obtained for gestational dating. This measurement should start at the fetal head/crown and extend to the caudal end/rump, excluding extremities and the yolk sac. The CRL is the most accurate measurement for dating pregnancies up to 10 weeks (Figures 3-14 and 3-15).

Table 3-1.	Gestational age via early embryonic size.	
Weeks of Gestation	**Early Embryonic Size (mm)**	**Gestational Age (Days)**
6–6½	1	43
	2	44
	3	45
7–7½	4	46
	5	47
	6	48
	7	49
	8	50
	9	51
	10	52
	11	53
	12	54
	13	55
	14	56
8–8½	15	57
	16	58
	17	59
	18	60
	19	61
	20	62
	21	63
	22	64
	23	65
	24	66
9	25	67

Reprinted with permission from Goldstein SR, Wolfson R: Endovaginal ultrasound measurement of early embryonic size as a means of assessing gestational age. J Ultrasound Med 13:27–31, 1994.

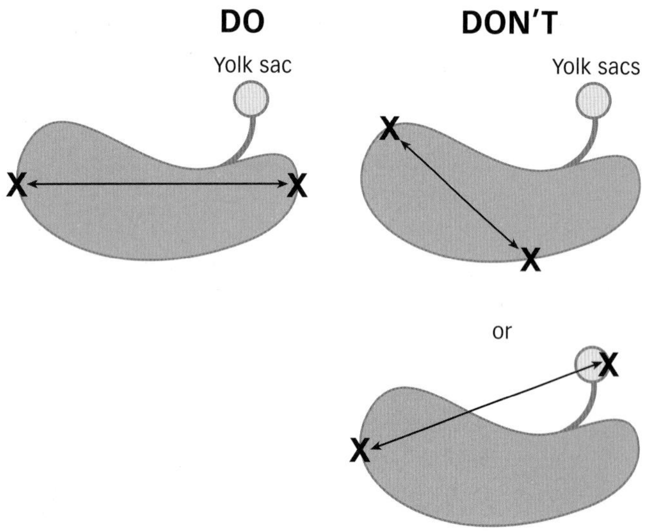

DO

Yolk sac

DON'T

Yolk sacs

or

Figure 3-14. *Correct way to measure the early crown-rump length.*

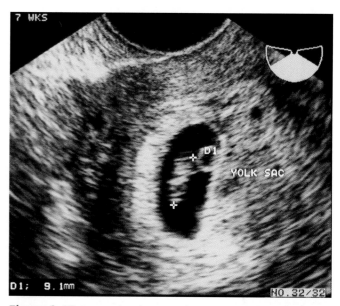

Figure 3-15. *Image showing an embryonic pole being measured (calipers).*

Table 3-2.   Sonographic visualization of embryonic/fetal anatomy.

Weeks' Gestation	Trans-abdominal	Mean Sac Diameter	FIRP	SIS	Trans-vaginal	Mean Sac Diameter	FIRP	SIS
3–4	Decidualized endometrium				Gestational sac	2–3 mm	>2000 mIU/ml	>1000 mIU/ml
5	Gestational sac	5 mm	>3600 mIU/ml	>1800 mIU/ml	Yolk sac/ double bleb sign	6–10 mm	>7200 mIU/ml	>3600 mIU/ml
5.5–6	Yolk sac/ double bleb sign	20 mm			Embryonic pole (2–4 mm) with cardiac activity	6–10 mm	>10,800 mIU/ml	>5400 mIU/ml
6–7	Embryonic pole with cardiac activity	20–25 mm				16 mm		

The following formulas can be used to calculate gestational age with an accuracy of ± 3–5 days (see also Tables 3-1 and 3-2):

- *Transabdominal ultrasound:* CRL (mm) + 6.5 = age in gestational weeks
- *Transvaginal ultrasound:* CRL (mm) + 42 = age in gestational days

If a gestational sac measures 2.0–2.5 cm (MSD), one should be able to identify a fetal pole with heart motion using transabdominal ultrasound. At approximately 8 weeks' gestation the gestational sac should fill half of the uterine cavity. Identification of a defined fetal pole should allow one to see cardiac activity. If the ultrasound system has M-mode capability, it is recommended that cardiac activity and fetal heart rate be documented with an M-mode tracing (Figure 3-16). Prior to 7–8 weeks, the normal range for embryonic heart rate is 90–115 beats per minute (bpm). By 9 weeks, however, the range for normal fetal heart rate is 140 bpm ± 20, and this range applies throughout the rest of the pregnancy (Table 3-3). Abnormally low embryonic/fetal heart rates in the first trimester may suggest impending pregnancy failure and warrant close monitoring. By 10 weeks the gestational sac should completely fill the uterine cavity. By 11 weeks the fetal spine begins to segment, giving the fetus the ability to curl. This may affect the accuracy of CRL measurements and accounts for the reason CRL is not used to date pregnancy after week 10 (although CRL is used throughout the first trimester for other purposes, particularly for nuchal translucency screening).

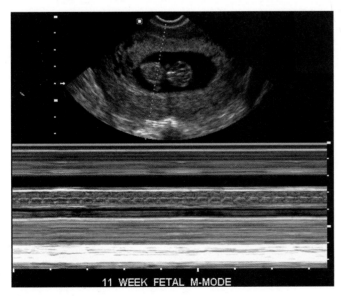

Figure 3-16. *Cardiac activity is demonstrated with M-mode sonography in this 11-week fetus.*

Table 3-3.   Normal embryonic and fetal heart rates.

Gestational Age	Normal Heart Rate (bpm)
< 7–8 weeks	90–115
≥ 9 weeks	140 ± 20*

*This remains the normal value through term.

Normal Changes Can Mimic Pathology

Developmentally, many changes occur during this time. One must be knowledgeable about these physiologic changes in order not to mistake them for pathologies. For example, the normal fetal primitive hindbrain (**rhomb-encephalon**) should not be mistaken for an abnormal fluid collection in the fetal head (**hydrocephaly**). The rhombencephalon is usually seen before 10 weeks and appears as a cystic structure in the cranium of the fetus (Figure 3-17).

Very early, at 5–6 weeks, the amnion lies in close proximity to the embryonic pole. Care must be taken not to mistake this for an abnormal nuchal translucency when screening a pregnancy for possible genetic anomalies (Figure 3-18). Between 8 and 12 weeks, there is very rapid growth of the fetal gut, and the abdomen is unable to accommodate the intestinal enlargement. In a normal developmental process known as **physiologic herniation**, the fetal midgut therefore herniates into the base of the umbilical cord, giving the appearance of an abdominal wall defect. Usually by the 12th week the abdomen has grown enough to accommodate the intestines as they involute back into their normal position. Care should be taken not to mistake normal physiologic herniation for an omphalocele or gastroschisis before 12 weeks' gestation (Figure 3-19).

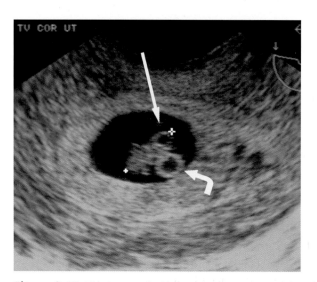

Figure 3-17. *This transvaginal image shows crown-rump length being measured. Note the cystic area in the crown portion, representing the rhombencephalon (straight arrow). The yolk sac is also shown (curved arrow).*

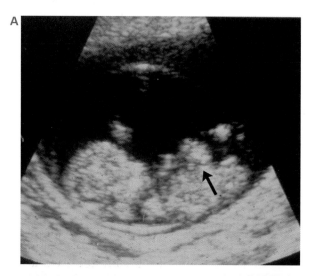

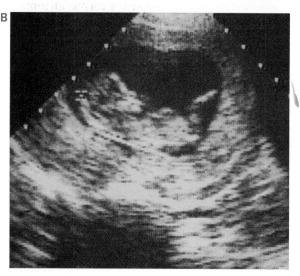

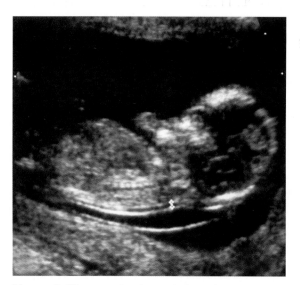

Figure 3-18. *Image showing nuchal translucency as opposed to the amnion. Reprinted with permission from Callen P: Ultrasonography in Obstetrics and Gynecology, 4th Edition. Philadelphia, Saunders, 2000, p 141, fig 5-54A.*

Figure 3-19. A *A 10-week fetus showing physiologic gut herniation (arrow).* **B** *A fetus at 12 weeks with bowel involuted back into the abdomen.*

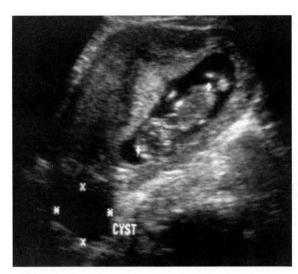

Figure 3-20. *Normal intrauterine pregnancy with a corpus luteum.*

Table 3-4.	Correlation of maternal beta-hCG levels with gestational age.
Weeks from the Last Menstrual Period	**Beta-hCG Levels (mIU/ml)**
3	5–50
4	3–426
5	19–7,340
6	1,080–56,500
7–8	7,650–229,000
9–12	25,700–288,000
13–16	13,300–254,000
17–24	4,060–165,400
25–40	3,640–117,000

Data from http://www.obfocus.com/questions/qanda7.htm.

In the early stage of pregnancy the corpus luteum cyst often can be identified sonographically. Progesterone produced by the corpus luteum is critical to the maintenance of the pregnancy prior to 6 weeks. After week 6 the trophoblastic cells of the developing placenta take over hormone production. The corpus luteum cyst regresses and is usually resolved by 12 weeks. Cysts that persist after 16 weeks require careful monitoring (Figure 3-20).

PREGNANCY TESTS AND HUMAN CHORIONIC GONADOTROPIN

Today's pregnancy tests are quite accurate in detecting **human chorionic gonadotropin** (**hCG**), a hormone produced by the trophoblastic cells that become the placenta. The main role of hCG is to stimulate the corpus luteum to produce progesterone, which maintains luteal function and sustains the pregnancy. Production of hCG begins approximately 8 days after conception, and samples can be obtained and evaluated through blood serum testing or urinalysis. With normal pregnancy, hCG levels rise exponentially until 8 weeks after the last menstrual period (6 weeks) by doubling every 48 hours. By 6 weeks of age, hCG peaks and levels off until delivery. Human chorionic gonadotropin helps maintain the activity of the corpus luteum, which is responsible for producing estrogen and progesterone, both critical to proper implantation and maintenance of the pregnancy up to 6 weeks.

There are two kinds of hCG, alpha-hCG and beta-hCG. Alpha-hCG is readily influenced by other hormones,

hematuria, and some medications (aspirin, for instance). Therefore measurements of alpha-hCG commonly produce high false-positive findings. Beta-hCG, on the other hand, is directly associated with pregnancy and gives us a qualitative or quantitative result. The qualitative measurement of beta-hCG simply indicates a positive or negative finding, whereas the quantitative measurement yields a numeric value that directly relates to the gestational age of the embryo (Table 3-4). The quantitative measurement of beta-hCG is very important to the sonography practitioner and **sonologist** when attempting to rule out a failed pregnancy. With a normal pregnancy, beta-hCG should double every 48 hours. Throughout this chapter we refer to these laboratory values and discuss how the practitioner can use this quantitative information in addition to the diagnostic information obtained from the ultrasound examination.

Beta-hCG levels can be reported using one of two different standards: the First International Reference Preparation (FIRP) or Third International Standard (3rd IS) and the Second International Standard (2nd IS or SIS). The FIRP tends to be more conservative than the 2nd IS and is therefore most commonly used. As a rule the number value of the 2nd IS is approximately one-half the FIRP value. Table 3-5 demonstrates the correlation between serum levels of beta-hCG and sonographic visualization of pregnancy.

Table 3-5.	Correlation of maternal beta-hCG levels with transvaginal ultrasound findings.	
Beta-hCG Levels (mIU/ml) (FIRP*)		**Ultrasound Findings**
1000		Gestational sac
7200		Yolk sac
10,800		Live embryo

*For the 2nd IS, divide these numbers by 2.

Data from Bree RL, Edwards M, Bohm-Velez M, et al: Transvaginal sonography in the evaluation of normal early pregnancy: correlation with HCG level. Am J Roentgenol 153:75–79, 1989.

COMPLICATIONS OF EARLY PREGNANCY

First trimester bleeding is common and occurs in 25% of all pregnancies. Of those, 20%–50% will spontaneously abort. If the bleeding is temporary, painless, spotty, and dark brown in color, it is usually due to implantation of the blastocyst (Figure 3-21). Upon implantation, there is some erosion and sloughing of endometrium. The brown color indicates old blood, not active bleeding. More worrisome causes of bleeding in the first trimester include abortion, ectopic pregnancy, and trophoblastic disease.

Abortion

Abortion, often referred to as **miscarriage**, is defined as the spontaneous termination of a pregnancy before the

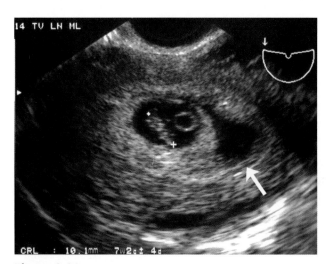

Figure 3-21. *Implantation bleed (arrow) noted adjacent to gestational sac.*

Box 3-1.	Sonographic signs that suggest an abnormal pregnancy.
	Sac too large and/or empty
	Sac too small for contents
	Poor decidual reaction (< 2 mm)
	Weak decidual echo amplitude
	Low implantation
	Irregular gestational sac/yolk sac shape
	Duplication or absence of yolk sac
	Crenated amnion

fetus can survive outside the uterus on its own, usually at 20 weeks. When an embryo dies, spontaneous abortion (SAB) usually occurs within 1–3 weeks. Etiologies include a failure in the development of the embryo (ovular defects) and maternal disorders such as endocrine abnormalities, hormonal factors, infections (TORCH), and incompetent cervix. Other factors that have been suggested when cause cannot be definitively determined include stress, male factors, and environmental influences. (Box 3-1 lists the key sonographic signs that suggest an abnormal pregnancy.) Sonographers use a variety of terms to describe abortions, including the following:

- Threatened
- Incomplete
- Spontaneous/complete
- Inevitable
- Habitual
- Missed/blighted ovum
- Elective

Threatened Abortion

A **threatened abortion** is signaled by the following symtoms:

- Positive pregnancy test
- Spotting/bleeding with closed cervix
- Cramping

Of patients presenting with these symptoms, half will have normal outcomes and half will have failed pregnancies. Factors that can affect outcomes include maternal age, smoking, caffeine and alcohol consumption, and luteal phase deficiency, as well as congenital uterine anomalies.

Box 3-2.	Rate of pregnancy loss varies with bleeding and gestational age.

Heartbeat at < 6 weeks with bleeding, 33% lost

Heartbeat at < 6 weeks without bleeding, 16% lost

Heartbeat at 7–9 weeks with bleeding, 10% lost

Heartbeat at 7–9 weeks without bleeding, 5% lost

Heartbeat at 9–11 weeks with bleeding, 4% lost

Heartbeat at 9–11 weeks without bleeding, 1%–2% lost

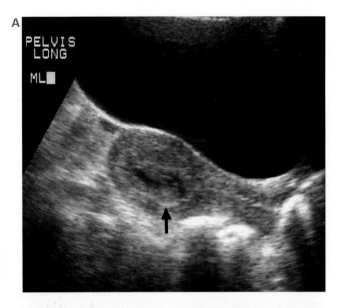

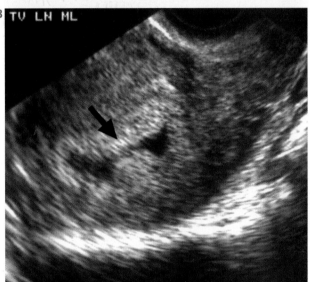

Figure 3-22. *Retained products of conception associated with an incomplete abortion:* **A** *Transabdominal study.* **B** *Transvaginal study.*

If a viable embryo/fetus is identified, the prognosis is more hopeful. Nevertheless, the rate of pregnancy loss with a positive heartbeat varies with gestational age and degree of vaginal bleeding (see Box 3-2). Heart rates of less than 85 bpm are worrisome but less reliable as a prognostic indicator in younger embryos.

Incomplete/Complete Abortion

A patient who presents with an **incomplete abortion** may have the same symptoms as a woman who has a threatened abortion in addition to the passage of clots and tissue. Sonographically, there are retained products of conception (RPOC) within the endometrial cavity. The sonographic appearance of these products varies greatly depending on the stage of pregnancy and what is retained (Figure 3-22). Clinically, the hCG levels fall slowly and may plateau, remaining weakly positive when a pregnancy test is performed. If the abortion is **complete (spontaneous)**, on the other hand, the endometrial cavity is empty and the hCG levels tend to fall rapidly.

Inevitable Abortion

If a patient presents with symptoms of a threatened abortion but also demonstrates a dilated cervix, the diagnosis is **inevitable abortion**. Membranes and/or fetal parts may be seen bulging into the endocervical canal (Figures 3-23 A and B).

Habitual Abortion

Two or more consecutive pregnancy losses prior to 20 weeks' gestation are defined as **habitual abortion**. The most common causes of habitual abortion are an incompetent cervix and luteal phase deficiency. An

incompetent cervix (Figure 3-23C) may be the result of congenital weakness due to exposure to diethylstilbestrol (DES). Other causes include cervical lesions and trauma from multiple invasive procedures (elective abortion/dilation and curettage) or multiparity.

Luteal phase deficiency is the inability of the corpus luteum cyst to produce an adequate amount of progesterone. The result is inadequate decidualization of the endometrium, which inhibits proper implantation. The corpus luteum cyst plays a critical role in sustaining early pregnancy for as long as 6 weeks, until the placenta takes over hormone production.

A

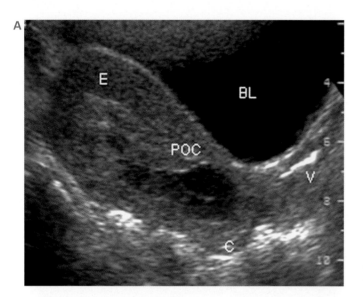

B

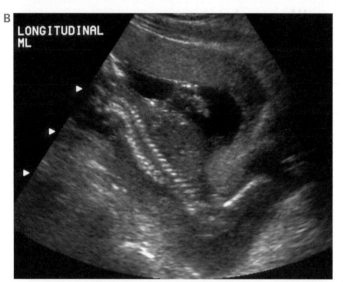

C

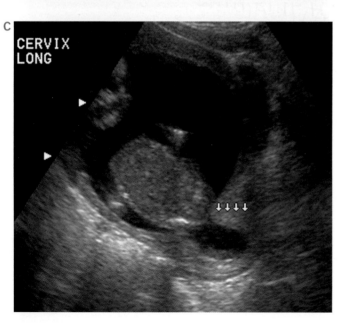

Figure 3-23. A *Longitudinal transabdominal image showing products of conception within the endocervical canal. The endometrial stripe can be seen in the fundal region of the uterus. E = endometrium, V = vagina, C = cervix, BL = bladder, POC = products of conception.* **B** *Longitudinal scan showing a fetus in breech position with its femur and pelvis within the endocervical and vaginal canal.* **C** *Second trimester pregnancy with incompetent cervix and inevitable abortion; the four short arrows are pointing toward bulging membranes within the endocervical canal.*

Missed Abortion, Anembryonic Gestation, and Blighted Ovum

These terms are often used (and misused) interchangeably. A **missed abortion** is defined as that experienced by a patient with a positive pregnancy test but a nonviable pregnancy that has failed to be expelled. The demise is "missed" clinically because the patient has had no symptoms of abortion. In the missed abortion the pregnancy began with an embryo, but somewhere along the way it died. Again, the sonographic appearance can vary depending on the stage of demise and degree to which the products of conception have degenerated (Figure 3-24).

The **blighted ovum** is an **anembryonic pregnancy** and a pathologic (not sonographic) diagnosis. Sonographically the examiner can appreciate a sac, but it is usually larger than normal and without a visible embryo. The examiner may identify a large empty sac with ultrasound but cannot know whether there was a tiny embryo

A

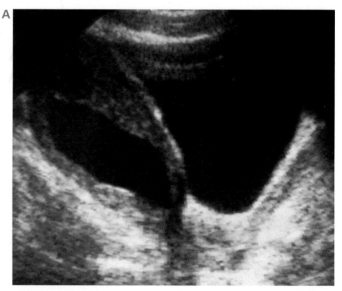

Figure 3-24. A *Longitudinal scan of a large intrauterine gestational sac showing no yolk sac or fetus. Following page:* **B** *Transverse image shows a large and irregularly shaped gestational sac containing a very tiny piece of tissue thought to have been the embryo (arrow). No heart motion was detected.*

Table 3-6.	Key findings in anembryonic gestations by transabdominal and transvaginal sonography.	

Transabdominal	Transvaginal
> 20 mm MSD with no yolk sac	> 13 mm MSD with no yolk sac
> 25 mm MSD with no embryo	> 18 mm MSD with no embryo

that died very early and has been resorbed (see Table 3-6). Therefore the blighted ovum is not a sonographic diagnosis. Most agree that the more recent term **failed pregnancy** should be used to eliminate any confusion over these misused terms.

Elective Abortion

The legal, deliberately induced termination of a pregnancy by a physician is called an **elective abortion**. Other terms include *therapeutic abortion* (TAB), *voluntary interruption of pregnancy* (VIP), *induced abortion*, and *termination of pregnancy* (TOP). State laws vary relative to the legal limits for termination.

Prior to 9 weeks' gestational age, an oral dose of the antiprogesterone mifepristone (RU486) can be given a few days before insertion of a prostaglandin pessary, which will induce cervical dilation and uterine contractions. This is referred to as **medical termination** of pregnancy and is 95% effective in inducing abortion. Between 9 and 12 weeks surgical termination is performed with a suction curettage. After 12 weeks dilation of the cervix and evacuation of the uterus (D&E) must be performed.

Sonographic Signs of Abnormal Pregnancy

Sonographers should watch for several signs of an abnormal and potentially abortive pregnancy:

- Sac too large and/or empty (Figure 3-25)
- Sac too small for contents (Figure 3-26)
- Poor decidual reaction, < 2 mm (Figure 3-27)
- Low implantation (Figure 3-27)
- Irregular sac/yolk sac shape (Figure 3-28)
- Duplication/absence of yolk sac (Figure 3-9D)
- Crenated amnion
- Subchorionic bleed (Figure 3-21)

Ectopic Pregnancy

An **ectopic pregnancy** is any pregnancy occurring outside the normal intrauterine location. It is a very serious condition that can affect future fertility and is considered the leading cause of maternal death in the United States. Fifty percent of women who have an ectopic pregnancy

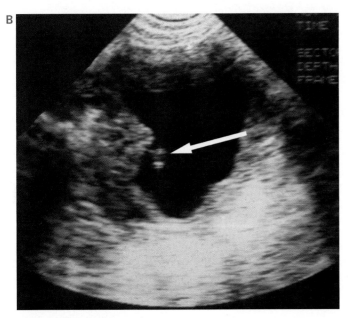

Figure 3-24, continued.

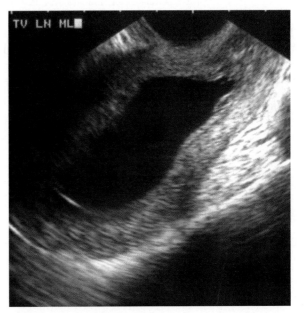

Figure 3-25. *Longitudinal intrauterine gestational sac fills the endometrial cavity, yet no fetus can be identified.*

A

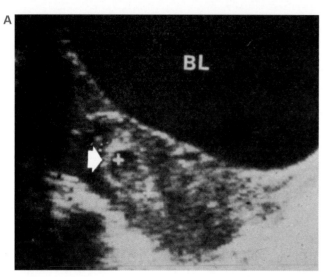

B

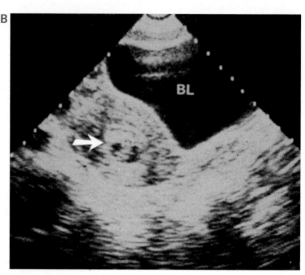

Figure 3-26. A and **B** *Both of these patients by dates were 7–8 weeks and presented with spotting. Although the fetuses (arrows) measured consistently with dates and showed cardiac activity, both sacs appeared small, crowding the fetuses. In both cases, the patients spontaneously aborted a few days after their sonograms. BL = bladder.*

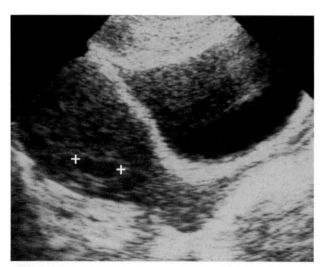

Figure 3-27. *Longitudinal transabdominal image shows a lowly implanted intrauterine gestational sac (calipers) with a poor decidual reaction. Ten weeks by good menstrual dates, this sac is too small and shows no internal contents.*

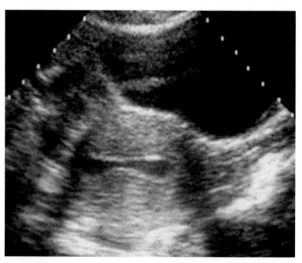

Figure 3-28. *Longitudinal image showing an irregular intrauterine gestational sac with no yolk sac or fetal parts.*

never achieve pregnancy again, while 10% experience a recurrent ectopic pregnancy. Ectopic pregnancies may occur in a variety of locations. The most common site is the ampullary portion of the fallopian tube, where fertilization usually occurs. Less commonly an ectopic pregnancy may be cornual/interstitial, cervical, ovarian, or abdominal (Figure 3-29A and Box 3-3). Risk factors include pelvic inflammatory disease (PID), use of an intrauterine contraceptive device (IUD), previous ectopic pregnancy, DES exposure, previous tubal reconstruction, fertility assistance, and advanced maternal age and parity (Box 3-4).

Clinical Presentation

Typically, patients with ectopic pregnancies present with a positive pregnancy test and the classic triad of pain (Figure 3-29B), bleeding, and adnexal mass. There are exceptions to all rules. Twenty percent of patients with ectopic pregnancies present with a history of normal menses and no amenorrhea, and they show no sonographic evidence of adnexal abnormality.

The tubal ectopic pregnancy is most common; therefore the adnexal mass corresponds with the position of the blastocyst within the fallopian tube. Prior to rupture the

Figure 3-29. A *The various incidences and locations of ectopic pregnancies. Reprinted with permission from Callen P: Ultrasonography in Obstetrics and Gynecology, 5th Edition. Philadelphia, Saunders, 2008, p 1029, fig 32-12. (Modified from Benson RC: Handbook of Obstetrics & Gynecology, 8th Edition. Los Altos, CA, Lange Medical Publications, 1983; and Schoenbaum S, Rosendorf L, Kappelman N, et al: Gray-scale ultrasound in tubal pregnancy. Radiology 127:757, 1978.)* **B** *Location of referred pain associated with ectopic pregnancy.*

A

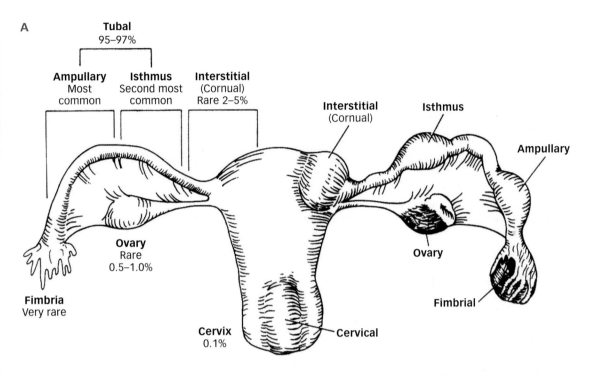

B

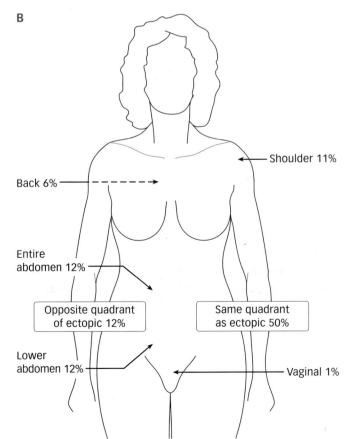

Box 3-3.	Sites of ectopic pregnancy.

Ampullary portion of the fallopian tube, where fertilization usually occurs (most common site)

Cornu/interstitium

Cervix

Ovary

Abdomen

Box 3-4.	Factors that increase the risk of an ectopic pregnancy.

Pelvic inflammatory disease (PID)

Intrauterine contraceptive device (IUD)

Previous ectopic pregnancy

Exposure to diethylstilbestrol (DES)

Previous tubal reconstruction

Fertility assistance

Increasing maternal age and parity

mass appears as a thick-walled cyst (i.e., the **tubal ring**) and is usually on the same side as the corpus luteum cyst (Figure 3-30A). If color flow imaging is applied, the ring will light up with color in what is sometimes referred to as the "ring of fire" (Figure 3-30B; see also Figures 3-30 C and D). Pain may be mild or severe, and its location depends on the site of the ectopic pregnancy and whether or not rupture has occurred. In most patients, tubal rupture occurs 3–5 weeks after the last menstrual period. In some cases the patient bleeds internally and the hemorrhage is not apparent (Figure 3-31A). In such cases other clinical signs may be present—pallor, weakness, low blood pressure, and weak pulse. Beta-hCG levels do not rise normally with ectopic pregnancies. They tend to rise more slowly and then plateau. It is diagnostically critical to have a quantitative beta-hCG level with which to correlate the ultrasound findings. If the hCG levels are high enough that a normal intrauterine gestational sac should be visible sonographically but the sonogram reveals an empty uterus, the diagnosis is ectopic pregnancy until proven otherwise.

Rupture

Free fluid in the pelvis, especially the posterior cul-de-sac, suggests rupture of an ectopic pregnancy. If rupture has occurred and there is active bleeding, blood can collect within the endometrial cavity. Surrounded by the decidualized endometrium, this fluid collection looks saclike (i.e., is a pseudosac) and care must be taken not to

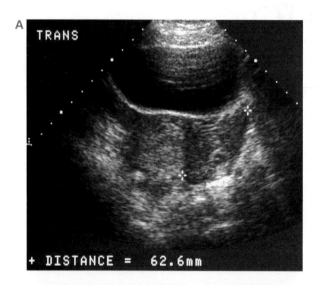

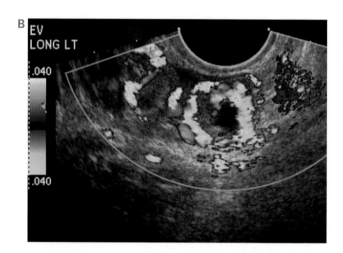

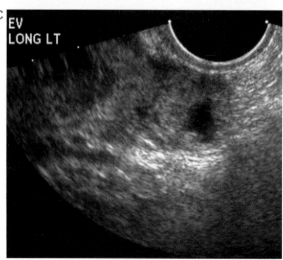

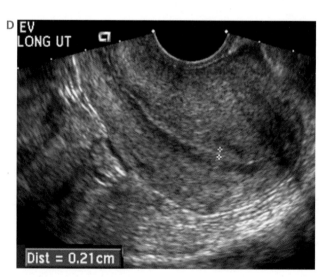

Figure 3-30. A Transverse transabdominal image of an empty uterus with a solid left adnexal mass extending along the iliopsoas margin (calipers) surgically proven to be a ruptured ectopic pregnancy. **B** Transvaginal evaluation of the adnexa demonstrates a tubal ring with color. **C** Tubal ring without color showing thick decidual reaction. **D** Image of the uterus shows no evidence of an intrauterine pregnancy.

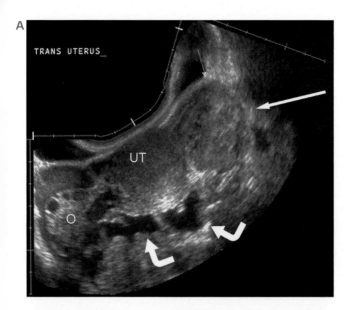

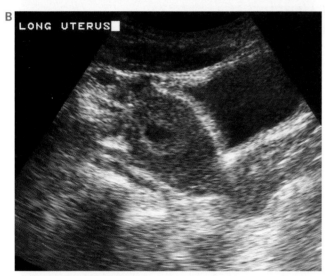

mistake it for a normal pregnancy (Figure 3-31B). Cul-de-sac fluid should increase one's suspicion of ectopic pregnancy, especially when accompanied by an empty uterus and a positive hCG. Adding an adnexal mass to these other findings boosts the risk of ectopic pregnancy to 85%–90% (Figures 3-31 C–E).

Cornual/Interstitial Ectopic Pregnancy

The **cornual** or **interstitial ectopic pregnancy** occurs where the fallopian tube inserts into the uterus. In this location part of the gestational sac is within the uterus and part is within the fallopian tube. The pregnancy can

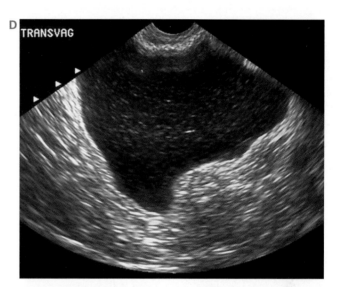

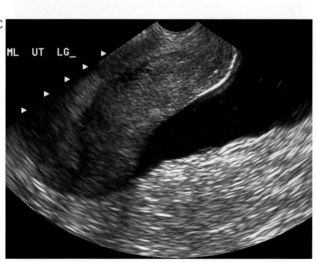

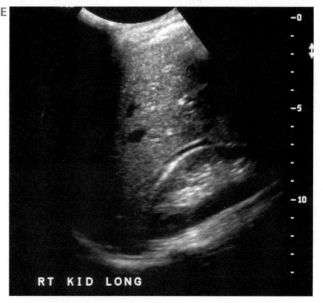

Figure 3-31. A *Transverse image through uterus showing a solid left adnexal mass (straight arrow), empty uterus, and normal right ovary surrounded by complex fluid (curved arrows). Ruptured left ectopic pregnancy. UT = uterus, O = ovary.* **B** *The saclike structure within the uterus is a pseudosac. There is no double decidual ring.* **C** *Blood from a ruptured ectopic pregnancy in the posterior cul-de-sac.* **D** *Large collection of blood in adnexa.* **E** *Fluid from ruptured ectopic pregnancy extending into Morison's pouch.*

A

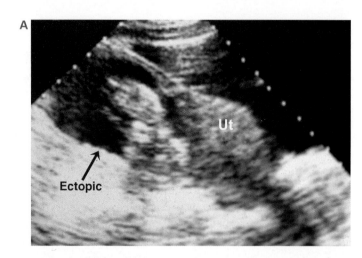

B

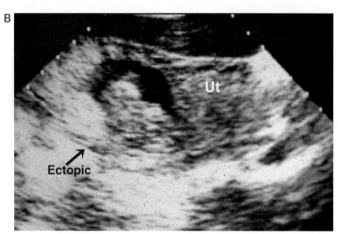

Figure 3-32. A *Longitudinal view of the uterus showing a gestational sac with a fetus at the superior aspect of the uterine fundus. Ut = uterus.* **B** *Transverse image showing the uterus with an interstitial ectopic pregnancy extending from the right horn of the uterus. Viable fetus within. Ut = uterus.*

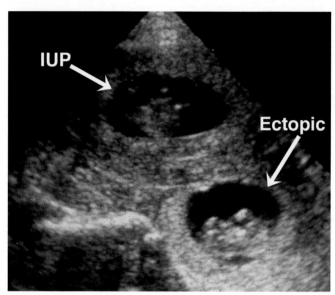

Figure 3-33. *Transverse uterus containing a viable intrauterine pregnancy with a viable ectopic pregnancy seen in the left cul-de-sac. IUP = intrauterine pregnancy.*

progress up to 3–4 months in this location because the uterus allows for greater expansion and the patient does not experience the same degree of pain, if any. Rupture of the uterus results in massive hemorrhage and is a life-threatening event. These pregnancies usually require a wedge resection of the cornu or a hysterectomy. Any time the gestational sac appears to be shifted to one side of the uterus, one should pay close attention to rule out a cornual ectopic pregnancy. It is essential to make certain that myometrium can be seen completely surrounding the products of conception (Figure 3-32).

Heterotopic Pregnancy
If an intrauterine gestational sac can be identified on ultrasound, the likelihood of an ectopic pregnancy is very low. Rarely, however, an ectopic pregnancy occurs in combination with a normal intrauterine pregnancy as a **heterotopic pregnancy**. The incidence of this occurring

is approximately 1 in 30,000. Heterotopic pregnancies are most commonly seen in patients who have undergone fertility assistance. In this population, the incidence is 1 in 7000. Once this condition is identified, an attempt is usually made to terminate the ectopic pregnancy while salvaging the intrauterine pregnancy. Early diagnosis can be difficult but, when identified, two-thirds of the surviving intrauterine pregnancies progress to term (Figure 3-33).

Cervical Ectopic Pregnancy
Sonographically, a **cervical ectopic pregnancy** (Figure 3-34) can be difficult to differentiate from an inevitable abortion, as the gestational sac is implanted within the endocervical canal. Color Doppler can assist in differentiating between the two. If the diagnosis is spontaneous abortion, there is usually a thin sonolucent rim around the sac and color flow is not detected because it is a failed pregnancy. The cervical ectopic pregnancy shows the color "ring of fire." The cervical location is rare, and the main predisposing risk factors are previous uterine curettage or prior cesarean scar. Initial treatment of choice is the injection of methotrexate and aspiration. The cervical ectopic pregnancy, although rare, can also be associated with uncontrollable hemorrhage, and half of these cases require hysterectomy. Massive hemorrhage is associated with attempts to evacuate these pregnancies, and total hysterectomy may be required if methotrexate treatment is unsuccessful.

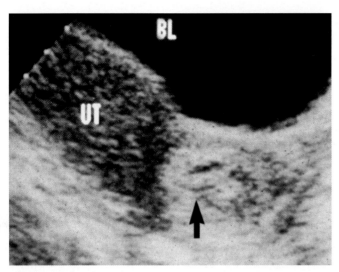

Figure 3-34. *Longitudinal transabdominal image showing a cervical ectopic pregnancy (arrow). UT = uterus, BL = bladder.*

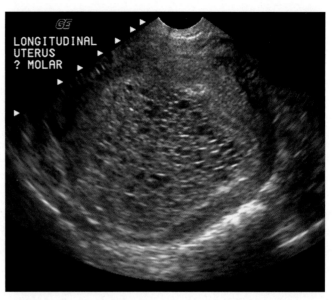

Figure 3-35. *Transvaginal image through a uterus containing molar tissue.*

Abdominal Ectopic Pregnancy

Also rare, **abdominal ectopic pregnancies** are sometimes referred to as **tubal abortions**. If a fertilized egg is expelled out of the tube into the pelvic cavity, where it communicates with the abdominal cavity, the zygote can migrate into the abdomen, attach itself to something vascular, and grow. Although unusual, term abdominal ectopic pregnancies producing live infants have been documented. Abdominal ectopics are usually diagnosed later in the pregnancy. Associated sonographic findings include an eccentric fetal position, oligohydramnios, difficulty seeing placental boundaries, and lack of a myometrial rim.

Gestational Trophoblastic Disorder/ Molar Pregnancy

Molar pregnancy is an abnormal pregnancy resulting from a pathologic ovum with proliferation of the epithelial covering of the chorionic villi accompanied by dissolution and cystic cavitation of the avascular stroma of villi. Although the cause for development of a molar pregnancy is not known, it has been proposed that the source may be the death of an embryo early in development. Embryonic circulation ceases but maternal circulation continues to nourish the trophoblastic cells while sustaining fluid transfer from the maternal blood into the chorionic villi. With no fetal circulatory mechanism, fluid builds up in the villi, giving rise to the hydropic changes within the placental tissues. First reported by Hippocrates, this anomaly was not suspected of originating from the trophoblastic cells of the chorion until 1895, when Felix Marchand published his theory. Proliferation of trophoblastic cells is controlled by paternal genomes, while embryonic growth is controlled by maternal genomes. Causes for the development of molar tissue include a duplicated chromosome within the sperm, fertilization of an ovum by two sperm, or lack of a chromosome in the ovum, each causing an excess of paternal genetic material.

Gestational trophoblastic disorder (**GTD**) denotes a group of interrelated diseases that involve hydatidiform, invasive, and partial moles. The condition appears to be mostly sporadic, but risk factors include history of a previous molar pregnancy and extremes of the reproductive years. All cases are associated with diffuse and marked edema of the placenta with cystic enlargement of the chorionic villi (Figure 3-35). Patients usually present large for gestational age (LGA) with marked elevation of hCG, lack of fetal heart tones, hyperemesis gravidarum, and pregnancy-induced hypertension (PIH). Bilateral ovarian theca-lutein cysts (the result of ovarian hyperstimulation) are seen in as many as 50% of cases (Figure 3-36). Following evacuation of the molar tissue, it may take 2–4 months for complete resolution of the cysts. Bleeding may be present, as well as hyperthyroidism. Molar pregnancies tend not to recur, and the prognosis for future pregnancies is quite favorable. See Chapter 16 for a case study involving molar pregnancy. The types, causes, and characteristics of molar pregnancies are described below.

A 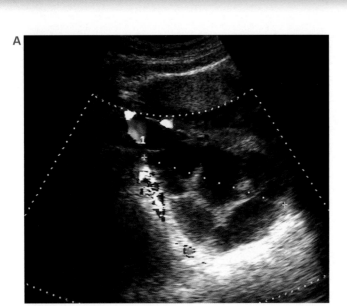 B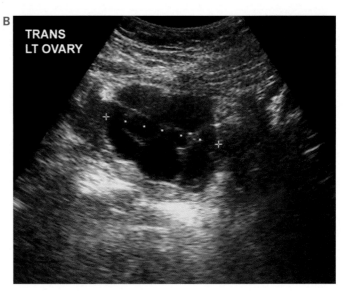

Figure 3-36. A and **B** Images showing hyperstimulation of both right and left ovaries associated with molar pregnancy.

A 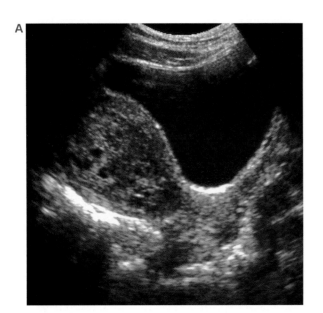 B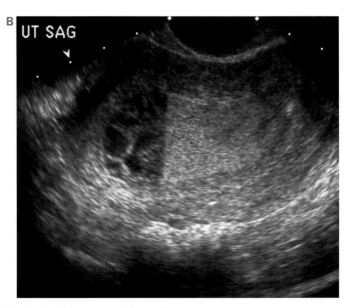

Figure 3-37. A Longitudinal transabdominal image showing very early hydropic changes consistent with a hydatidiform mole. **B** Longitudinal transvaginal image showing very early hydropic changes consistent with a hydatidiform mole.

Hydatidiform Mole (Complete)

A **complete hydatidiform mole** is considered benign and is thought to result from the fertilization of an empty egg; therefore a fetus never develops. This completely androgenic conceptus is characterized by rapid overgrowth and hydrops of the placental tissues. The sonographic appearance has been described as a "bunch of grapes" (Figure 3-37). Those predisposed to hydatidiform moles include women of low socioeconomic status under 20 and over 40 years of age and those with protein and folic acid deficiencies. In 1%–2% of patients with complete moles, there is an associated fetus as the result of dizygotic twinning.

Hydatidiform Mole (Partial/Incomplete)

Fertilization of a single egg by two sperm cells results in a **partial mole**. This form of mole is associated with a **triploid pregnancy** and a chromosomally abnormal fetus. Although the mole is benign, the fetus has too many chromosomes, one entire set of extra chromosomes. The

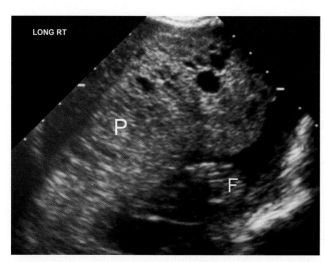

Figure 3-38. *Image showing a thick placenta with molar changes. Fetal parts are seen surrounded by amniotic fluid. P = placenta, F = fetus.*

condition is almost always lethal. The clinical presentation differs somewhat from that of a complete mole, simulating a missed or incomplete abortion. One sees focal cystic changes in the placenta, and the gestational sac reveals a transverse to anterior/posterior dimension greater than 3:2. If the pregnancy progresses, the fetus may have multiple malformations and signs of intrauterine growth restriction (Figure 3-38). Although rare, in some cases two conceptions can occur, one developing normally while the other develops into GTD. In this situation there would be a normal fetus with the coexisting mole, which would be even rarer than the one previously discussed.

Invasive Mole

Fewer than 1% of moles are invasive, growing through the decidua and into the myometrium and associated vasculature. Other names for an invasive mole include **chorioadenoma destruens**, **gestational trophoblastic neoplasm** (**GTN**), **gestational trophoblastic tumor** (**GTT**), and **placental site trophoblastic tumor** (**PSTT**).

An invasive mole is usually diagnosed after evacuation of a molar pregnancy, an abortion, or term delivery when there is persistent, often severe, hemorrhage. Although considered malignant, invasive moles rarely metastasize and are considered highly curable. Sonographic diagnosis can be difficult, as this is usually a postpartum or pathologic diagnosis and beyond sonographic resolution. These are thought to follow the hydatidiform mole in 50% of cases, while 25% develop after a therapeutic abortion and 25% after delivery of a term fetus.

Table 3-7. Staging of choriocarcinoma.

Stage	Criterion
I	Confined to uterus
II	Metastasis to pelvis/vagina
III	Metastasis to lung
IV	Distant metastases

Choriocarcinoma

More prevalent among Asians, choriocarcinoma is a highly malignant mole that metastasizes rapidly to the lung (80%), vagina (30%), pelvis (20%), brain and liver (10%), and bowel, kidney, and spleen (< 5%). Like chorioadenoma destruens (invasive mole), choriocarcinomas may follow a mole (50%), an abortion (30%), a normal pregnancy (20%), and occasionally an ectopic pregnancy (3%). The primary tumor can be quite small (2.5–8 mm). Diagnosis and staging can be accomplished using pelvic sonography, beta-hCG levels, chest radiographs, and chest/abdomen/brain computed tomography. Staging of choriocarcinoma is shown in Table 3-7. Patients should be monitored with serial measurements of hCG levels until hCG is undetectable and the regression of theca-lutein cysts can be documented sonographically.

SCANNING TIPS, GUIDELINES, AND PITFALLS

1. Transvaginal scanning provides the best detail for evaluating an early intrauterine pregnancy. Appendix C contains sample evaluation forms and clinical data sheets.

2. Take care not to mistake the normal amnion, early in pregnancy, for a thickened nuchal translucency.

3. Maternal ovaries must always be evaluated in the first trimester whether scanning vaginally or transabdominally.

4. It is always prudent to perform a transabdominal survey when performing a vaginal evaluation in order not to miss anatomy and masses that may extend beyond the field of view for the high-frequency vaginal transducer.

5. One can evaluate a subchorionic bleed by comparing it to the volume of the gestational sac (as measured by the prolate ellipse method of (length × width × height × 0.52). If the size of the bleed is less than a quarter of the size of the gestational sac (determined by eyeballing), the pregnancy has a good chance of progressing. If the size of the bleed is greater than half of the sac, the finding is worrisome for abortion.

6. A retroflexed uterus can be confusing on clinical examination as well as sonographic examination. On clinical examination, the fundus of the uterus may feel like a cul-de-sac mass and subjectively make the uterus feel small for the expected gestational age. Sonographically, it might be mistaken for an ectopic pregnancy in the cul-de-sac. When scanning transvaginally, the imager must ascertain the relationship of the cervix, the lower uterine segment of the uterus, the body, and the fundus. By doing so, the examiner can easily avoid this mistake (Figure 3-39).

7. An eccentric sac location can be worrisome for an ectopic pregnancy. Conditions that might make one suspect cornual ectopic include a pregnancy within one horn of a bicornuate uterus and a uterine fibroid causing lateral displacement of the gestational sac. If a thick rind of myometrium can be seen surrounding the pregnancy, the pregnancy is not cornual ectopic (Figure 3-40).

8. An overdistended bladder can cause artifactual flattening of a normal intrauterine gestational sac, making it look abnormal.

9. **Pseudocyesis** is a condition that leads a woman to believe that she is pregnant when she is not. This is seen both in patients who want to be pregnant so badly that they convince themselves they are and in patients who fear becoming pregnant and believe they are. In both cases, the patient mentally convinces

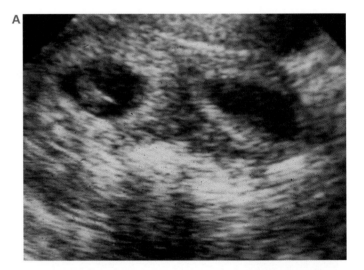

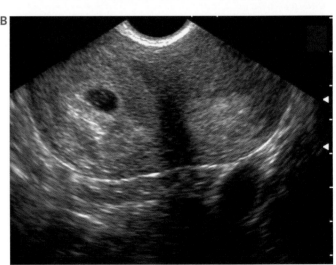

Figure 3-39. *Linear array image showing a retroflexed uterus with a gestational sac containing a fetus in the fundal portion. One can follow the endocervical/ endometrial canal indicated by the arrow.*

Figure 3-40. A *Transverse image through a bicornuate uterus with a viable intrauterine pregnancy in the right horn. The left horn shows decidual reaction with blood contained within the endometrial canal simulating another gestational sac.* **B** *Intrauterine pregnancy in the right horn with normal thick decidual reaction in the left side.*

her body that she is pregnant. Menses will cease, her abdomen will begin to enlarge, and she will claim to have symptoms including breast tenderness, nausea, and quickening. The sonographic examination, however, reveals a normal uterus and ovaries.

10. When a patient presents with pain during the first trimester, ectopic pregnancy is always a concern. Other conditions that cause pain include round ligament pain, degenerating fibroids, hemorrhagic ovarian cysts, and urinary tract infections.

REFERENCES

Callen PW (ed): *Ultrasonography in Obstetrics and Gynecology*, 5th Edition. Philadelphia, Saunders Elsevier, 2008.

De Lange M, Rouse GA: *OB/GYN Sonography: An Illustrated Review*. Pasadena, CA, Davies Publishing, 2004.

Goldstein C, Hagen-Ansert SL: First-trimester complications. In Hagan-Ansert SL (ed): *Textbook of Diagnostic Ultrasonography*, 7th Edition. St. Louis, Elsevier Mosby, 2012, pp 1081–1102.

Hickey J: *Essentials of Obstetrics and Gynecology: A Comprehensive Sonographer's Guide*, 2nd Edition. Forney, TX, Pegasus Lectures, 2008.

Johnson KE: *Human Developmental Anatomy*. The National Medical Series for Independent Study. Media, PA, Harwal, 1988.

Levi CS, Lyons EA: The first trimester. In Rumack CM, Wilson SR, Charboneau JW (eds): *Diagnostic Ultrasound*, 4th Edition. St. Louis, Elsevier Mosby, 2011, pp 1072–1118.

Miller BF, Keane CB: *Encyclopedia and Dictionary of Medicine, Nursing and Allied Health*, 7th Edition. Philadelphia, Saunders, 2005.

Moore KL, Persaud TVN: *Before We Are Born*, 8th Edition. Philadelphia, Saunders Elsevier, 2011.

Sauerbrei EE, Nguyen KT, Nolen RL: *A Practical Guide to Ultrasound in Obstetrics and Gynecology*, 2nd Edition. Philadelphia, Lippincott-Raven, 1998.

Spitz JL: The normal first trimester. In Hagan-Ansert SL (ed): *Textbook of Diagnostic Ultrasonography*, 7th Edition. St. Louis, Elsevier Mosby, 2012, pp 1064–1080.

SELF-ASSESSMENT EXERCISES

Questions

1. Fertilization usually occurs in which portion of the fallopian tube?
   A. Interstitial
   B. Cornual
   C. Isthmus
   D. Ampulla
   E. Fimbria

2. The first structure that can be seen sonographically within the gestational sac is the:
   A. Primary yolk sac
   B. Secondary yolk sac
   C. Amnion
   D. Embryonic disc
   E. Vitelline duct

3. The maternal surface of the placenta is called the:
   A. Decidua basalis
   B. Decidual reaction
   C. Decidua vera
   D. Decidua parietalis
   E. Decidua capsularis

4. A missed abortion would most likely present clinically as:
   A. Bleeding with cramping
   B. Abdominal pain with or without bleeding
   C. Large for gestational age
   D. Hyperemesis gravidarum
   E. Asymptomatic

5. Physiologic herniation of the fetal midgut should resolve by week:
   A. 4
   B. 6
   C. 8
   D. 10
   E. 12

6. Of the following, which is the most common site for an ectopic pregnancy?

   A. Cornual

   B. Ampullary

   C. Ovarian

   D. Cervical

   E. Abdominal

7. Of the following ovarian conditions, which is most commonly associated with molar pregnancy?

   A. Theca-lutein cysts

   B. Corpus luteum cyst

   C. Polycystic ovaries

   D. Multicystic ovary

   E. Hemorrhagic follicular cyst

8. At 5–10 weeks, the secondary yolk sac is considered abnormal if it measures less than:

   A. 2 mm

   B. 3 mm

   C. 4 mm

   D. 5 mm

   E. 6 mm

9. Once the fertilized egg has reached the 12–16 cell stage, it is referred to as the:

   A. Ovum

   B. Zygote

   C. Blastomere

   D. Morula

   E. Blastocyst

10. An embryo becomes a fetus at week:

    A. 4

    B. 6

    C. 8

    D. 10

    E. 12

11. If the First International Reference Preparation (FIRP) hCG level is 4000, the Second International Standard (2nd IS) would be approximately:

    A. 1000

    B. 2000

    C. 4000

    D. 6000

    E. 8000

12. Of the following, which would be an indication for an abnormal pregnancy?

    A. Fundal implantation of gestational sac in uterus

    B. Defined double decidual ring around the intra-uterine gestational sac

    C. Embryo with calcified yolk sac

    D. Round or oval gestational sac within the uterus

    E. Double yolk sac within an intrauterine gestational sac

13. This patient presents with a beta-hCG level of 5730, right-lower-quadrant pain, and bright red spotting. This history and the transverse image shown here suggest that the most likely diagnosis is:

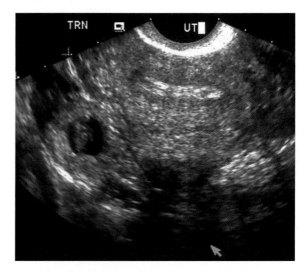

    A. Ectopic pregnancy

    B. Hemorrhagic corpus luteum

    C. Round ligament pain

    D. Threatened abortion

    E. Trophoblastic disease

14. This patient presents with bleeding and cramping. Her pregnancy test is weakly positive. This transvaginal image suggests:

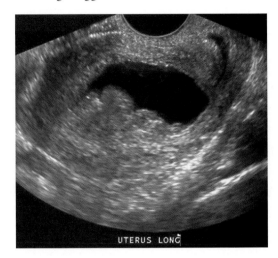

A. Ectopic pregnancy

B. Molar pregnancy

C. Incomplete abortion

D. Normal intrauterine pregnancy

E. Pseudocyesis

15. This patient presents large for gestational age and bleeding. Her pregnancy titers are extremely high. No fetal heart tones can be heard. Judging from this transverse image through the uterus, the diagnosis is most likely:

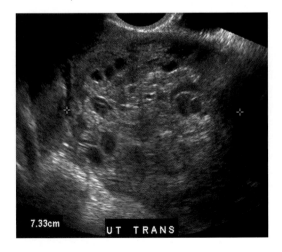

A. Ectopic pregnancy

B. Molar pregnancy

C. Incomplete abortion

D. Twin demise

E. Pseudocyesis

16. To what is the thin arrow pointing?

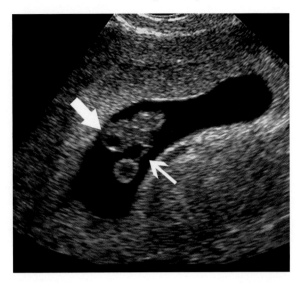

A. Yolk sac

B. Umbilical cord

C. Vitelline duct

D. Amnion

E. Fetal arm

17. To what structure is the bold arrow pointing?

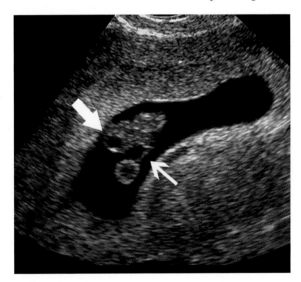

A. Yolk sac

B. Fetal stomach

C. Enlarged ventricle

D. Rhombencephalon

E. Primitive heart

18. There is an abnormal finding on this image. What is it?

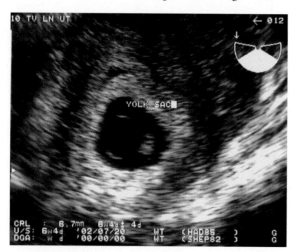

A. Embryonic hydrocephaly

B. Abdominal wall defect

C. Molar changes in placenta

D. Absent limbs

E. Abnormal yolk sac

19. The amnion and chorion usually fuse by week:

A. 6

B. 8

C. 10

D. 12

E. 14

20. For as long as 10 weeks, the normal gestational sac should grow:

A. 1–2 mm/day

B. 2–3 mm/day

C. 4–5 mm/day

D. 3–4 mm/day

E. 5–6 mm/day

Answers

See Appendix F on page 609 for answers and explanations.

The Second and Third Trimesters: Basic and Targeted Scans

Joe Rodriguez, RT, RDMS, * *Kathryn A. Gill, MS, RT, RDMS, FSDMS,* *
and Misty H. Sliman, BS, RT(R)(S), RDMS * ***

OBJECTIVES

After completing this chapter you should be able to:

1. Explain the differences between the basic and targeted ultrasound examinations.

2. List the images required to document the fetal anatomic survey during basic and targeted scans.

3. Describe how to perform an amniotic fluid index and list the normal parameters.

4. List the four fetal measurements used to determine gestational age and describe the anatomy used to identify the appropriate level for measurement.

5. Discuss the abnormalities that can be associated with oligohydramnios and polyhydramnios.

6. Discuss the high-yield anatomic areas for identifying fetal anomalies.

7. Explain the clinical indications for a targeted scan.

8. List the additional cardiac views performed during a targeted scan.

9. Describe some of the findings suggesting that a fetus might be chromosomally abnormal.

CHAPTER 3 DESCRIBED HUMAN DEVELOPMENT and sonographic monitoring from conception to the end of the first trimester at gestational week 12. This chapter considers the second and third trimesters (weeks 13–27 and 28–40) and introduces the concepts of the basic and targeted scans, including their purposes and technique. The **basic scan** (covered in Part 1 of this chapter), formerly referred to as a **level I scan**, requires a full fetal anatomic survey as well as documentation of the lower uterine segment, amniotic fluid volume, placental location, fetal position and heart motion, and maternal adnexal findings. As with any sonographic evaluation, an examination protocol, if followed, ensures that the study is complete and as an added benefit

---

*Authors of Part 1: The Basic Scan; **Author of Part 2: The Targeted Scan.

Box 4-1.	**Images required for the basic scan.**

Uterine cervix (long axis)

Placenta (long axis and transverse)

Spine (long axis)

Amniotic fluid

Four extremities

Three-vessel cord

Cerebral ventricles

Thalami

Cerebellum/cisterna magna

Four-chamber heart

Stomach/umbilical vein

Kidneys

Cord insertion

Bladder

Box 4-2.	**Additional images required for the targeted scan.***

Forward projection of frontal horns of ventricles

Coronal view of face (maxilla, mandible, zygomatic arches, nasal area)

Binocular distance

Nasal bone length

Nuchal fold

Fetal neck

Short-axis heart views, inflow and outflow tracts, ductus and aortic arch

Diaphragm

Gastrointestinal patterns

Long bones (femur/humerus, ulna/radius, tibia/fibula)

Hands and feet

Cord insertion into placenta

Doppler evaluation (middle cerebral artery, cord)

*The targeted scan requires these images in addition to all of the images required in the basic scan.

allows the practitioner to complete the study in a timely manner. By determining the fetal position sonographically, the examiner can systematically obtain images from the fetal head to the rump. The fetal survey should include the brain, spine, heart, stomach, kidneys, cord insertion into the fetal abdomen, bladder, and four extremities. In contrast, the **targeted scan** (see Part 2 of this chapter) requires additional images in high-risk pregnancies. Boxes 4-1 and 4-2 show how the basic and targeted scans differ.

PART 1: THE BASIC SCAN

Uterine Survey

Before the practitioner begins taking images, he or she should perform a survey of the uterus to establish the following:

1. That the pregnancy is intrauterine
2. The fetal number
3. The fetal lie
4. The placental localization
5. The amniotic fluid volume, by subjective assessment

Once the fetal position is determined (cephalic, breech, or transverse and whether the head is on the left or right), it is easier to know where to begin the anatomic survey. Starting with the fetal head and working down is one way

to image all the fetal parts systematically. This method makes remembering what has already been imaged easier and makes interpretation of the images easier for the sinologist as well. Establish your examination protocol and follow it with every patient you scan. By doing so you will find that you reduce the time required for your study because you are not just "fishing" and waiting for the anatomy to move under your transducer.

By imaging the **lower uterine segment**, we are able to determine that the fetus is intrauterine, document the fetal presenting part, and rule out placenta previa (attachment of the placenta to the lower area of the uterus, which can cause bleeding before or during delivery; see Figure 4-1). The longitudinal view of the placenta can usually be seen well on the side opposite from where the fetus lies. For example, if the fetus is in a cephalic presentation and lies on the maternal left, go to the maternal right where extremities and fluid can be seen; from that view you will also be able to image whether the placenta is anterior or posterior (Figures 4-2 A and B). Fetal position can also give clues as to whether the placenta is anterior or posterior. A fetus lying on the posterior portion of the

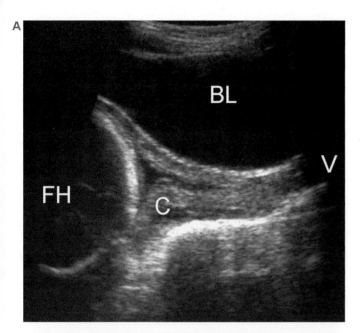

Figure 4-1. A *Longitudinal scan through the lower uterine segment showing the fetal head presenting against the cervix and the maternal bladder. The fetal position is cephalic. FH = fetal head, C = cervix, BL = bladder, V = vagina* **B** *Longitudinal image demonstrating breech presentation with the fetal legs presenting. L = leg, FH = fetal head, P = placenta.* **C** *Longitudinal image through the lower uterine segment demonstrating a total placenta previa. V = vagina, C = cervix, P = placenta, FB = fetal body, BL = maternal bladder.*

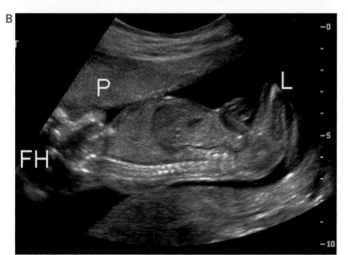

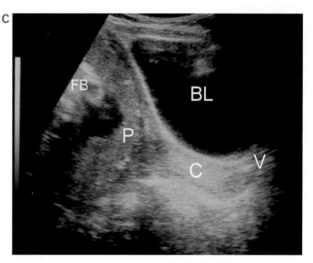

Figure 4-2. A *Longitudinal image demonstrating a fundal anterior placenta, fetal extremities, and umbilical cord (arrow) within a pocket of amniotic fluid. P = placenta, E = extremities* **B** *Longitudinal image of a fundal posterior placenta, fetal extremity, and a large pocket of amniotic fluid. Note the three-vessel cord (Mickey Mouse sign) indicated by the arrow. P = placenta, E = extremity, AF = amniotic fluid. (Figure continues . . .)*

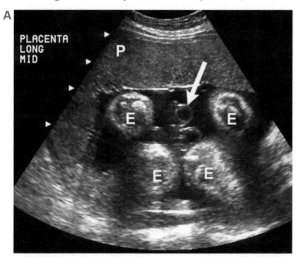

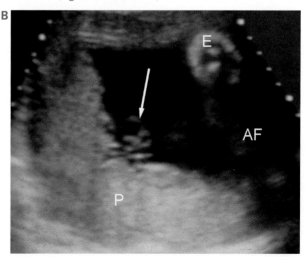

uterus is most likely to be accompanied by an anterior placenta. A fetus in close proximity to the anterior uterine wall is likely to show a posterior placenta (Figures 4-2 C and D). Fetal position must be documented as **cephalic** (head presenting), **breech** (rump or foot presenting), or **transverse** (shoulder presenting). An **oblique lie** denotes a cross between any two of those positions. If the fetus is breech, specifying the type of breech is particularly helpful in near-term pregnancies, as it may alter the management of the delivery. Various breech positions are shown in Figure 4-2E. Other, less common positions exist.

Figure 4-2, continued. C *Transverse image of the fetal abdomen against the anterior uterine wall. The placenta is posterior. Note the fetal stomach, gallbladder (straight arrow), and adrenal gland (curved arrow). P = posterior, S = stomach.* **D** *Long-axis view of the entire fetal spine. The spine is against the anterior uterine wall while the placenta is posterior. P = placenta.* **E** *Drawing demonstrating various fetal positions and presentations.*

C
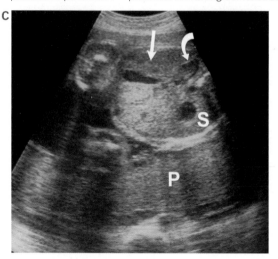

D
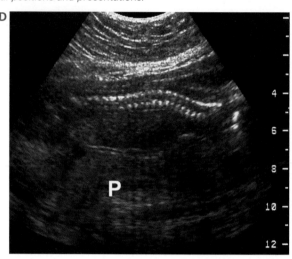

E

Fetal Positions

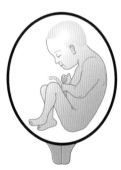
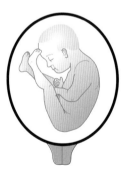
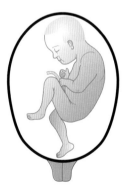

Cephalic	Complete/full breech	Frank/rump breech	Footling breech

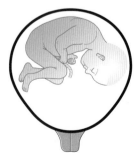
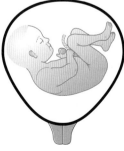
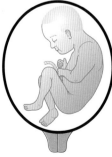
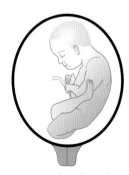

Transverse with head maternal left	Transverse with head maternal right	Incomplete breech/ foot below buttocks	Incomplete breech/ knee below buttocks

Anatomic Survey

The fetal anatomic survey includes imaging the major organ systems. Performing an ultrasound examination between 16 and 26 weeks' gestation allows one to image all the organs included in the survey as well as to predict a relatively accurate due date (± 1½ weeks). Although fetal organs may be seen earlier than listed, the following list indicates when organs are readily identified with sonography.

- Bladder: 10 weeks
- Extremities: 10 weeks
- Brain anatomy: 12–14 weeks
- Stomach: 14 weeks
- Kidneys: 15–17 weeks
- Four-chamber heart: 16–18 weeks
- Spine: 16–18 weeks (complete ossification after 18 weeks)
- Gallbladder: 20 weeks

Spine

Longitudinal imaging is best to identify symmetry and length of the spine and to image the spinal canal. In the longitudinal plane the spinal canal can be identified as a hypoechoic area in the central portion of the spine (Figure 4-3A). Coronal views are also used to visualize the bulging or widening of the posterior ossification points and the skin line (Figure 4-3B). Because of the length of the spine and the twisting of the fetal abdomen, distortions of the spine can occur, giving the appearance of questionable findings. Meticulous scanning of the entire spine in one continuous motion in both the longitudinal and transverse planes is essential to avoid confusion.

By 16 gestational weeks the three **ossification** (bone formation) centers of the vertebral bodies can be visualized sonographically. These ossification centers are best visualized in a transverse plane. Two of the ossification centers (**laminae**) are positioned posterior to the spinal canal, and the third (**centrum**) is anterior, becoming the vertebral body (Figure 4-3C). In the third trimester the complete echogenic vertebral body can be visualized in the transverse plane. Transverse imaging is best to identify any bulging of the posterior ossification centers, which would indicate a spinal defect. When evaluating for spinal

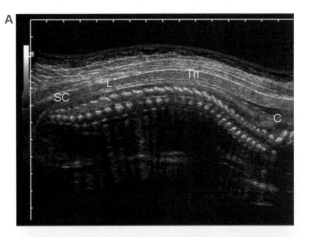

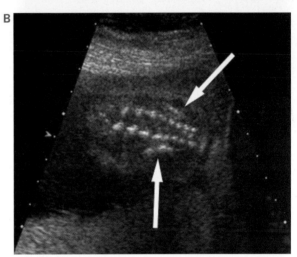

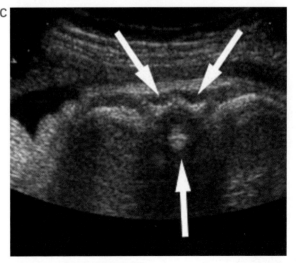

Figure 4-3. A *Long-axis view of the entire fetal spine. C = cervical, Th = thoracic, L = lumbar, SC = sacrum/coccyx.* **B** *Coronal view of the lumbosacral region of the fetal spine. Iliac wings are indicated by the arrows. The coronal view is probably the best view to eliminate defects of the posterior ossification points. The posterior ossification points should be aligned parallel to each other and the central echo from the spinal cord should be seen between the posterior ossification points. In addition, the iliac wings are an excellent landmark in the lower spine to confirm proper angulation.* **C** *This image nicely demonstrates the three ossification centers (arrows) that represent the early fetal spine. The two posterior ossification points should be parallel or angled toward each other.*

defects, one should also be concerned with defects that affect the soft tissue surface of the back (Figures 4-4 A and B). Keep in mind that ossification of the **lumbosacral** spine is not complete until after 18 weeks. Some spinal defects might be difficult to appreciate prior to this time. Transverse sections of the fetal spine should be seen as one images the fetal organs transversely; therefore it is not usually necessary to take additional transverse spinal images unless a suspicious region is encountered.

The rest of the fetal anatomic survey can be easily done if one starts at the top of the fetal head and scans transverse to the fetus all the way down to the rump (Figure 4-4C).

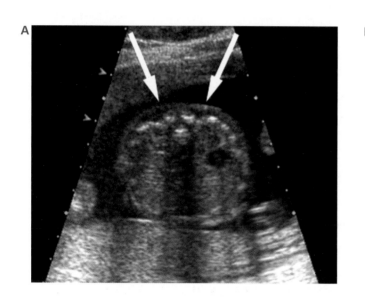

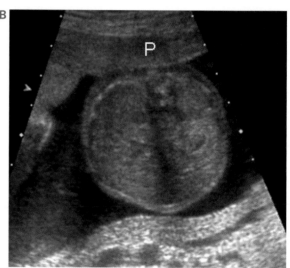

Figure 4-4. A *This transverse image of the fetal abdomen and spine shows the normal skin line (arrows). Defects at the skin line can occur without affecting the ossification points. For this reason the skin line should be scanned to eliminate any dimpling or other skin line defects. Although this can be difficult if the fetal position and amniotic fluid levels are not optimum, the sonographer should make every possible attempt to view this area.* **B** *In this transverse image, the posterior fetal body is in intimate contact with a portion of the anterior placenta, which can obscure a small superficial wall defect. The sonographer can decrease the pressure applied by the transducer, change the angle of the transducer, or place the patient in a decubitus position to move the fetus away from the placenta. Occasionally, the fetus voluntarily moves during the course of the procedure. P = placenta.* **C** *How to document the fetal anatomic survey.*

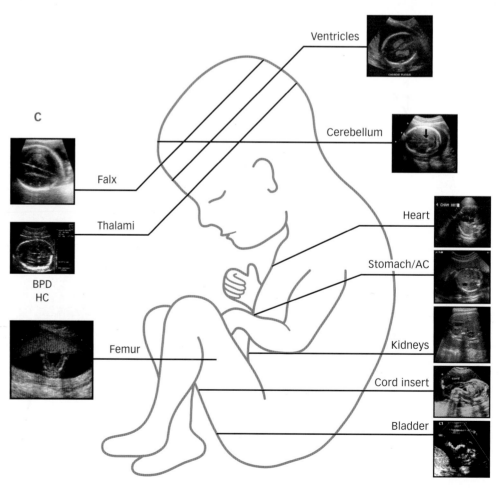

Head

One method of performing the fetal anatomic survey is to start with the head and work your way down the fetus. This system is easy to follow once you have established the fetal position in the uterus. The first image should be that of the **falx**—the fold of dura mater separating the cerebral hemispheres—and the lateral ventricles of the brain. Lateral ventricles are seen on either side of the falx. The side closest to the transducer can be the most difficult to see because of the ring-down artifact (Figure 4-5A). In the early second trimester, the lateral ventricles appear quite prominent, as there is little cerebral cortex. By the inexperienced practitioner this may be mistaken for hydrocephalus. The echogenic **choroid plexus** (the structure in the brain where cerebrospinal fluid is produced), also prominent at this gestational age, should be situated between the medial and lateral walls of the ventricles.

After 18 weeks' gestation, the choroid plexus serves as a landmark for visualizing the atrium of the lateral ventricles (Figure 4-5B). A ventricular measurement just distal to the choroid plexus can be obtained at this level. This measurement remains constant throughout the second and third trimesters of pregnancy. Measurements should not exceed 10 mm, with the average measurement being 7–8 mm (Figure 4-5C).

The **thalami** are two mid-level oval structures on either side of the midline just anterior and superior to the cerebellum. The thalami are the standard landmarks used to localize the proper level for obtaining the biparietal diameter (BPD) and head circumference (HC) measurements (Figure 4-6A). At this level one will also see the slitlike third ventricle between the thalami and the cavum septum pellucidum anteriorly situated between the frontal horns of the lateral ventricles (Figure 4-6B).

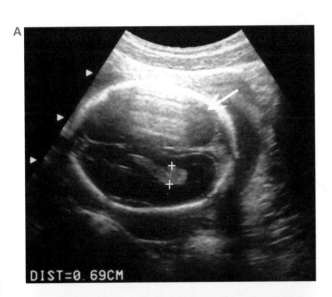

A

DIST=0.69CM

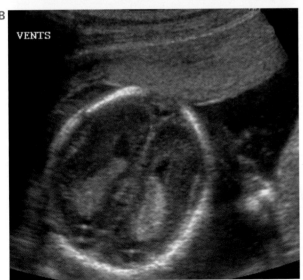

B

VENTS

Figure 4-5. A *The normal hypoechoic lateral ventricle can be seen containing the normal echogenic choroid plexus (calipers), which fills a good portion of the lateral ventricle. The ventricle closest to the transducer is rarely seen because of reverberation artifacts from the fetal skull (arrows). **B** Imaging the skull from the anterior or posterior projection allows the sonographer to view the lateral cranial structures symmetrically. It should be noted that in the third trimester this view is not easily obtained because of the ossification of the fetal skull. **C** Early in the second trimester, the lateral ventricles (calipers) appear to occupy much of the cranium, but as the fetal skull and brain grow the ventricles remain consistent in size throughout pregnancy.*

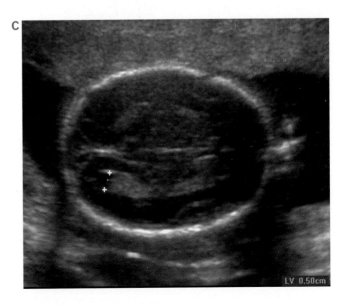

C

LV 0.50cm

Just inferior to the thalami are the **cerebral peduncles**. These arrowhead-shaped structures are seen anterior to the posterior fossa, where the cerebellum and cisterna magna are seen. The **cisterna magna**, part of the subarachnoid space, is visualized in the posterior fossa between the cerebellum and the occipital bone (Figure 4-6C). It is common to see small septations within the cisterna magna. The cisterna magna should not measure more than 10 mm from cerebellar border to the inner

aspect of the occipital bone. A cisterna magna measuring more than 10 mm is suggestive of a Dandy-Walker malformation. A cisterna magna less than 2 mm is abnormal and might be suggestive of an Arnold-Chiari II malformation. The **nuchal** (neck) thickness can be measured at this same level (Figure 4-6D).

The **cerebellum** (the region of the brain responsible for motor control) is located in the posterior fossa.

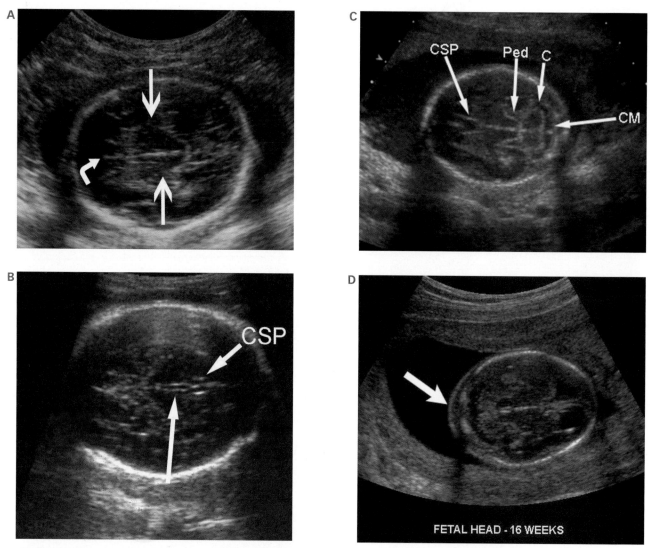

Figure 4-6. A *Inferior to the lateral ventricles are the cerebral thalami (arrows), which appear as hypoechoic triangles on either side of the midline echo. At this level, the cavum septum pellucidum is also visible (curved arrow).* **B** *This image through the thalami nicely demonstrates the third ventricle and the cavum septum pellucidum. CSP = cavum septum pellucidum.* **C** *The cerebral peduncles are just inferior to the thalami and will point to the cerebellum and cisterna magna. The cisterna magna or posterior fossa is an elongated fluid-filled compartment directly behind the cerebellum and in front of the cranial wall. It does not communicate with any other structure and its shape can be altered by extrinsic or outside pressure. Normal septations can be seen running through it. Enlargement of or failure to identify this structure should alert the sonographer to a possible abnormality. Ped = peduncles, C = cerebellum, CM = cisterna magna.* **D** *Nuchal thickness (arrow) demonstrated at the level of the cerebellar peduncles. Following page:* **E** *The two round hypoechoic cerebellar hemispheres are seen just anterior to the cisterna magna and lateral to the midline. They should be symmetrical. Measuring the cerebellum can be done for estimation of gestational age or to check for trisomy.*

Sonographically, the cerebellar lobes are hypoechoic and the echogenic vermis of the cerebellum is seen between the cerebellar lobes (Figure 4-6E). The transverse linear diameter of the cerebellum corresponds closely to the gestational age of the fetus up to 20 weeks. After that the diameter is approximately 2 cm at 30 weeks and 3.2 cm at 40 weeks. Figure 4-7 shows the proper way to measure the cerebellum and cisterna magna. (See also Table 9 in Appendix A.)

Heart

The **four-chamber view** of the heart is the minimum standard to which all sonographers adhere on a routine obstetric screening ultrasound (Figure 4-8A). The heart lies at an oblique angle, with its apex pointing toward the left side of the fetus. Because of the position of the heart within the chest cavity, the right ventricle will be seen directly beneath the anterior chest wall and the left atrium will be posterior, closest to the fetal spine (Figure 4-8B).

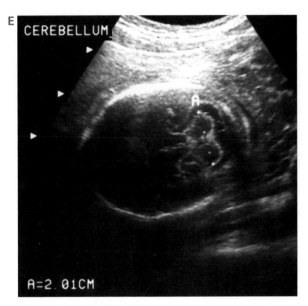

Figure 4-6, continued.

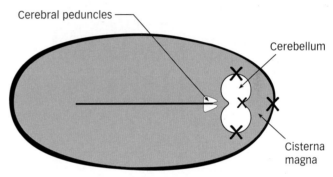

Figure 4-7. *The proper way to perform cerebellar and posterior fossa measurements.*

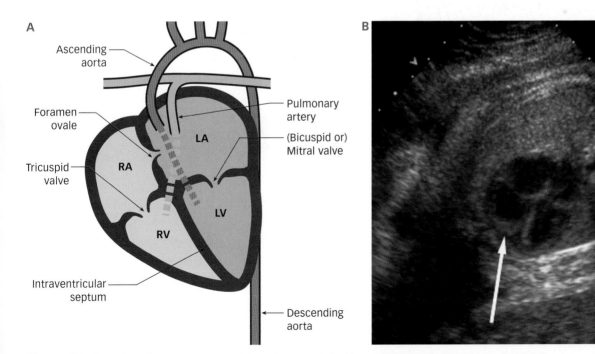

Figure 4-8. A *Fetal cardiac anatomy. RA = right atrium, LA = left atrium, RV = right ventricle, LV = left ventricle.* **B** *Although more sophisticated views of the fetal heart are being advocated, the four-chamber view remains the standard all sonographers should include in a routine obstetric study. In this projection the four chambers are nicely outlined and the right ventricle can be identified by the moderator band (arrow) in the lower portion of the ventricle. The right ventricle is slightly larger than the left ventricle. (Figure continues . . .)*

C

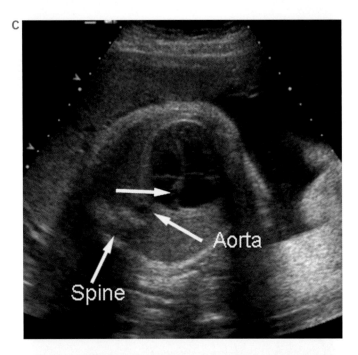

D

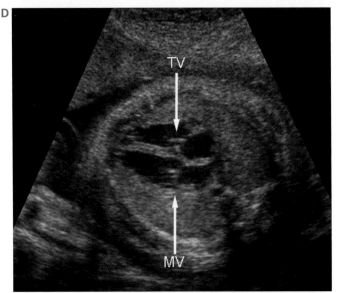

E

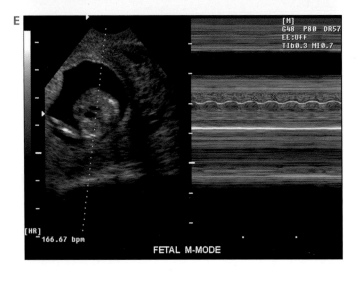

Figure 4-8, continued. C *The foramen ovale (arrow) is a normal opening in the atrial septum that closes after birth. This normal opening is easily seen in the second and early third trimesters but becomes more difficult later in the pregnancy. It should be noted that the best way to evaluate both the atrial and ventricular septa is with the ultrasound beam perpendicular to the septal wall.* **D** *This four-chamber view shows both the tricuspid and mitral valves. TV = tricuspid valve, MV = mitral valve.* **E** *This dual image shows placement of the cursor over the fetal heart in order to obtain an M-mode tracing to document fetal viability and calculate fetal heart rate.*

The right ventricle can be differentiated from the left ventricle because it has more **trabeculae** (fibromuscular support bands) than the left ventricle and the moderator band will be seen at the apex (Figure 4-8C). The ventricles and atria should be symmetrical in size, and the heart as a whole should occupy one-third of the chest cavity. Two interventricular valves allow blood to flow from the atrial into the ventricular cavities. On the right side is the **tricuspid valve** and on the left side is the **bicuspid** or **mitral valve** (Figure 4-8D). It is recommended that an M-mode tracing be obtained to document fetal heart rate, as that information can be useful to the referring clinician as well (Figure 4-8E). A normal fetal heart rate should fall within the range of 140 beats per minute (bpm) ± 20. A fetal heart rate of more than 180 bpm constitutes **tachycardia** and one that is less than 100 bpm, **bradycardia**. Causes of tachycardia and bradycardia are noted in Boxes 4-3 and 4-4; however, sonography practitioners must remember that fetal heart rates respond to activity the same as our heart rates respond to exercise. If a fetus is

Box 4-3.	Causes of tachycardia.
	Supraventricular origin
	Atrial flutter
	Atrial fibrillation
	Caffeine/sugar

Box 4-4.	Causes of bradycardia.
	Manual compression (transient)
	Focal myometrial contraction
	Heart block

Figure 4-9. A *The fluid-filled stomach is seen at the same level as the umbilical vein. These are landmarks for identifying the proper location for abdominal circumference measurements. Adrenal glands (arrow) can also be seen at this level. S = stomach, UV = umbilical vein.* **B** *The normal distended fetal gallbladder can be seen on the right side of the umbilical vein and stomach. Its appearance is similar to the adult gallbladder and is easily identified. GB = gallbladder, UV = umbilical vein, S = stomach, AD = adrenal glands, SP = spine.* **C** *Occasionally, debris can be seen within the fetal stomach (arrow). This can be from the fetus swallowing normal vernix or it may be associated with meconium or in utero bleeding.*

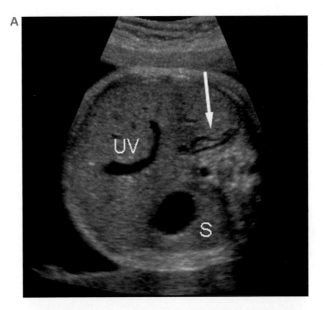

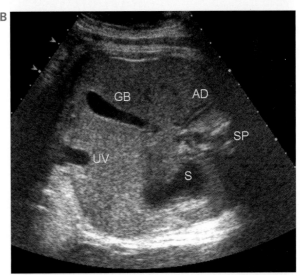

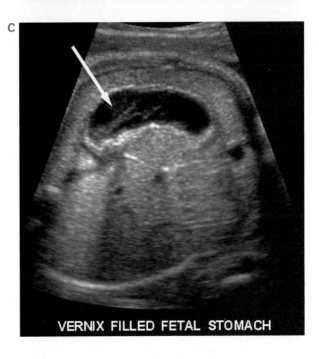

in an active sleep state, the heart rate will be faster than it is when the fetus is in an inactive sleep state. Heart rhythms that change slowly and regularly are much less worrisome than those that abruptly change before your eyes. Still, any change should be monitored and documented.

Stomach

The fetal stomach can be seen as early as 10 weeks' gestation and will be consistently imaged as fetal swallowing improves at approximately 14 weeks' gestation. Sonographically, the stomach is seen as a rounded, fluid-filled structure on the left side of the fetal abdomen. The stomach and gallbladder should be the only fluid-filled organs seen in the fetal upper abdomen. The stomach will be imaged on the same plane as the umbilical vein and the left branch of the portal vein, both of which are used as landmarks to identify the correct plane for measuring the abdominal circumference (Figure 4-9A; refer to Table 10 in Appendix A). Care should be taken not to mistake the fetal gallbladder for the umbilical vein. The gallbladder can be imaged from 20 weeks' gestation and will lie to the right of midline, while the umbilical vein is located midline and can be seen at the abdominal cord insertion site (Figure 4-9B). During an obstetric ultrasound examination, fluid is usually seen within the lumen of the stomach. If a fluid-filled stomach cannot be identified, it may indicate esophageal atresia or an interruption of the swallowing reflexes. Sometimes, debris can be seen within the stomach and can be associated with swallowed vernix, meconium, or blood (Figure 4-9C). The fetal adrenal glands can also be seen at this level and are routinely imaged during the third trimester. They are extremely prominent in the fetus and have a sonographic appearance different from that of the kidneys. Sonographically, the adrenal gland cortex is hypoechoic and the medulla is echogenic. They have a flat shape, however, and lie oblique to the spine (Figure 4-10).

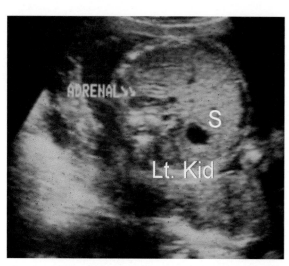

Figure 4-10. *Adrenal glands can be mistaken for kidneys, as they have a similar internal architecture; however, adrenal glands are flat and lie oblique to the spine, while kidneys are more rounded. S = stomach, Lt. Kid = left kidney.*

Kidneys

Fetal kidneys begin producing fetal urine at 13–15 weeks' gestation, and by 16–18 weeks' gestation the major component of amniotic fluid is fetal urine. When amniotic fluid levels are low, one of the primary concerns is that the kidneys may not be functioning properly. Since amniotic fluid is critical to fetal lung development, fetal kidney function must be ascertained. Fetal kidneys should be routinely identified by 15–17 weeks' gestation. They lie adjacent to the lumbar spine just inferior to the adrenal glands. They are bean-shaped and can be identified as round structures on transverse images. During the early second trimester the fetal kidneys may be somewhat difficult to appreciate because they blend in with surrounding tissues, in which case reducing the dynamic range to enhance the contrast of the image can help to better delineate the fetal kidneys. Sonographically, the kidneys appear as rounded, slightly hypoechoic structures adjacent to the fetal spine. The kidneys are of a medium-level reflectivity, and the renal sinus pelvis appears as a sonolucent slit within the central portion of the kidney (Figure 4-11A). By mid–second trimester the pelvicaliceal system becomes visible by ultrasound. In the third trimester there is an increasing amount of perinephric fat around the kidneys, making them more visible with ultrasound (Figure 4-11B). Because there is very little fat within the fetal kidneys, the sonographically hypoechoic renal pyramids appear very prominent and should not be confused with hydronephrosis or cysts (Figure 4-11C). Fetal kidney length is closely related to gestational age up to 30 weeks. (See Table 11 in Appendix A.)

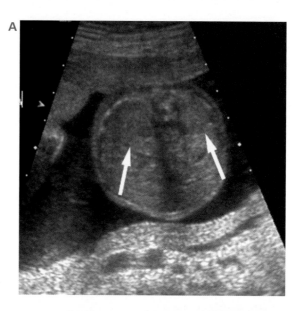

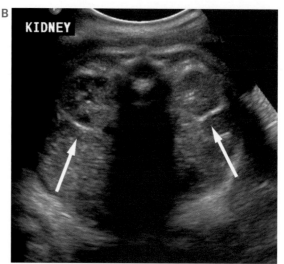

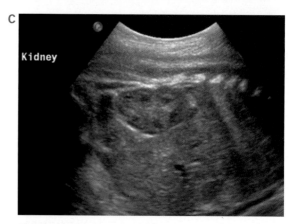

Figure 4-11. A *In this transverse scan, the second trimester fetus demonstrates the fetal kidneys just lateral to the spine (arrows). In the second trimester the kidneys tend to be isoechoic to the surrounding structures because of the lack of perinephric fat.* **B** *In the third trimester the perinephric fat becomes more prominent, creating a bright halo affect around the kidney and making the kidney outline more prominent (arrows).* **C** *In this longitudinal scan of a third trimester pregnancy the echogenic perinephric fat clearly outlines the characteristic shape of the kidney.*

Cord Insertion

The **umbilical cord** consists of two umbilical arteries that spiral around one larger umbilical vein. The arteries carry deoxygenated blood from the fetus to the placenta; the vein carries oxygenated blood from the placenta to the fetus (Figure 4-12A). The umbilical arteries arise from the **hypogastric arteries** to carry deoxygenated blood from the fetus to the placenta. As the arteries ascend from the fetal pelvis, they course along the lateral borders of the urinary bladder (Figures 4-12 B and C). The umbilical vein enters the fetus and courses upward in a cephalic direction to join the left branch of the portal vein (Figure 4-12D). A transverse image across the normal umbilical cord demonstrates the Mickey Mouse

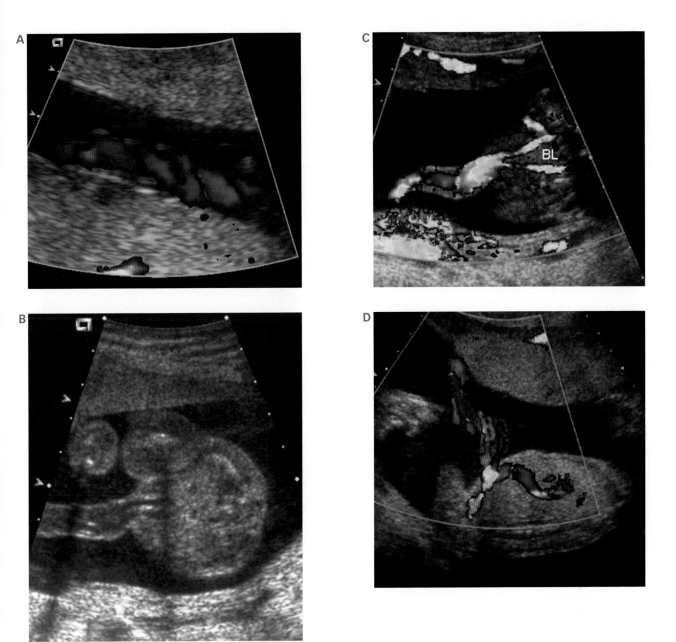

Figure 4-12. A *The cord is formed by one large umbilical vein and two smaller umbilical arteries that spiral around the vein. Longitudinal imaging identifies the spiral configuration of the three vessels that comprise the umbilical cord. Color Doppler can be used to appreciate the vessels more clearly.* **B** *The umbilical cord insertion into the fetal abdomen is demonstrated. This will be seen just superior to the fetal bladder. Abdominal wall defects such as the gastroschisis and omphaloceles occur at this level.* **C** *Confirming a three-vessel umbilical cord within the amniotic fluid can be a challenging proposition in the third trimester or with oligohydramnios. In these cases, a normal three-vessel umbilical cord can be confirmed by imaging the two umbilical arteries lateral to the fetal urinary bladder. BL = bladder.* **D** *In this longitudinal scan the umbilical vein can be seen extending superiorly to connect with the left branch of the portal vein, while the umbilical arteries are seen going inferiorly toward the iliac arteries.*

configuration (Figure 4-13A). The larger vessel, the umbilical vein, forms Mickey's head, while the two smaller vessels (the umbilical arteries) form his ears, producing the iconic **Mickey Mouse sign**. The umbilical vessels are encased in a viscous gelatinous material called **Wharton's jelly**. Although focal thickening of Wharton's jelly has been associated with omphaloceles, it has frequently been reported in normal fetuses (Figures 4-13 B–D). The sonographer must pay attention to the fetal anterior abdominal wall to exclude any abdominal wall defects such as omphaloceles and gastroschisis.

Although umbilical cord length can be quite variable, the umbilical cord at term averages approximately 60 cm in length, is 1–2 cm in diameter, and has as many as 40 spirals. It is covered by the amnion. Nuchal cords are the most common cord entanglement problems that occur. A **nuchal cord** is defined as one that completely encircles the fetal neck (Figure 4-14).

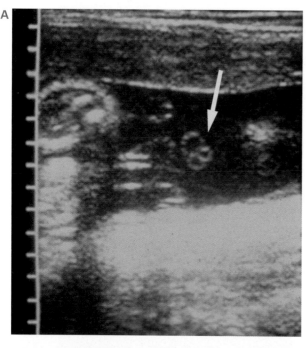

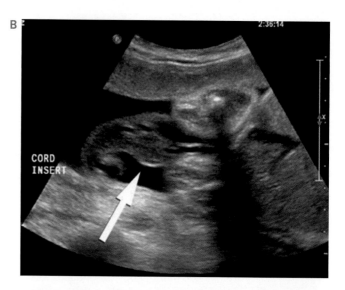

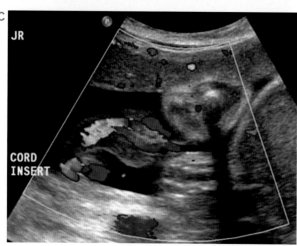

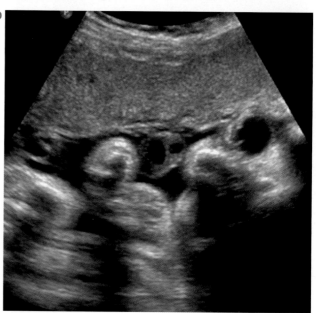

Figure 4-13. A *This image demonstrates a transverse slice through the umbilical cord, demonstrating the Mickey Mouse sign (arrow).* **B** *Wharton's jelly is a gelatinous substance that encases the three umbilical vessels within the umbilical cord. It is usually equally distributed throughout the cord but can sometimes be clumped in one area, creating a focal "mass effect" in the cord. This image demonstrates a focal clumping at the cord insertion (arrow).* **C** *Color Doppler can be used to identify the umbilical cord vessels as they course their way through the focal thickening of the cord.* **D** *A cross-sectional image at the level of the thick Wharton's jelly presents this view, which may be confused with an abnormal umbilical cord.*

Bladder

The fetal urinary bladder can be visualized by ultrasound at 10–12 menstrual weeks and empties and fills approximately every 30 minutes. Normally it can be seen filling and emptying throughout the course of an ultrasound examination. Failure to image the urinary bladder during an ultrasound examination should alert the sonographer to the possibility of a urinary tract problem. Because urinary tract disorders in a fetus can be life-threatening, it is essential that the sonographer do everything possible to identify the urinary bladder. The urinary bladder wall is very thin, and usually neither it nor the ureters are appreciated unless they are distended (Figure 4-15A). The fetal urinary bladder lies anteriorly in the midline and changes in size with filling and urination. A cystic area in the pelvis that does not change in size and/or is off center requires further investigation (Figures 4-15B and 4-16A).

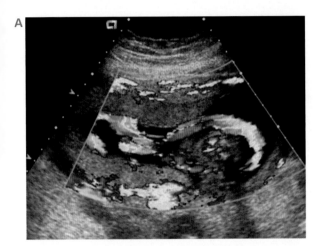

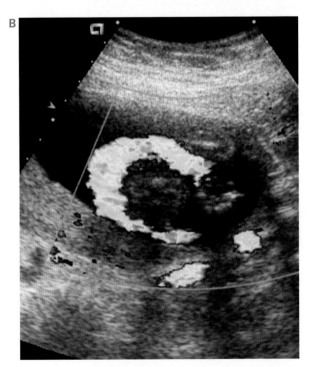

Figure 4-14. A *Color Doppler should be used to identify the position of the cord within the uterus. The cord is long and flexible, and an active fetus can easily become entangled or create a knot within the cord. In this scan the cord is seen wrapped around the fetal neck, creating a nuchal cord. To be classified as a true nuchal cord the cord must be seen encircling the entire neck and the ends of the cord should be seen crossing each other.* **B** *Although the majority of the cord is seen encircling the fetal neck in this scan, one can see that the circle is open on the left side of the scan, indicating that this is not a true nuchal cord but rather a case of the umbilical cord being draped over the fetal neck.*

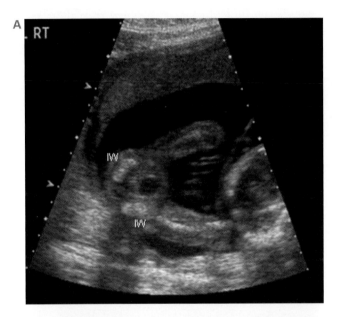

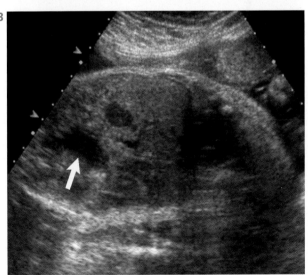

Figure 4-15. A *The fetal urinary bladder is seen as a cystic round or oval structure within the pelvic region. On a transverse scan, the echogenic pelvic iliac wings are useful landmarks for identifying the proper scanning plane. IW = iliac wings.* **B** *The full urinary bladder (arrow) is identified as a round cystic mass within the pelvic region on a longitudinal scan.*

Extremities

Guidelines require documentation of all four fetal extremities and a measurement of the femur length for gestational age. Typically, this involves identifying the **femurs** (thigh bones) in the legs (Figures 4-16 A and B) and the **humeri** (long bones in the forearms running from shoulder to elbow) in the arms (Figures 4-16 C and D). The distal extremities should show two bones, the **ulna** and **radius** in the arm and the **tibia** and **fibula** in the leg. Although basic guidelines do not require documentation of hands and feet specifically, parents love to see these and they can provide information for potential chromosomal abnormalities (Figures 4-16 E and F).

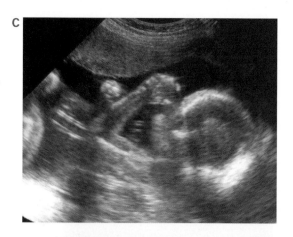

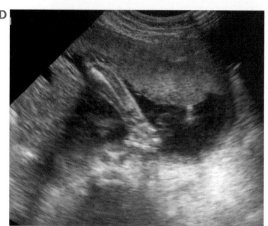

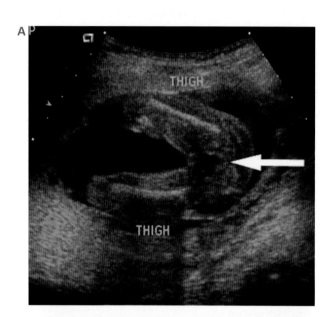

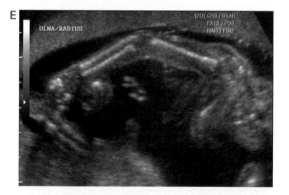

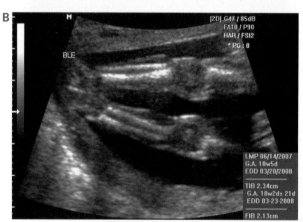

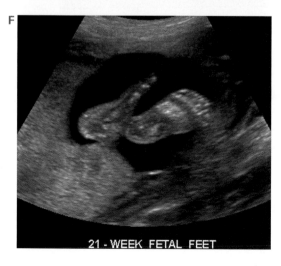

Figure 4-16. A *A smaller urinary bladder can be seen 37 minutes after scanning the image in Figure 4-15A. Fetuses fill and empty their bladders approximately every 30 minutes. Knowing this helps the examiner rule out a normal urinary bladder to identify a cystic tumor. At the level of the bladder (arrow), one is very close to the lower extremities, the femurs in particular.* **B** *Example of the full lower extremity.* **C–E** *Images showing arms and hands.* **F** *Both fetal feet are demonstrated in this image.*

Biometry to Determine Age and Assess Normality

Biparietal Diameter and Head Circumference

The **biparietal diameter** (**BPD**) and **head circumference** (**HC**) are the most commonly used measurements for dating pregnancies in the second and third trimesters (refer to Table 12 in Appendix A; modern instruments automatically make the calculation of age based on the sonographic measurement). Both BPD and HC are most accurate during the second trimester and less accurate in the third trimester.

Fetal head measurements should be taken in an axial scanning plane, at the level of the **thalamus** (the symmetrical structure at the brain's midline responsible for relaying information to the cortex), the frontal horns, and the cavum septum pellucidum. Head shape should be oval and the measurement should be taken from the outer edge of the parietal bone in the near field of the image to the inner edge of the parietal bone in the far field of the image, a method referred to as the **leading edge** or **outer edge to inner edge** method (Figure 4-17). Visible skin and hair are not included in the measurement.

Head shape can affect the accuracy of the biparietal diameter measurement in estimating weeks of gestation. When the normality of the fetal head shape is in question, the **cephalic index** (**CI**) should be calculated to determine if the fetal head shape is typical. If not, biparietal diameter

dating is not reliable. The cephalic index is calculated by dividing the biparietal diameter by the occipital frontal diameter (OFD) and multiplying that by 100 for a percentage:

$$CI = BPD/OFD \times 100$$

The normal range for the cephalic index is 78% ± 8%. If the cephalic index is less than 70%, the fetal head is **dolichocephalic**, too long and narrow. Dolichocephaly can be the result of crowding, molding, or normal variation. A cephalic index that is greater than 86% indicates **brachycephaly**, a head that is too broad and round. This head shape is one that is bothersome, as chromosomal abnormalities, including Down syndrome, can be associated with it. If the cephalic index is abnormal, the biparietal diameter measurement is unreliable for dating purposes and must be eliminated before measurement averages are calculated for average gestational age.

The head circumference measurement, on the other hand, is not affected by head shape. Head circumference is calculated as follows (modern instruments with computer-generated ellipse capability determine head circumference automatically):

$$HC = (BPD + OFD) \times 1.62$$

where 1.62 is the correction factor for ellipses (the fetal head is ellipsoid) when measuring from the outer edge of the parietal bone in the near field to the inner edge in the

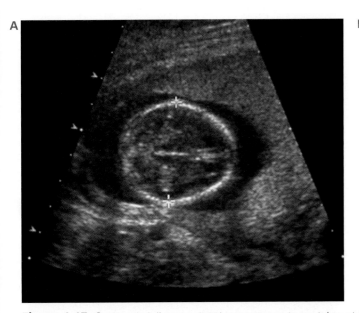
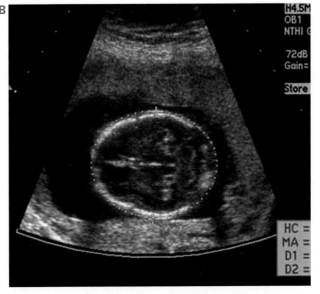

Figure 4-17. A *Biparietal diameter (BPD) measurements are taken at the level of the hypoechoic thalamus and the cavum septum pellucidum. The fetal head should be oval in shape. Calipers are placed at the leading edge from outer skull table (anterior) to inner skull table (posterior).* **B** *The head circumference is taken at the same level as the BPD. The ellipse should enclose the outer skull tables.*

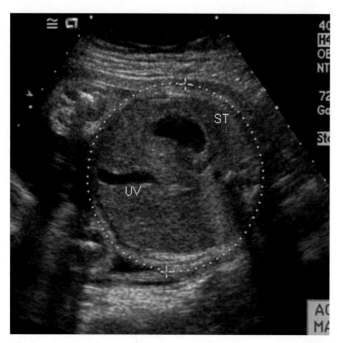

Figure 4-18. *The abdominal circumference measurement is taken at the level of the fetal stomach and umbilical vein. The abdomen shape should be as round as possible and the calipers should enclose the skin line. ST = stomach, UV = umbilical vein.*

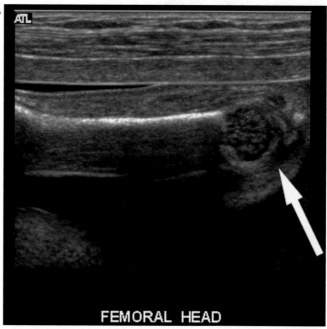

FEMORAL HEAD

Figure 4-19. A *The femur length should include only the shaft or diaphysis of the bone and should not include the femoral head (arrow). Following page:* **B** *The femur is a long echogenic structure within the fetal thigh whose length is a critical measurement. Improper angulation can foreshorten the length; therefore care should be taken to obtain the most accurate measurement (calipers).*

far field. Note that if the measurement were made from outer edge to outer edge, the correction factor would be 1.57—a figure found in some standard references, including Callen (see References)—rather than 1.62.

Abdominal Circumference

As with head circumference, modern instruments with computer-generated ellipse capability determine **abdominal circumference** (**AC**) automatically based on the sonographic measurements. The abdominal circumference also can be calculated:

$$AC = (APD + TAD) \times 1.57$$

where APD is anterior/posterior diameter, TAD is transverse abdominal diameter, and 1.57 is the correction factor.

The abdominal circumference should be taken at the level of the stomach and the junction of the umbilical vein and the left branch of the portal vein (the **J** or **hockey stick sign**; Figure 4-18). These landmarks ensure that the measurement is taken through the fetal liver, where the abdominal circumference diameter will be its largest. The shape of the abdomen should be round. Care should be taken when scanning the fetal abdomen because the

abdominal girth can change easily with outside pressure. Even fetal breathing increases and decreases the abdominal circumference. Unlike the measuring technique for the cephalic index, the abdominal circumference measurement should include fetal skin by placing the calipers or ellipse along the outer perimeter of the abdomen. At the same level as the umbilical vein and stomach, one can appreciate the adrenal glands and gallbladder. The adrenal glands are very prominent in the fetus and newborn and have the appearance of flat kidneys because of the echogenic central medulla and the hypoechoic cortex. Although images of the gallbladder are not required as part of the basic guidelines, its nonvisualization could be suggestive of cystic fibrosis.

Femur Length

The femur length measurement is the most accurate measurement for dating in the third trimester. (Refer to Table 13 in Appendix A.) The measurement is of the diaphysis and should not include the femoral head or the distal **epiphysis**. Both the femoral head and the epiphysis can make the distal ends of the femur pointed; therefore one should make sure the ends of the femur flare are blunted for proper measurements (Figure 4-19). The normal

B

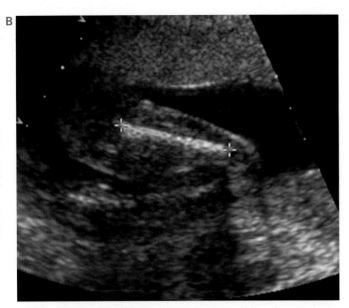

Figure 4-19, continued.

femur and humeral measurements are very close in size and each can be measured for dating purposes. If fetal position precludes adequate visualization of the femur, the humerus can be measured instead. (See Appendix A, Table 14 for multiple fetal parameters used in assessing gestational age.)

Gender

Gender identification is not required to meet the basic guidelines, but it is a common request made of sonography practitioners. Many argue that this can now be done in the first trimester by identifying the phallic projection and determining whether it points toward the head or feet. If it points upward the fetus will be male, and if it points downward the fetus will be female. Although this first trimester technique has been touted by experts in the field, the authors of this chapter do not recommend making a gender diagnosis until after 16 weeks. The reason for this delay is twofold: First, gender determination is not anatomically complete until 16 weeks, and second, making sex determinations in the first trimester requires a high level of expertise (Figure 4-20). Many mothers develop a strong maternal bond based on fetal gender when that information is provided. When a mistake is made, the emotional effect can be quite devastating. Experienced practitioners become very good at identifying gender when fetuses cooperate, but caution is advised for those with limited expertise.

A

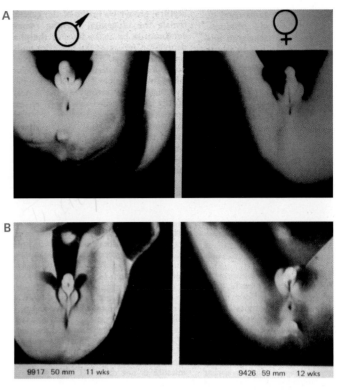

B

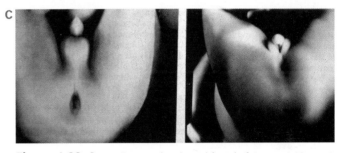

9917 50 mm   11 wks   9426 59 mm   12 wks

C

Figure 4-20. **A** Specimens of male and female fetuses at 10 weeks' gestation. **B** Specimens of male and female fetuses at 11 and 12 weeks. **C** Specimens of male and female fetuses at 14½ weeks. (Males are on the left in all three images.)

In the second trimester, diagnosing a male is fairly easy if the fetus is cooperative. We look for the erect penis between the fetal thighs (Figure 4-21A) or the classic **turtle sign**, which represents the penis (turtle's head) and the scrotum (turtle shell; see Figure 4-21B). Females, however, can be difficult to identify even among cooperative fetuses. One should look for the labia; however, in early pregnancies three small lines that represent the borders of the labia will be visualized. **Labia**, when imaged completely, will look like a butterfly—two labia with a hypoechoic space in between (Figure 4-21C). Some refer to this as the **hamburger** or **Big Mac sign**. In the third trimester of pregnancy, the labia can be easily identified.

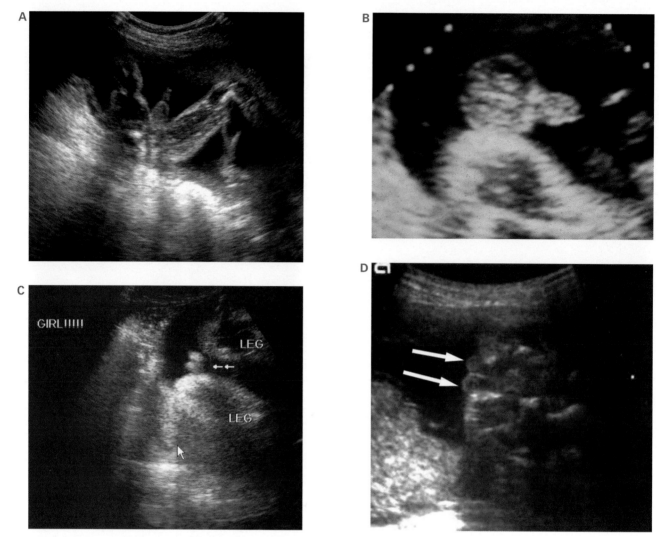

Figure 4-21. A *When fetuses are developed enough and cooperate, determining gender is fairly easy, as in the case of this male.* **B** *The genitalia of a male fetus, showing the classic "turtle sign." The turtle's shell is the scrotum and the turtle's head is the penis.* **C** *The labia (tandem arrows) of this female fetus are well demonstrated.* **D** *The labia in this image are somewhat prominent (arrows) and should not be mistaken for a scrotum.*

Because fetuses receive hormone stimulation from the mother, female fetuses may have enlarged labia that can simulate a scrotum (Figure 4-21D). This is why the split between the labia should be demonstrated for females and both scrotum and penis demonstrated for males. Another technique one might try is the **jiggle test**. In response to patting on the maternal abdomen, a scrotum will jiggle like gelatin. Swollen labia will not jiggle.

Amniotic Fluid

Amniotic fluid—the clear, yellowish liquid in the amniotic sac that surrounds the fetus—is essential for the protection of the fetus, to help regulate body temperature, and to allow space for the fetus to move within the uterine cavity. Fetal movement aids in development of the muscles and skeletal structures. Amniotic fluid is also critical to fetal lung development. Approximately one-third of the water in the amniotic fluid is replaced each hour. In the first and second trimesters, the amniotic fluid volume should increase, and by the third trimester the fluid maintains a constant level. In the late third trimester we begin to see a gradual decrease in amniotic fluid.

Amniotic fluid can be evaluated by **eyeballing**, by the **four-quadrant amniotic fluid index** (**AFI**), and by the **single-deepest-pocket** (**SDP**) **method**. Eyeballing involves subjective assessment and requires experience. The quantitative AFI and SDP methods provide measurements, removing some responsibility for determining

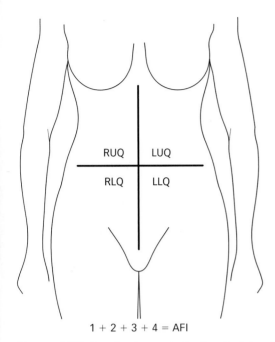

Figure 4-22. *Drawing demonstrating how to determine the amniotic fluid index (AFI). The largest anterior/posterior fluid pocket is measured in each uterine quadrant then added together for the AFI. RUQ = right upper quadrant, LUQ = left upper quadrant, RLQ = right lower quadrant, LLQ = left lower quadrant.*

Box 4-5.	Interpreting amniotic fluid indices.

Four-quadrant method, normal ranges:

Phelan et al.: 13 cm ± 5 cm

Rutherford et al.: > 5 cm and < 20 cm

Jeng et al.: > 8 cm and < 24 cm

Single deepest pocket (Manning et al.):

< 1 cm = oligohydramnios

1–2 cm = decreased fluid

2–8 cm = normal

> 8 cm = mild polyhydramnios

> 12 cm = moderate polyhydramnios

> 16 cm = severe polyhydramnios

abnormal findings from the sonographer but still requiring proper technique.

With the four-quadrant AFI, the uterine cavity is divided into four quadrants, and the deepest pocket of fluid in each is measured. The pockets must be void of fetal body parts and umbilical cord. Measurements of the four pockets are summed (Figure 4-22), and an interpretation of normal amniotic fluid, oligohydramnios, or polyhydramnios depends on the measurement standard used; several exist (Box 4-5). Table 15 in Appendix A correlates normal fluid levels with gestational age.

Polyhydramnios, too much amniotic fluid, can be associated with fetal anomalies, maternal metabolic disorders, and multiple gestations. It has been suggested that if there is enough fluid to accommodate multiple fetal trunk cross sections at various levels of the uterine cavity, the amount is excessive (Figure 4-23). Similarly, a fetus with enough room to stretch its legs straight and extend its arms above the head has too much fluid. With the SDP method, a deepest pocket, void of fetal body parts, > 8 cm suggests polyhydramnios (Box 4-6).

Oligohydramnios is defined as too little or not enough amniotic fluid (Figure 4-24). Causes include intrauterine fetal demise, bilateral renal abnormalities, intrauterine

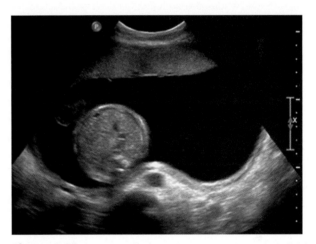

Figure 4-23. *This scan demonstrates too much amniotic fluid (polyhydramnios) around the fetal abdomen.*

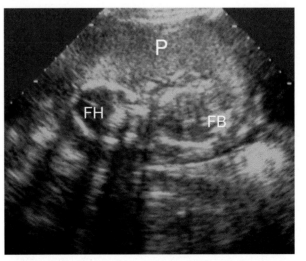

Figure 4-24. *In this severe case of oligohydramnios, no fluid is seen separating the anterior placenta from the fetus and posterior uterine wall. This fetus had bilateral renal agenesis. P = placenta, FH = fetal head, FB = fetal body.*

Box 4-6.	Conditions associated with polyhydramnios.

Maternal metabolic disorders

Multiple gestations

Central nervous system anomalies

Gastrointestinal obstructions

Chromosomal anomalies

Box 4-7.	Conditions associated with oligohydramnios.

Fetal demise

Bilateral renal disorders

Intrauterine growth restriction

Premature rupture of membranes (PROM)/post dates

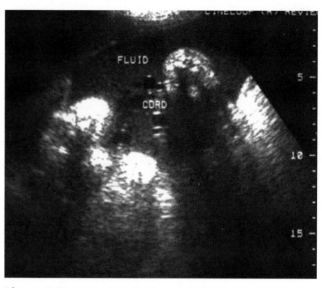

Figure 4-25. *Meconium-filled amniotic fluid.*

growth restriction, and premature rupture of membranes. Post-term pregnancies are at an increased risk for oligohydramnios. Oligohydramnios makes fetal imaging difficult (Box 4-7).

Sonography practitioners must be aware that amniotic fluid levels can be affected by a number of circumstances and that fluid levels can change abruptly within a 24-hour period. **Vernix** can be seen late in the third trimester as echogenic particles floating in the amniotic fluid. Vernix is sebum, desquamated epithelial cells, and shed hair that covered the skin of the fetus. This finding is normal and should not cause alarm. **Meconium**, however, refers to fetal bowel contents. Fetuses do not expel meconium in utero unless they are in distress. It will cause the amniotic fluid to appear gray and hazy and should be considered an ominous sign (Figure 4-25).

PART 2: THE TARGETED SCAN

If for any reason a physician determines that a pregnancy is high-risk, a **targeted scan** is often warranted to increase the rate of detecting and diagnosing possible fetal malformation during pregnancy. While basic scan protocols are still the gold standard for the evaluation of the fetus, a targeted scan is more focused and is often directly overseen by a perinatologist or even a pediatric cardiologist.

Targeted scans require more elaborate imaging of most of the same anatomy evaluated in the basic scan, with careful attention to the precise assessment of dimensions, positions, and involvement of fetal structures.

Because the targeted scan is designed to fit the patient's clinical history and/or the possibility of a specific fetal anomaly, no two targeted scans will be exactly the same, nor is it likely that tailored examinations will include everything discussed in this chapter. Sonographers responsible for targeted scans are rarely surprised by a perinatologist's request to measure, image, and evaluate nontraditional components of the fetal anatomy.

Indications

The potential indications for targeted scanning are many and change with time and medical progress. Currently, the indications for targeted scanning include the following:

- Smoking
- Teratogen exposure
- Exposure, including prolonged exposure, to certain chemicals, prescriptions, and/or treatments
- Drug abuse
- Advanced maternal age (AMA)
- Asthma
- Sexually transmitted diseases
- Maternal infection
- Rh sensitization

- Diabetes
- Hypertension
- Family history
- Multiple gestations
- Physical battery during pregnancy
- History of previous fetal anomalies
- Present fetal anomalies
- Uterine abnormalities
- Habitual abortion

These indications are just a few of the reasons a pregnancy may be considered at risk and therefore require one or more targeted scans during the gestational period.

Protocols

Protocols vary among practitioners and institutions. Some of the structures listed in this chapter may be evaluated as part of every targeted scan, while others may never be evaluated during the course of a sonographer's career. When performing a targeted scan, the most seasoned sonographer may struggle with some of the more tedious and specialized views. Therefore, even though a targeted scan is specifically designed to increase the odds of identifying anomalies, that goal is undermined if the sonographer fails to follow protocols and remain vigilant.

Head and Neck

Head: Circle of Willis The majority of all major structures of the fetal head are included in the basic protocols for obstetric imaging. In addition, Doppler examination of the circle of Willis is often incorporated into targeted scanning. The **circle of Willis** is a ring of arteries made up of the posterior cerebral arteries, posterior communicating arteries, middle cerebral arteries, and anterior communicating arteries that serves as a safety mechanism for blood flow through the fetal (and, later, adult) brain (Figure 4-26A). The congenital absence of one of the vessels may be of no clinical significance because the circle of Willis so effectively redirects blood through the remaining vessels that feed the entire brain. Thorough imaging and Doppler analysis of the circle of Willis have proven to help detect and assess intrauterine growth restriction (IUGR), vein of Galen aneurysms, and even fetal anemia (Figures 4-26 B–E). See Chapter 12 for further information about Doppler analysis.

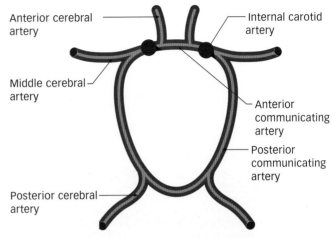

Circle of Willis

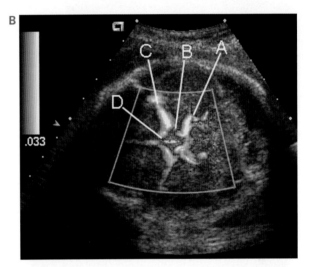

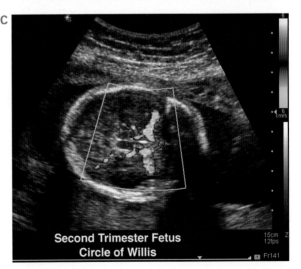

Second Trimester Fetus
Circle of Willis

Figure 4-26. A *The circle of Willis.* **B** *Transverse image with power Doppler color imaging at the level of the circle of Willis. A = posterior cerebral artery, B = posterior communicating artery, C = middle cerebral artery, D = anterior cerebral artery.* **C** *Transverse image with traditional color Doppler imaging at the level of the circle of Willis in the fetal head. (Figure continues . . .)*

Figure 4-26, continued. D *Spectral analysis of the blood flow velocities within the middle cerebral artery, part of the circle of Willis.* **E** *Middle cerebral artery pulsatility index. Reprinted with permission from Harrington K, Carpenter RG, Nguyen M, et al: Changes observed in Doppler studies of the fetal circulation in pregnancies complicated by pre-eclampsia or the delivery of a small-for-gestational-age-baby. I. Cross-sectional analysis. Ultrasound Obstet Gynecol 6:19, 1995.*

D

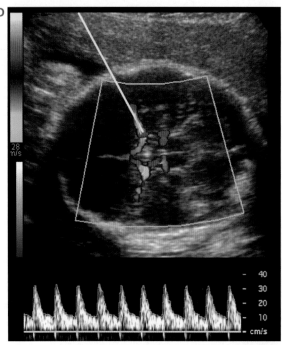

E

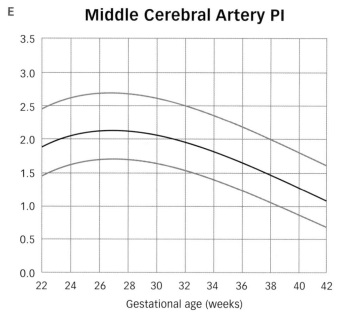

Neck The fetal neck is evaluated for position, mass, adjacent blood flow, and overall appearance. The fetal neck contains many small structures that are often overlooked until an abnormality arises. In a relaxed state, the fetus tends to tuck its chin to the thorax. If the head and neck are seen to be hyperextended for a prolonged period, further investigation is warranted to determine the cause. By imaging the fetal profile, the practitioner can often determine correct position (Figure 4-27).

Chromosomal abnormalities such as Turner syndrome and various central nervous system abnormalities influence the fetal neck. When the central nervous system is compromised, the swallowing mechanism of a prenatal fetus is often affected. As a result, polyhydramnios occurs. Therefore a targeted scan will look for fetal swallowing movements of the tongue and esophagus in the fetal neck. Knowledge of the physiologic mechanism involving swallowing development may allow identification of altered swallow-related movements in the fetus with malformations of the digestive tract or neurological disorders.

Nuchal Translucency The area of sonolucent thickening posterior to the neck in all fetuses is termed **nuchal translucency** (**NT**). This area is seen as a very small sono-

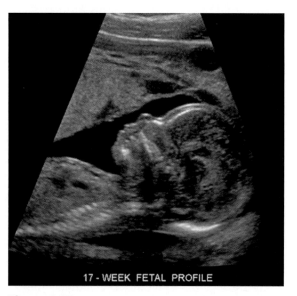

17 - WEEK FETAL PROFILE

Figure 4-27. *Longitudinal image through the midline of the fetus in a relaxed position demonstrates an appropriate fetal profile.*

lucent/anechoic space in the first trimester of pregnancy and relates to the skin and lymph tissue. Because it is so small, correct evaluation is difficult and error is common. Therefore high-resolution equipment and magnification are imperative to obtain the most accurate measurements in the first trimester fetus. When obtaining this measurement, the examiner should take care to exclude the soft

Conventional Measurement

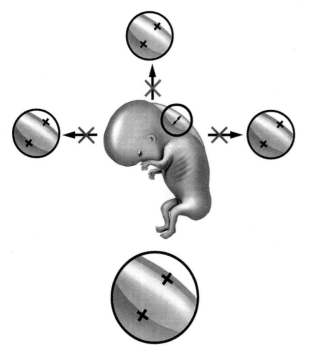

A

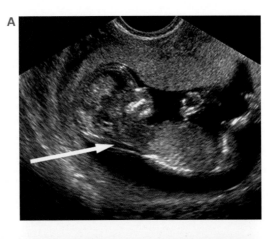

B

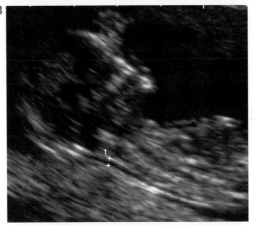

Figure 4-28. *Nuchal translucency with insets showing incorrect and correct (large inset) caliper placement. Reprinted with permission from Callen P:* Ultrasonography in Obstetrics and Gynecology, *4th Edition. Philadelphia, Saunders, 2000, p 40, fig 3-2.*

tissue adjacent to this space and to measure only the "gap" (Figure 4-28). For the best possible screening technique, sonographers should obtain nuchal translucency measurements between the 11th and 14th weeks of gestation using the **crown-rump length** (**CRL**). At 11 weeks the CRL should be 45 mm; at 14 weeks it should be 84 mm (Figure 4-29A). From gestational weeks 11 to 14, normal nuchal translucency is 1.0 to 2.5 mm, and measurements exceeding 3.0 mm are considered abnormal (Figures 4-29 B and C). Nevertheless, it must be borne in mind that measurements may vary slightly with flexion and extension of the fetal neck ($\pm$ 0.4–0.6 mm) and that an accurate true sagittal image of the fetal spine is imperative (Figure 4-29D).

C

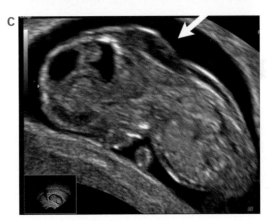

Figure 4-29. A *Longitudinal first trimester scan through the fetal midline, demonstrating the area of the nuchal translucency (arrow).* **B** *Longitudinal midline of a 13-week and 3-day fetus with measurement of the nuchal translucency (calipers).* **C** *Longitudinal image through the midline of the fetus demonstrating an abnormal nuchal translucency (arrow).* **D** *Nuchal translucency/crown-rump length chart. Adapted from Nicolaides KH, Sebire NJ, Snijders JM:* The 11–14 Week Scan: The Diagnosis of Fetal Abnormalities. *New York, Parthenon, 1999, p 19, fig 9.*

D

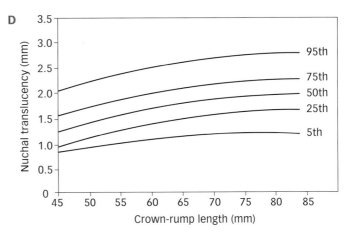

Nuchal Fold This measurement is of the skin thickness from the occipital bone of the fetal cranium to the outer edge of the fetal skin constitutes measurement of the **nuchal fold** (Figure 4-30). The nuchal fold should be measured between 15 and 20 weeks at the level of the cerebellum when imaging the fetal head transversely. In a normal fetus the thickness of the nuchal fold should not exceed 5 mm when maternal age < 35 years. Measurements exceeding 5 mm are thought to be a risk factor for trisomy 21, Down syndrome, and in such cases patients are often offered amniocentesis to determine the karyotype of the fetus. Care must be taken in measuring the nuchal thickness at the appropriate level, as slightly incorrect angles can create the illusion of a thick nuchal fold measurement. Although nuchal thickening may persist after 20 weeks' gestation in Down syndrome patients, regression is common in both chromosomally normal and abnormal fetuses. Amniocentesis is the only definitive means of determining the chromosomally abnormal fetus. Other considerations for nuchal folds that are found to exceed the normal range for thickness include Turner syndrome, cystic hygroma, fetal hydrops, and human miscalculation.

Face With many central nervous system and chromosomal abnormalities there can be associated facial abnormalities. Therefore it is especially important to visualize the face of the fetus in detail. Coronal, transverse, and longitudinal views of the fetal face are usually warranted when completing a targeted scan. The most common facial anomalies include the various cleft defects of the lip and palate. The nose and lips are easily imaged with a coronal view of the fetal face (Figure 4-31), and this view aids greatly in the detection of a median, bilateral, or unilateral cleft lip. While three-dimensional (3D) imaging adds no real diagnostic value in detecting the surface defects of the face, cleft defects that are just under the surface of the normal lip are better identified with 3D

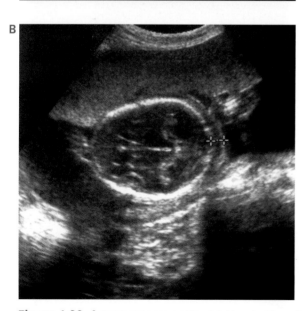

Figure 4-30. A *Transverse scan of the fetal head with nuchal fold thickness measurement (calipers).* **B** *Transverse image of the fetal head demonstrating fetal cerebellum and area of nuchal fold (calipers).*

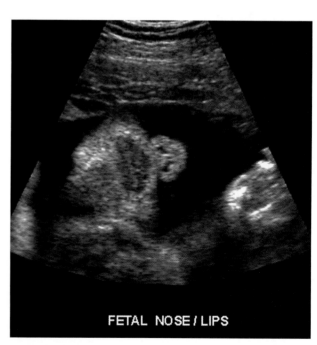

Figure 4-31. *Coronal image of the fetal face indicating the normal appearance of the nose and lips.*

imaging (Figure 4-32). Detection and determination of severity of the cleft palate when the lip is normal have been quite difficult with conventional two-dimensional (2D) imaging (Figure 4-33A). With the angle manipulation and reconstruction that 3D offers, a real alternative for evaluation of the palate and associated malformations is available to the practitioner (Figure 4-33B).

Profile. While the basic scan does not include images of the fetal face, sonographers often image the fetal profile for the mother, as it is an image she can clearly identify. Facial and profile images are taken mostly for the parents, and other facial images are often not included in the basic

examination itself. Care should be taken, however, to really look at the fetal face, as it can be a high-yield area for signs of anomalies.

Frontal bossing and micrognathia are very specific and sonographically identifiable abnormalities of the profile that are often missed because they can be so subtle. Fetuses usually are free-floating, relaxing comfortably within the uterus of the mother. Therefore the fetal face should be facing forward and not looking over its right or left shoulder unless position is altered by forces such as the placenta, fetal extremities, or nuchal cord. The overall appearance of the profile should be of great consideration,

A 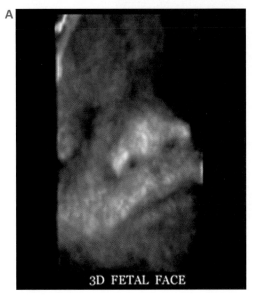 **B**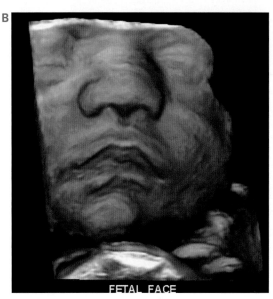

Figure 4-32. A *3D image of the fetal face showing a normal appearing nose and lips.* **B** *Normal fetal face using 3D imaging technology.*

A 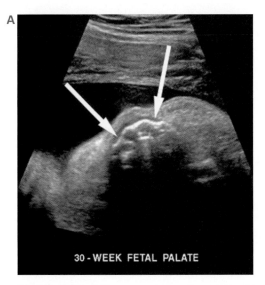 **B**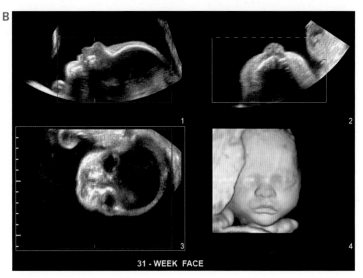

Figure 4-33. A *Transverse image through the fetal palate (arrows).* **B** *3D image of the fetal face showing planes for analysis and reconstruction.*

as many structures can be imaged, measured, and evaluated for possible screening and subsequent diagnosis of fetal abnormalities (Figure 4-34).

Nasal Bone. The length of the nasal bone can be useful in the evaluation of pregnancies at risk for **aneuploidy** (the state of having chromosomes in a number that is not an exact multiple of the haploid number), particularly trisomy 21 (Down syndrome). The sonographer must obtain a good midline fetal profile image in order to best demonstrate this minuscule bone sonographically.

A short or absent nasal bone will alter the profile of the face, making it appear flattened. (Refer to Table 16 in Appendix A.) This finding should raise concern and warrant a more thorough investigation of the face. For screening purposes, several studies and reports have stated that the optimal time frame for obtaining nasal bone length is between 11 and 14 weeks' gestation (Figure 4-35).

Orbits. The fetal orbits can provide information about facial abnormalities. The **zygomatic arches** (cheek bones) form the floor of the orbit and should be at the

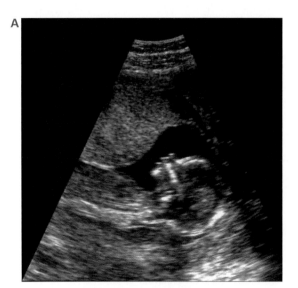
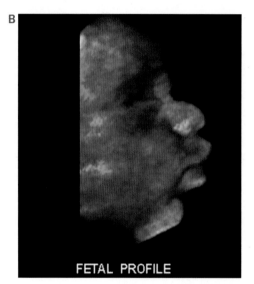

Figure 4-34. A *Longitudinal image through the fetal midline demonstrating a normal appearing profile.* **B** *3D image of the fetal profile.*

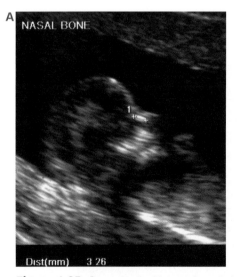
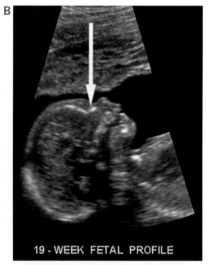
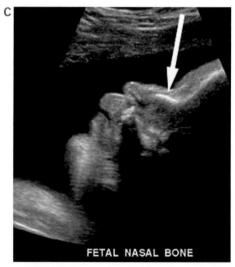

Figure 4-35. A *Longitudinal image through the fetal midline showing nasal bone length measurements (calipers) in the first trimester.* **B** *Sagittal image of the fetal profile demonstrating the presence of the second trimester nasal bone (arrow).* **C** *Longitudinal midline image of the nasal bone (arrow) of a third trimester fetus.*

same level on each side, allowing the orbit to take on a normal rounded shape. The binocular distances are usually not taken in the coronal plane because of the potential for imprecision. Instead, a transverse projection through the fetal orbits provides a good perspective from which the orbits can be measured with accuracy. Three measurements can be performed: the binocular distance, the orbital diameter, and the interorbital distance; these aid in the detection of conditions that affect the orbits. The **binocular distance (BOD)**, also called the **outer orbital distance (OOD)**, is obtained by measuring from the lateral wall of one orbit to the lateral edge of the other (Figure 4-36A). Binocular measurements can change throughout pregnancy and should be balanced carefully with accurate fetal gestational ages (see Table 17 in Appendix A). The **orbital diameter (OD)** is the measurement of each orbit separately (see Table 18 in Appendix A). Using the inner bony surfaces of the orbit, the practitioner can measure the orbital diameter, which has been considered to be even more accurate than the binocular distance (Figure 4-36B). An abnormally small orbit is referred to as **microphthalmia**; bilateral microphthalmia can be associated with fetal alcohol syndrome. In this condition, usually only one of the fetal orbits is affected. The distance between the orbits is called the **interorbital** (also known as the **interocular**) **distance (IOD**; Figure 4-36C). Generally, the distance between the orbits should closely approximate the diameter of a single normal orbit. An IOD that is too great suggests **hypertelorism**, and an IOD that is too small signals **hypotelorism**.

Eye/Globe. While imaging the fetal orbits, the practitioner can identify other structures, including the eyelids, the lenses, and the hyaloid arteries of the eye. The fetal eyelids can be seen bilaterally with a coronal projection of the fetal face (Figure 4-37). The normal appearance of the lens is identified by its highly echogenic rim with

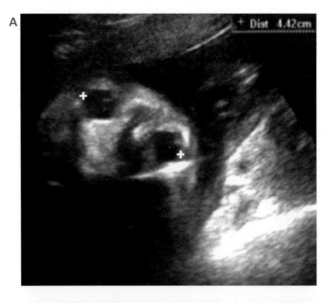

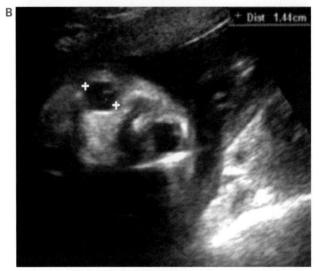

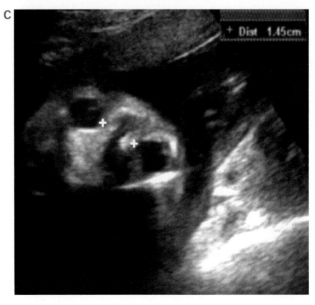

Figure 4-36. A *Transverse image through the fetal head demonstrating the fetal orbits with a binocular distance (BOD) measurement (calipers).* **B** *Transverse image through the fetal head demonstrating the fetal orbital diameter (OD) measurement (calipers).* **C** *Transverse image through the fetal head demonstrating the fetal orbits with an interorbital distance (IOD) measurement (calipers).*

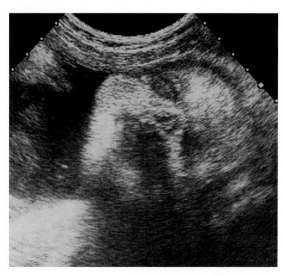

Figure 4-37. *Coronal image through the fetal face demonstrating the eyelids of the side close to the transducer.*

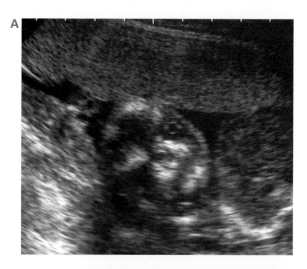

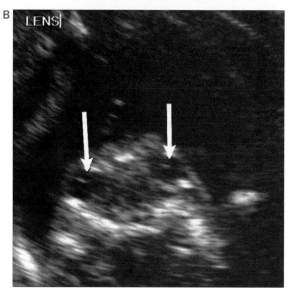

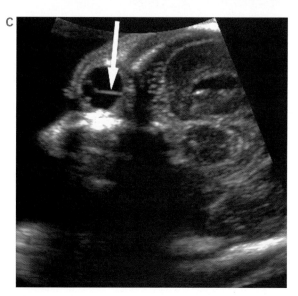

Figure 4-38. A *Coronal image of the lens of the fetal eye.* **B** *Transverse image through the fetal orbits indicating the lenses (arrows) of the eyes bilaterally.* **C** *Coronal image through the orbit of a 26-week fetus demonstrating Cloquet's canal (arrow). However, a patent hyaloid artery is a possibility.*

a characteristic anechoic center visualized within the anterior chamber of the eye. The lens can be identified in the coronal and transverse scanning planes of the fetal face (Figures 4-38 A and B). In addition, when the fetus is awake and alert, lid and eye movement is common and can be an indicator of fetal well-being. If one or both lenses cannot be visualized in any plane, congenital absence of the eye (**anophthalmia**) must be considered. If any portion of the central area of the lens appears to be echogenic, congenital cataracts could be suggested. Ever-increasing technological advancements allow us to see more detailed anatomy. For example, the **hyaloid artery** is a tributary of the ophthalmic artery. The hyaloid artery feeds the lens to aid in its development early in the gestational period. **Cloquet's canal**, the remnants of the hyaloid artery, may be recognized sonographically connecting to the back of the lens within the eye of a fetus (Figure 4-38C).

Other Facial Bones. The remainder of the facial bones, which consist of the maxilla and mandible, are also evaluated. Measurements are not routinely performed unless there is obvious facial asymmetry. The overall bony structure is usually compared with the contrasting region by imaging the face in the coronal plane. If the right and left sides of the face look the same, then the maxilla and mandible are thought to be characteristically normal. However, **mandible length** (**ML**) has been proven to be useful in the determination of micrognathia in some fetuses (Figure 4-39; refer to Table 19 in Appendix A). **Micrognathia** is an abnormally small chin and **retrognathia** is a recessed chin due to posterior displacement of the mandible. While the fetal profile subjectively evaluates

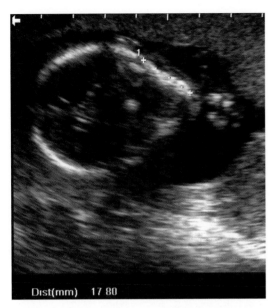

Figure 4-39. *Transverse image through the fetal jaw demonstrating the fetal mandible with a mandibular measurement (calipers).*

the mandible for these facial defects, fetal position and transducer placement can mask minor irregularities.

Ears. Evaluation of the size, shape, position, and overall appearance of the fetal ears can be helpful when performing in-depth sonography on those considered at risk for aneuploidy. Babies born with specific chromosomal abnormalities have smaller ears (**microtia**) that are often lower than the ears of those of normal karyotype. Although ear position is somewhat subjective, the most superior portion of the ear normally approximates the level of the top of the fetal orbit (Figure 4-40A). Also, there is a direct relationship between the fetal ear length and the gestational age in a fetus; therefore ear lengths can be an indicator for microtia and related chromosomal abnormalities (Figures 4-40 B and C; refer to Table 20 in Appendix A). Three-dimensional sonography promises an even better fetal ear evaluation (Figure 4-40D).

A
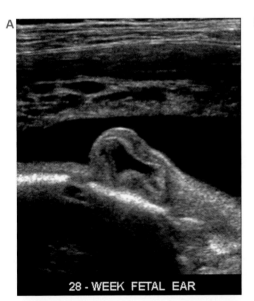
28 - WEEK FETAL EAR

C
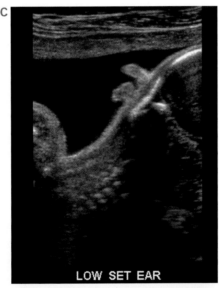
LOW SET EAR

B
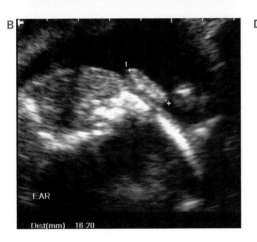
EAR
Dist(mm) 16 20

D
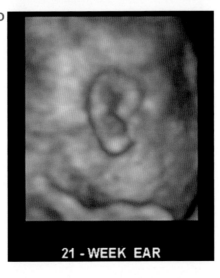
21 - WEEK EAR

Figure 4-40. A *Parasagittal image of a fetal ear.* **B** *Coronal image of the fetal ear with measurement (calipers).* **C** *Coronal image of an abnormal appearing shape of the fetal ear.* **D** *3D image demonstrating the fetal ear.*

Heart

Many high-risk perinatal units incorporate fetal echocardiography into targeted scans. Because fetal echocardiography is time-consuming, it is often reserved for patients who have risk factors that would indicate a full targeted echocardiogram overseen by a pediatric cardiologist. Restricting the scan to a more limited evaluation of the heart still has many benefits without losing high predictive value. The American Institute of Ultrasound in Medicine has suggested incorporating additional cardiac views into basic scan protocols when time and circumstances allow so sonographers can become comfortable performing them. Some of these views are discussed in this section.

Sonographically, the fetal heart is best evaluated between 18 and 34 weeks' gestation. However, the later the scan is performed, the more difficult it will be to obtain images because of shadowing from the fetal skeleton. High-resolution equipment and transducers are essential when evaluating the fetal heart. Careful attention must also be taken to ensure that high frame rates are imposed without the loss of detail. Understanding fetal circulation and normal detailed anatomy is very important when performing a targeted scan. Armed with this extensive knowledge, the practitioner can evaluate the heart more completely and tailor the examination to specific abnormalities while determining that all structures are functioning properly. Figure 4-41 shows the structural anatomy and direction of flow within a normal fetus.

Inflow Tracts Deoxygenated circulating blood returning from the periphery of the fetus enters the fetal heart at the right atrium through the **inflow tracts**: the **superior vena cava (SVC)** and **inferior vena cava (IVC)**. Blood returns

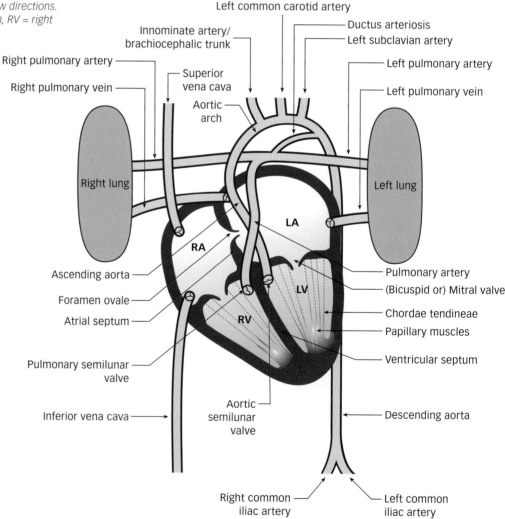

Figure 4-41. *The heart with flow directions. RA = right atrium, LA = left atrium, RV = right ventricle, LV = left ventricle.*

Left common carotid artery

Innominate artery/ brachiocephalic trunk

Ductus arteriosis

Left subclavian artery

Right pulmonary artery

Left pulmonary artery

Right pulmonary vein

Superior vena cava

Left pulmonary vein

Aortic arch

Right lung

Left lung

LA

RA

Ascending aorta

Pulmonary artery

Foramen ovale

(Bicuspid or) Mitral valve

LV

Atrial septum

Chordae tendineae

Papillary muscles

RV

Ventricular septum

Pulmonary semilunar valve

Inferior vena cava

Aortic semilunar valve

Descending aorta

Right common iliac artery

Left common iliac artery

from the head and upper extremities into the right atrium of the heart through the superior vena cava. The passage of oxygenated blood from the umbilical vein spills through the inferior vena cava via the ductus venosus into the right atrium (Figure 4-42). The walls of the superior vena cava and inferior vena cava are not very dense and therefore often go unnoticed sonographically. A long-axis view to the right of fetal midline demonstrates these vessels, resembling the long horns of a bull, with the right atrium portraying the bull's head (Figure 4-43).

Chambers of the Heart When evaluating the chambers, one must be sure that the fetal heart is positioned correctly in the thorax. Normal position will have the apex of the heart pointing toward the left side of the fetus at a 45 degree angle with the true sagittal plane, with the base of the heart pointing to the fluid-filled stomach. The chamber that is positioned closer to the fetal spine is the **left atrium**. In contrast, the **right ventricle** lies just beneath

the anterior chest wall (Figure 4-44). The **five-chamber view** of the heart is often imaged as a four-chamber view; therefore it does not require much manipulation of the transducer to achieve. Angle upward to bring the aorta into the center of the screen. The circle within the very center of the four-chamber heart is actually not a chamber at all but a **short-axis**, or transverse, view of the ascending aorta (Figure 4-45). The aortic valve and the left ventricular outflow tract are seen in the five-chamber view.

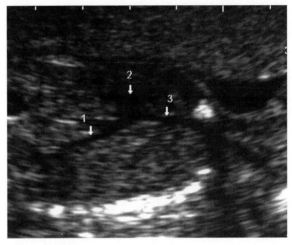

Figure 4-43. *Longitudinal image of the right atrium with identification of the inflow tracts. 1 = inferior vena cava, 2 = right atrium, and 3 = superior vena cava.*

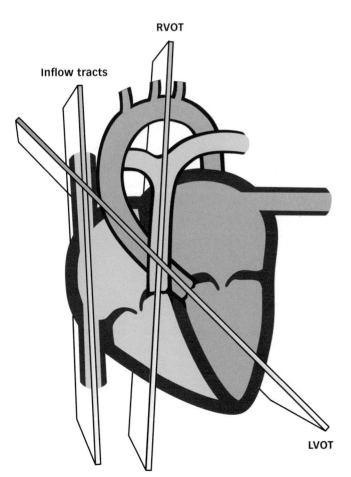

Figure 4-42. *Heart with scan planes. RVOT = right ventricular outflow tract, LVOT = left ventricular outflow tract.*

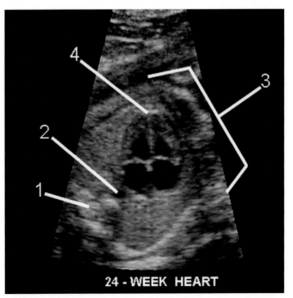

Figure 4-44. *Transverse image through the fetal thorax demonstrating a four-chamber heart. 1 = fetal spine, 2 = abdominal aorta, 3 = anterior portion of the fetal thorax, 4 = apex of the heart.*

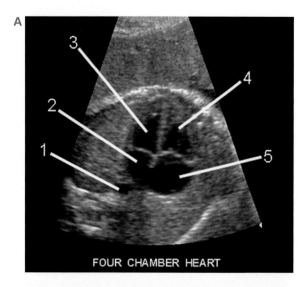

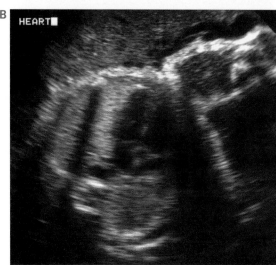

Figure 4-45. **A** *Transverse image through the fetal thorax demonstrating a four-chamber heart. 1 = abdominal aorta/descending aorta, 2 = left atrium, 3 = left ventricle, 4 = right ventricle, 5 = left atrium.* **B** *Transverse image through the fetal heart demonstrating a five-chamber view of the fetal heart. The circular area within the center is a portion of the aortic root/ascending aorta.*

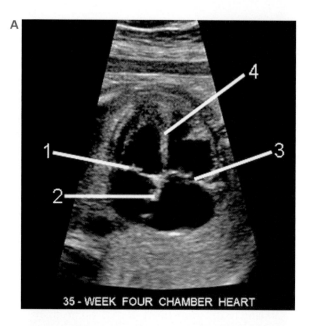

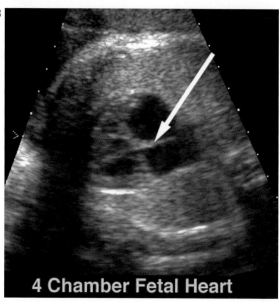

Figure 4-46. **A** *Transverse image through the fetal thorax demonstrating a four-chamber heart. 1 = bicuspid or mitral valve, 2 = incomplete atrial septum due to the foramen ovale, 3 = tricuspid valve, 4 = ventricular septum with some dropout.* **B** *Transverse view through the fetal thorax with a more perpendicular beam axis to the atrial septum (arrow). The atrial septum appears to more continuous in appearance.*

Atrial Septum The **atrial septum** is the muscular division between the right and left atria of the heart. **Atrial septal defects** are some of the most common cardiac defects and difficult to diagnose sonographically. There are instances when the atrial septum may not be completely visualized even when normal; therefore several images must be taken (Figure 4-46). The reason the atrial septum is one of the most difficult images to obtain has to do with the foramen ovale (see "Foramen Ovale" section below).

Ventricular Septum The **ventricular septum** is the true separation located between the left and right ventricles. It is a 3D structure, and often several images are required

to definitively rule out a ventricular septal defect (VSD). It is important to sweep slowly through the ventricles to evaluate the ventricular septum in detail. A beam perpendicular to the long axis of the septum is best for the evaluation of the ventricular septum. This is usually obtained in the same plane as the left ventricular outflow tract (Figure 4-47A). Four- and five-chamber views are not well suited to the evaluation of the ventricular septum because of dropout, which is caused by the beam

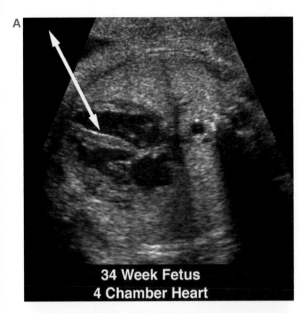

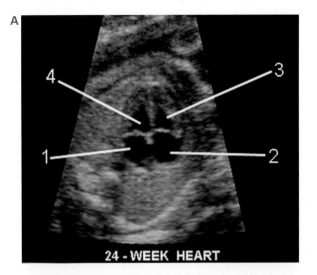

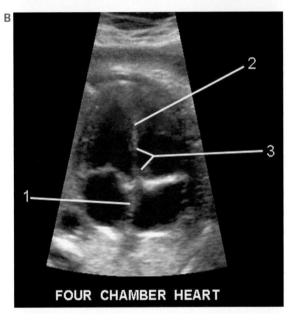

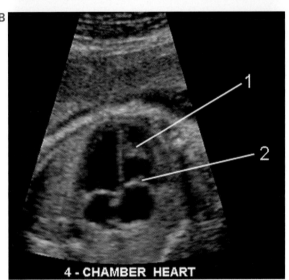

Figure 4-47. A *Transverse view through the fetal thorax with a more perpendicular beam axis to the ventricular septum (arrow). The ventricular appears to more continuous in appearance.* **B** *Transverse image through the fetal thorax with a more apical transducer placement providing a beam angle that is more parallel to the ventricular septum, therefore demonstrating a pseudo–ventricular septal defect due to dropout. 1 = atrial septum, 2 = ventricular septum, 3 = pseudo–ventricular septal defect.*

Figure 4-48. A *Transverse image through the fetal thorax demonstrating a four-chamber heart. 1 = left atrium, 2 = right atrium, 3 = right ventricle, 4 = left ventricle.* **B** *Transverse image through the fetal thorax demonstrating the heart with 1 = papillary muscles, 2 = chordae tendineae.*

being parallel to the septum itself. This artifact can mask real ventricular septal defects and also produce a pseudo–ventricular septal defect (Figure 4-47B).

Valves Two types of valve control the flow of blood through the heart, the atrioventricular and the semilunar valves. These valves open and close in pairs, giving two distinctive sounds to the heartbeat during **systole** (contraction) and **diastole** (relaxation) of the heart.

Atrioventricular Valves. The **atrioventricular valves** (**AV valves**) consist of the tricuspid valve and bicuspid valve. The **tricuspid valve** is located between the right atrium and the right ventricle of the heart. This valve contains three leaflets or cusps; the bicuspid valve has only two. During fetal circulation, blood that has entered the left atrium from the right atrium passes through the **bicuspid** (**mitral**) **valve** into the left ventricle (Figures 4-41 and 4-48A). The atrioventricular valves allow a transfer of blood in only one direction, normally from the atria to the ventricles. These are controlled by a process of muscular contractions that pull on a network of complex chords called **chordae tendineae** (Figures 4-41 and 4-48B). The chordae tendineae are connected to the posterior surfaces of the atrioventricular valves and function to open and close the leaflets. During ventricular systole, the **papillary muscles** contract, pulling on these chords. This causes the valves to open during the diastolic phase of cardiac relaxation. This pulling and subsequent valve opening allows blood to flow from the atria to the ventricles. Subsequently, the papillary muscles begin to relax, which permits the atrioventricular valves to close. The chordae tendineae also function to inhibit the leaflets from opening in the wrong direction, as happens with valve prolapse. At the junction of the papillary muscles and the chordae tendineae, a bright echogenic focus in the fetal heart is often considered to be a normal variant due to the density of the junction. With high-resolution systems, however, these are seen as soft tissue within the ventricles. Normality should not be assumed automatically. There are pathologies and tumors that can appear similar.

Semilunar Valves. Two **semilunar valves** (**SL valves**) control the outward flow of blood from the heart through the pulmonary and aortic arteries. The **pulmonary semilunar valve** controls blood flow from the right ventricle into the pulmonary artery. In addition blood is pushed through the **aortic semilunar valve** into the ascending aorta (Figures 4-41, 4-42, 4-49, and 4-53B). Contraction of the ventricles during systole opens the semilunar valves, allowing blood to move into the pulmonary artery and aorta. During diastole the ventricles of the heart relax and the semilunar valves close, stopping blood flow into the great vessels. These valves are identified when imaging the fetal outflow tracts; separated images are not required unless fetal echocardiography has been ordered.

Foramen Ovale In adult circulation, blood leaves the right atrium and passes through the tricuspid valve into the right ventricle. In the fetus, however, only some of the blood is delivered directly into the right ventricle. The fetus does not breathe in the maternal womb; instead it receives needed oxygen from a transfer of gases within the placenta from its mother through the umbilical vein. Therefore there are no requirements for the fetal blood to circulate, in great quantities, through the fetal respiratory system. Consequently, much of the blood normally bypasses the fetal lungs by passing through an oval-shaped opening in the atrial septum. This passageway is the **foramen ovale** and is located between the right and left atria (Figures 4-41 and 4-50). The foramen ovale should always open into the left atrium because of flow direction and blood pressure. It also closes after birth in most babies. When it remains patent instead, it is considered an atrial septal defect.

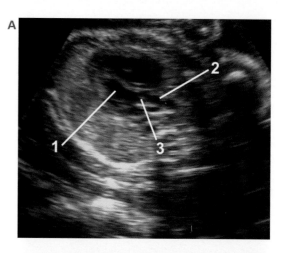

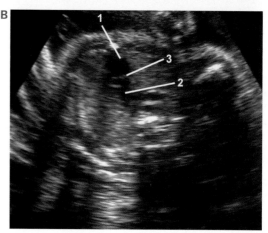

Figure 4-49. A *Transverse image through the fetal thorax demonstrating the aortic semilunar valve within the left ventricular outflow tract. 1 = left ventricle, 2 = ascending aorta, 3 = aortic semilunar valve.* **B** *Transverse image through the fetal thorax demonstrating the pulmonary semilunar valve within the right ventricular outflow tract. 1 = right ventricle, 2 = pulmonary artery, 3 = pulmonary semilunar valve.*

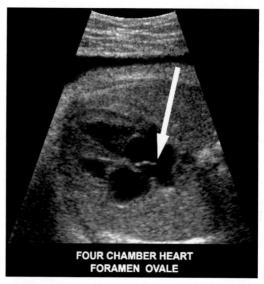

FOUR CHAMBER HEART
FORAMEN OVALE

Figure 4-50. *Transverse image of the fetal thorax demonstrating a four-chamber view of the fetal heart. The foramen ovale (arrow) is imaged normally opening into the left atrium.*

Outflow Tracts Outflow tracts—often termed the **great vessels**—should appear symmetrical. Although they are not routinely measured, measurements are warranted when the outflow tracts appear to be prominent or different in lumen diameter. Accurate gestational age must be determined before vessels can be considered abnormal because great vessel diameters vary with gestational age. The right and left ventricular outflow tracts normally cross each other and should never be seen as parallel. If they are imaged in a parallel configuration, this finding is conclusive for a conotruncal abnormality. The great vessels can also be transposed; **transposition of the great vessels (TGV)** describes the aorta abnormally connected to the right ventricle and the pulmonary artery abnormally connected to the left ventricle. While a large percentage of structural cardiac abnormalities can be detected when imaging a four-chamber view of the heart, more anoma-

lies can be detected when inflow tracts, outflow tracts, ductal arch, and aortic arch are included in the evaluation of the fetal heart.

Right Ventricular Outflow Tract. Blood passes through the pulmonary semilunar valve into the **pulmonary artery**, otherwise known as the **right ventricular outflow tract** (**RVOT**; see Figures 4-41 and 4-42). Sonographically, the walls of the RVOT are not very prominent, making this great vessel darker in appearance, resembling a vein. The RVOT delivers deoxygenated blood to the lungs. The pulmonary trunk branches into the right and left pulmonary arteries, as well as a fetal division termed the **ductus arteriosus** (Figures 4-41 and 4-51). The deoxygenated blood, which is primarily from the superior vena cava, mixes with the oxygenated blood from the aorta.

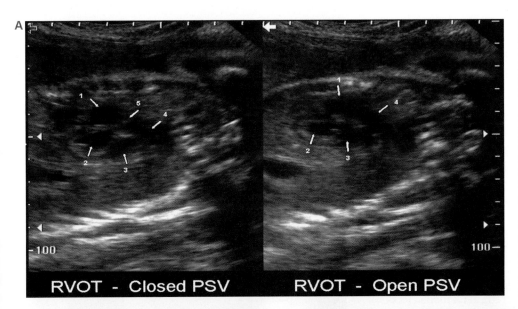

RVOT - Closed PSV   RVOT - Open PSV

Figure 4-51. A *Split image of the right ventricular outflow tract (RVOT) with the left image revealing the pulmonary semilunar valve in the closed position and the right image showing an open pulmonary semilunar valve. 1 = right ventricle, 2 = left ventricle, 3 = left atrium, 4 = RVOT/pulmonary artery, 5 = pulmonary semilunar valve closed.* **B** *Transverse image of the fetal thorax demonstrating a short-axis view of the fetal thorax with clear picture of the RVOT with its right and left pulmonary branches. 1 = right ventricle, 2 = left ventricle, 3 = left atrium, 4 = RVOT/pulmonary artery, 5 = left pulmonary artery, 6 = right pulmonary artery.* **C** *Short-axis view of the fetal heart demonstrating color flow analysis of the RVOT with its branches.*

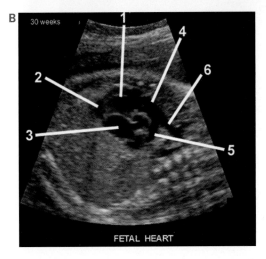

FETAL HEART

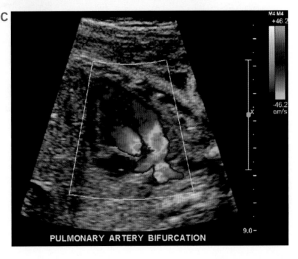

PULMONARY ARTERY BIFURCATION

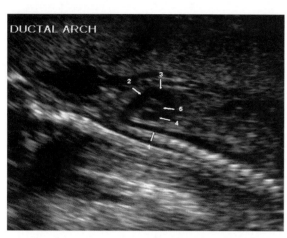

Figure 4-52. *Longitudinal image through the fetal thorax with the spine visualized posteriorly. Image is demonstrating the ductal arch with a flattened appearance of the superior boarder resembling a hockey stick. 1 = descending aorta, 2 = ductus arteriosus, 3 = pulmonary artery/right ventricular outflow tract, 4 = left atrium, 5 = aorta.*

Ductal Arch. The **ductus arteriosus** is the natural communication between the pulmonary artery (RVOT) and the descending aorta in a fetus. The ductus arteriosus allows even more blood to bypass the fetal lungs and remain in circulation throughout the body (Figure 4-41). Sonographically, the ductal arch resembles a hockey stick (Figure 4-52). This curve is composed of the RVOT, ductus arteriosus, and descending aorta, forming a more flattened appearance than seen with the candy cane–shaped aortic arch. In comparison, the ductal arch does not have any branches that extend from its superior border. After birth, the ductus arteriosus closes to allow blood to circulate through the lungs, and the collapsed remnant of the ductus arteriosus becomes the ligamentum arteriosum. If this developmental process does not occur and the ductus arteriosus remains as a **patent ductus arteriosus (PDA)**, the baby often becomes **cyanotic** (blue baby) as a result of the decreased oxygen within the bloodstream.

Left Ventricular Outflow Tract. Oxygen-rich blood passes through the aortic semilunar valve into the ascending aorta, otherwise known as the **left ventricular outflow tract** (**LVOT**; see Figures 4-41 and 4-42). The LVOT and the largest view of the left ventricle are seen best in the same plane. Consequently a large segment of the ventricular septum can also be seen at this level. The LVOT is easily and consistently recognized sonographically because of the dense tissue that makes up its walls (Figure 4-53).

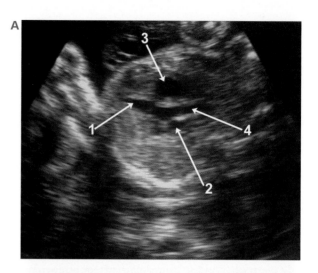

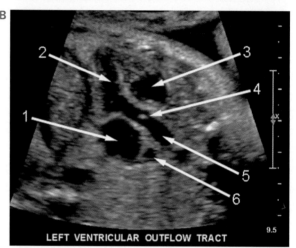

LEFT VENTRICULAR OUTFLOW TRACT

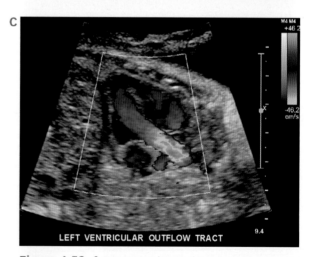

LEFT VENTRICULAR OUTFLOW TRACT

Figure 4-53. A *Transverse image through the fetal thorax demonstrating a long-axis view of the left ventricular outflow tract (LVOT) with the aortic semilunar valve in the open position. 1 = left ventricle, 2 = left atrium, 3 = right ventricle, 4 = LVOT/ascending aorta.* **B** *Apical view of the fetal heart demonstrating the long-axis view of the LVOT/ascending aorta with the aortic semilunar valve in a closed position. 1 = left atrium, 2 = left ventricle, 3 = right ventricle, 4 = aortic semilunar valve, 5 = LVOT/ascending aorta, 6 = pulmonary artery.* **C** *Long-axis view of the fetal LVOT demonstrating color flow analysis.*

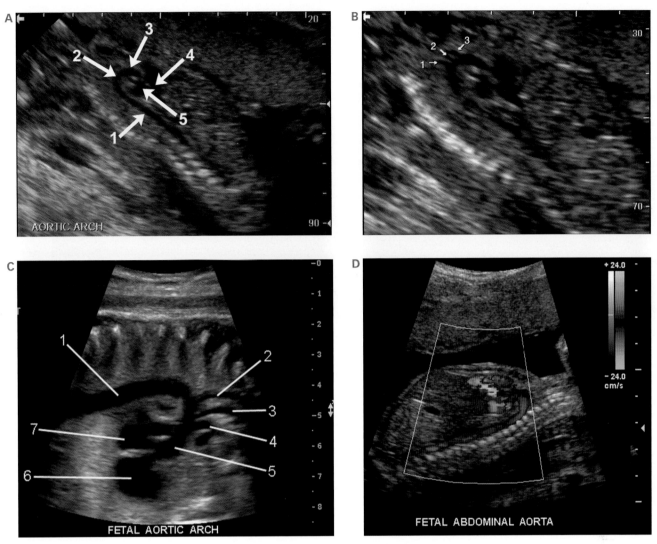

Figure 4-54. A *Longitudinal image of the aortic arch within the fetal thorax. 1 = descending aorta, 2 = aortic arch, 3 = ascending aorta, 4 = left ventricle, 5 = left atrium.* **B** *Longitudinal image of the aortic arch with branches extending off the superior border. 1 = left subclavian artery, 2 = left common carotid artery, 3 = innominate artery/brachiocephalic trunk.* **C** *Longitudinal image of the aortic arch with branches. 1 = descending aorta, 2 = left subclavian artery, 3 = left common carotid artery, 4 = innominate artery/brachio-cephalic trunk, 5 = ascending aorta, 6 = left ventricle, 7 = left atrium.* **D** *Longitudinal image of the aortic arch demonstrating color flow analysis.*

Aortic Arch. As the LVOT courses superiorly in the fetal thorax, it then curves to the right to form a prominent **aortic arch** that extends into the descending aorta, which passes posterior to the left atrium (Figure 4-41). This arch is visualized best in long axis and looks like a candy cane or walking stick with a tight narrow curve (Figure 4-54A). From the top of the arch arterial branches can often be identified and documented. These three arterial branches include the innominate artery, the **left common carotid artery**, and the left subclavian artery (Figures 4-54 B–D).

Analysis of the Heart When imaging the fetal heart, the practitioner can take advantage of various modalities, such as M-mode, spectral Doppler, 2D, 3D, and 4D imaging, in order to visualize many parts of the heart. Nevertheless, real-time imaging with M-mode tracings is the initial means of evaluating the heart. Real-time imaging can be used to assess normal chamber size, valve motion, cardiac wall movement, and wall thicknesses. Many linear measurements can be obtained to evaluate structure size across gestational ages (Figures 4-55 A and B; Table 4-1).

Figure 4-55. A *M-mode analysis through the right and left ventricles of the fetal heart. 1 = left ventricle, 2 = right ventricle, 3 = exterior wall of the right ventricle, 4 = chamber of the right ventricle, 5 = ventricular septum, 6 = chamber of the left ventricle, 7 = exterior wall of the left ventricle.* **B** *M-mode analysis through the right and left atria of the fetal heart. 1 = left atrium, 2 = right atrium, 3 = exterior wall of the right atrium, 4 = chamber of the right atrium, 5 = atrial septum, 6 = chamber of the left atrium, 7 = exterior wall of the left atrium.* **C** *Fetal heart rate chart. Adapted with permission from Callen P:* Ultrasonography in Obstetrics and Gynecology, *4th Edition. Philadelphia, Saunders, 2000, p 416, fig 13-59.*

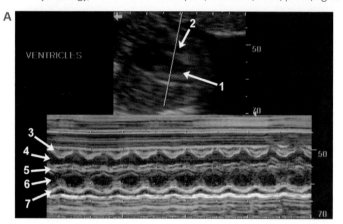
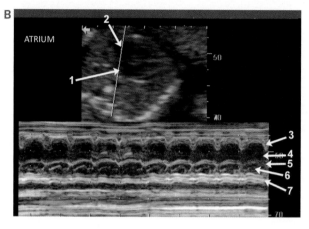

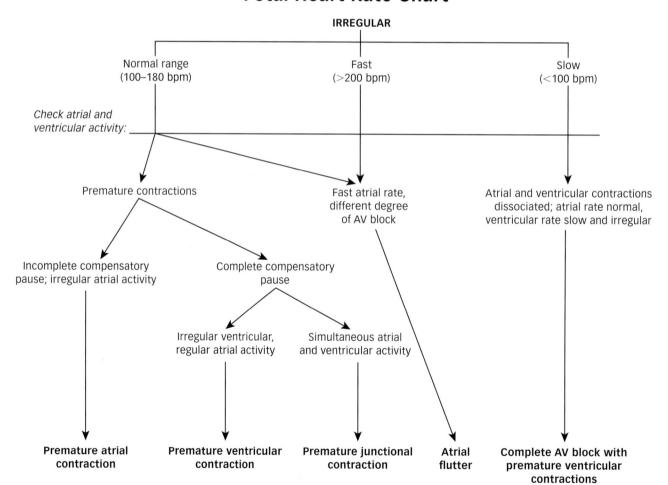

Table 4-1. Fetal heart protocol for the targeted scan.

Views	Documented on Image
Four-chamber view	Right ventricle, left ventricle, right atrium, left atrium, tricuspid valve, mitral valve, and foramen ovale
Five-chamber view	Right ventricle, left ventricle, right atrium, left atrium, tricuspid valve, mitral valve, foramen ovale, and ascending aorta in center
Inflow tracts (long horns of bull)	Right atrium, inferior vena cava, and superior vena cava
Right ventricular outflow tract (RVOT)	Right ventricle, pulmonary semilunar valve, pulmonary artery, and right atrium
Left ventricular outflow tract (LVOT)	Left ventricle, aortic semilunar valve, ascending aorta, and left atrium
Atrial septum	Right atrium, foramen ovale opening into the left atrium, and left atrium
M mode	Samples through the atria and ventricles
Ventricular septum	Left ventricle, right ventricle, left atrium, and LVOT
Ductal arch	RVOT with descending aorta (hockey stick)
Aortic arch	Ascending aorta, right common carotid artery, left common carotid artery, brachiocephalic artery, descending aorta, left ventricle, and left atrium (candy cane)

Arrhythmias (abnormal heart rhythms) are common and can be assessed easily with real-time scanning, M-mode imaging, and spectral Doppler analysis. Arrhythmias vary in severity and type, including premature ventricular contraction, premature atrial contraction, atrial flutter, and atrioventricular block. Of these, premature ventricular contraction is considered one of the most common types in a fetus and is diagnosed with the aid of sonography. With **premature ventricular contractions** (**PVCs**) and **premature atrial contractions** (**PACs**), the ventricles or the atria contract too soon, which creates the appearance of the heart skipping a beat. **Atrial flutter** is an abnormal heart rhythm in which the atria of the heart contract much more frequently than the ventricles. Therefore the atrial heart rate can be tachycardic while the ventricular rate can appear normal or even bradycardic. If there is an **atrioventricular block** (**AV block**) the atrial rhythm may be normal but the ventricular rate is often bradycardic (Figure 4-55C).

Targeted scans require that several M-mode tracings be taken separately through the atria and ventricles to fully evaluate the heart rhythm and structures. The perinatal sonographer should be knowledgeable of correct M-mode placement so that evaluation and measurements can be obtained. Sonographers should be aware of their technique when scanning the fetal heart. Even the slightest pressure on the fetal chest can slow or even stop the fetal heart rate. Easing up on transducer pressure allows the heart to resume a normal rhythm immediately. Focal myometrial contractions can have the same effect on fetal heart rate.

Abdominal Vasculature

Observing the vasculature can prove to be very useful when performing targeted sonographic examinations. There are times when visualizing abdominal vessels will help you evaluate and even locate organs in the abdominal cavity. For example, coronally the renal arteries arise from the aorta (see Box 4-8 and Figure 4-56). Imaging the renal arteries can be very useful for the evaluation of renal variants. Pelvic **ectopic kidneys** (abnormally positioned kidneys), **crossed renal ectopia** (displacement of one kidney to the opposite side, with or without fusion), and unilateral or bilateral **renal agenesis** (failure of kidney development) can be difficult to appreciate in a fetus. If a kidney is present, there will be a feeding arterial vessel,

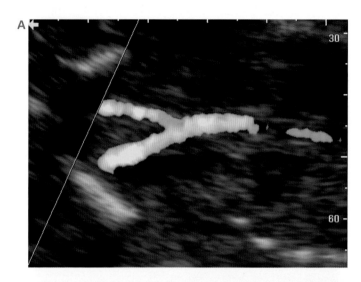

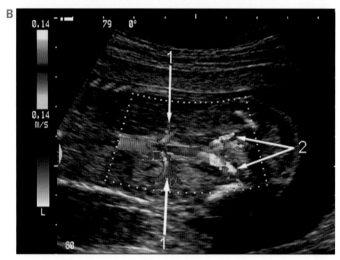

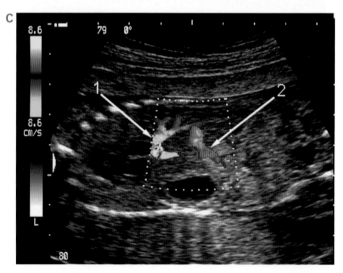

Figure 4-56. A *Power Doppler color image of the distal aorta demonstrating the aortic bifurcation.* **B** *Color Doppler coronal image of the aorta demonstrating the renal arteries branching from the lateral portion of the aorta along with distal aortic bifurcation. 1 = right and left renal arteries with branches, 2 = common iliac arteries.* **C** *Color Doppler demonstrating branching hepatic veins along with the intra-abdominal portion of the umbilical vein/portal vein. 1 = hepatic veins, 2 = umbilical vein/portal vein.*

Box 4-8.   Abdominal vasculature that can be imaged with some consistency.

Aortic bifurcation

Renal arteries

Hepatic veins

Celiac axis

Superior mesenteric artery

Inferior mesenteric artery

and color/power Doppler will demonstrate it nicely. In cases of renal agenesis, the renal vessels will also be absent. Finally, vessels with slower blood flow velocities often are better visualized with power Doppler imaging.

Thorax and Abdomen

The overall sizes and shapes of the thorax and the abdomen are easily compared by obtaining longitudinal images of the fetus just inferior to the fetal profile (Figure 4-57A). If the fetal thorax appears to be smaller than the abdomen, clinical considerations include dwarfism, pulmonary hypoplasia, and macrosomia (Figure 4-57B; refer to Table 21 in Appendix A).

The fetal lungs can be evaluated bilaterally with the diaphragm, stomach, and liver imaged in a longitudinal scanning plane (Figures 4-57 C and D). With just a few images, many potential problems can be ruled out and assessed. Herniation of any of the abdominal contents into the fetal thorax can be lethal. An organ or organs found within the fetal thorax can affect normal lung development. A left diaphragmatic hernia often pushes the heart against the right side wall of the thorax. At a few academic institutions, intrauterine surgery is possible. If too much of the diaphragm is absent, surgery is not usually a viable consideration; however, this decision will be made by the institutions involved with fetal surgery. In a fetus with a congenital diaphragmatic hernia, one may be asked to attempt to determine what percentage of the diaphragm is still present, as this information may be needed for management options.

Fetal liver and spleen measurements and volume calculations have been found to relate to the age of the gestation (refer to Tables 22 and 23 in Appendix A) and can be helpful in determining the effects of erythroblastosis fetalis in Rh-sensitized fetuses (Figure 4-58). Knowledge of the fetal presenting part and correct interpretation of

Figure 4-57. A *Longitudinal image of a fetus demonstrating a normal appearing thorax shape. 1 = abdomen, 2 = thorax.* **B** *Transverse image through the fetal thorax demonstrating a thoracic circumference (calipers).* **C** *Longitudinal image demonstrating the left hemidiaphragm separating the fetal thorax and abdomen on the left side of the fetus. Note that there is no evidence of abnormal fluid collection in the fetal thorax or fetal abdomen. 1 = heart, 2 = lungs, 3 = left hemidiaphragm, 4 = stomach.* **D** *Longitudinal image demonstrating the right hemidiaphragm separating the fetal thorax and abdomen on the right side of the fetus. Note that there is no evidence of abnormal fluid collection in the fetal thorax or abdomen. 1 = lungs, 2 = right hemidiaphragm, 3 = liver.*

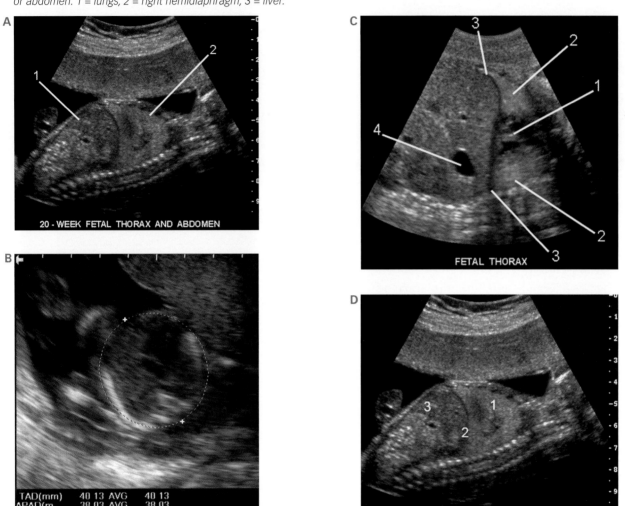

Figure 4-58. A *Longitudinal image of the fetal abdomen with a length measurement of the fetal liver (calipers). Also noted on this image is the fetal right kidney (arrow).* **B** *Transverse image of the fetal abdomen with a length measurement of the fetal spleen (calipers).*

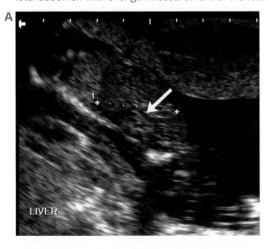

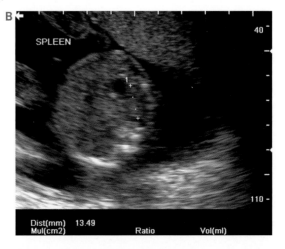

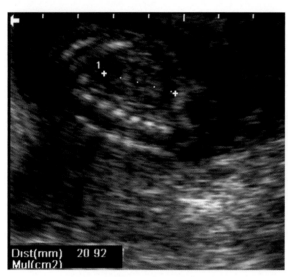

Figure 4-59. *Coronal image of the fetal abdomen with a length measurement of the fetal kidney (calipers).*

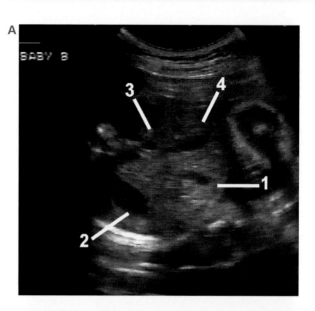

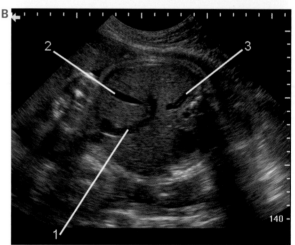

Figure 4-60. A *Transverse view through the fetal abdomen. 1 = umbilical vein, 2 = stomach, 3 = abdominal/descending aorta, 4 = gallbladder.* **B** *Transverse view through the fetal abdomen demonstrating the normal appearance of the right adrenal gland. 1 = umbilical vein, 2 = gallbladder, 3 = right adrenal gland.*

the positions of the fetal heart, stomach, liver, spleen, and gallbladder can allow situs inversus to be ruled out or confirmed (Figures 4-59 and 4-60). The normal arrangement of these organs is defined as **situs solitus** or **normal situs**. **Situs inversus** (or **transversus**) is a condition in which the organs of the thorax and/or abdomen are arranged in a reversed position. The heart normally is positioned to the left side of the body, termed **levocardia**, but when the fetal heart is positioned to the right side of the thorax the term is **dextrocardia**. While situs inversus can be a normal variant and the function of the affected organs may be normal, there can also be associated abnormalities. Starting at 20 weeks the fetal gallbladder is readily identified in the same plane as the umbilical vein and stomach. If the gallbladder is not visualized at all (e.g., in views such as those in Figure 4-60), cystic fibrosis might be a consideration.

Adrenal Glands The adrenal glands are not usually evaluated with measurements but are easily identified in the fetus because of their normally prominent size. A normal adrenal gland has a hypoechoic cortex with a hyperechoic centrally located medulla. In the transverse plane the fetal adrenal gland should be somewhat flattened and oval in appearance (Figure 4-60B). In a longitudinal scanning plane, the adrenal is more triangular in appearance. With renal agenesis, the adrenal gland will fall into the renal fossa. Nevertheless the sonographer should be able to differentiate between the two because the echo pattern of the kidney—mid-level reflectivity with a hypoechoic pelvis—differs from that of the adrenal gland as described above. When pathology of the adrenal gland exists, usu-

ally the gland enlarges and the echogenic center becomes less noticeable. This adrenal gland can then resemble a fetal kidney and be mistaken for one. (Refer to Table 24 in Appendix A for normal measurements often seen in association with the fetal adrenal glands.)

Bowel Echogenic bowel in a fetus remains a focus of interpretation with higher-frequency transducers. We are able to distinguish small bowel from large bowel, as small bowel is centrally positioned and large bowel can be seen surrounding the small bowel. Hyperechoic bowel that is as echogenic as bone is associated with an increased incidence of fetal abnormalities. Cystic fibrosis, cytomegalovirus (CMV), intrauterine growth restriction (IUGR), and chromosomal abnormalities such as Down syndrome

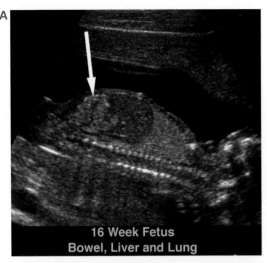

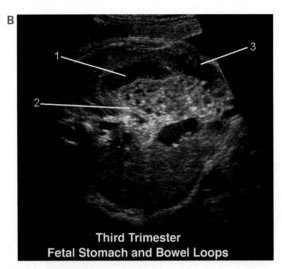

Figure 4-61. A *Longitudinal image through fetal midline demonstrating normal appearing bowel (arrow) in the lower abdominal cavity.* **B** *Transverse image through the fetal abdomen demonstrating the fetal stomach and mildly dilated loops of bowel. This would also be a good image to take possible small bowel diameters along with a very good diameter of the descending colon. 1 = stomach, 2 = small bowel, 3 = descending colon.*

are all considerations when echogenic bowel is reported (Figure 4-61). With bowel obstruction, dilated loops of bowel within the fetal abdomen will be seen and increasing peristaltic movement will be evident. This finding warrants measurements of the bowel. An internal luminal diameter greater than 7 mm is considered abnormal. (Refer to Tables 25 and 26 in Appendix A.)

Cord

The umbilical cord of the fetus is seen and evaluated thoroughly in basic scanning protocols. Differentiating and imaging floating umbilical cord from the cord at its

insertion into the fetal abdomen are required as well as imaging the umbilical arteries at the level of the fetal bladder and the umbilical vein within the fetal liver. When blood vessels are visualized on either side of the bladder, the sonographer must be careful not to assume that these vessels are the two umbilical arteries (Figures 4-62 A and B). The iliac/femoral arteries are also at this level and can easily be mistaken for umbilical arteries. The umbilical arteries will be immediately adjacent to the fetal bladder and with careful scanning can be visualized ascending into the umbilical cord (Figure 4-62C). The iliac/femoral arteries are more lateral in location.

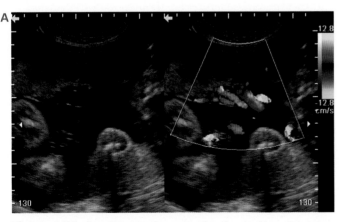

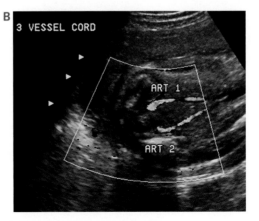

Figure 4-62. A *Split image demonstrating the cord insertion into an anterior placenta with confirmation using evaluation with color Doppler. This area must be identified and imaged during real-time scanning in percutaneous umbilical blood sampling procedures.* **B** *Image demonstrating 2D and color evaluation of the two umbilical arteries at the level of the fetal bladder, suggesting a three-vessel umbilical cord intra-abdominally. ART = artery. (Figure continues . . .)*

Figure 4-62, continued. C *Power Doppler imaging demonstrating two-vessel umbilical arteries at the level of the fetal bladder.* **D** *Transverse section through the fetal neck showing the nuchal umbilical cord.* **E** *Longitudinal image through the fetus demonstrating the clinching of the umbilical cord during examination. 1 = hand, 2 = umbilical cord, 3 = male genitalia.*

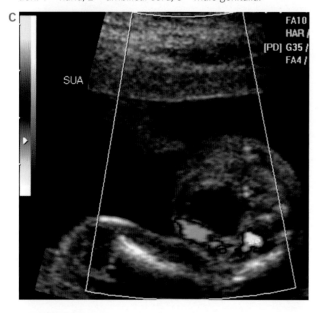

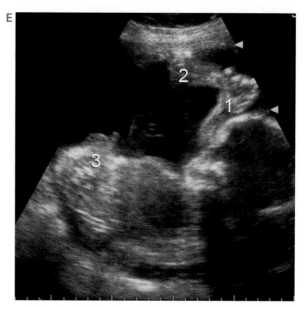

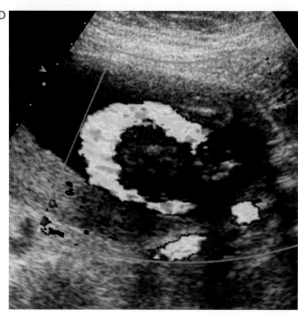

In some high-risk conditions, an invasive procedure may be necessary in order to attempt to evaluate and treat a developing fetus. Percutaneous umbilical blood sampling (PUBS) can aid in the proper diagnosis of fetal complications during pregnancy. While there are many invasive procedures with which a perinatal sonographer assists, such as chorionic villus sampling (CVS), amniocentesis, and vesicocentesis, PUBS procedures prove to be more challenging. This procedure is performed by inserting a needle into the umbilical vein at the placental cord insertion, which is the most stationary and reliable place for the perinatologist to insert the needle. Once proper placement of the needle is confirmed, blood is withdrawn and tested. Therapeutic treatment can be administered at this time as well. If the fetus has an infection, antibiotics can be delivered and, as in cases of Rh sensitization, blood transfusions can be administered.

Fetuses that are found with a nuchal cord or clinching the umbilical cord can have decelerations in the heart rate that can be observed during a fetal **nonstress test**. Patients with a nonreactive stress test may be sent to the sonography laboratory for a biophysical profile (Figures 4-62 D and E). Often these fetuses are thought to be in distress, and a biophysical profile can determine fetal well-being (see Chapter 8).

Bilateral Long Bones

When evaluating arms and legs, the practitioner should identify the presence or absence of bones in the extremities. When any form of skeletal variant is recognized, all long bones of the fetus should be carefully measured and documented. With a systematic approach, one can easily identify all long bones. For the lower extremities, the sonographer should scan in an axial scanning plane through the pelvis and identify the iliac bones. The proximal portion of the diaphysis of the femur will then be seen. The probe should then be rotated to find the long axis of the shaft of the femur. The lower leg can then be identified and the bones evaluated. The tibia can be differentiated

Figure 4-63. A *Long-axis view of the tibia (calipers) seen posterior to the fibula in the lower portion of the fetal leg.* **B** *Long-axis view of the fibula (calipers) seen anterior to the tibia in the calf of the fetal leg.* **C** *Long-axis view of the humerus (calipers) seen adjacent to the forearm and hand of this fetus. 1 = hand, 2 = forearm, 3 = scapula.* **D** *Long-axis view of the ulna (calipers) seen adjacent to the upper arm of this fetus. 1 = humerus, 2 = scapula.* **E** *Long-axis view of the radius (calipers) seen posterior to the ulna of the fetal forearm.*

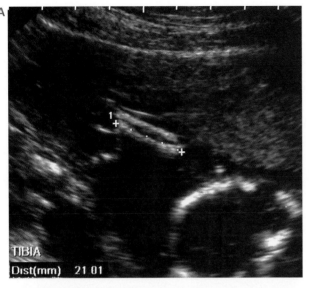

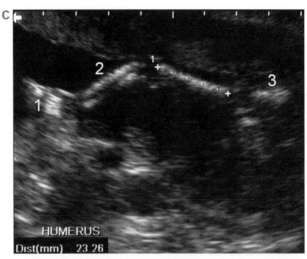

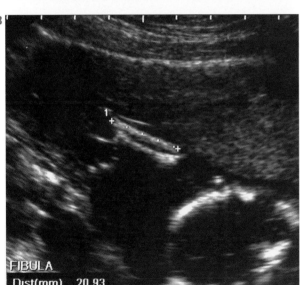

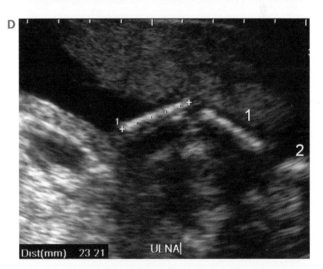

from the fibula because the tibia is more proximal to the knee and the fibula extends to the ankle. The probe must be turned 90 degrees to evaluate the foot.

To evaluate the upper extremities, the practitioner should begin in a long-axis scanning plane through the thorax. Scanning laterally, one identifies the scapula. The head of the humerus articulates with the glenoid cavity of the scapula, and the proximal portion of the diaphysis of the humerus is identified. By rotating the probe, the practitioner can visualize the shaft of the humerus. The ulna is visualized by sliding lower on the arm into the elbow. The radius will extend into the wrist (Figure 4-63).

Long bones are not limited to the extremities. The fetal clavicle, ribs, and scapula are considered long bones and can be measured to identify anomalies of the skeletal system as well as gestational age (Figure 4-64; refer to Tables 27, 28, and 29 in Appendix A).

Clavicle

Because of the normal curvature of the clavicle from the sternum to the shoulder, a transverse view of the fetus is usually warranted in order to visualize the longest plane for evaluation (Figure 4-65). The estimated fetal gestational age in weeks is approximately equal to the length of the clavicle, and clavicular length does not appear to be affected by growth restriction. There is evidence that clavicular length can be of use in detecting some congenital anomalies that specifically affect the clavicles. Because the fetal shoulders are the most difficult for the mother

to deliver vaginally, clavicular measurements can also be a very useful tool in determining delivery options for some births. For various reasons, cesarean section may be warranted by increased fetal size (**macrosomia**) and/or decreased maternal pelvic girth. If a vaginal delivery is attempted, there may be increased risk for shoulder dystocia, a circumstance in which the head is delivered but the shoulders lodge behind the mother's pubic bone. (Refer to Table 30 in Appendix A.)

Hands and Feet

Evaluation of the hands and feet is included in a targeted sonogram. Position of the hands and feet and the presence of any fetal posturing should be included in the evaluation (Figures 4-66 A and B). Fetuses do not have much muscular control; therefore in the normal fetus the hands stay in a relaxed position with the fingers somewhat

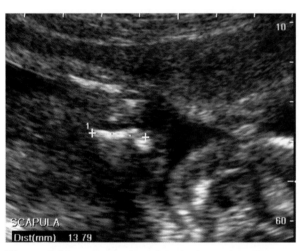

Figure 4-64. *Long-axis view of the fetal scapula (calipers).*

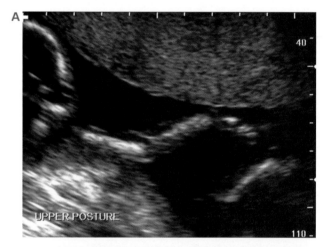

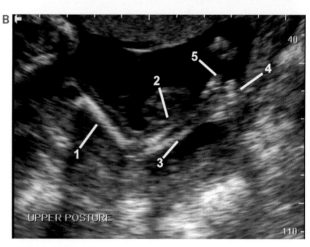

Figure 4-66. A *Long-axis view of the fetal arm in a relaxed position.* **B** *Coronal view of the fetal arm demonstrating a normal appearing posture. 1 = humerus, 2 = radius, 3 = ulna, 4 = hand, 5 = thumb. Note that the radius is on the same side of the arm as the fetal thumb. (Figure continues . . .)*

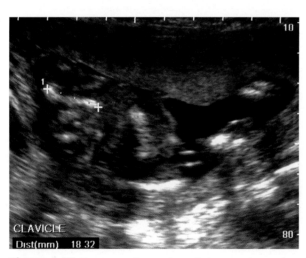

Figure 4-65. *Transverse image through the superior portion of the fetal thorax demonstrating a long-axis view of the fetal clavicle (calipers).*

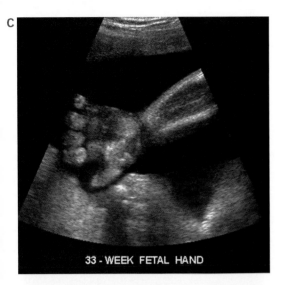

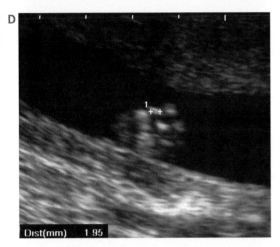

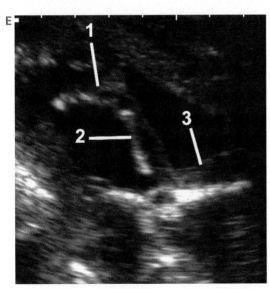

bent and close in proximity. The proximal, middle, and distal phalanges can be visualized when the hand is open (Figure 4-66C). Hypoplasia or lack of the middle phalanx of the fifth digit causes clinodactyly of the fifth digit and is associated with trisomy 21 (Figure 4-66D).

The fetal foot should be in a relaxed position, facing the anterior surface of the fetus. Fetuses do not have the control necessary to point the toes for long periods of time; therefore the ankle should be flexed, allowing the foot to be at approximately a 90 degree angle to the lower leg. The foot should be seen in profile, with the femur and the tibia image in the same plane (Figure 4-66E). Because of variations of the foot itself, foot measurements should be taken from the longest toe to the heel (Figure 4-67; refer to Tables 31 and 32 in Appendix A). Although foot measurements can be taken late in the first trimester, these measurements are more accurate during the second trimester

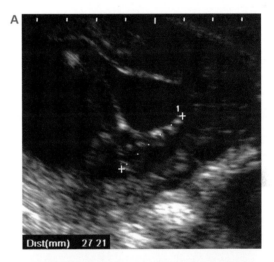

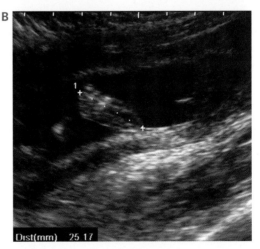

Figure 4-66, continued. C *Coronal image of the fetal lower arm and hand with five fingers well demonstrated.* **D** *Coronal image of a portion of the fetal hand demonstrating the middle phalanx of the fifth digit or pinky (calipers).* **E** *Sagittal image of the fetal leg demonstrating the proper alignment and therefore normal posture of the lower leg. 1 = foot, 2 = fibula, 3 = femur.*

Figure 4-67. A *Sagittal image of the fetal foot with proper placement of calipers for length measurement evaluation.* **B** *Plantar view of the fetal foot with measurement obtained from the longest (second) toe to the fetal heel. (Figure continues . . .)*

C

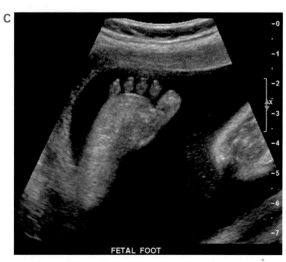

Figure 4-67, continued. C *Plantar view of the fetal foot with five toes well demonstrated.*

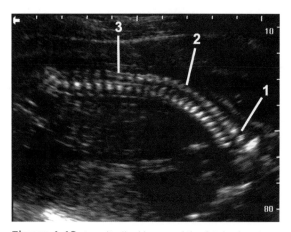

Figure 4-68. *Longitudinal image of the fetal spine. 1 = seven cervical vertebrae, 2 = twelve thoracic vertebrae, 3 = five lumbar vertebrae.*

because of increased fetal size and decreased movement. The femur/foot ratio during the second trimester is approximately 1:1. This ratio is important because it can be used to evaluate for skeletal dysplasias.

Spine

When spinal defects are visualized, it is important to identify exactly which of the fetal vertebrae are affected. The sonographer must be able to count the vertebrae (Figure 4-68). There are seven **cervical vertebrae** contained within the fetal neck. There are 12 **thoracic vertebrae** in the fetal thorax, which provide a base for rib attachment and protect many vital organs of the thorax and abdomen. Five **lumbar vertebrae** in the lower back form the lumbar spine, which is thought to be the strongest portion of the spine, providing the majority of support

for the entire body. The **sacrum** is the triangular pelvic portion, composed of five fused vertebrae and four fused bones that make up the smaller **coccyx** at the end of the vertebral column. While most neural tube defects affect the lumbar-sacral area, meticulous scanning of the entire spine can provide the exact location and specific number of vertebrae that are involved in a defect, so that severity, management, and treatment options can be considered while preparing the parents for possible fetal outcomes.

Measurement Comparisons

Standard obstetric measurements are useful in determining gestational age and estimating fetal weight and delivery dates. Nevertheless, comparisons can be made of the basic fetal measurements that allow the sonographer to assess the proportions of a fetus and possibly identify growth malformations earlier (see Boxes 4-9 and 4-10; Appendix A, Tables 33–34; Appendix C, second and third trimester data sheets).

Box 4-9.	**Growth malformations.**
	Skeletal dysplasias
	Symmetrical intrauterine growth restriction
	Asymmetrical intrauterine growth restriction
	Microcephaly
	Brachycephaly
	Dolichocephaly
	Hydrocephalus
	Macrosomia

Box 4-10.	**Ratios for comparison.**
	Biparietal diameter/occipital frontal diameter (BPD/OFD)
	Head circumference/abdominal circumference (HC/AC)
	Femur length/biparietal diameter (FL/BPD)
	Femur length/head circumference (FL/HC)
	Femur length/abdominal circumference (FL/AC)
	Resistivity index (RI)
	Pulsatility index (PI)
	Systolic/diastolic ratio (S/D ratio)
	Growth percentiles

SCANNING TIPS, GUIDELINES, AND PITFALLS

The Basic Scan

1. Uterine survey: Before images are obtained, a quick general survey of the uterus should be performed to establish fetal lie and identify location of the placenta. This can be done by "blessing the uterus." We call it this because of the scan motion performed to quickly look at the uterine environment. Start midline, at the symphysis pubis, and slide the transducer straight up the maternal midline until you reach the fundus of the uterus. You are, of course, paying attention to the anatomy seen while performing this maneuver (Figure 4-69). Upon reaching the fundus, slide back down to mid-uterus and then slide to one side (maternal right for example), again observing anatomy in that area. Once you reach the lateral uterus, slide to the opposite side. You have just "blessed the uterus," sonographically speaking, and know where the fetus lies (whether on the maternal right or left and whether cephalic, breech, or transverse), how many fetuses there may be, and where the placenta is (anterior, posterior, fundal, and/or low). Now you are ready to start taking images. Begin at the fetal head—regardless of where the head may be in the uterus—and work your way down the fetus in a systematic and orderly manner.

2. Four-chamber heart: For best results, the probe should be placed below the level of the heart and the beam should be angled cephalad toward the apex of the heart. This will cause the beam to enter from the base of the heart and image upward through the atria. If you are at the level of the fluid-filled stomach and umbilical vein, simply tilt the transducer toward the fetal head and the four-chamber view will appear.

Figure 4-69. *The "bless the uterus" technique of uterine survey to establish fetal lie. Here the fetus is cephalic with arms and legs on maternal left.*

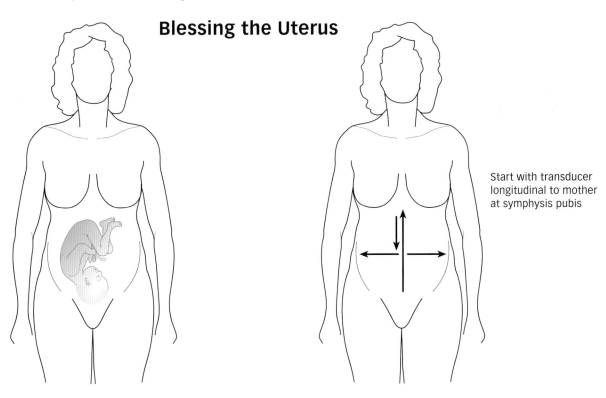

Blessing the Uterus

Start with transducer longitudinal to mother at symphysis pubis

1. Start midline at symphysis pubis = head
2. Slide up middle to uterine fundus then back down to mid-uterus = chest / arm / body
3. Slide to maternal right = fetal spine
4. Slide to maternal left = fetal extremities

3. Umbilical cord: On occasion a focal thickening of Wharton's jelly close to the abdominal wall may mimic an abdominal wall defect. This can be ruled out by identifying the umbilical vessels as they insert into the fetal abdomen.

4. Femur/humerus length measurement is a somewhat confusing concept because we do not actually measure the entire length of these long bones. Care should be taken to measure the shaft or diaphysis of the bone only and not to include the heads or condyles, which are somewhat hypoechoic. Because these parts of the bone do not ossify until after birth, they are not consistently recognized sonographically. Distal epiphyseal centers do not usually appear until after 30 weeks' gestation (Figure 4-70).

5. When trying to obtain the femur length, locate the transverse fetal bladder and then rotate the transducer about 45 degrees toward the fetus's anterior abdomen; the femur should begin to elongate in view. Another method is to image the lumbosacral spine longitudinally and rotate 90 degrees toward the fetus's anterior abdomen.

6. Imaging the three-vessel umbilical cord in cross section (to locate the Mickey Mouse sign) can be difficult. When in doubt, use color Doppler or power Doppler to identify the two umbilical arteries on either side of the fetal bladder and to confirm that there are indeed three vessels.

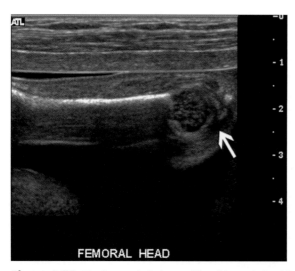

Figure 4-70. *The hypoechoic femoral head (arrow) should not be included when measuring the femur length.*

7. Be careful to ensure that it is the umbilical arteries, at the level of the fetal bladder where the umbilical cord inserts into the abdomen, that are being imaged. The iliac arteries lie lateral to the umbilical arteries and can easily be mistaken for them.

8. When attempting to identify fetal sex, start with the transverse fetal bladder. Angle slightly inferior to the bladder and you will be in the general vicinity of the fetal genitalia.

9. Fetal bradycardia can be induced by pressing the transducer heavily over the fetal chest while imaging. If you notice a slowing of the heartbeat while you are scanning, ease up on your pressure to see if the rhythm returns to a normal rate.

10. When determining the amniotic fluid index using the four-quadrant method or when assessing the angle of the fetal head in the uterus (especially in cases of asynclitism, when there is a lateral deflection of the fetal head, or absence of parallelism between the presenting part of the fetus and the pelvic planes), it is important to hold the transducer perpendicular to the uterus. If your patient is in a straight supine position, you will also be perpendicular to the table; however, if the patient must roll to one side or the other, some adjustment of the transducer placement will be necessary. Therefore make sure you are perpendicular to the uterus (Figure 4-71). If one places the transducer along the lateral edge of the uterus, the fluid pocket imaged may not be in the quadrant intended. Figure 4-72 shows how the sound beam is directed when the transducer is placed laterally. Scanning from the patient's lateral right side may actually cause you to image a fluid pocket on the left.

11. Documenting both fetal kidneys on one image is easy if you place the transducer right on top of the fetal spine. If the fetus is lying on its side and you set the transducer over the fetal abdomen, the anterior kidney will be nicely demonstrated but the posterior kidney will be lost behind the shadow of the spine. If you place the transducer on the spine, the shadow will be projected between the kidneys, showing both nicely (Figure 4-73).

12. Fetal adrenal glands are normally prominent and should not be mistaken for kidneys. In transverse view, the adrenal glands will be more ovoid in shape, whereas kidneys will be rounded.

Angle of Asynclitism

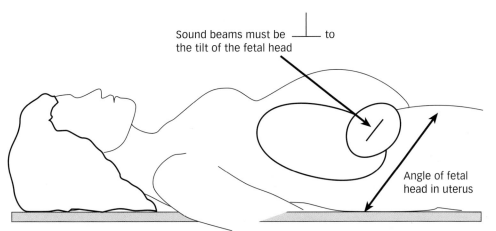

Sound beams must be ⊥ to the tilt of the fetal head

Angle of fetal head in uterus

Figure 4-71. *How to determine the angle of asynclitism of the fetal head.*

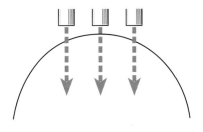

Proper position for measuring AFI fluid pockets

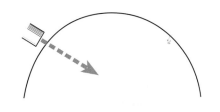

Improper for measuring AFI fluid pockets

Figure 4-72. *Proper transducer placement for measuring amniotic fluid pockets within quadrants.*

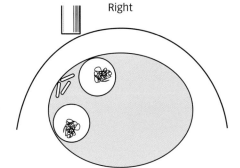

Right   Wrong

Figure 4-73. *How to avoid spine shadowing when imaging both fetal kidneys.*

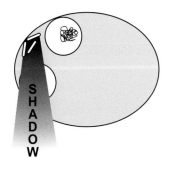

Right

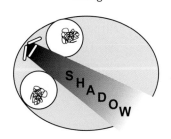

Wrong

SHADOW

SHADOW

A

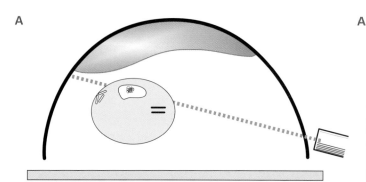

B

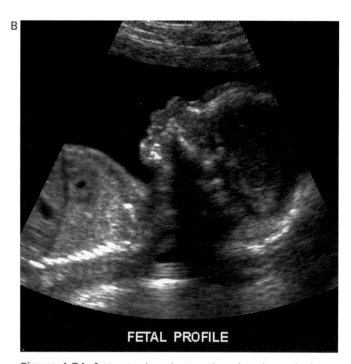

FETAL PROFILE

Figure 4-74. A *How to place the transducer in order to obtain a fetal profile view.* **B** *Profile of the fetal face and chest.*

13. To get the profile of a fetus, the fetus must be face up or lying on one side. If the fetus is lying on the maternal right, go to the opposite side (maternal left) and scan longitudinally to the fetus. Your sound beam must be directed from underneath the fetus up toward the anterior maternal abdomen (Figure 4-74).

14. When evaluating the fetal spine that is against the placenta or uterine wall, one should try to get the fetus to move. Spinal defects may be compressed or obscured from view if the fetus is pressed against surrounding structures.

The Targeted Scan

15. From the normal four-chamber heart view, slightly rotate the transducer toward the fetal right shoulder to image the left ventricular outflow tract (LVOT).

A

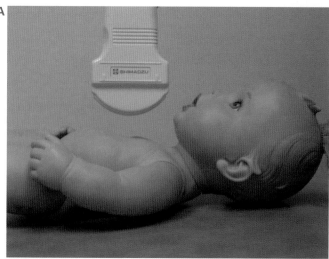

B

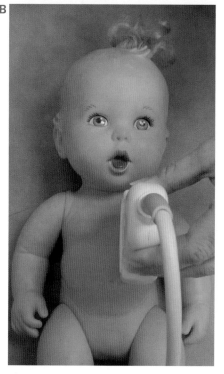

Figure 4-75. A *Image showing placement of the transducer longitudinally over the fetal thorax. This is a good position for imaging aortic and ductal arches with only slight manipulation of the transducer.* **B** *Image demonstrating slight movement to the fetal left side in order to document the aorta and aortic arch longitudinally. (Figure continues . . .)*

16. While imaging the LVOT, angle the transducer slightly toward the fetal head to obtain the right ventricular outflow tract (RVOT).

17. When imaging the longitudinal view of the fetal spine, angle slightly to the right of the fetal spine to obtain a longitudinal view of the aortic arch (Figures 4-75 A and B).

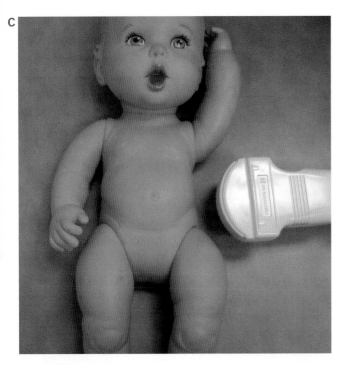

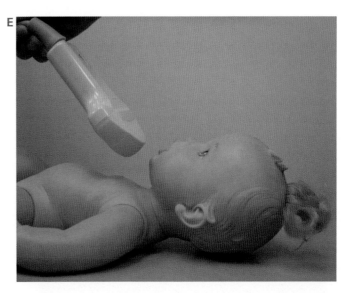

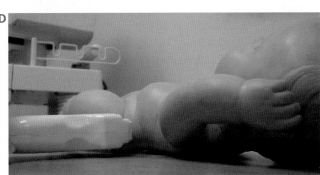

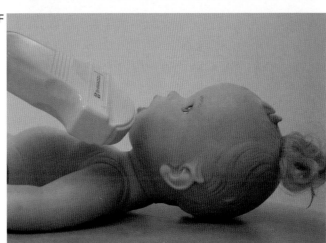

Figure 4-75, continued. C *Transducer location to image the aortic bifurcation, renal arteries, and kidneys bilaterally in the fetal coronal plane.* **D** *Transducer position demonstrating the beam's more posterior location in a fetus, which is needed to image the aortic bifurcation, renal arteries, and kidneys bilaterally in the coronal plane.* **E** *Image demonstrating a transverse beam angle that is parallel to the long axis of the fetal mandible.* **F** *Image demonstrating an oblique beam angle that is perpendicular to the long axis of the fetal mandible. (Figure continues . . .)*

18. Images of the aortic bifurcation, renal arteries, and kidneys bilaterally can be visualized while imaging the fetus in the coronal plane with the beam angle positioned more posteriorly (Figures 4-75 C and D).

19. Images of the fetal mandible can be obtained by manipulating the transducer so the ultrasound beam is perpendicular or parallel to the long axis of the mandible. Transverse or oblique views may be required depending on fetal position within the uterus (Figures 4-75 E and F).

20. To evaluate the fetal profile and all other associated structures, locate the fetal spine and then move the transducer to the completely opposite position to obtain a sagittal view of the fetal face. For example, if you obtain long-axis images of the fetal spine from the mother's right side, the maternal left side is where you should start to image the fetal profile (Figures 4-75 G and H).

21. Coronal images of the fetal head and face can be obtained with many different positions of the transducer on the fetal head. Beam angles can originate from the fetal right side, left side, top of the head, and/or area of the fetal chin. Figures 4-75 I and J depict the many possibilities that offer the same results.

G

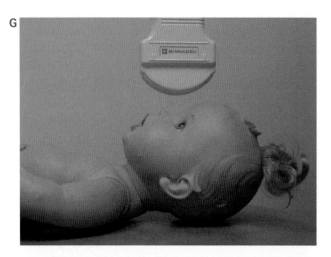

H

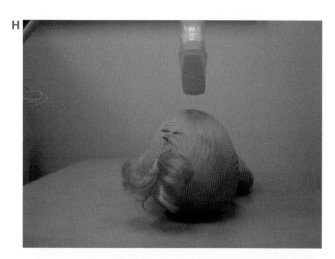

I

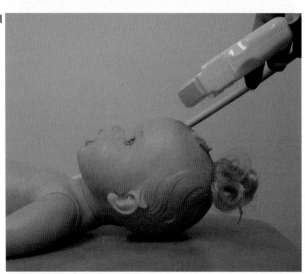

J

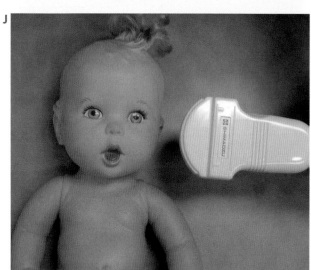

Figure 4-75, continued. G *Beam placement to the fetal midline to effectively image the profile in the sagittal plane.* **H** *Beam placement to the fetal midline to effectively image the profile in the sagittal plane.* **I** *Transducer placed in order to get a coronal image of the fetal face.* **J** *Image demonstrating beam direction from the fetal left side in order to obtain a coronal image of the fetal face. Following page:* **K** *Transducer placement to scan the fetal orbits transversely.* **L** *Beam position and angle to image the fetal nose and lips coronally.* **M** *Transducer position to image the long axis of the fetal clavicle.* **N** *Beam position to scan the fetal palette.*

22. Rotate the transducer 90 degrees from the midline of the fetal face to obtain a transverse scanning plane. It is important to be truly transverse to the fetal orbits—not just the head—in order to measure them correctly (Figure 4-75K).

23. To image the fetal nose and lips for evaluation of cleft defects in the coronal scanning plane, slide the probe to the tip of the fetal nose and then angle back into the lips (Figure 4-75L).

24. To image and measure the clavicle, position the transducer high in the fetal thorax with a slight oblique rotation (Figure 4-75M).

25. Imaging the roof of the fetal mouth can often prove to be very difficult, and 2D imaging of the fetal pal-

ate is not routinely successful without the use of 3D imaging. However, if the mouth is opened wide at any point, diagnostic images can be obtained thanks to amniotic fluid enhancement of the defect (Figure 4-75N).

26. Unlike scanning the abdomen, which requires angling the transducer through a sonic window rather than sliding the transducer, obstetric scanning technique requires larger movements and chasing the fetus to obtain quality images.

27. Be patient! Fetuses may be lying in positions that are not necessarily good for imaging, so you may not be able to complete an entire examination in the allotted time. (See Table 4-2.)

Figure 4-75, continued.

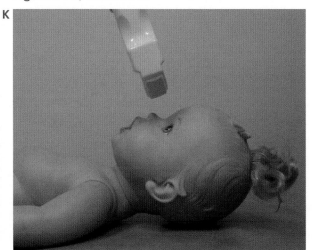

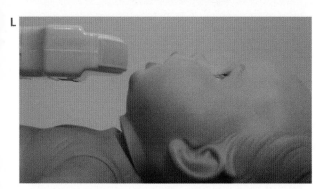

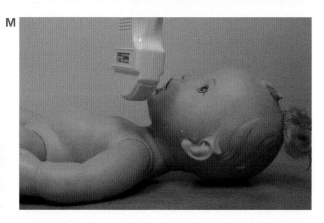

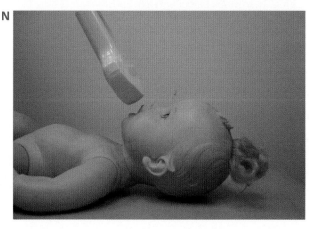

Table 4-2. Pitfalls.

Category	Pitfalls
Fetal	Fetal position
	Oligohydramnios
	Polyhydramnios
	Placental position
	Early gestational age
	Late gestational age
	Fetal movement
Maternal	Maternal obesity
	Fibroid uterus
	Previous scarring from cesarean section
	Maternal movement/breathing
Other	Resolution of equipment
	Transducer frequency
	High-resolution zoom
	Caliper calibration
	Sonographer experience and skill level

REFERENCES

Benson CB, Doubilet PM: Fetal measurements: normal and abnormal fetal growth. In Rumack CM, Wilson SR, Charboneau JW, et al (eds): *Diagnostic Ultrasound*, 4th Edition, Volume 2. Philadelphia, Elsevier Mosby, 2011, pp 1457–1464.

Bisset RAL, Khan AN, Thomas NB: *Differential Diagnosis in Obstetrics and Gynecologic Ultrasound*, 2nd Edition. Philadelphia, Elsevier, 2002.

Callen PW (ed): *Ultrasonography in Obstetrics and Gynecology*, 5th Edition. Philadelphia, Saunders Elsevier, 2008.

Craig M: *Pocket Guide to Ultrasound Measurements*. Philadelphia, Lippincott, 1988.

DuBose T: *Fetal Sonography*. Philadelphia, Saunders, 1996.

Goldberg B, McGahan J: *Atlas of Ultrasound Measurements*, 2nd Edition. Philadelphia, Mosby, 2006.

Jeng CJ, Jou TJ, Wang KG, et al: Amniotic fluid index measurement with the four-quadrant technique during pregnancy. J Reprod Med 35:674–677, 1990.

Maizels M, Cuneo B, Sabbagha RE: *Fetal Anomalies: Ultrasound Diagnosis and Postnatal Management.* New York, Wiley-Liss, 2002.

Manning FA, Hill LM, Platt LD: Quantitative amniotic fluid volume determination by ultrasound: antepartum detection of intrauterine growth retardation. Am J Obstet Gynecol 139:254–258, 1981.

McGahan JP, Porto M: *Diagnostic Obstetrical Ultrasound.* Philadelphia, Lippincott, 1994.

Nicolaides K, Sebire N, Snijders J: *The 11–14 Week Scan: The Diagnosis of Fetal Abnormalities.* New York, Parthenon, 1999.

Phelan JP, Smith CV, Broussard P, et al: Amniotic fluid volume assessment with the four-quadrant technique at 36–42 weeks' gestation. J Reprod Med 32:540–542, 1987.

Rutherford SE, Phelan JP, Smith CV, et al: The four-quadrant assessment of amniotic fluid volume: an adjunct to antepartum fetal heart rate testing. Obstet Gynecol 70:353, 1987.

Sabbagha RE: Diagnostic accuracy of targeted imaging for fetal anomalies. In Chervenak FA, Isaacson GC, Campbell S (eds): *Ultrasound in Obstetrics & Gynecology,* Volume 2. Boston, Little Brown, 1993.

Sauerbrei EE, Nguyen KT, Nolan RL: *A Practical Guide to Ultrasound in Obstetrics and Gynecology,* 2nd Edition. New York, Lippincott Williams & Wilkins, 1998.

Spitz JL: Sonography of the second and third trimesters. In Hagan-Ansert SL (ed): *Textbook of Diagnostic Ultrasonography,* 7th Edition. St. Louis, Elsevier Mosby, 2012, pp 1103–1141.

SELF-ASSESSMENT EXERCISES

Questions

Part 1: The Basic Scan

1. All of the following are considered functions of amniotic fluid *except*:

   A. To maintain fetal body temperature

   B. To act as a shock absorber

   C. To ensure normal fetal lung development

   D. To ensure normal development of the musculo-skeletal system

   E. To provide nourishment

2. Of the following cranial structures, which is the landmark for locating the atria of the lateral ventricles?

   A. Periventricular vasculature

   B. Choroid plexus

   C. Cavum septum pellucidum

   D. Corpus callosum

   E. Cisterna magna

3. Which of the following structures is not among those measured for gestational age?

   A. Cerebellum

   B. Ocular diameters

   C. Cisterna magna

   D. Clavicle

   E. Foot

4. Which of the following statements is *not* true for the spine?

   A. Splaying at the base of the skull is normal.

   B. The lemon and banana signs indicate spina bifida.

   C. Ossification of the lumbosacral region is not complete until after 18 weeks.

   D. Transversely, one can see one posterior and two anterior ossification centers.

   E. Imaging the spine is part of the basic scan.

5. When imaging the fetal heart, the valve seen between the left atrium and left ventricle is the:

   A. Aortic

   B. Pulmonary

   C. Tricuspid

   D. Foramen ovale

   E. Mitral

6. Of the following cardiac anomalies, which can be easily missed on the four-chamber view?

    A. Situs inversus

    B. Epstein anomaly

    C. Transposition of the great vessels

    D. Hypoplastic left ventricle

    E. Endocardial cushion defect

7. Which part of the heart lies closest to the anterior chest wall?

    A. Left atrium

    B. Left ventricle

    C. Right atrium

    D. Right ventricle

    E. Aortic arch

8. Of the following images, which would not be required to meet the basic guidelines?

    A. Four-chamber view of heart

    B. All four fetal extremities

    C. Umbilical cord insertion into fetal abdomen

    D. Three-vessel cord

    E. Fetal hands and feet

9. The cephalic index is performed to identify:

    A. Head shape

    B. Hydrocephalus

    C. Growth restriction

    D. Gestational age

    E. Brain volume

10. Of the following, which would *not* be associated with polyhydramnios?

    A. Spina bifida

    B. Fetal demise

    C. Intestinal obstruction

    D. Dwarfism

    E. Anencephaly

Part 2: The Targeted Scan

11. A targeted scan is ordered to evaluate a pregnancy for:

    A. Gender

    B. Anomalies

    C. Multiple gestation

    D. Placental location

    E. All of the above

12. Measured between the 11th and 14th gestational week, the nuchal translucency is considered normal if it ranges from:

    A. 0.5 to 5.0 mm

    B. 1.0 to 4.0 mm

    C. 1.5 to 3.5 mm

    D. 1.0 to 3.0 mm

    E. 1.0 to 2.5 mm

13. Of the following choices, which anomaly cannot be seen on profile view of the fetal face?

    A. Cleft lip

    B. Hypotelorism

    C. Frontal bossing

    D. Micrognathia

    E. Prominent occiput

14. The atrioventricular valves of the fetal heart include the:

    A. Tricuspid valve

    B. Bicuspid valve

    C. Semilunar valve

    D. A and B

    E. B and C

15. Another name for situs inversus is:

    A. Situs solitus

    B. Situs transversus

    C. Levocardia

    D. Organomegaly

    E. None of the above

16. Echogenic bowel can be seen with all of the following *except*:

    A. Cytomegalovirus

    B. Cystic fibrosis

    C. Down syndrome

    D. Bowel obstruction

    E. All of the above

17. Hypoplasia of the middle phalanx of the fifth digit of the hand will cause:

    A. Clinodactyly

    B. Syndactyly

    C. Down syndrome

    D. Adactyly

    E. A and B

18. Targeted scans are usually overseen by which physician specialist?

    A. Radiologist

    B. Obstetrician

    C. Pediatrician

    D. Pathologist

    E. Perinatologist

19. The nuchal fold is best evaluated between:

    A. 11 and14 weeks

    B. 15 and 20 weeks

    C. 24 and 28 weeks

    D. 30 and 35 weeks

    E. Timing does not matter.

20. The normal nuchal fold should not exceed:

    A. 2 mm

    B. 3 mm

    C. 4 mm

    D. 5 mm

    E. 6 mm

21. The nuchal fold thickness measurement is taken at the level of the:

    A. Cerebral ventricles

    B. Thalami

    C. Falx

    D. Third ventricle

    E. Cerebellum

22. The right ventricle, pulmonary semilunar valve, pulmonary artery, and right atrium are demonstrated in the:

    A. Four-chamber view

    B. Five-chamber view

    C. Right ventricular outflow tract

    D. Left ventricular outflow tract

    E. Aortic arch

23. The following structure resembles a candy cane when imaged:

    A. Aortic arch

    B. Ductal arch

    C. Inflow tracts

    D. Pulmonary arteries

    E. Atrioventricular valves

24. A fetal chest that is smaller than the fetal abdomen could be due to:

    A. Dwarfism

    B. Pulmonary hypoplasia

    C. Macrosomia

    D. None of the above

    E. All of the above

25. If the gallbladder is not visualized, the cause may be:

    A. Sickle cell anemia

    B. Fetal hydrops

    C. Cystic fibrosis

    D. Intrauterine growth restriction

    E. Erythroblastosis fetalis

Answers

See Appendix F on page 610 for answers and explanations.

The Placenta and Umbilical Cord

Jim Baun, BS, RDMS, RVT, FSDMS, and Kathryn A. Gill, MS, RT, RDMS, FSDMS

OBJECTIVES

After completing this chapter you should be able to:

1. Describe placental circulation and hemodynamics as they relate to the mother and fetus.

2. List and define the placental variants and explain how they might adversely affect the pregnancy.

3. Identify the sonographic characteristics of placental aging and explain the grading system.

4. Discuss the pitfalls of diagnosing placenta previa.

5. Explain how cord length can affect the fetus and outcome of pregnancy.

THROUGHOUT HISTORY MAN HAS BEEN CURIOUS about the placenta and has believed its value included supernatural and medicinal properties. In 3400 BC, Egyptians thought the placenta represented the eternal soul, and the Chinese are just one of many cultures believing that ingestion of placenta can cure ailments such as delirium, weakness, loss of willpower, and pinkeye. Even today's alternative medicine options promote this practice. Several websites offer recipes for preparing placenta, including placenta lasagna, pizza, stew, and pâté.

The placenta plays a critical role in the growth, development, and maturation of a normal, healthy pregnancy, and sonography plays an important role in evaluating the placenta. As part of a comprehensive sonographic examination of a second or third trimester pregnancy, the placenta should be evaluated for the following:

1. Size and shape

2. Number

3. Texture

4. Location relative to the internal cervical os

EARLY PLACENTAL DEVELOPMENT

The endometrium responds to hormone stimulation in preparation for receiving a fertilized egg. Upon ovulation, the corpus luteum produces progesterone, which induces the secretory changes in the endometrium. **Decidua**—the term for the uterine lining following conception—is the functional layer of the endometrium that "falls away" after delivery. Changes in the endometrium may be seen in both intrauterine and ectopic pregnancies.

A

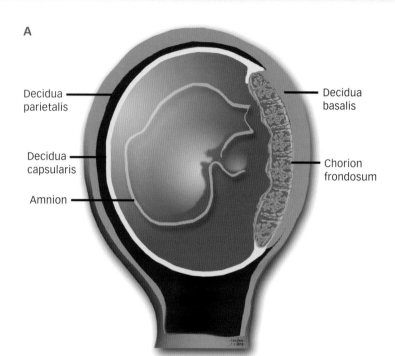

Decidua parietalis

Decidua capsularis

Amnion

Decidua basalis

Chorion frondosum

Figure 5-1. A *Parts of the decidual lining of the endometrial cavity and fetal membranes.* **B** *Early intrauterine gestational sac demonstrating the deciduas and double decidual ring. The arrow is pointing to the intrauterine gestational sac. DC = decidua capsularis, DP = decidua parietalis.*

B

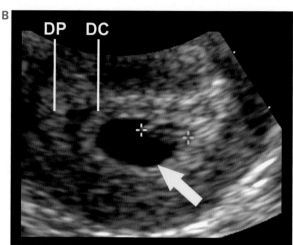

DP   DC

The site where the blastocyst implants in the endometrium is called the **decidua basalis**, which ultimately develops into the maternal portion of the placenta. The layer of decidua that is stretched out into the uterine cavity and closes over and surrounds the blastocyst and chorionic sac is called the **decidua capsularis**. An avascular area of the decidua capsularis develops into the **smooth chorion**, or chorionic membrane. As the pregnancy grows, the chorionic membrane surrounds the nonplacental portion of the uterine cavity and fuses with the amniotic membrane. The decidua lining the remaining part of the uterine cavity is called the **decidua parietalis**, or **decidua vera** (Figure 5-1).

At the site of implantation, chorionic villi surround the entire gestational sac. The **syncytiotrophoblast** erodes endometrial tissues (capillaries, glands, and connective tissue), allowing maternal blood to seep out and surround implanted villi, establishing a primitive uteroplacental circulation. This bushy part of the chorion that interweaves with the decidua basalis is the **chorion frondosum**, or **villous chorion** or **chorionic villus** (Figure 5-2A). Sonographically, the chorion frondosum appears as a thickened, echogenic area adjacent to the gestational sac at the site of implantation (Figure 5-2B). As the decidua capsularis balloons out into the uterine cavity, it comes to lie directly

adjacent to the decidua parietalis. This **apposition** of the two layers of decidua gives rise to the **double decidual sac sign**—a useful and accurate sonographic finding for identifying a normal intrauterine gestation and excluding ectopic pregnancies (Figures 5-2 C and D).

The smooth chorion arises from the decidua capsularis. Each blastocyst develops one chorion. As the uterine lining is stretched out into the uterine cavity, the decidua capsularis loses its vascularity and becomes greatly thinned and attenuated. It eventually contacts and fuses with the decidua parietalis, obliterating the uterine cavity. The cellular decidual components degenerate and eventually disappear, leaving only the membrane-like chorion. Occasionally, the chorion does not fuse completely with the decidua parietalis, leaving small, focal detached areas that fill with blood. These structures, called **subchorionic hematomas**, are frequently imaged sonographically during the first trimester (Figure 5-3A). The chorion is divided into the *smooth chorion* and the *villous chorion*. The villous chorion forms the fetal portions of the placenta. The portion of the chorionic wall related to the placenta is called the **chorionic plate** (Figure 5-3B). It typically contains the chorionic vascular structures that can be seen on the fetal surface of the placenta.

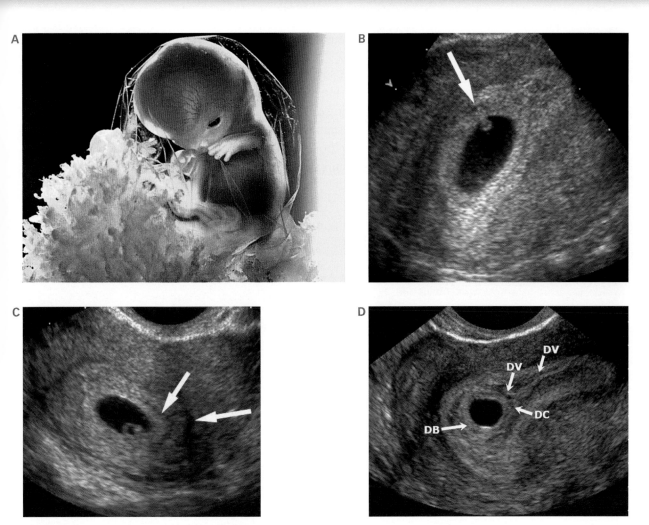

Figure 5-2. A *Chorionic villus.* **B** *Arrow shows thickened ridge of chorion where the early placenta is developing.* **C** *Double sac sign (arrows).* **D** *Longitudinal image of an early intrauterine gestational sac. DB = decidua basalis, DC = decidua capsularis, DV = decidua vera.*

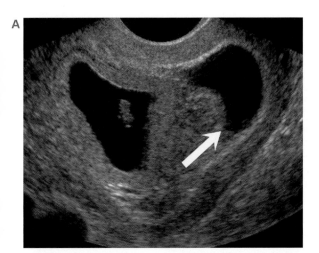
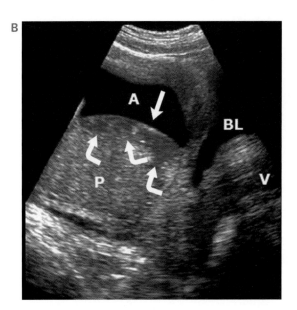

Figure 5-3. A *Transvaginal image of early intrauterine pregnancy with a subchorionic bleed indicated by the arrow.* **B** *Longitudinal image through the lower uterine segment of a second trimester gestation. The curved arrows demonstrate the subchorionic space while the straight arrow shows the chorionic plate. BL = maternal bladder, A = amniotic fluid, P = placenta, V = vagina.*

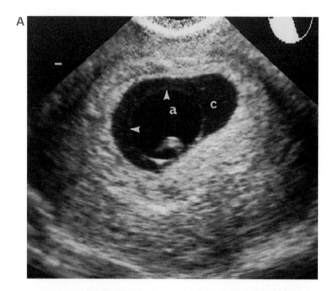

AMNIOTIC BANDS AND SHEETS

Usually by 12 weeks but certainly by 16 weeks, the chorion and amnion fuse (Figure 5-4). Episodes of bleeding during pregnancy or invasive procedures such as amniocentesis may force the amnion and chorion apart (chorio-amnio separation; Figure 5-5). If rupture occurs, the result is **amniotic band syndrome**. **Amniotic**

Figure 5-4. A *Early intrauterine gestational sac demonstrating the amniotic membrane (a) and chorionic cavity (c).* **B** *Early gestation demonstrating the amnion (arrow). Note that the yolk sac (YS) lies between the amnion and chorion. Growth shows the amnion (arrow) expanding toward the chorion (C).* **C** *Between 12 and 16 weeks, the amnion (arrows) fuses with the chorion and is no longer identified as a separate structure.*

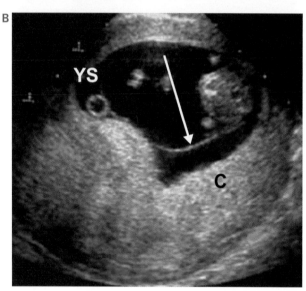

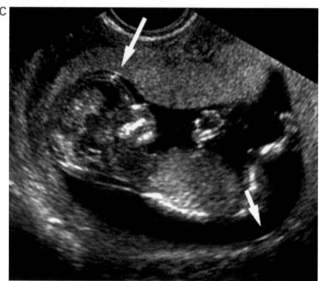

Figure 5-5. A *Membrane (arrow) seen anterior to placenta (P) represents separation of the amnion from the chorion.* **B** *Bleeding during pregnancy can force the amnion (arrow) and chorion (curved arrow) to separate, resulting in an amniotic band.*

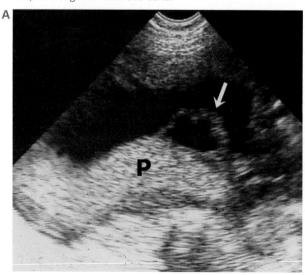

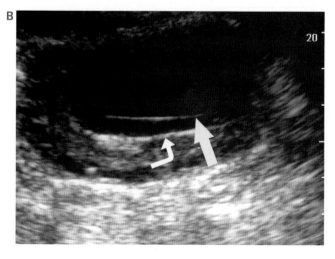

bands are thin strands of tissue that can attach to and wrap around fetal parts, causing constrictures, deformities such as clefts, and amputations (Figure 5-6).

Amniotic sheets are thought to relate to folds of amnion and chorion across a uterine synechia (Figure 5-7A). They look different from amniotic bands because they are thicker and have a free edge that is often globular. Unlike amniotic bands, amniotic sheets are considered benign (Figures 5-7 B and C). Nevertheless, care should still be taken to confirm that fetal movement is not restricted.

A

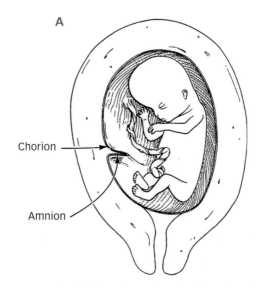

B

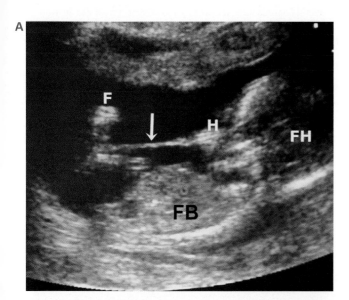

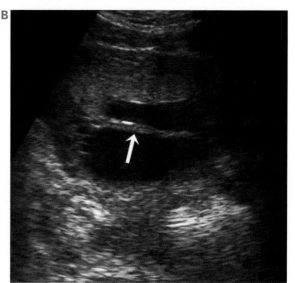

C

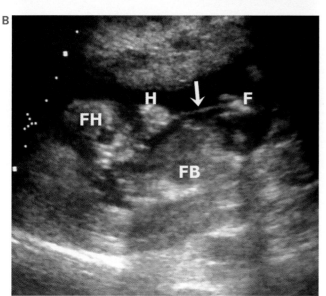

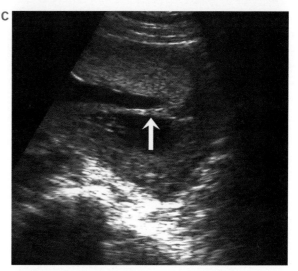

Figure 5-6. A and **B** *The amniotic band (arrow) can attach to fetal parts and cause structural anomalies and restrict fetal movement. FH = fetal head, FB = fetal body, F = foot, H = hand.*

Figure 5-7. A *Amniotic sheets are thought to be amnion and chorion folded over a uterine synechia. Reprinted with permission from Nelson LH: Ultrasonography of the Placenta—A Review. Laurel, MD, AIUM, 1994, p 42.* **B** and **C** *Thick strands represent amniotic sheets (arrow) resulting from scarring of the uterine cavity.*

PLACENTAL ANATOMY AND PHYSIOLOGY

The placenta is a highly vascular, discoid organ critical to the developing fetus (Figure 5-8A). It possesses three main functions (Box 5-1):

1. It metabolizes substances that serve as sources of nutrients and energy for the embryo/fetus.

2. It transports gases, nutrients, hormones, electrolytes, antibodies, and waste products to and from the fetus.

3. It secretes endocrine proteins such as human chorionic gonadotropin (hCG) and **human chorionic somatomammotropin** (**hCS**), both of which are essential for the maintenance and growth of the pregnancy.

The placenta can lose as much as 30% of its surface area and still maintain adequate function.

Box 5-1. Placental functions.
Nutrients to fetus*
Exchange of gases*
Hormones
Antibodies
Waste excretion*

*Three main functions of the placenta.

Table 5-1 correlates the thickness of the placenta with gestational age. Typically, the placenta measures 2–4 cm in thickness (anteroposterior diameter) and weighs about 600 grams at birth. Nevertheless, there is enormous variability in the actual size and shape of a placenta, and

A

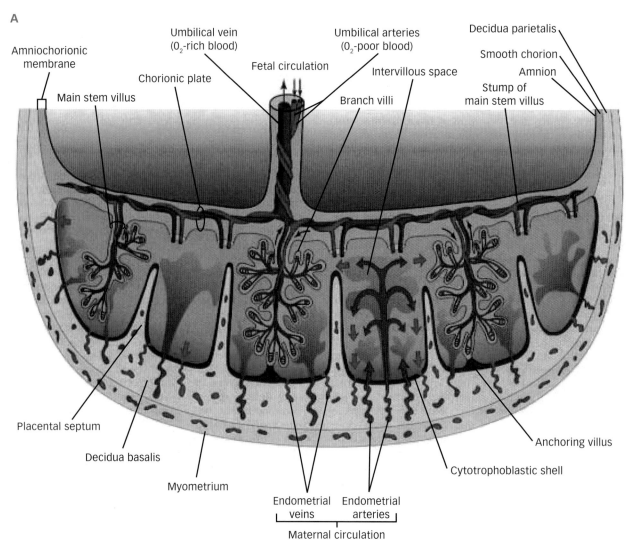

Figure 5-8. A *Drawing of the placenta. Used with permission from Moore KL, Persaud TVN:* The Developing Human: Clinically Oriented Embryology, *8th Edition. Philadelphia, Saunders Elsevier, 2008, p 116. (Figure continues . . .)*

Table 5-1.	Placental thickness correlated with gestational age.	
Gestational Age (Weeks)	Mean Thickness (cm)	± 2 SD
10	1.15	0.8–1.55
15	1.8	1.15–2.3
20	2.05	1.2–2.8
25	2.5	1.8–3.2
30	3.0	1.8–3.6
35	3.25	2.5–4.0
40	3.35	2.5–4.2

Box 5-2. Conditions associated with large placenta.

Diabetes
Rh sensitization
TORCH infections
Syphilis
Triploidy

Box 5-3. Conditions associated with small placenta.

Intrauterine growth restriction
Abnormal placentation (membranous)
Pre-eclampsia
Severe insulin-dependent diabetes
Chronic infection
Chromosomal abnormalities

the size relates directly to uteroplacental circulation. However, a placenta should not measure more than 4–5 cm at term. Factors that may contribute to placental morphologic variations include race, altitude, pathologic circumstances of implantation, underlying maternal co-morbidity, and maternal habits such as smoking. A large, fluffy placenta is usually the result of villous edema and hyperplasia. Placental enlargement is associated with fetal hemolytic disease, maternal diabetes, and severe maternal anemia (Figure 5-8B and Box 5-2). Abnormally small placentas are associated with intrauterine growth restriction (IUGR), pre-eclampsia, severe insulin-dependent

diabetes, chronic infection, and chromosomal abnormalities (Box 5-3).

The placenta is considered a maternal-fetal structure because of the apposition or fusion of fetal organs to maternal tissue for the purpose of physiologic exchange. Functionally and anatomically, the placenta is divided into two portions, maternal and fetal.

Maternal Portion

The maternal portion of the placenta constitutes less than 20% of placental weight. It is composed of compressed sheets of decidua basalis (placental septa) that project into pools of maternal blood and divide the placental body into the lobular **cotyledons**. Into each of these cotyledons project one or two stem villi and their many branch villi. The intervillous space is a large, blood-filled space that surrounds the chorionic villus. It is derived from the coalescence of lacunar networks that are found in the embryonic chorion frondosum. Maternal blood enters the intervillous space from the endometrial spiral arteries and is drained by the endometrial veins, which are found over the entire surface of the decidua basalis. The branch villi are continuously bathed with the maternal blood that is circulating in the intervillous space. It is at this level that the essential transfer of oxygen, nutrients, hormones, waste products, and other substances takes place (Figure 5-8C).

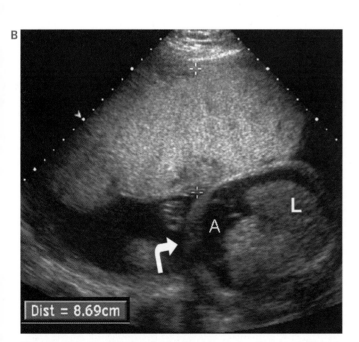

B

Dist = 8.69cm

Figure 5-8, continued. B *Thickened anterior placenta (calipers) at 8.6 cm. Note that the fetal abdomen also shows evidence of hydrops, demonstrating skin edema (arrow) and abdominal ascites (A). L = liver. (Figure continues . . .)*

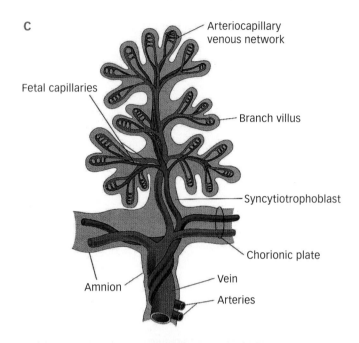

C

Arteriocapillary venous network

Fetal capillaries

Branch villus

Syncytiotrophoblast

Chorionic plate

Amnion

Vein

Arteries

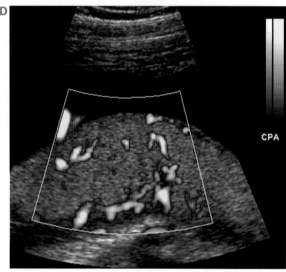

D

CPA

Figure 5-8, continued. C *Drawing of a stem chorionic villus and its arterio-capillary-venous system. The arteries carry poorly oxygenated fetal blood and waste products from the fetus, whereas the vein carries oxygenated blood and nutrients to the fetus. Used with permission from Moore KL, Persaud TVN: The Developing Human: Clinically Oriented Embryology, 8th Edition. Philadelphia, Saunders Elsevier, 2008, p 117.* **D** *Normal posterior placenta showing vascularization.*

Fetal Portion

The primary functional units of the placenta are fetal structures called villi. The large surface area created by the multiple convolutions of each villus provides the blood/cellular membrane contact necessary for the transfer of metabolic products between fetus and mother (see Figure 5-8C). The placental membrane is a two- to three-cell-thick covering over the small branches of the villus that regulates the transfer of some substances from the

maternal serum into the fetal bloodstream. The placental membrane acts as a true barrier only to molecules of a certain size, configuration, and charge. Some metabolites, toxins, and hormones, though present in the maternal circulation, do not pass through the placental membrane in sufficient concentrations to affect the embryo or fetus. However, most drugs and other substances in the maternal plasma pass through the placental membrane and enter the fetal plasma, including heparin and certain types of bacteria.

PLACENTAL CIRCULATION AND HEMODYNAMICS

A large volume of maternal arterial blood flow into the placenta is required to adequately perfuse the rapidly growing fetus. Therefore, in an average pregnancy, maternal blood volume increases by 45%–50% by term. Uterine arterial flow increases to accommodate this increased volume, and at about 14 weeks' gestation the appearance of end-diastolic flow velocities in an umbilical arterial Doppler spectral waveform indicates the establishment of continuous intervillous circulation. Blood flowing into the low-pressure intervillous spaces via the spiral arteries demonstrates pulsatile but low-resistance flow patterns throughout gestation using Doppler ultrasound techniques. (See Chapter 12.)

Maternal Placental Circulation

The blood in the intervillous space is temporarily outside the maternal circulatory system. It enters the intervillous space through 80 to 100 spiral endometrial arteries in the decidua basalis. These vessels discharge into the intervillous space through gaps in the cytotrophoblastic shell. The blood flow from the spiral arteries is pulsatile and propelled in jet-like fountains by the maternal blood pressure (Figure 5-8D). The welfare of the embryo and fetus depends on the adequate bathing of the branch villi with maternal blood more than on any other factor. Significant reductions of uteroplacental circulation may result in fetal hypoxia and intrauterine growth restriction.

Fetal Placental Circulation

Poorly oxygenated blood leaves the fetus and passes through the umbilical arteries to the placenta. At the site of attachment of the cord to the placenta, these arteries divide into a number of radially disposed chorionic arteries that branch freely in the chorionic plate before entering the chorionic villi. The blood vessels form an extensive arterio-capillary-venous system within the chorionic villi, which brings the fetal blood extremely close to the maternal blood. This system provides a very large area for the exchange of metabolic and gaseous products between the maternal and fetal bloodstreams.

The well-oxygenated fetal blood in the fetal capillaries passes into thin-walled veins that follow the chorionic arteries to the site of attachment of the umbilical cord, where they converge to form the umbilical vein. This large vessel carries oxygen-rich blood to the fetus (Figure 5-9).

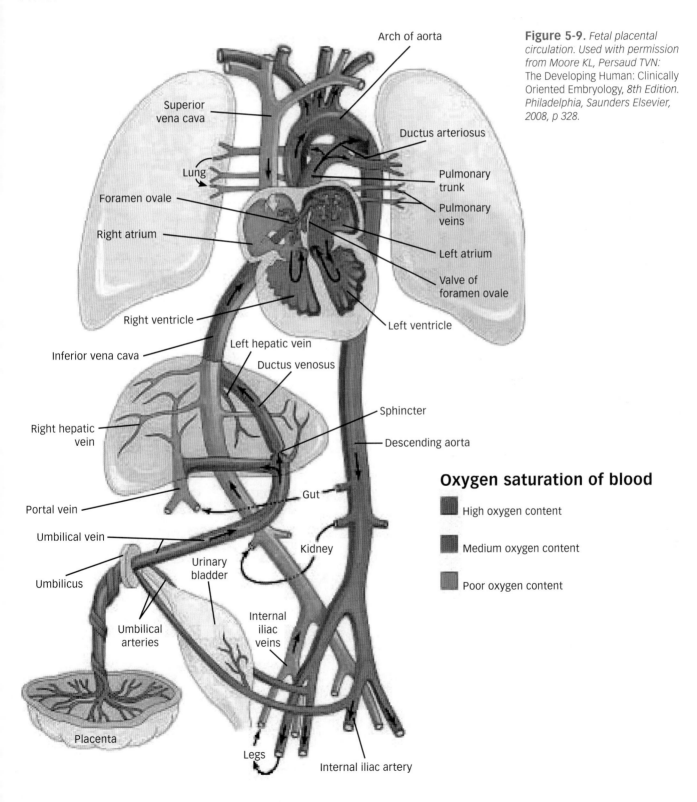

Figure 5-9. *Fetal placental circulation. Used with permission from Moore KL, Persaud TVN:* The Developing Human: Clinically Oriented Embryology, *8th Edition. Philadelphia, Saunders Elsevier, 2008, p 328.*

Oxygen saturation of blood

High oxygen content

Medium oxygen content

Poor oxygen content

PLACENTAL LOCATION

The placenta can attach itself anywhere within the uterine cavity and this position should be reported with some degree of detail. For example, a placenta that wraps around the lateral aspect of the uterus can appear to be both anterior and posterior when scanning the uterus in the long axis (Figures 5-10 A and B). One should also be aware that uterine growth can cause a previously reported low placenta to appear to have moved or changed position. This is referred to as **placental retraction** (Figure 5-10C). With uterine growth, the placenta is pulled and stretched, which causes some thinning at the edges and gives the appearance that it moves away from its original low position. Another explanation is trophotropism: The placenta may grow in areas of optimal myometrial perfusion and atrophy in areas that are not well vascularized. For these reasons, a **low-lying** or **marginal placenta** should be checked later in the pregnancy to confirm its position.

PLACENTAL GRADING

Structural, or maturational, changes occur within the placenta as it ages. A method of **placental grading** based on sonographically observable changes was devised to help assess fetal lung maturity. Paramount among the changes that can be observed with sonography is the development of small areas of calcific degeneration in the basal plate or within the placental cotyledons. While subsequent studies have demonstrated that statistical correlation between placental grade and lung maturity is generally poor, the identification of a mature placenta in the second or early third trimester may indicate impending placental insufficiency or may predict other postnatal morbidity such as respiratory distress syndrome, especially in the presence of underlying maternal medical complications.

The sonographic criteria used to grade a placenta appear in Figure 5-11A. In cases where different areas of the placenta exhibit different degrees of maturity, the area that appears most mature is graded and reported (Figures 5-11 B–F).

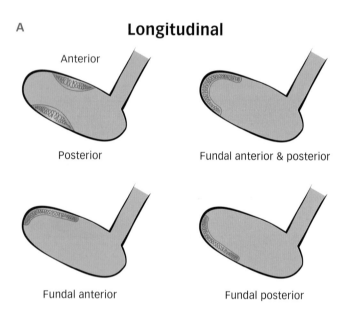

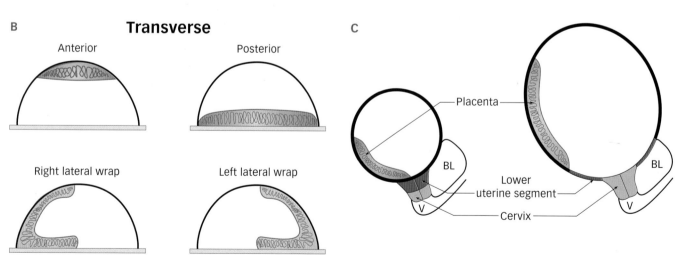

Figure 5-10. A *Placental locations as seen in the longitudinal plane.* **B** *Placental locations as seen in the transverse plane.* **C** *Due to the differential growth rate of the uterus during pregnancy, an early low-lying placenta can appear to change position by the third trimester. BL = maternal bladder, V = vagina.*

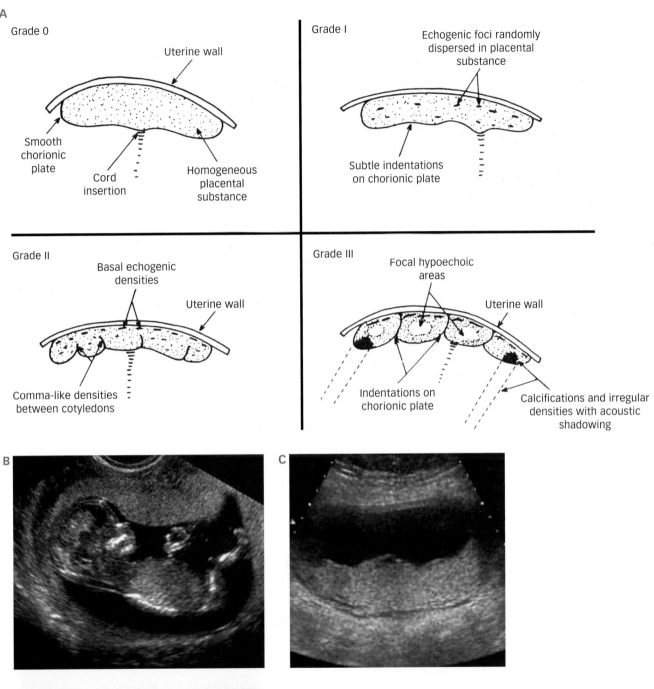

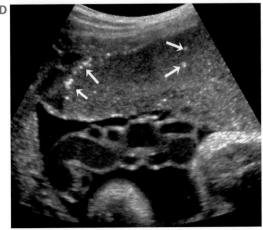

Figure 5-11. A *Grannum's placental grading starts with grade 0 (late first to early second trimester), with a smooth echo pattern of the parenchyma, no calcifications of the chorionic/basal plate, and no indentations of the chorionic plate. Grade I (mid-second to early third trimester) displays diffuse, randomly distributed calcifications (2–4 mm) and subtle indentations of the chorionic plate. Grade II (late third trimester to delivery) is characterized by dot-dash calcifications parallel to the basal plate and larger indentations of the chorionic plate. Finally, grade III (39 weeks to postdelivery) displays larger calcifications and indentations of the basal plate. Reprinted with permission from Grannum PA, Berkowitz RL, Hobbins JC: The ultrasonic changes in the maturing placenta and their relation to fetal pulmonic maturity. Am J Obstet Gynecol 133:915, 1979.* **B** *Anterior grade 0 placenta showing smooth homogeneous echo pattern and smooth chorionic plate.* **C** *This posterior grade I placenta demonstrates undulation of the chorionic plate, making it appear broken, and there is mild heterogenicity of the placenta.* **D** *This anterior placenta shows bright echogenic foci scattered throughout the placenta and especially along the basal area (arrows), typical of grade II. (Figure continues . . .)*

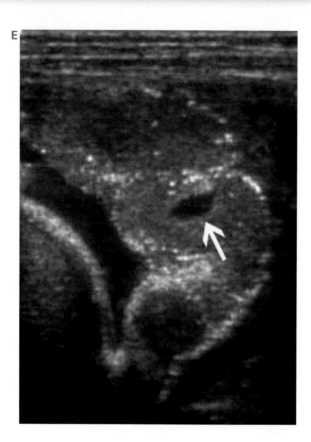

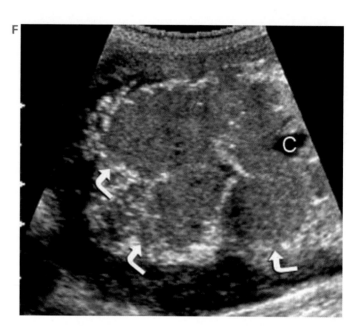

Figure 5-11, continued. E *This grade III placenta shows distinct lobulations with areas of calcification and cystic degeneration (arrow).* **F** *A grade III placenta showing areas of cystic degeneration (C) and distinct lobulations (curved arrows) outlined by hyperechoic calcific changes.*

Early placental aging, as demonstrated by the presence of calcifications within the placenta, may be related to many factors, including cigarette smoking, maternal age, parity, and other maternal morbidity. Women who demonstrate placental calcification on sonography at 34–36 weeks have an increased risk of delivering infants of low birth weight, in poor condition at birth, and at risk for perinatal death. In patients with underlying medical conditions such as diabetes or **hypertension** (essential or pregnancy-induced hypertensive disorder [PIHD]) and in patients at increased risk for intrauterine growth restriction, placental grading can provide important information about the status and potential outcome of the pregnancy.

FIBRIN DEPOSITION

Maternal blood pooling in the subchorionic and perivillous spaces is normal. Examination with high-frequency transducers will reveal slow flow. Over time, fibrin deposits develop. These appear sonographically beneath the chorionic plate (subchorionic; Figure 5-12A) or within the placenta around individual villi (perivillous). (A large

subchorionic hematoma is referred to as a **Breus mole**.) Intervillous thromboses contain both fetal and maternal blood and range in size from just a few millimeters to several centimeters. Thromboses usually develop in the mid-placental region and may be described as *maternal lakes* (Figure 5-12 B and C). They are associated with an enlarged placenta, and there is an increased incidence with Rh incompatibility, suggesting that sensitization might result.

Decidual septal cysts are rare but occur in the same general vicinity between the cotyledons of the placenta. Cysts and thromboses can look similar sonographically (Figure 5-13). Thrombus, however, changes with time, including the development of fibrinous strands and plaque formation. These lesions may sometimes be responsible for elevation of **maternal serum alpha-fetoprotein** (**MSAFP**).

Placental infarctions are the result of ischemic necrosis of placental villi caused by interference with maternal blood flow to the intervillous space. Often part of the normal aging process, placental infarctions are usually peripheral in location. If uteroplacental circulation is

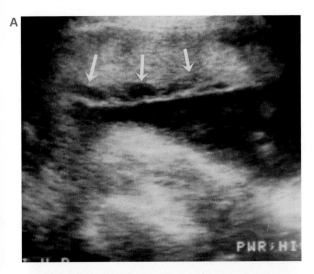

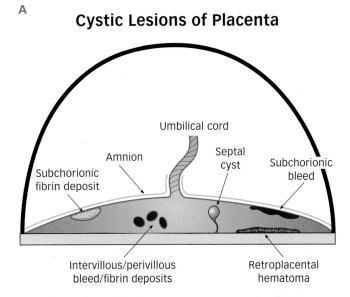

Cystic Lesions of Placenta

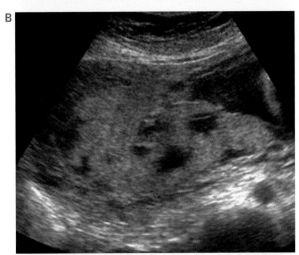

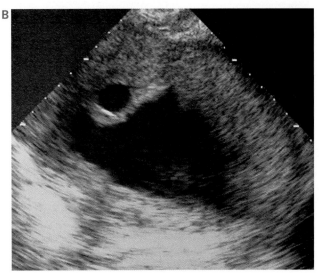

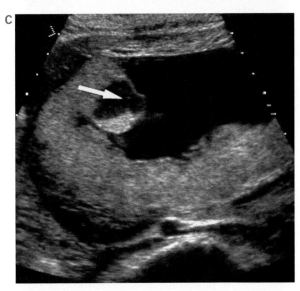

Figure 5-13. A *Various locations for cystic lesions of the placenta.* **B** *Placental cyst is well-defined and shows no internal fibrinous strands that would suggest thrombosis.*

Figure 5-12. A *Along the edge of this anterior placenta are multiple subchorionic fibrin deposits (arrows).* **B** *Intervillous thromboses or maternal lakes are usually located more centrally in the placenta.* **C** *A placental venous lake showing some debris and a septation (arrow) within.*

otherwise normal, there are rarely any fetal complications. Placental infarctions occur more commonly with eclampsia/pre-eclampsia. When this condition is severe, placental insufficiency may occur. Infarctions are often difficult to image with ultrasound as they appear more echogenic rather than hypoechoic unless there is associated active hemorrhage.

Intraplacental lesions are frequently encountered during sonographic examination. Most are associated with collections of blood or clots. There is some overlap in describing these blood formations, and their sonographic appearances can be very similar.

PLACENTAL VARIANTS

Placenta Extrachorialis

Placenta extrachorialis is a placenta in which the membranous chorion does not extend to the edge, forming a ring that may be completely or partially circumferential. As many as 20% of delivered placentas show partial extrachorionic regions where the attachment of the fetal membranes to the chorionic plate forms a ring. There are two types, the *circummarginate* and the *circumvallate* (Figures 5-14 A–C).

Circummarginate Placenta

With the **circummarginate placenta**, the ring formed by the attachment of membranes is flat. This type of placenta extrachorialis may be quite difficult to identify sonographically and has no clinical significance.

Circumvallate Placenta

The **circumvallate placenta**—the second type of placenta extrachorialis—has a small central chorionic ring that is folded and surrounded by thickened amnion and chorion (Figure 5-14D). This fold can be seen best in the second trimester and may predispose the patient to early placental separation from the uterine wall, antepartum bleeding, preterm labor, and perinatal mortality. A circumvallate placenta should be included in a differential diagnosis for vaginal bleeding in the second trimester with a normally implanted placenta.

A key sonographic feature of circumvallate placenta is an infolding of the fetal membrane upon the fetal surface of the placenta during the middle of the second trimester (Figure 5-14E). By the third trimester, only a bright border at the periphery of the placenta is demonstrable.

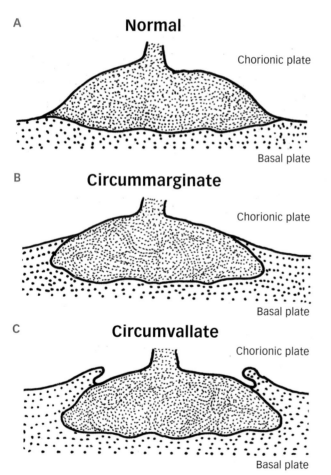

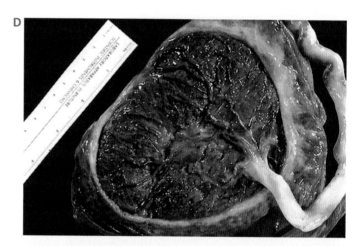

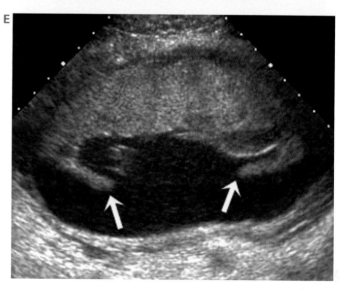

Figure 5-14. A *Normal placental attachment.* **B** *Circummarginate placenta.* **C** *Circumvallate placenta.* **D** *Specimen of a circumvallate placenta.* **E** *Anterior circumvallate placenta shows the folds at the edge bilaterally (arrows).*

Accessory Lobes

Due to alterations in the mechanisms of early placentation, three placental variants can occur—the *bipartite*, *succenturiate*, and *annular placentas*.

Bipartite Placenta

The **bipartite placenta** is divided into two lobes, relatively equal in size but united by primary vessels and chorionic membranes (Figure 5-15A). Localization of the cord insertion helps to identify the main placental lobe. Identification of the extra lobe is necessary to help reduce the risk of postpartum bleeding and infection. Intrauterine rupture of connecting membranes and vessels may result in massive fetal bleeding and death. And the presence of connecting membranes and vessels over the **internal os** (opening of the cervix into the uterus) may result in serious bleeding complications during labor and delivery.

Succenturiate Placenta

The **succenturiate placenta** is a lesser variant with a smaller accessory lobe of placental tissue attached to the main lobe by vessels and membranes. Like patients with bipartite placenta, patients with succenturiate lobe are at increased risk for vasa previa and postpartum bleeding (Figures 5-15 B–D).

Annular Placenta

Annular placenta/placenta membranacea is a thin ring-shaped placenta that attaches circumferentially to the myometrium. This anomaly is rare, occurring in only 1 of 3300 deliveries. Associated complications include placenta previa, prenatal hemorrhage, intrauterine growth restriction, and preterm delivery.

Figure 5-15. A *Bipartite placenta.* **B** *Specimen of a succenturiate lobe.* **C** *Succenturiate lobe of placenta noted along posterior wall while the main placenta is anterior. Color shows vessel attachment.* **D** *Bipartite placenta showing vascular attachments (arrows).*

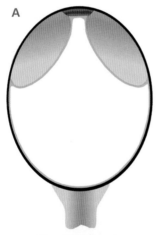

A

Bipartite placenta

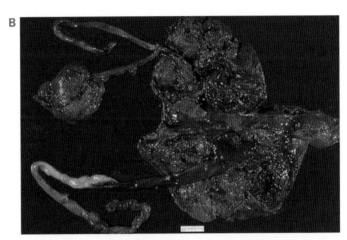

B

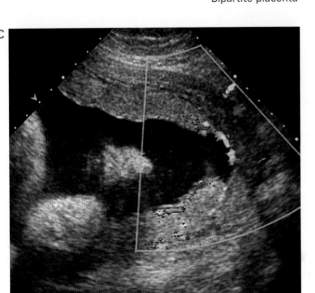

C

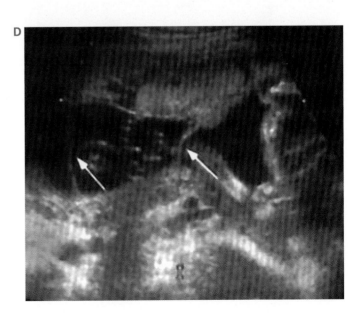

D

Placenta Previa

In **placenta previa**, a portion of the placenta covers the internal cervical os. There are several classifications of this condition:

- *Complete*: Bulk of placenta covers the entire internal cervical os.
- *Partial*: Part of the internal cervical os is covered by placenta.
- *Marginal*: Placenta encroaches upon but does not cover the internal cervical os.
- *Low-lying*: Lower edge of placenta extends into lower uterine segment within 2 cm of the internal cervical os (Figure 5-16A).

There are a number of risk factors associated with placenta previa, including advanced maternal age, multiple D&C procedures, multiparity, and previous c-section, each of which triples one's risk (Box 5-4). Why this is so

is unclear, but it is thought to be associated with scarring of the internal uterine surface and poorly vascularized endometrium. Also, studies have suggested that patients who have had a previous transverse c-section incision are at greater risk for placenta previa than those having a vertical incision, as the placenta favors attaching to the site of the prior incision. Clinical complications include potential hemorrhage from the large retroplacental blood vessels at the time of labor and delivery requiring a c-section delivery.

The cardinal clinical symptom for placenta previa is "painless" vaginal bleeding. Other causes for spotting during pregnancy include cervicitis, cervical polyps, and a bloody show prior to the onset of normal labor.

True placenta previa cannot be diagnosed sonographically prior to 34–36 weeks unless more than one-third of the placental mass covers the internal cervical os (Figure 5-16B). Because of placental retraction, marginal and

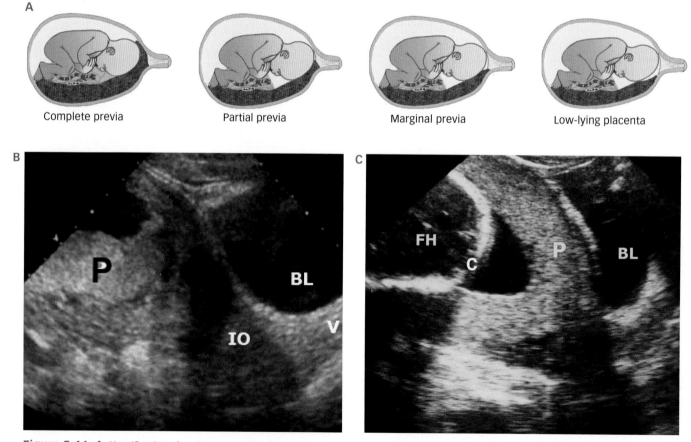

A

Complete previa   Partial previa   Marginal previa   Low-lying placenta

B

P   BL
IO   V

C

FH   C   P   BL

Figure 5-16. A *Classifications for placenta previa.* **B** *Posterior placenta previa. BL = maternal bladder, IO = internal os region, V = vagina, P = placenta.* **C** *Example of a total placenta previa. Note that the fetal head (FH) is not in close proximity to the crucial triangle. C = cervix, P = placenta, BL = maternal bladder.*

low-lying placentas diagnosed in the second trimester should be re-evaluated near term to confirm the initial diagnosis. Special attention to the lower uterine segment—imaging the cervix, maternal bladder, and sacral prominence (**crucial triangle**)—will assist in diagnosing placenta previa (Figure 5-16C). By the late third

trimester, the fetal presenting part should come in close proximity to this crucial triangle. An eccentric fetal lie should initiate the search to rule out placenta previa (Figures 5-17 A and B).

Pitfalls of diagnosing placenta previa include imaging with an overdistended maternal bladder, lower uterine segment myometrial contractions, and vasa previa. An overdistended maternal bladder can compress the anterior portion of the lower uterine segment against the posterior portion while elongating the cervix. This can give the appearance of placenta previa (Figure 5-17C). Postvoid imaging is recommended in these cases to verify the diagnosis. Contractions in the lower uterine segment can have the same effect (Figure 5-17D). **Vasa previa** is the term used to describe the velamentously inserted

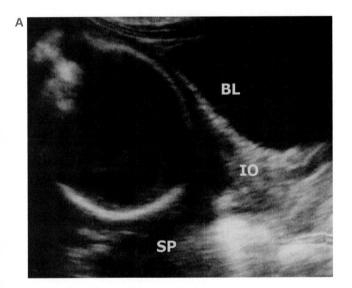

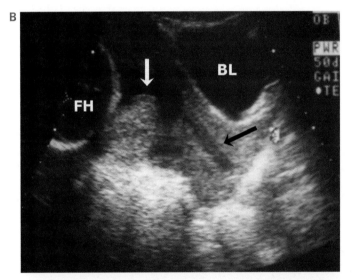

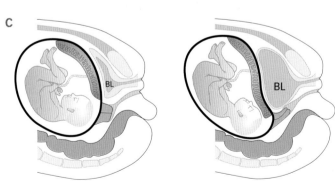

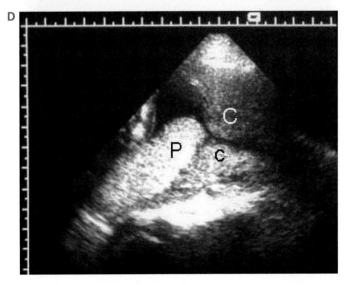

Figure 5-17. A *Longitudinal view of the lower uterine segment demonstrating the crucial triangle. BL = bladder, IO = internal os, SP = sacral prominence.* **B** *Longitudinal image of the lower uterine segment demonstrating a marginal posterior placenta. Note the hypoechoic endocervical canal (black arrow) and the placental edge (white arrow). BL = maternal bladder, FH = fetal head.* **C** *Schematic of a false placenta previa due to an overdistended maternal bladder (BL).* **D** *Anterior lower uterine segment contraction. P = placenta, C = contraction, c = cervix.*

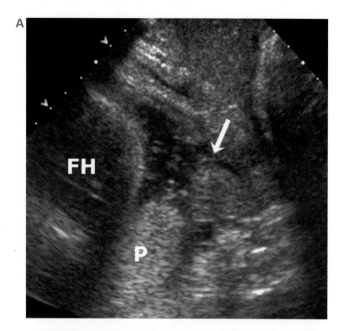

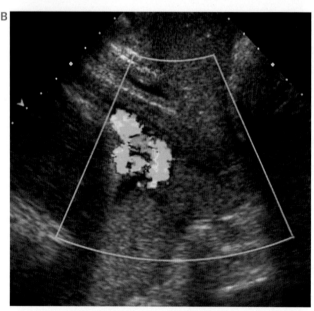

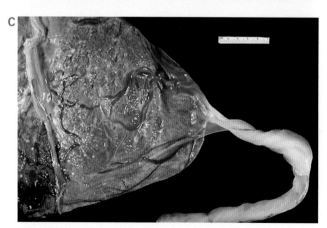

Figure 5-18. A *Internal cervical os demonstrated by arrow with loops of umbilical cord seen between fetal head (FH) and os. P = placenta.* **B** *Same image with color applied to demonstrate cord.* **C** *Specimen of a velamentous cord insertion.*

cord vessels that precede presenting fetal parts. This too requires delivery by c-section as a vaginal delivery would cause serious cord compression (Figure 5-18).

Placental Abruption

The premature separation of the placenta from the uterine wall is referred to as **placental abruption**, **placenta abruptio**, or **abruptio placentae**. Intrauterine bleeding occurs in all cases and, if severe, fetal and/or maternal death may occur. The perinatal mortality rate can be as high as 25%. Risk factors include advanced maternal age, cigarette smoking, maternal vascular/renal disease, maternal hypertension, trauma, short umbilical cord, cocaine abuse, submucosal fibroids, placenta previa, uterine anomalies, and premature rupture of membranes (Box 5-5). Hemorrhages are classified as *apparent* or *concealed*, and clinical signs depend on the type of abruption (Figure 5-19A). Patients may have no symptoms, or they may present with signs of acute hemorrhage and shock. The apparent hemorrhage is usually a clinical diagnosis. Symptoms include vaginal bleeding with severe abdominal pain, a rigid, board-like uterus, and elevated maternal blood pressure. The **concealed abruption** occurs in about 20% of cases, and the hemorrhage is confined to the uterine cavity (Figure 5-19B). The detachment of the placenta may be complete and the consequences severe. Other more severe clinical signs include evidence of fetal distress, hypovolemic shock, and disseminated intravascular coagulopathy (DIC).

An abruption is pathologically graded from 0 to 3 as defined in Box 5-6. Sonographic findings vary depending on type, size, location, and age of blood clot. The

Box 5-5.	Associated risks for placental abruption.
	Advanced maternal age
	Smoking
	Cocaine abuse
	Trauma
	Maternal disease (hypertension, renal, vascular)
	Short umbilical cord
	Submucosal fibroids
	Uterine anomalies
	Placenta previa
	Premature rupture of membranes

most common is that of a mass or fluid collection at the margin of the placenta, which causes elevation of the placental edge. There may be bulging of the placenta in the region of the abruption, causing it to look thickened. Bleeding into the amniotic fluid causes the fluid to appear speckled on sonography. Fresh blood collections associated with the abruption placenta will be echo-free and then complex to solid as clot develops, finally resuming its echo-free character as liquefaction occurs. An abruption may resolve spontaneously and appear as a normal placenta (Figures 5-19 C and D).

Box 5-6.	Grading system for placental abruption.

Grade 0 = Asymptomatic (diagnosed by clot in placenta after delivery)

Grade 1 = Vaginal bleeding with changes in maternal vital signs

Grade 2 = Maternal symptoms + fetal distress

Grade 3 = Severe fetal distress/negative fetal heart tones (−FHTs)

Figure 5-19. A *Types of placental abruption.* **B** *Concealed and external hemorrhage.* **C** *Hypoechoic area of bleeding between the placenta (P) and myometrium (M) associated with placental abruption.* **D** *Anterior placenta (P) demonstrating an area of abruption (A). Note how the placenta droops at the level of the hematoma.*

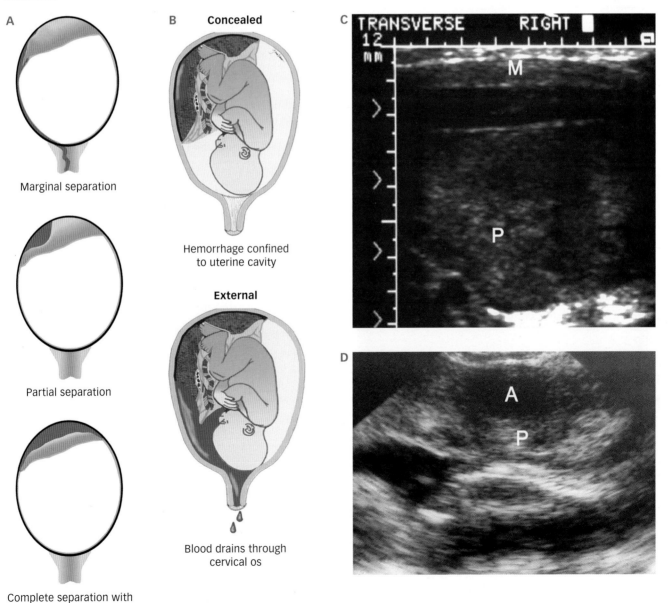

A

Marginal separation

Partial separation

Complete separation with concealed hemorrhage

B   **Concealed**

Hemorrhage confined to uterine cavity

External

Blood drains through cervical os

C   TRANSVERSE   RIGHT
12
mm
M

P

D

A

P

Abnormalities of Adherence

Deficiency of decidua during implantation may cause placental villi to adhere to the myometrium. These adhesions are referred to as *placenta accreta*, *increta*, and *percreta* (Figure 5-20A):

1. **Placenta accreta** is the condition in which placental villi penetrate the decidua but do not invade the myometrium. It is usually the result of a defect in or the absence of the decidua basalis. It is the most common abnormality of adherence (60%) and the least severe.

2. **Placenta increta** involves further penetration of the villi into the myometrium but not the serosa.

3. **Placenta percreta**, a condition in which the villi penetrate through both the myometrium and serosa, may result in uterine rupture.

There can be variable degrees of adherence, classified as *focal*, *partial*, or *complete*. Focal adherence indicates that only a small localized area of the placenta is invasive, while partial or complete adherence indicates that more or all of the placenta is affected. In some cases the placenta may attach to other organs, such as the bladder or rectum.

Although these conditions are considered rare, there seems to be an increase in incidence thought to be due to the increased number of c-sections performed.

Predisposing factors for placenta accreta, increta, and percreta include previous cesarean section, placenta previa, D&C, grand multiparity, endometritis, submucosal fibroids, synechiae (Asherman syndrome), advanced maternal age, and adenomyosis (Box 5-7). Placenta accreta occurs with placenta previa in about 10% of cases. Additional risk factors include smoking and hypertension.

Box 5-7.	**Predisposing factors for abnormalities of placental adherence.**
	Synechiae (Asherman syndrome)
	Previous D&C
	Previous c-section
	Previous placenta previa
	Grand multiparity
	Submucosal fibroids
	Endometritis
	Adenomyosis
	Advanced maternal age
	Smoking
	Hypertension

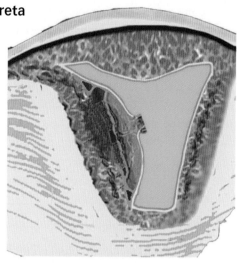

A Placenta Accreta

Villi attach to myometrium

No invasion

Placenta Increta

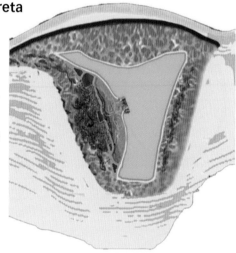

Villi invade uterine wall

Penetrate uterine muscle

Placenta Percreta

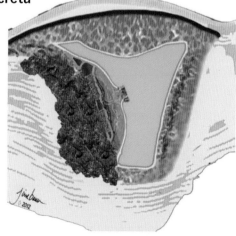

Penetration of uterine wall

Attachment to other organs

Figure 5-20. A *The various types of placental attachments. Following page:* **B** *Example of placenta increta. There is no delineation between placenta and myometrium as the placenta has grown into the myometrium. P = placenta.* **C** *Increased color Doppler flow in retroplacental space with extension into (increta) (straight arrows) or through myometrium (percreta) (curved arrow).*

Prenatally, there may be no apparent clinical signs, or there can be associated maternal hemorrhage in the third trimester as well as abnormally high beta-hCG and maternal alpha-fetoprotein levels in the second trimester. If hemorrhage occurs, there is an increased risk of maternal and fetal morbidity and mortality. Total hysterectomy is usually necessary with deep invasion of the placenta because the placenta cannot be delivered normally and hemorrhage will ultimately result in extensive postpartum bleeding.

Sonographic diagnosis is difficult and depends on the type of adherence. Criteria include:

- Absence of normal-appearing retroplacental space with loss of venous Doppler flow—accreta

- Reduction in the appearance of myometrial thickness—accreta

- Loss of the hyperechoic serosal border

- Myometrium appears thicker and more echogenic—increta (Figure 5-20B)

- Increased color Doppler flow in retroplacental space with extension into (increta) or through myometrium (percreta) (Figure 5-20C)

- Multiple venous lakes

Although sonography can be used to evaluate the placental attachment, MRI is more helpful in identifying the specific type of invasion.

Conservative treatments include medical management with methotrexate, angiographically directed embolization, and surgical wedge resection. A newer method is an operative technique in which a vertical incision is made and the uterus turned inside out so the placenta can be manually removed.

Chorioangioma

Occurring in approximately 1 out of 100 deliveries, the **chorioangioma** is a vascular (angiomatous) tumor of the chorion that can be microscopic or several centimeters in size. It is considered the most common tumor of placental origin, and it is benign. It is usually located along the fetal surface of the placenta and can vary in appearance from solid and homogeneous to complex. Doppler and color flow findings also vary.

When chorioangiomas are large (>5 cm), complications may occur, such as polyhydramnios and fetal circulatory and cardiopulmonary disorders (Table 5-2).

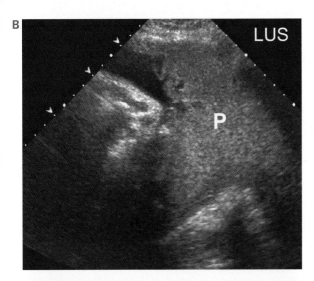

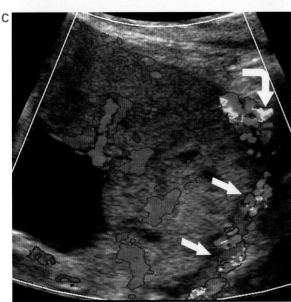

Figure 5-20, continued.

Table 5-2.   Complications of chorioangioma.

Fetal	Maternal
Congestive heart failure	Polyhydramnios
IUGR	Toxemia
Nonimmune hydrops	Preterm labor
Hemangioma	Thrombocytopenia
Anemia	Elevated maternal serum alpha-fetoprotein

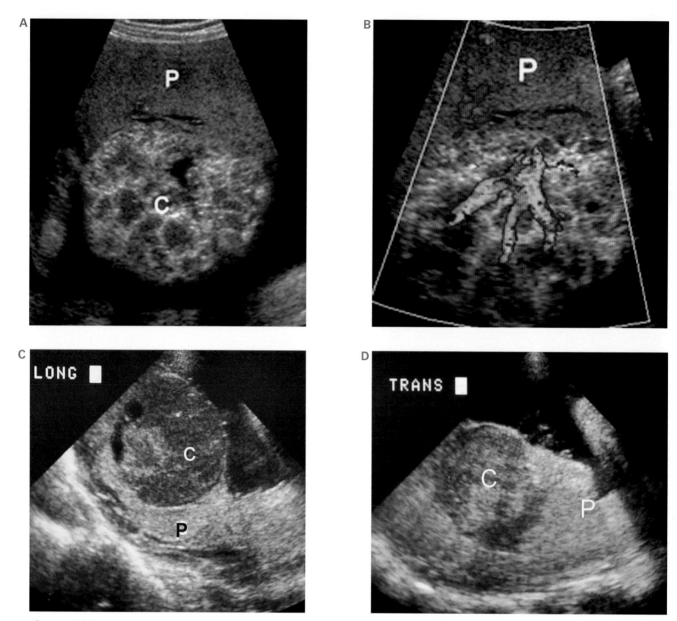

Figure 5-21. *Chorioangioma of the placenta without (**A**) and with (**B**) color. P = placenta, C = chorioangioma. Longitudinal (**C**) and transverse (**D**) images of a chorioangioma.*

Chorioangiomas may also be associated with placental abruption, intrauterine growth restriction, preterm labor, and an elevated alpha-fetoprotein (Figure 5-21).

CORD ABNORMALITIES

The **umbilical cord** is formed by the fusion of the body stalk and the yolk stalk. The **body stalk** contains the umbilical vessels and allantois, while the **yolk stalk** contains the vitelline vessels and vitelline (omphalomesenteric) duct (Figure 5-22A). The normal umbilical cord contains two arteries and one vein that allow for transport of blood between the fetus and the fetal portion of the placenta (Figures 5-22 B–C). The larger umbilical vein carries oxygenated blood; the two smaller arteries carry deoxygenated blood. Average length is 55 cm (range = 30–120 cm), with a maximum transverse diameter of no more than 2 cm. Cord edema (Figure 5-23) can be associated with Rh isoimmunization, respiratory distress, transient tachypnea, macerated stillbirth, and placental abruption. The entire cord is covered by amnion, and the vessels are surrounded by **Wharton's jelly**, which helps protect the cord from compression.

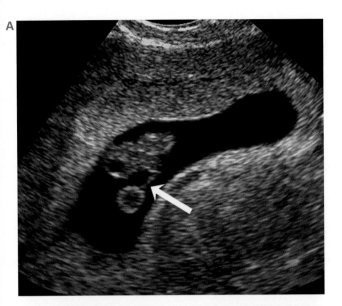

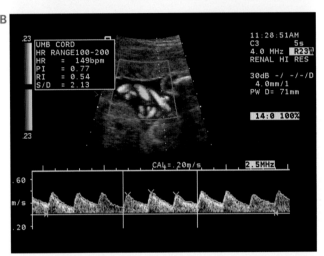

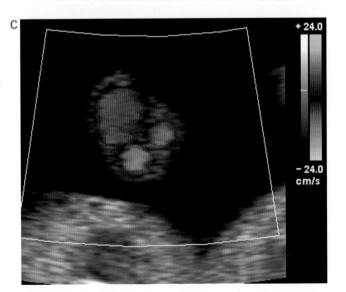

Figure 5-22. A *Vitelline duct (arrow) connecting the yolk sac to the embryo.* **B** *Doppler waveform of a normal umbilical artery demonstrating low-resistance flow.* **C** *Transverse image of three-vessel umbilical cord showing two small arteries and one large vein creating the "Mickey Mouse" appearance.*

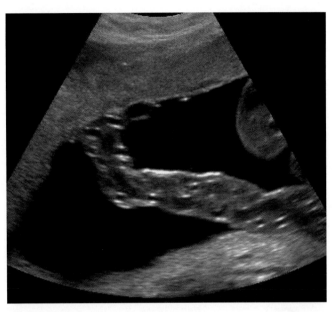

Figure 5-23. *Edematous umbilical cord.*

Box 5-8.	Abnormalities associated with single umbilical artery (SUA).

Trisomies 13 & 18

Genitourinary (GU) anomalies

Cardiac anomalies

CNS anomalies

Abdominal wall defects

VACTERL syndrome

Sirenomelia

Intrauterine growth restriction (IUGR)

Single Umbilical Artery

Absence of an umbilical artery—or **single umbilical artery** (**SUA**)—is believed to occur in 1% of all live births. Single umbilical artery is frequently referred to as a **two-vessel cord**. It may be caused by:

- Primary agenesis of one of the arteries
- Secondary atrophy of a previously present artery
- Persistence of the original, single embryonic artery

By itself, a two-vessel cord does not put the fetus at risk. However, single umbilical artery may be associated with other anomalies in as many as 20%–60% of cases (Box 5-8). For this reason, prenatal discovery of an absent umbilical artery (Figure 5-24) should prompt a thorough survey of the fetal anatomy.

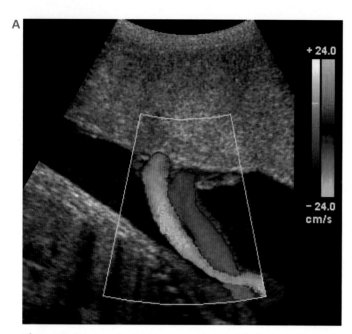

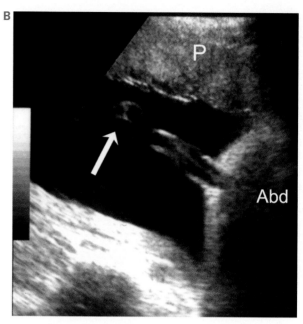

Figure 5-24. *Longitudinal two-vessel cord with (**A**) and without (**B**) color. Cord insertion into the fetal abdomen demonstrates only two vessels. Note the transverse cross-section (arrow). Abd = fetal abdomen, P = placenta.*

A multivessel cord (>3 vessels) is far rarer than the single umbilical artery, but it too has been associated with anomalies, as well as conjoined twinning.

Short Cord

If the umbilical cord is abnormally short (<35 cm), a number of complications may arise. The fetus may not be able to descend normally during labor, and as it attempts to do so the cord may become stressed and compressed, affecting the fetal heart rate, causing placental abruption, or both.

The severest complication associated with a short or absent cord is the **limb–body wall complex** (**LBWC**). This anomaly is characterized by a lethal exteriorization of the thoracoabdominal contents due to a lack of closure of the anterior abdominal wall. This occurs very early and results from abnormal folding and fusion of the body folds. The amnion adheres to the fetal surfaces and disrupts normal development. Also known as **body stalk anomaly**, **short umbilical cord syndrome**, and **cyllosoma**, limb–body wall complex has gross effects incompatible with life (Figure 5-25A). See Chapter 7 for additional information on limb–body wall complex.

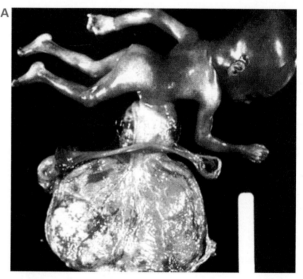

Figure 5-25. A *Body stalk anomaly. Following page:* **B** *First trimester (12 weeks) fetus showing adherence to the placenta typical of the limb–body wall complex due to absence or severe shortening of the umbilical cord.* **C** *Fetal organs are shown outside the abdominal cavity (torso) in this fetus with limb–body wall anomaly.* **D** *Second trimester fetus adhering to the anterior placenta (P). Note the hyperextension of the head and the fused single lower limb (arrow). FH = fetal head. The diagnosis was limb–body wall with sirenomelia.* **E** *Body stalk anomaly. P = placenta, A = abdominal contents.*

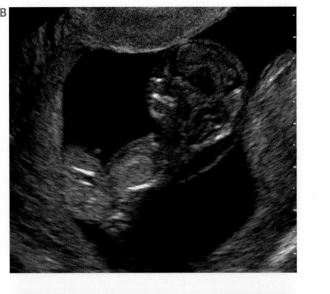

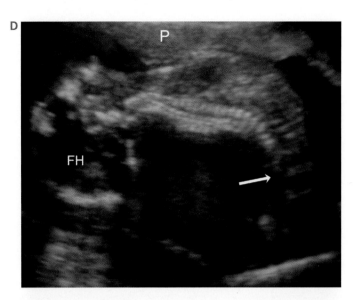

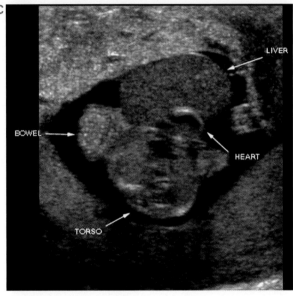

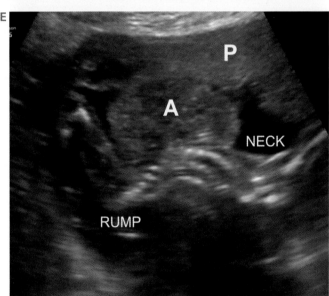

Figure 5-25, continued.

Sonographic findings include varying degrees of herniation of liver and abdominal viscera, including ectopia cordis, musculoskeletal deformities, and abnormalities of the central nervous system. The fetus or fetal parts appear to adhere to the placenta (Figures 5-25 B–E).

Long Cord

Complications resulting from an abnormally long umbilical cord (>80 cm) include true or false knots, prolapse, and the nuchal cord (Figure 5-26A).

False knots presenting as a focal bulge are simply folded loops of cord and rarely associated with complications. True knots, however, can lead to obstruction of blood flow to the fetus and consequent demise. True knots are not routinely identified sonographically but, when imaged, have the appearance of a cloverleaf (Figure 5-26B).

Cord prolapse results when compression of the umbilical cord cuts off the blood supply to the fetus. This is a life-threatening event for the fetus. Predisposing factors include fetal malpresentation, polyhydramnios, premature rupture of membranes (PROM), multiple gestations, and cephalopelvic disproportion.

A

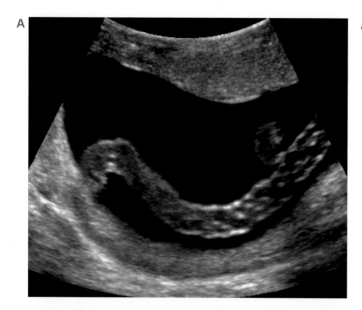

B

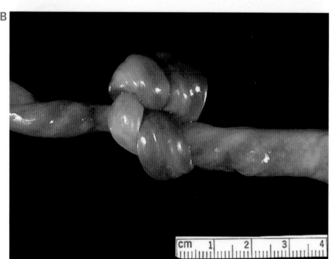

Figure 5-26. A *Long umbilical cord.* **B** *Cord knot.*

A

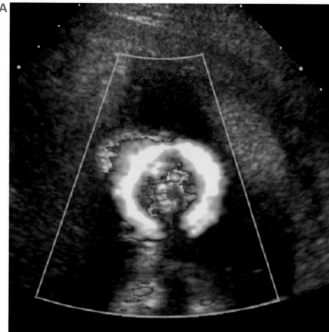

B

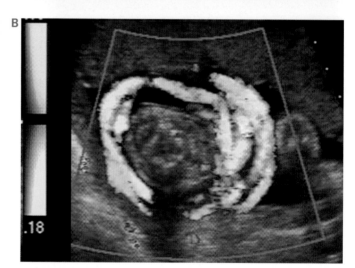

Figure 5-27. A *and* **B** *Nuchal cord demonstrated with color Doppler.*

Nuchal cord—wrapping of the umbilical cord around the fetal neck—occurs in about 25% of deliveries. Nuchal cord is rarely associated with fetal complications, and some clinicians prefer that it not be documented in the sonography report (Figure 5-27).

Umbilical Venous Thrombosis

Torsion, knotting, or compression of the umbilical cord may cause venostasis and ultimately **umbilical venous thrombosis**. Because occlusion of the umbilical vein prevents normal perfusion, fetal death almost always occurs. It occurs more frequently in fetuses of diabetic mothers

and in fetuses with nonimmune hydrops. Sonographic findings include increased echogenicity in the lumen of umbilical vessels and absence of Doppler signals within an umbilical vessel (Figure 5-28).

Cystic Structures

Cystic lesions of the umbilical cord may simply be the result of localized deposition and/or degeneration of the Wharton's jelly surrounding the cord. Aneurysms and

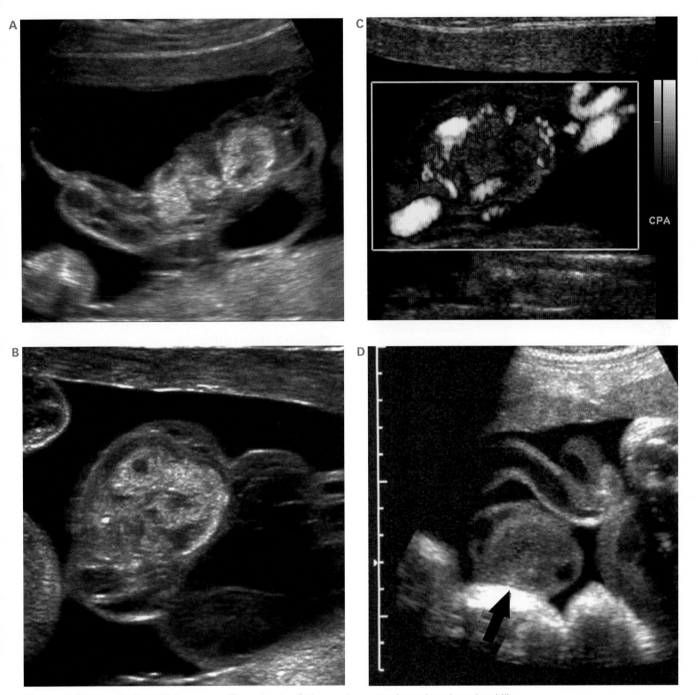

Figure 5-28. *Longitudinal (**A**), transverse (**B**), and color (**C**) image demonstrating a thrombosed umbilical cord presenting as a cord mass.* **D** *Umbilical cord cyst (arrow) adjacent to a normal transverse section showing three vessels.*

varices also can present as cystic masses or cord enlargement. These tend to thrombose and therefore require close monitoring. Color Doppler can assist in verifying whether or not the cyst is pathologically obstructing blood flow within the cord.

True Cysts

True cysts of the cord originate primarily from two developmental sources, the vitelline (omphalomesenteric) duct and the allantoic duct. The distinction between the two can only be made histologically. True cysts are not

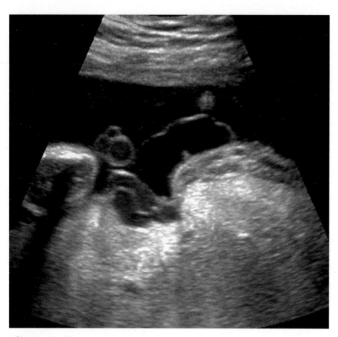

Figure 5-29. *Umbilical cord cyst.*

common, usually do not interfere with fetal circulation, and most often resolve spontaneously (Figure 5-29).

Vitelline/Omphalomesenteric Duct Cyst

The **vitelline** (**omphalomesenteric**) **duct cyst** of the umbilical cord is caused by the persistence and dilatation of the embryonic vitelline/omphalomesenteric duct. The cystic lesions are generally located close to the fetus and vary greatly in size. See Chapter 3 for additional information on the vitelline/omphalomesenteric duct.

The Allantoic Duct Cyst

The **allantoic cyst** is the cystic dilatation of the primitive embryonic allantois. It may be associated with other abnormalities of the genitourinary tract, including obstructive uropathy.

Abnormal Insertions

With normal developmental rotation of the embryo, the yolk sac and connecting stalk will be positioned opposite the implantation site, resulting in the central location of the umbilical cord insertion. Normal cord insertion into the placenta should be found in the middle of the placenta (Figure 5-30A). Further growth and development of the placenta cause the placenta to grow toward the areas of myometrium with the greatest blood supply, while the areas of lesser perfusion atrophy. When this happens, the cord occasionally inserts differently. This event, which leads to the unusual cord insertion, is referred to as **trophotropism**. Trophotropism is another explanation accepted for normal placental retraction (Figure 5-30B).

A

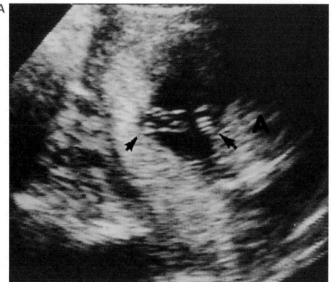

B

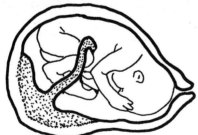

Central insertion—normal

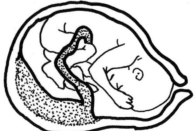

Marginal insertion
"battledore placenta"

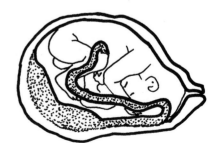

Velamentous insertion

Figure 5-30. A *Normal cord insertion (arrows) into a fundal placenta and fetal abdomen (A).*
B *Classifications for cord insertions.*

Battledore Placenta

The **battledore placenta** is one where the umbilical cord inserts at the edge of the placenta. This is sometimes referred to as a *marginal cord insertion*. It usually is of no clinical significance (Figure 5-30B).

Velamentous Insertion

Velamentous insertion differs from the marginal insertion because the attachment of the cord is to the membranes rather than to the placental mass, and attachment is at some distance from the fetal surface. Although rare, this condition carries significant risk of fetal morbidity and mortality. The cord is less protected and may be damaged during delivery. Because there are vessels that run between the membranes, there is a greater risk of cord shearing and positioning across the internal cervical os (vasa previa). Other associated complications include intrauterine growth restriction and preterm birth. Identification of vasa previa warrants delivery by cesarean section. (See Figure 5-31.)

Cord Masses

Solid tumors of the umbilical cord are rare and include the hemangioma and teratoma/dermoid. They usually occur at the cord insertion site and may be associated with an elevated AFP. An umbilical cord hematoma can be diffuse or focal and solid or cystic, depending on the age of the process. Causes include mechanical trauma between fetal/maternal tissues, cord knots/torsion, or traction on a

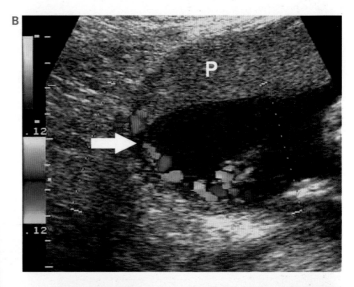

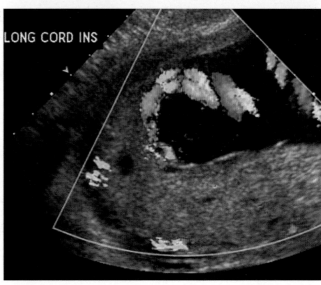

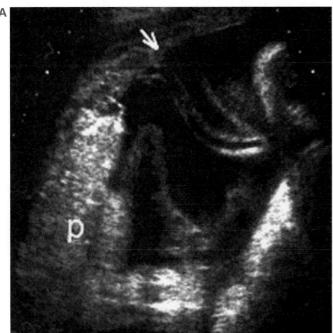

Figure 5-31. A *Velamentous insertion. P = placenta.* **B** *Color Doppler demonstrates cord insertion at periphery of placenta (arrow), P = placenta.* **C** *Color image of a long cord insertion.*

shortened cord. The incidence of umbilical cord hematoma seems to have increased as the numbers of invasive procedures, such as percutaneous blood sampling (PUBS), have increased (see Chapter 15). Cord hematomas carry a poor prognosis with a very high perinatal loss (50%), warranting close clinical follow-up (Box 5-9).

Box 5-9.	Cord abnormalities detectable with sonography.
	Knots (true & false)
	Nuchal
	SUA and multiple vessels
	Enlarged
	Absence
	Cysts
	Tumors
	Thrombosis
	Hematoma
	Patent urachus

SCANNING TIPS, GUIDELINES, AND PITFALLS

1. If a single umbilical artery (SUA) is suspected, be sure to scan the entire length of the cord, paying special attention to the cord insertion into the fetal abdomen. Sometimes the cord will show two vessels at one end but three at the other. Color Doppler can help to verify the two arteries surrounding the fetal bladder. If two arteries are noted at the fetal origin, the risk of associated fetal anomalies is very low—the same as that for normal three-vessel cords (Figure 5-32).

2. Although vaginal ultrasound can provide an excellent view of the cervix and internal cervical os, this technique is not recommended when placenta previa is suspected. An alternative technique is to scan the patient transperineally or translabially. The perspective is the same, but the technique does not necessitate instrumentation of the vagina (Figure 5-33).

3. When there is a suspicion of placenta previa, it is recommended that pre- and postvoid images be taken to rule out pseudo–placenta previa caused by overdistention of the maternal bladder.

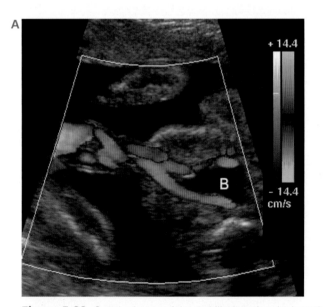
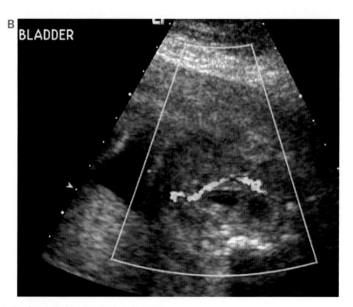

Figure 5-32. A Color image of the umbilical cord at the insertion into the fetal abdomen. Color demonstrates the two umbilical arteries surrounding the fetal bladder, which verifies a three-vessel cord. B = fetal bladder. **B** Color image showing a single umbilical artery at the level of the fetal bladder.

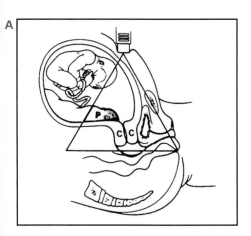

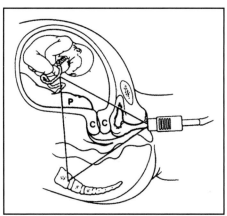

Figure 5-33. A *Schematics of translabial scan planes. Reprinted with permission from the American Journal of Roentgenology C = cervix, P = placenta.* **B** *Normal with fetal head (H) at internal os. B = maternal bladder.* **C** *Drawing of marginal placenta.* **D** *Translabial image of low-lying placenta. FH = fetal head, P = placenta.* **E** *Drawing of partial placenta previa.* **F** *Translabial image of partial placenta previa. C = cervix.*

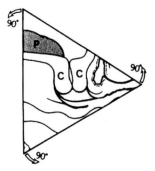

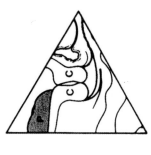

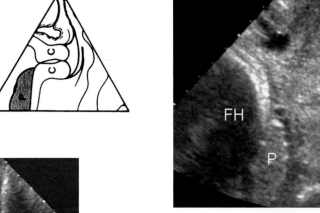

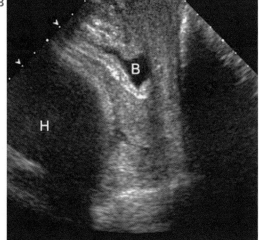

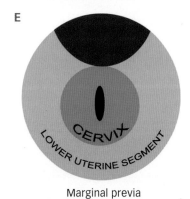

Marginal previa

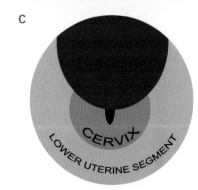

Partial previa

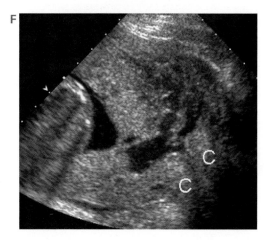

Figure 5-34. *Synechia vs. septum (coronal plane).*

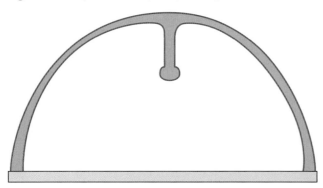

Synechia

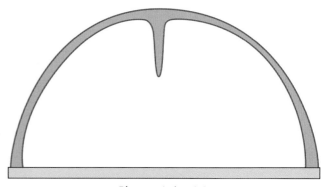

Bicornuate/septate

4. Scanning across the septum of a bicornuate, septated, or subseptate uterus can create the appearance of a **synechia**. The septation, however, will be centrally located, and the shelf-like membrane will extend from anterior myometrium and point toward the posterior myometrium. Unlike the synechia, which has a bulbous free edge, the septum tapers to a point (Figure 5-34).

5. The vascular venous bed behind a normal placenta is often quite prominent, with a posterior placenta, and can make one think the placenta is abrupted. Placental abruption is almost always clinically symptomatic. Placental abruption is not likely in the asymptomatic patient (Figure 5-35).

6. The circumvallate placenta can also appear to be separated from the uterine wall, and although this anomaly predisposes a patient to placental abruption, the diagnosis is not likely in the asymptomatic patient. Additional scanning along the periphery of the placenta will show the infolded portion as a thick linear band of placental tissue parallel to the chorionic surface with amniotic fluid trapped within the fold.

7. When measuring the placenta, one should obtain the measurement through the mid portion. Calipers should be placed perpendicularly from the chorionic plate extending to the basilar plate. Do not include the vascular retroplacental vessels, myometrium, fibroids, or focal myometrial contractions. Avoid using too much pressure while scanning because compression can affect the measurement. Special attention is necessary to obtain the correct axis when measuring the fundal placenta (Figure 5-36).

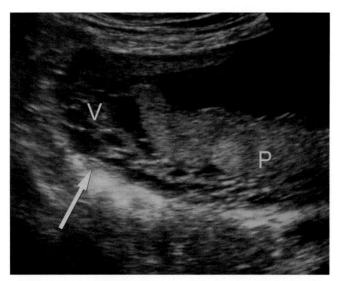

Figure 5-35. *Longitudinal placenta demonstrating engorged vessels in the retroplacental space, giving the appearance of an abruption (arrow). V = vessels, P = placenta.*

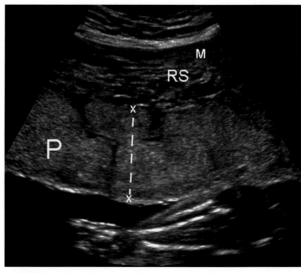

Figure 5-36. *Sonogram showing proper position of calipers (Xs) when measuring the placenta (P). Do not include the retroplacental vascular space (RS). M = myometrium.*

REFERENCES

Benirschke K: Normal early development. In Creasy RK, Resnick R (eds): *Maternal-Fetal Medicine: Principles and Practice*, 3rd Edition. Philadelphia, Saunders, 2008, pp 37–46.

Bey M, Dott A, Miller JM Jr: The sonographic diagnosis of circumvallate placenta. Obstet Gynecol 78 [Part 2]:515–517, 1991.

Bradley WG, Fiske CE, Filly RA: The double sac sign of early intrauterine pregnancy: use in exclusion of ectopic pregnancy. Radiology 143:223–226, 1982.

Brown HL, Miller JM, Khawali O, et al: Premature placental calcification in maternal cigarette smokers. Obstet Gynecol 71:914–917, 1988.

DeCherny AH, Nathan L, Goodwin TM: *Current Obstetric and Gynecologic Diagnosis and Treatment*, 10th Edition. New York, McGraw-Hill, 2006.

De Lange M, Rouse GA: *Ob/Gyn Sonography: An Illustrated Review*. Pasadena, CA, Davies, 2004.

Feldstein VA, Harris RD, Machin GA: Ultrasound evaluation of the placenta and umbilical cord. In Callen PW (ed): *Ultrasonography in Obstetrics and Gynecology*, 5th Edition. St. Louis, Saunders Elsevier, 2008, pp 721–757.

Finberg HJ: Umbilical cord and amniotic membranes. In McGahan JP, Porto M (eds): *Diagnostic Obstetrical Ultrasound*. Philadelphia, Lippincott, 1994, pp 104–133.

Fleischer AC, Finberg HJ, Graham DF: Sonography of the umbilical cord and intrauterine membranes. In Fleischer AC, Manning F, Jeanty B, et al (eds): *Sonography in Obstetrics and Gynecology, Principles and Practice*, 5th Edition. Stamford, CT, Appleton and Lange, 1996, pp 203–222.

Fleischer AC, Toy E, Lee W, et al: *Obstetrics and Gynecology: Principles and Practice*, 7th Edition. New York, McGraw-Hill, 2011.

Foy PM: The placenta. In Hagan-Ansert SL (ed): *Textbook of Diagnostic Ultrasonography*, 7th Edition. St. Louis, Elsevier Mosby, 2012, pp 1220–1237.

Gielchinsky Y, Mankuta D, Rojansky N, et al: Perinatal outcome of pregnancies complicated by placenta accreta. Obstet Gynecol 104:527–530, 2004.

Hagan-Ansert SL: The umbilical cord. In Hagan-Ansert SL (ed): *Textbook of Diagnostic Ultrasonography*, 7th Edition. St. Louis, Elsevier Mosby, 2012, pp 1238–1248.

Hung T, Shau W, Hsieh C, et al: Risk factors for placenta accreta. Obstet Gynecol 93:545–550, 1999.

Lyons AS, Petrucelli RJ: *Medicine: An Illustrated History*, Revised Edition. New York, Harry N. Abrams, 1997.

Montan S, Jorgensen C, Svalenius E, et al: Placental grading with ultrasound in hypertensive and normotensive pregnancies: a prospective, consecutive study. Acta Obstet Gynecol Scand 164:477–480, 1987.

Moore KL, Persuad TVN, Torchia MG: *The Developing Human: Clinically Oriented Embryology*, 9th Edition. Philadelphia, Elsevier Saunders, 2012.

Nelson LH: *Ultrasonography of the Placenta: A Review*. American Institute of Ultrasound in Medicine, 1994.

Nishijima K, Shukunami K, Arikura S, et al: An operative technique for conservative management of placenta accreta. Obstet Gynecol 105:1201–1203, 2005.

Proud J, Grant AM: Third trimester placental grading by ultrasonography as a test of fetal well-being. Br Med J 294:1641–1644, 1987.

Spirt BA, Gordon LP: The placenta and cervix. In McGahan JP, Porto M (eds): *Diagnostic Obstetrical Ultrasound*. Philadelphia, Lippincott, 1994, pp 83–102.

Spirt BA, Gordon LP: Sonography of the placenta. In Fleischer AC, Manning F, Jeanty B, et al (eds): *Sonography in Obstetrics and Gynecology, Principles and Practice*, 5th Edition. Stamford, CT, Appleton and Lange, 1996, pp 174–202.

Yeh HC: Sonographic signs of early pregnancy. Crit Rev Diagn Imaging 28:181–211, 1988.

SELF-ASSESSMENT EXERCISES

Questions

1. A normal term placenta should not measure more than:

   A. 1–2 cm

   B. 2–3 cm

   C. 3–4 cm

   D. 4–5 cm

   E. 5–6 cm

2. Of the following conditions, which would *not* be associated with a thick, hydropic placenta?

   A. Infections

   B. Intrauterine growth restriction

   C. Fetal hydrops

   D. Gestational diabetes

   E. Triploidy

3. "Decidua" refers to the:

   A. Endometrium

   B. Myometrium

   C. Perimetrium

   D. Uterine cavity

   E. None of the above

4. A vascular tumor of the chorion is referred to as a:

   A. Angioma

   B. Hemangioma

   C. Chorioangioma

   D. Angiomyoma

   E. Angiosarcoma

5. Which of the following statements is *not* true of placental circulation?

   A. The spiral arteries demonstrate low-pressure flow throughout pregnancy.

   B. Deoxygenated blood leaves the fetus by way of the umbilical vein.

   C. During pregnancy, fetal and maternal blood do not mix.

   D. Inadequate blood flow to the uterus can result in fetal hypoxia and intrauterine growth restriction (IUGR).

   E. The umbilical vein provides oxygenated blood to the fetus while the arteries return deoxygenated blood.

6. Which term would best describe this placenta?

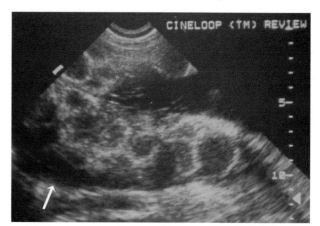

   A. Grade I

   B. Grade II

   C. Grade III

   D. Triploidy

   E. Abruptio

7. To what is the arrow pointing in the image in question 6?

   A. Placental cyst

   B. Abruptio placentae

   C. Submucous fibroid

   D. Retroplacental vessels

   E. Ascites

8. In this transverse image of pregnant uterus, which would best describe the placental location?

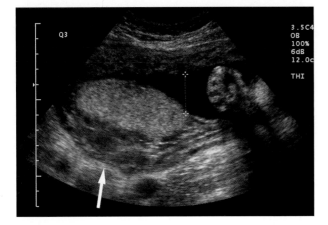

   A. Anterior

   B. Posterior

   C. Fundal

   D. Lateral

   E. Previa

9. To what is the arrow pointing in the image of an asymptomatic patient above?

   A. Abruptio placentae

   B. Myometrial contraction

   C. Retroplacental space

   D. Subchorionic hematoma

   E. Submucous fibroid

10. A placenta that has two equal lobes connected by vessels is called:

    A. Bipartite placenta

    B. Succenturiate lobe

    C. Circumvallate placenta

    D. Membranous placenta

    E. Lobar placenta

11. This patient presented with painless vaginal bleeding that was bright red. The most likely diagnosis is:

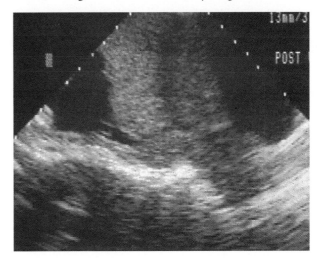

    A. Abruption placenta

    B. Placenta previa

    C. Marginal placenta

    D. Incompetent cervix

    E. Degenerating fibroid

12. When the placenta invades the myometrium and penetrates the serosa it is called:

    A. Placental abruption

    B. Placenta previa

    C. Placenta accreta

    D. Placenta percreta

    E. Placenta increta

13. Which of the following anomalies could be the result of a ruptured amniotic band?

    A. Alobar holoprosencephaly

    B. Situs inversus

    C. Duodenal atresia

    D. Renal agenesis

    E. Facial clefts

14. The placental edge should be at least which of the following distances from the internal cervical os to be considered in satisfactory position?

    A. 0.5 cm

    B. 1.0 cm

    C. 1.5 cm

    D. 2.0 cm

    E. 2.5 cm

15. The placenta's primary functions include all of the following *except*:

    A. Provides an interchange for gases

    B. Provides nutrients to the fetus

    C. Protects the fetus from infection

    D. Allows for transfer of antibodies and hormones

    E. Allows for waste excretion

Answers

See Appendix F on page 610 for answers and explanations.

Ultrasound of the Cervix during Pregnancy

Pamela M. Foy, MS, RDMS, FSDMS

OBJECTIVES

After completing this chapter you should be able to:

1. Explain how to image and properly measure cervical length in the pregnant patient.

2. Describe the sonographic features of cervical dilatation and associated funneling of intact membranes.

3. Discuss the differences between the Shirodkar and McDonald procedures.

4. List conditions associated with preterm cervical dilatation.

5. Describe the differences among transvaginal, transabdominal, and transperineal/translabial scanning techniques.

THE SONOGRAPHIC EVALUATION OF THE CERVIX has become part of the obstetric examination in many imaging centers. Improved probe technology has led to an expanding list of indications for the pregnant patient. Historically, the cervix was evaluated transabdominally during pregnancy, but transvaginal and transperineal imaging have become the techniques of choice because of superior image quality, reproducibility, and visualization of the cervix.

Women with the following problems may benefit from an ultrasound examination of the cervix:

1. Women with suspected cervical incompetence

2. Women with symptoms of preterm labor in current pregnancy

3. Asymptomatic pregnant women with risk factors for preterm birth

4. Women with suspected placenta previa or low-lying placenta (see also Chapter 5)

5. Women with suspected cervical pregnancy

Although asymptomatic pregnant women without risk factors for **preterm birth** (**PTB**) whose cervical length falls below the 10th percentile have been found to have an increased risk of preterm birth, it is not yet clear that this information can be used to improve the outcome of pregnancy. Studies have shown that the relative risk of premature delivery increases approximately 1.5 times for each 5 mm decrease in cervical length as measured by transvaginal sonography.

ANATOMY

The cervix, the cylindrical fibrous portion of the uterus, extends from the inferior end of the body or corpus of the uterus at the constricted isthmus to the superior portion of the vagina. The cervix protrudes into the superior part of the vagina and opens into it through the external cervical os. The internal cervical os is the opening of the cervix into the **uterine isthmus**. The cavity between these two openings—the **cervical canal**—is approximately 35 mm in length. The attachment of the vagina to the cervix divides the cervix into supra- and infravaginal segments. The blood supply of the uterus is derived primarily from the uterine arteries (Figure 6-1A), which are branches of the **internal iliac arteries** (Figure 6-1B). The uterine arteries course along the lateral aspect of the cervix.

Various cervical lengths have been reported transabdominally in a normal pregnancy, but this technique tends to produce measurements significantly longer than those recorded with either transvaginal or transperineal probes. In transabdominal studies of 100 pregnant and 50 nonpregnant women, Ayers et al. found that the average cervical length for the nonpregnant cervix was 25 mm compared to 37 mm for the pregnant cervix. The cervical measurements obtained in this study were rarely more than 60 mm. The reproducibility of these measurements is limited. A good rule of thumb for the pregnant cervix is it should never measure less than 3 cm.

CERVICAL LENGTH MEASUREMENTS

Many physicians rely on a **digital examination** of the cervix and an ultrasound examination of the cervix as these tests are complementary with important information gained from each. A digital examination of the cervix provides useful clinical information about dilation of the external cervical os, **effacement**, and station of the presenting part. The position of the cervix (anterior, mid, or posterior) and consistency (soft, medium, or firm) can also be determined digitally. However, the supravaginal portion of the cervix is difficult to evaluate digitally, especially in a closed cervix. The length of the vaginal portion of the cervix usually comprises about 50% of the

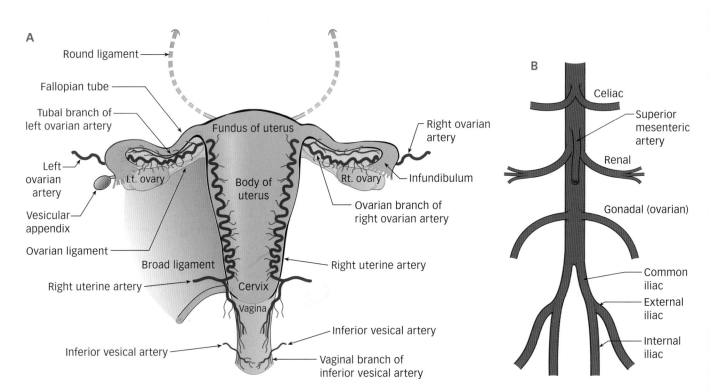

Figure 6-1. A *The uterine vasculature and the relationship of the cervix to the uterus and vagina.* **B** *The uterine arteries are branches of the internal iliac arteries; the gonadal arteries originate from the aorta.*

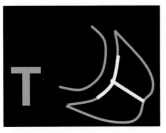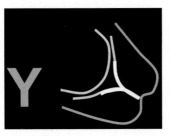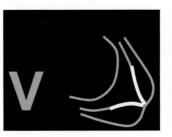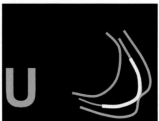

Figure 6-2. *Process of cervical effacement as viewed sonographically. Based on Zilianti M, Azuaga A, Calderon F, et al: Monitoring the effacement of the uterine cervix by transperineal sonography: a new perspective. J Ultrasound Med 14:719–724, 1995.*

total cervical length. Therefore, digital evaluation of the length of the cervix is subjective and may be inconsistent. In contrast, sonographic measurement of cervical length generates images that can be standardized, avoiding the subjectivity of the digital examination.

Cervical length can be obtained sonographically by measuring with electronic calipers the distance from the internal cervical os to the external cervical os. Cervical length by ultrasound may vary depending on the technique used. The longest cervical measurements are usually obtained with the transabdominal technique. This measurement is influenced by maternal bladder fullness. The effect of maternal bladder filling can therefore not be estimated or controlled for by standardizing the apparent volume of urine in the maternal bladder.

In 1995, Zilianti et al. nicely demonstrated the process of effacement of the uterine cervix sonographically (Figure 6-2). From the beginning of labor the cervical canal shortens progressively and a funnel-shaped internal cervical os (ICO) occurs until complete cervical effacement is achieved. As the length of the cervix shortens, noticeable changes occur at the internal cervical os. The letters T Y V U illustrate the cervical changes. Progressive changes occur in the superior portion of the cervix (ICO), whereas the inferior part, the external cervical os (ECO), maintains the same characteristics it has at the beginning of labor. Effacement usually precedes dilatation in both **primiparous** and **multiparous** patients. While these changes have been described in women actively in labor, changes of the internal cervical os can be routinely visualized in women with **preterm labor** (**PTL**) and incompetent cervix. The dilated os is visualized with sonography as **funneling** when the amniotic sac protrudes into the endocervical canal. Funneling can be a subjective finding and false positives can arise with transabdominal

and transvaginal scanning—transabdominally from bladder overdistention and from contractions of the lower uterine segment, transvaginally from undue pressure on the cervix from the transducer. Criteria for documenting funneling have been described, including (see Figure 6-3):

1. Funnel width—dilatation of the internal cervical os
2. Funnel length—length of a line that connects the apex of the funnel to the superior edge of the base of the funnel
3. Functional length—cervical length distal to the funnel extending to the external cervical os

The functional cervical length—the length of the cervix distal to the funnel—has been the most consistently measured and has been related to the risk of preterm birth in virtually every study.

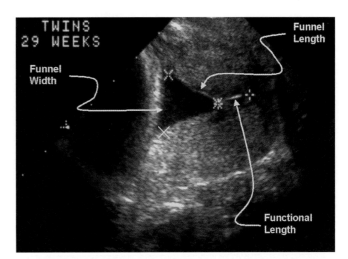

Figure 6-3. *Transvaginal image of the cervix demonstrating how to measure the functional length of the cervix, funnel width, and funnel length. Reprinted with permission from Zilianti M, et al: Monitoring the effacement of the uterine cervix by transperineal sonography: a new perspective. J Ultrasound Med 14:719–724, 1995.*

CERVICAL INCOMPETENCE

Cervical incompetence, or passive premature cervical dilation, is a leading cause of second trimester pregnancy loss. It is marked by painless dilation and effacement of the cervix with bulging and later rupture of the membranes. In order for the diagnosis to be established, the patient must have had a prior second trimester pregnancy loss or a delivery of an early preterm fetus. Common causes of incompetent cervix are congenital weakness and prior trauma to the cervix, frequently from prior obstetric lacerations and less commonly from gynecologic procedures such as **D&C** (**dilatation and curettage**) or **cone biopsy** (removal of a thin or thick cone-shaped piece of abnormal cervical tissue). Uterine anomalies as well as DES (diethylstilbestrol) exposure have been associated with congenital structural changes of the cervix. When the diagnosis of incompetent cervix is not clearly evident by the patient's history, weekly digital assessment of the cervix between 18 and 24 weeks' gestation has become customary. Digital surveillance lacks precision and places great weight on the examiner's somewhat subjective assessment of cervical length, position, dilation, and consistency. The ultrasound features typical of cervical incompetence are more reproducible and include:

1. Cervical length < 20 mm (Figure 6-4)

2. Funneling—bulging of the membranes into the cervical canal (Figure 6-5)

3. Open internal cervical os > 20 mm in width

4. **Hourglass membranes**—fetal membranes prolapsed through the external cervical os (Figure 6-6)

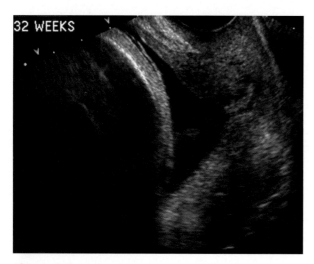

Figure 6-4. *Transvaginal long-axis view of cervix. Functional cervical length is 10 mm and funnel length is 27 mm.*

CERCLAGE

Obstetricians have searched for a surgical procedure that may strengthen the cervix. In 1955, Shirodkar placed a submucosal band at the internal cervical os to manage cervical incompetence. This technique was performed during pregnancy and required anterior displacement of the bladder with submucosal dissection. The **Shirodkar cerclage** ("stitch" or "suture") can be left in place for subsequent pregnancies provided a c-section is performed. Several years later, McDonald described the use of a purse-string technique that could also be used during pregnancy (Figure 6-7). The **McDonald purse-string**

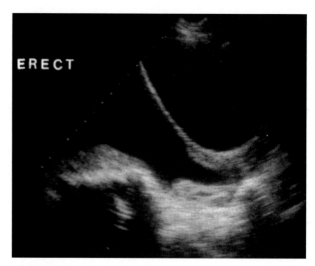

Figure 6-5. *Transabdominal image displaying funneling. The fetal membranes can be seen bulging into the cervical canal.*

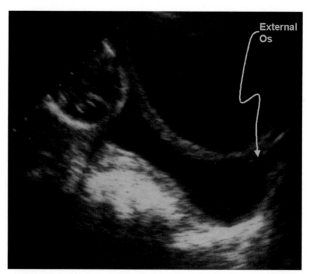

Figure 6-6. *Transabdominal image of "hourglass membranes." The fetal membranes are prolapsed through the external cervical os (arrow).*

technique has proven to be as successful as the Shirodkar cerclage and involves considerably less dissection. It has a high rate of success and low rate of complications.

These techniques may be used prophylactically or emergently depending on when the diagnosis is made. In women with a classic history of painless dilation in a previous pregnancy before 26 weeks, prophylactic placement of a cerclage is often performed at 10–15 weeks' gestation. Complications of a prophylactic cerclage include bleeding, infection, and slippage of the cerclage into the distal portion of the cervix. Cerclage may be placed emergently in women who present with advanced dilatation of the internal cervical os with bulging membranes. Different techniques are available to the obstetrician to elevate the membranes out of the surgical field. It is very uncommon

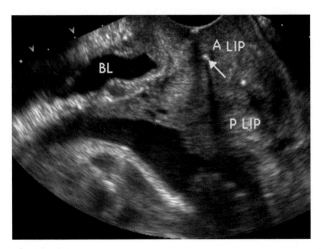

Figure 6-7. *Transvaginal long-axis view of cervix with McDonald stitch. BL = maternal bladder, A LIP = anterior lip, P LIP = posterior lip.*

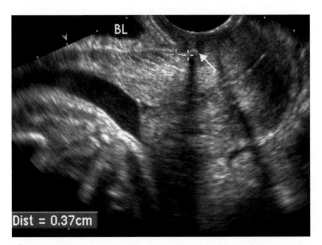

Figure 6-8. *Transvaginal image of cervix with a McDonald cerclage. Stitch that shadows (arrow) is seen in the anterior lip of the cervix. One should always evaluate the placement of the stitch relative to the maternal bladder (BL).*

to perform a cerclage after 26 weeks' gestation due to the risk of inducing ruptured membranes or preterm labor.

Cerclage sutures are not usually placed under sonographic guidance. However, some physicians are now performing a transvaginal examination during the operative procedure to evaluate the stitch's position before leaving the operating room. Best results are expected when the stitch is within the middle or upper third of the cervix (Figure 6-8). It is important to make certain that the placement of the stitch in the anterior lip of the cervix is not so high that it compromises the maternal urethra or urinary bladder. Periodic vaginal sonography should be performed to reassess the stitch position and evaluate for funneling.

PRETERM LABOR AND PREMATURE BIRTH

Premature birth is a major cause of perinatal morbidity and mortality. About 12.5% of US births—500,000 per year—are preterm. Most of these births occur after 32 weeks' gestation, when the outcome is expected to be very good. However, about 2% of preterm births occur before 32 weeks' gestation. Infants born at 24 weeks' gestation have a 10%–15% chance of survival. At 26 weeks' gestation the rate of survival is 80%, and at 28 weeks' gestation it is greater than 90%. Premature infants have a higher incidence of developmental delay, visual and hearing impairment, chronic lung disease, and cerebral palsy. The neonatal mortality rate is higher for males than for females.

Prematurity is considered a multifactorial problem and can include preterm labor, premature rupture of membranes, pre-eclampsia, abruptio placentae, multiple gestation, placenta previa, fetal growth restriction, excessive or inadequate amniotic fluid volume, fetal anomalies, **amnionitis**, and incompetent cervix. Maternal medical problems, including diabetes, asthma, drug abuse, and pyelonephritis, may all lead to preterm delivery. (See Box 6-1.) These clinical disorders can be divided into two broad categories called *spontaneous* or *indicated preterm births.* Approximately 75% of preterm births occur spontaneously after preterm labor or preterm premature rupture of membranes. Indicated preterm births follow medical or obstetric disorders that place the fetus at risk (maternal hypertension, diabetes, placenta previa or abruption, IUGR).

Risk for preterm delivery is associated with maternal characteristics such as ethnic origin, age, cigarette smoking, and drug abuse. Historical risk factors can include

Box 6-1.	Preterm delivery: a multifactorial problem.

Preterm labor

Premature rupture of membranes

Pre-eclampsia

Abruptio placentae

Multiple gestation

Placenta previa

Fetal growth restriction

Excessive or inadequate AFV

Fetal anomalies

Amnionitis

Incompetent cervix

Maternal medical problems, e.g., diabetes, asthma, pyelonephritis, drug abuse

Crohn's disease

cervical cone biopsy, cervical laceration, DES exposure in utero, previous second trimester pregnancy loss, uterine anomalies, and myomas. Painless dilation of the internal cervical os can be present in patients without identifiable risk factors.

A multicenter ultrasound study conducted by the Maternal-Fetal Medicine Units Network of the National Institute of Child Health and Human Development (NICHD) found that the degree of cervical shortening and the magnitude of endocervical funneling were correlated with the risk of preterm birth as a continuum rather than an all-or-nothing phenomenon. In this study, cervical length measurements of 2915 women were obtained transvaginally at 24 and 28 weeks' gestation. Cervical length at the 75th percentile was 40 mm, at the 50th percentile 35 mm, at the 25th percentile 30 mm, at the 10th percentile 26 mm, at the 5th percentile 22 mm, and at the 1st percentile 13 mm. These results demonstrate an inverse relationship between cervical length measurement and the relative risk of preterm delivery. Other studies have confirmed results of the NICHD study.

Multiple Gestation

Some women with multiple gestations seem to do well, while others have difficulty with preterm labor. The literature on the care of multiple gestations is contradictory. Some recommend bed rest (at home or in the hospital), home uterine activity monitoring, oral tocolytics, and/or cerclage. Identification of twin gestations at low risk

for preterm birth can allow physicians to be selective in choosing interventions to prevent prematurity.

More ultrasound data are available on women with possible incompetent cervix and risk of preterm birth than on normal subjects. Several studies indicate that:

1. The range of cervical length prior to 20 weeks is considerably greater than that for measurements made after 20 weeks.

2. After 20 weeks' gestation, the cervical length appears to shorten with increasing gestational age. Median values at 24–28 weeks are 35–40 mm and after 32 weeks, 30–35 mm.

3. Cervical effacement begins at the internal cervical os. This process, called funneling in the second and early third trimesters, is effacement in progress.

These findings are consistently associated with an increased risk of preterm birth: before 32 weeks' gestation an internal os funnel that is approximately 40%–50% or more of the total cervical length and a cervical length that is less than the 10th (26 mm) to 25th (30 mm) percentiles.

While there is a relationship between short cervix and preterm birth, an effective intervention has not yet been found. Cervical sonography can be helpful for women who are thought to be at risk for preterm birth by excluding those with a long cervix from unnecessary treatment.

Placenta Previa

Implantation of the placenta over the internal cervical os is defined as placenta previa. (See Chapter 5.) There are three recognized variations of placenta previa: total, partial, and marginal (Figure 6-9). In **total** (or **complete**) **placenta previa** the internal cervical os is completely covered by placenta (Figure 6-10). **Partial placenta previa** occurs when there is partial occlusion of the internal cervical os by the placenta. **Marginal placenta previa** is characterized by the encroachment of the placenta into the margin of the internal cervical os (Figure 6-11A). This does not cover the os. A **low-lying placenta** is defined as a placental edge that comes within 2 cm of the internal cervical os but does not cover it. Among the many factors associated with placenta previa are advanced maternal age and previous cesarean delivery. Together, these factors increase the risk that the placenta will advance beyond the normal basal plate and invade the myometrium.

Gestational age at the time of the ultrasound examination greatly influences the incidence of placenta previa. At 17

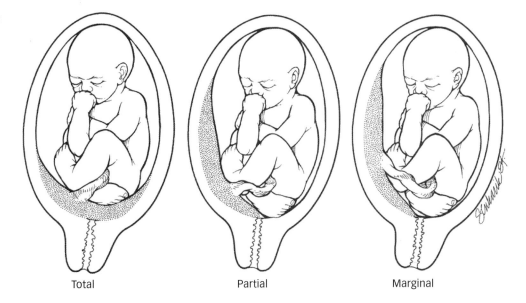

Figure 6-9. *The three variations of placenta previa: total, partial, and marginal. Reprinted with permission from Benedetti TJ: Obstetric hemorrhage. In Gabbe SG, Niebyl JR, Simpson JL (eds): Obstetrics: Normal and Problem Pregnancies, 2nd Edition. St. Louis, Elsevier, 1991. See Chapter 5 for detailed information about the placenta.*

Total   Partial   Marginal

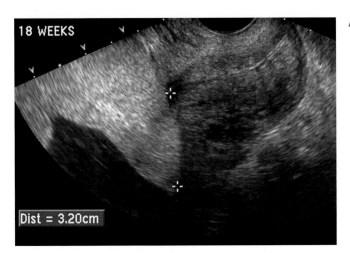

Figure 6-10. *Long-axis transvaginal view of cervix at 18 weeks' gestation—complete placenta previa. Anterior placenta is covering the internal cervical os by 3.2 cm (between + markers).*

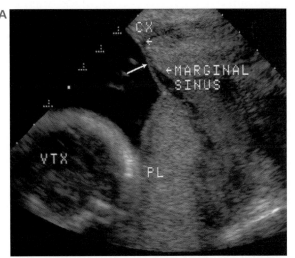

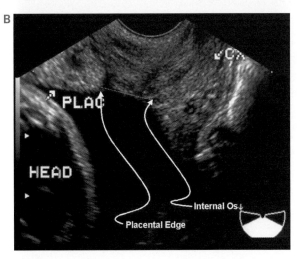

weeks' gestation, evidence of placental tissue covering the cervical os transabdominally will be found in 5%–6% of all pregnant women; however, more than 90% of these will resolve by term. While this observable fact has been termed **placental migration**, in reality it is the result of changes in architecture secondary to atrophy in areas where placental attachment encountered limited blood supply (trophotropism). Differential growth of the lower uterine segment during the second and third trimesters has been another explanation for this observation.

A transvaginal ultrasound during the second trimester that reveals placental tissue extending past the internal cervical os by 10 mm warrants a vaginal scan of the cervix for placental localization late in the third trimester (Figure 6-11B, a low-lying placenta).

Figure 6-11. A *Long-axis view of cervix—marginal previa. Patient presented with unexplained bleeding. Membrane can be seen extending from posterior placenta to internal cervical os.* **B** *One can routinely measure transvaginally from the edge of the placenta (arrow) to the internal cervical os (arrow) in this image depicting a low-lying placenta..*

CERVICAL PREGNANCY

In an ectopic pregnancy, implantation occurs at a site other than within the endometrium. A rare life-threatening form of ectopic pregnancy is a **cervical pregnancy**. This occurs in approximately 1 in 8500 deliveries. Cervical pregnancies are seen more frequently in women who have a previous uterine scar (C/S) and/or prior curettage of the uterus for retained products of conception. Painless vaginal bleeding during the first trimester is usually the first indication of a cervical pregnancy.

Sonographic demonstration of a gestational sac within the cervix inferior to the internal cervical os is highly suggestive of a cervical pregnancy (Figure 6-12). Depending on the gestational age, one may see only a gestational sac, a gestational sac with a yolk sac, or a gestational sac with a yolk sac and embryo. **Color Doppler** can reveal trophoblastic flow with a cervical pregnancy. Missed abortion (no fetal cardiac activity) should have an irregular sac shape, and the gestational sac location will change on serial ultrasounds. A nabothian cyst or inclusion cyst could be mistaken for a cervical pregnancy, but the ultrasound appearance is usually distinctive for this entity as this cyst will not be seen within the cervical canal.

As the majority of women with cervical pregnancy are in their childbearing years, the current trend is to preserve their reproductive function. Treatment options vary depending on the clinical state of the patient. Early diagnosis with diagnostic ultrasound can allow for nonsurgical medical treatment. Nonsurgical treatment may include but is not limited to systemic methotrexate administration and local intrasac potassium chloride (KCl) injections. Selective uterine artery embolization is also being utilized to treat cervical pregnancy. Total abdominal hysterectomy is usually recommended only for second and third trimester cervical pregnancies or to control life-threatening hemorrhage.

TECHNIQUE

The cervix can be visualized with transvaginal, transabdominal, or transperineal sonography. The transvaginal technique is more frequently performed by obstetric imagers and in recent years has become the standard for assessing cervical length. The transperineal and transabdominal techniques have been more commonly performed by radiologic imagers.

Transvaginal Sonography

Transvaginal probes are typically 5.0–7.5 MHz. These probes are covered with a protective transducer cover. Gel is placed between the probe cover and the transducer. With the maternal bladder empty, the patient is placed in the dorsal lithotomy position with her feet in stirrups. Sterile gel should be routinely used on the exterior of the probe cover. The transducer should be inserted along the posterior wall of the vagina, as the urethra is anterior to the vagina and is quite sensitive to pressure. The probe should be placed in the anterior fornix. Pressure applied to the cervix should be minimal to maintain contact between the probe and the cervix (Figure 6-13). *It is important to wait at least 30 seconds before measuring the cervix to allow the cervix time to adjust to a probe within the vagina.*

A true long-axis view of the cervix should be obtained, keeping in mind that it often does not lie exactly in the midline sagittal plane of the mother's body. It is often necessary to rotate the shaft of the probe to find the true long axis. One also needs to angle the probe anterior and posterior to ascertain the position of the cervix. Once the cervix is located, a real-time sweep should be performed from the midline of the cervix to the lateral aspect of both sides of the cervix. The uterine vessels will be seen at the lateral borders of the cervix, frequently at the level of the

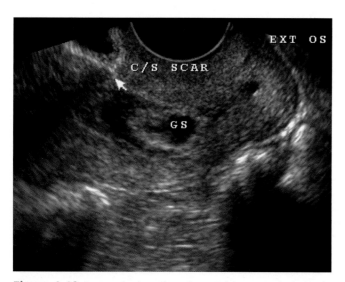

Figure 6-12. *Long-axis view of cervix containing a cervical ectopic pregnancy. Abbreviations: C/S SCAR = c-section scar, EXT OS = external os, GS = gestational sac.*

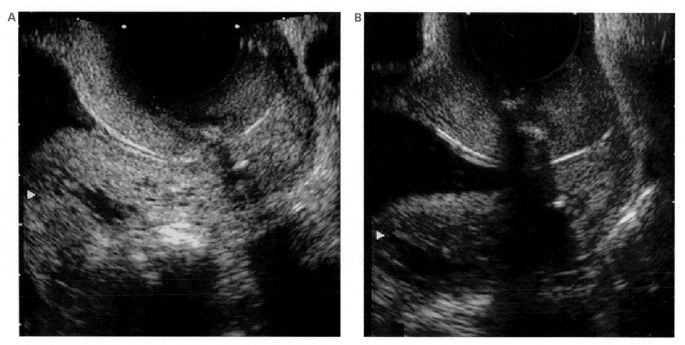

Figure 6-13. *When scanning transvaginally, it is important to avoid applying pressure to the cervix.* **A** *With pressure on the cervix, the cervical canal appears closed.* **B** *With probe in distal vagina, a large funnel can be visualized extending to cerclage stitch.*

internal cervical os. The endovaginal probe's field of view should be set at the widest angle permitted by the manufacturer during the exam.

The optimal length of time for the ultrasound examination of the cervix has not been determined. A brief examination lasting less than five minutes is often insufficient to detect possible changes in cervical length. One should record and measure the cervical length on three images. The first measurement is often longer than subsequent measurements. The electronic calipers are placed at the junction of

the anterior and posterior cervical walls at the internal and external cervical os (Figure 6-14). If the cervical length is curved, multiple sets of calipers may be needed to measure the entire cervical canal length accurately (Figure 6-15). The shortest cervical measurement obtained should be recorded. This measurement is the most reproducible and

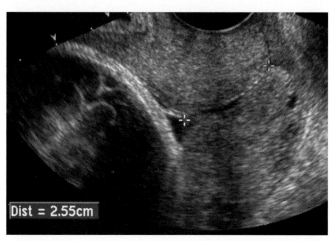

Figure 6-14. *Long-axis view of cervix with transducer placed in anterior fornix. Calipers are placed at internal and external os. Posterior wall of vagina is seen.*

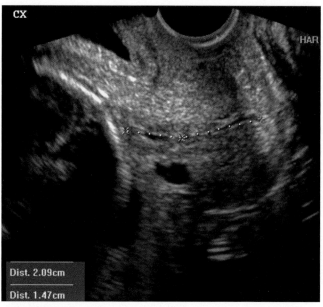

Figure 6-15. *Transvaginal long-axis view of cervix. Two linear measurements should be summed to determine the length of this curved cervix.*

has the best sensitivity and predictive value for assessing the risk of preterm birth. Applying suprapubic and fundal pressure with your hand at the end of the study can help to establish the shortest cervical length and to observe any funneling at the internal cervical os.

Transabdominal Sonography

Before vaginal probe technology, **transabdominal** sonography was the most commonly used technique to evaluate the uterine cervix in the 1970s and early 1980s. While the cervix can be demonstrated in most patients during the first trimester and early second trimester, cervical visualization is often poor during the later weeks of pregnancy. This may be due to maternal body habitus or the presenting fetal part overlying the cervix. Scanning technique is critical because the volume of urine in the maternal bladder is not predictably related to the total volume of urine in the fetal/maternal system and thus can compress the opposing cervical walls to a variable degree. Scanning after partial emptying of the maternal bladder can give a more accurate assessment of cervical length and cervical changes. (See Figure 6-16.) If the maternal bladder is too empty, the cervix may be impossible to see or, if seen, may appear shorter and bulkier. In reality, it is extremely difficult for pregnant women to partially empty their bladders.

In order to image the cervix transabdominally, the imager needs to scan in a long-axis plane just superior to the symphysis pubis. Angling a 3.5 or 5.0 MHz curvilinear probe inferiorly under the symphysis pubis will give the best visualization of the cervix.

Transperineal/Translabial Sonography

The **transperineal** and **translabial** approaches customarily use commercially available 3.5 MHz phased array or curvilinear transducers. Probe preparation includes placing a protective cover over the transducer (gel between cover and transducer) and then covering with sterile gel. With the patient in the supine position, the maternal bladder empty, and hips abducted, the transducer is placed on the perineum in a sagittal orientation between the labia minora just posterior to the urethra. Probe position and angle are adjusted under ultrasound visualization to optimize imaging the cervix. The internal cervical os and upper cervix are routinely visualized with this approach. However, the external cervical os may be obscured by overlying bowel gas within the rectum. Turning women into a lateral decubitus position may help to reduce this pitfall.

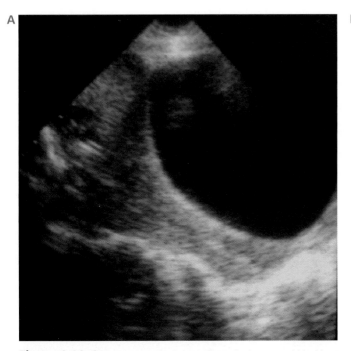

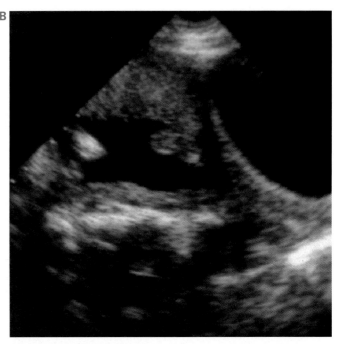

Figure 6-16. A *Image reveals an overdistended maternal bladder transabdominally. The cervix is elongated and the placenta appears to be covering the internal cervical os with partial emptying of the maternal bladder.* **B** *Image reveals that the placenta is not covering the internal cervical os and that the cervix is shorter in length.*

SCANNING TIPS, GUIDELINES, AND PITFALLS

Transvaginal Sonography

Tips

1. The maternal bladder should be empty.
2. The probe is inserted into the vagina and can be directed into the anterior fornix.
3. When a sagittal image of the cervix is obtained, relax probe pressure until the image begins to blur, and then apply pressure for the best image.
4. In the long-axis scanning plane of the cervix, the cervix is usually displayed in a horizontal plane on image.

Pitfalls

5. A probe inserted too far can compress the cervix, resulting in the measurement of a falsely elongated cervical length.
6. The external cervical os may be suboptimally visualized as a result of near-field reverberation artifact.

Transabdominal Sonography

Tips

7. The maternal bladder should be full.
8. Angle the probe inferiorly under the symphysis pubis.
9. In the long-axis scanning plane of cervix, the cervix is usually displayed in a vertical plane on image.

Pitfalls

10. An overdistended bladder may compress the cervix, making it appear elongated.
11. In the third trimester fetal parts lying over the cervix can obscure the cervix.

Transperineal Sonography

Tips

12. The maternal bladder should be empty.
13. Image the cervix in a sagittal scanning plane.
14. In long-axis scanning plane of cervix, the cervix is usually displayed in a horizontal plane on the image.

Pitfalls

15. If the external cervical os is obscured by bowel gas, try scanning the patient in the lateral decubitus position (right and left) or elevate the patient's hips and buttocks on a thick pad or pillow.

REFERENCES

Ayers JW, DeGrood RM, Compton AA, et al: Sonographic evaluation of cervical length in pregnancy: diagnosis and management of preterm cervical effacement in patients at risk for preterm delivery. Obstet Gynecol 71:939–944, 1988.

Berghella V, Daly SF, Tolosa JE, et al: Prediction of preterm delivery with transvaginal ultrasonography of the cervix in patients with high-risk pregnancies: does cerclage prevent prematurity? Am J Obstet Gynecol 181:809–815, 1999.

Berghella V, Kuhlman K, Weiner S: Cervical funneling: sonographic criteria predictive of preterm delivery. Ultrasound Obstet Gynecol 10:161–166, 1997.

Berghella V, Tolosa JE, Kuhlman K, et al: Cervical ultrasonography compared with manual examination as a predictor of preterm delivery. Am J Obstet Gynecol 177:723–730, 1997.

Carr DB, Smith K, Parsons L, et al: Ultrasonography for cervical length measurement: agreement between transvaginal and translabial techniques. Obstet Gynecol 96:554–558, 2000.

The Columbus Dispatch: A long way until Labor Day. Monday, January 24, 2000.

Cook CM, Ellwood DA: The cervix as a predictor of preterm delivery in "at-risk" women. Ultrasound Obstet Gynecol 15:109–113, 2000.

Cowan-Bennett C, Richards DS: Patient acceptance of endovaginal ultrasound. Ultrasound Obstet Gynecol 15:52–55, 2000.

Francois KE, Foley MR: Antepartum and postpartum hemorrhage. In Gabbe SG, Niebyl JR, Galan H, et al: *Obstetrics: Normal and Problem Pregnancies*, 6th Edition. New York, Churchill Livingstone, 2012, Chapter 19.

Goldstein C, Hagen-Ansert SL, Vander Werff BJ: The sonographic and Doppler evaluation of the female pelvis. In Hagan-Ansert SL (ed): *Textbook of Diagnostic Ultrasonography*, 7th Edition. St. Louis, Elsevier Mosby, 2012, pp 955–977.

Guzman ER, Forster JK, Vintzileos AM, et al: Pregnancy outcomes in women treated with elective versus ultrasound-indicated cervical cerclage. Ultrasound Obstet Gynecol 12:323–327, 1998.

Guzman ER, Rosenberg J, Houlihan C, et al: A new method using vaginal ultrasound and transfundal pressure to evaluate asymptomatic incompetent cervix. Obstet Gynecol 83:248–252, 1994.

Heath VCF, Souka AP, Erasmus I: Cervical length at 23 weeks of gestation: the value of Shirodkar suture for the short cervix. Ultrasound Obstet Gynecol 12:318–322, 1998.

Heath VCF, Southall TR, Souka AP, et al: Cervical length at 23 weeks of gestation: prediction of spontaneous preterm delivery. Ultrasound Obstet Gynecol 12:312–317, 1998.

Heath VCF, Southall TR, Souka AP, et al: Cervical length at 23 weeks of gestation: relation to demographic characteristics and previous obstetric history. Ultrasound Obstet Gynecol 12:304–311, 1998.

Hertzberg BS, Bowie JD, Weber TM, et al: Sonography of the cervix during the third trimester of pregnancy. AJR 157:73–76, 1991.

Hertzberg BS, Kliewer MA, Farrell TA, et al: Spontaneously changing gravid cervix: clinical implications and prognostic features. Radiology 196:721–724, 1995.

Hertzberg BS, Livingston E, et al: Ultrasonographic evaluation of the cervix: transperineal versus endovaginal imaging. J Ultrasound Med 20:1071–1078; quiz 1080, 2001.

Hibbard JU, Tart M, Moawad AH: Cervical length at 16–22 weeks' gestation and risk for preterm delivery. Obstet Gynecol 96:972–978, 2000.

Iams JD: Opinion: cervical sonography. Ultrasound Obstet Gynecol 10:156–160, 1997.

Iams JD: Premature birth. In Quilligan EJ, Zuspan FP (eds): Handbook of Obstetrics, Gynecology, and Primary Care. St. Louis, Mosby-Year Book, 1998.

Iams JD: Preterm birth. In Gabbe SG, Niebyl JR, Simpson, JL (eds): Pocket Companion to Accompany Obstetrics Normal and Problem Pregnancies, 4th Edition. New York, Churchill Livingstone, 2002.

Iams JD, Golderberg RL, Meis PJ, et al: The length of the cervix and the risk of spontaneous delivery. N Engl J Med 334:567–572, 1996.

Iams JD, Paraskos J, Landon MB, et al: Cervical sonography in preterm labor. Obstet Gynecol 84:40–46, 1994.

Imesis HM, Albert TA, Iams, JD: Identifying twin gestations at low risk for preterm birth with a transvaginal ultrasonographic cervical measurement at 24 to 26 weeks' gestation. Am J Obstet Gynecol 177:1149–1155, 1997.

Jackson GM, Ludmir J, Bader TJ: The accuracy of digital examination and ultrasound in the evaluation of cervical length. Obstet Gynecol 79:214–218, 1992.

Lauria MR, Smith RS, Treadwell MC, et al: The use of second-trimester transvaginal sonography to predict placenta previa. Ultrasound Obstet Gynecol 8:337–340, 1996.

Lockwood C, Kuczynski E: Opinion: markers of preterm delivery risk. Ultrasound Obstet Gynecol 12:301–303, 1998.

Mahony BS, Nyberg DA, Luthy DA, et al: Translabial ultrasound of the third-trimester uterine cervix. J Ultrasound Med 9:717–723, 1990.

Mashiach S, Admon D, Oelsner G, et al: Cervical Shirodkar cerclage may be the treatment modality of choice for cervical pregnancy. Hum Reprod 17:493–496, 2002.

Mason GC, Maresh MJA: Alterations in bladder volume and the ultrasound appearance of the cervix. Br J Obstet Gynaecol 97:457–458, 1990.

O'Brien JM, Allen AA, Barton JR, et al: Intravaginal saline as a contrast agent for cervical sonography in the obstetric patient. Ultrasound Obstet Gynecol 13:137–139, 1999.

Poder L: Ultrasound evaluation of the uterus. In Callen PW: Ultrasonography in Obstetrics and Gynecology, 5th Edition. Philadelphia, Saunders Elsevier, 2008, pp 919–941.

Rizzo G, Capponi A, Angelini E, et al: The value of transvaginal ultrasonographic examination of the uterine cervix in predicting preterm delivery in patients with preterm premature rupture of membranes. Ultrasound Obstet Gynecol 11:23–29, 1998.

Robinson JN, Economy KE, Feinberg BR, et al: Cervical hydrosonography in pregnancy to assess cervical length by transabdominal ultrasound. Obstet Gynecol 96:1023–1025, 2000.

Sarti DA, Sample WF, Hobel CJ, et al: Ultrasonic visualization of a dilated cervix during pregnancy. Radiology 130:147, 1979.

Smith CV, Anderson JC, Matamoros A, et al: Transvaginal sonography of cervical width and length during pregnancy. J Ultrasound Med 11:465–467, 1992.

Smith RS, Lauria CH, et al: Transvaginal ultrasonography for all placentas that appear to be low-lying or over the internal cervical os. Ultrasound Obstet Gynecol 9:22–24, 1997.

Sonek J, Shellhaas C: Cervical sonography: a review. Ultrasound Obstet Gynecol 11:71–78, 1998.

Souka AP, Heath V, Flint S: Cervical length at 23 weeks in twins in predicting spontaneous preterm delivery. Obstet Gynecol 94:450–454, 1999.

Su YN, Shih JC, Chiu WH, et al: Cervical pregnancy: assessment with three-dimensional power Doppler imaging and successful management with selective uterine artery embolization. Ultrasound Obstet Gynecol 14:284–287, 1999.

Taipale P, Hiilesmaa V: Sonographic measurement of uterine cervix at 18–22 weeks' gestation and the risk of preterm delivery. Obstet Gynecol 92:902–907, 1998.

Taipale P, Hiilesmaa V, Ylöstalo P: Transvaginal ultrasonography at 18–23 weeks in predicting placenta previa at delivery. Ultrasound Obstet Gynecol 12:422–425, 1998.

To MS, Skentou C, Cicero S, et al: Cervical assessment at the routine 23-weeks' scan: problems with transabdominal sonography. Ultrasound Obstet Gynecol 15:292–296, 2000.

Ushakov FB, Elchalal U, Aceman PJ, et al: Cervical pregnancy: past and future. Obstet Gynecol Surv 52:45–49, 1997.

Whittle WL, Fong KW, Windrim R: Cervical ultrasound and preterm birth. In Rumack CM, Wilson SR, Charboneau JW, et al (eds): *Diagnostic Ultrasound*, 4th Edition. St. Louis, Elsevier Mosby, 2011, pp 1528–1536.

Wong G, Levine D, Ludmir J: Maternal postural challenge as a functional test for cervical incompetence. J Ultrasound Med 16:169–175, 1997.

Yang JH, Kuhlman K, Daly S, et al: Prediction of preterm birth by second trimester cervical sonography in twin pregnancies. Ultrasound Obstet Gynecol 15:288–291, 2000.

Zemmlyn S: The length of the uterine cervix and its significance. J Clin Ultrasound 9:267, 1981.

Zilianti M, Azuaga A, Calderon F, et al: Monitoring the effacement of the uterine cervix by transperineal sonography: a new perspective. J Ultrasound Med 14:719–724, 1995.

SELF-ASSESSMENT EXERCISES

Questions

1. During pregnancy the normal cervical length should not measure less than:

   A. 1 cm

   B. 2 cm

   C. 3 cm

   D. 4 cm

   E. 5 cm

2. The best technique for measuring the cervix is:

   A. Transabdominal sonography

   B. Transperineal sonography

   C. Translabial sonography

   D. Transvaginal sonography

   E. Digital exam

3. When the uterine cervix begins to dilate, the functional cervical length:

   A. Gets longer

   B. Gets shorter

   C. Becomes more echogenic

   D. Becomes ill-defined

   E. Is unchanged

4. When intact fetal membranes are seen into the endo-cervical canal, it is called:

   A. Funneling

   B. Engorgement

   C. PROM

   D. Preterm labor

   E. Bulging

5. Obliteration of the cervix when associated with the process of labor is:

   A. Funneling

   B. Engorgement

   C. Atrophy

   D. Degeneration

   E. Effacement

6. A cerclage procedure performed at the internal cervical os that requires a c-section at delivery is called:

   A. McDonald's procedure

   B. Shirodkar cerclage

   C. Valsalva maneuver

   D. Digital examination

   E. Effacement

7. Which one of the following conditions would *not* be an indication for a cerclage procedure?

   A. Incompetent cervix

   B. Preterm labor

   C. Quadruplet gestation

   D. Habitual abortion

   E. Placenta previa

8. The uterine arteries branch off of the:

   A. Aorta

   B. Gonadal arteries

   C. Common iliac arteries

   D. Internal iliac arteries

   E. External iliac arteries

9. This transabdominal image of the cervix reveals:

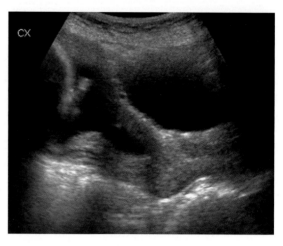

   A. Normal cervical length

   B. Funnel with a shortened cervical length

   C. Fetus in a cephalic presentation

   D. Normal amount of amniotic fluid

   E. No evidence of funneling

10. This transvaginal image of the cervix reveals:

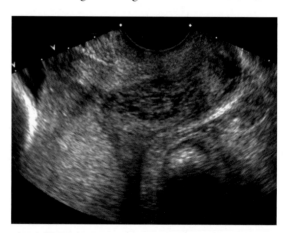

   A. Posterior placenta that completely covers the internal cervical os

   B. Anterior placenta that completely covers the internal cervical os

   C. Posterior placenta that partially covers the internal cervical os

   D. Anterior placenta that partially covers the internal cervical os

   E. Normal placenta

Answers

See Appendix F on page 611 for answers and explanations.

Anomalies Associated with Polyhydramnios

Kathryn A. Gill, MS, RT, RDMS, FSDMS

OBJECTIVES

After completing this chapter you should be able to:

1. Define polyhydramnios and explain why many anomalies are associated with it.
2. List fetal anomalies that contribute to polyhydramnios.
3. Describe the sonographic findings associated with those anomalies that can be seen with polyhydramnios.
4. Explain methods to improve visualization of the fetus in the setting of polyhydramnios.
5. Discuss the maternal effects of polyhydramnios.

SOME OF THE ANOMALIES DISCUSSED in this chapter may present with normal or even low amniotic fluid levels as there can be associated abnormalities, fetal and maternal, that contribute to the amniotic fluid volume. Nevertheless, in an attempt to help practitioners develop a mental file that will assist them in categorizing anomalies in association with fluid levels, the anomalies discussed in this chapter are the ones most likely to be seen in the presence of **polyhydramnios**—excessive amniotic fluid volume.

POLYHYDRAMNIOS

Amniotic fluid levels are influenced by several factors, including inflow from the maternal circulation across the amnion, inflow from the placental surface, and inflow from the fetal respiratory and genitourinary tracts. During the first half of pregnancy (up to 20 weeks' gestation) much of the amniotic fluid comes from maternal circulation. During the second half, amniotic fluid consists mostly of fetal urine, with a small part supplied by the fetal respiratory system as the result of breathing. Fetal swallowing is the main cause of fluid loss. Normally the fluid is replaced by circulation through the fetal kidneys and excretion as fetal urine.

Amniotic fluid is at maximum volume—approximately 800 ml—usually around 33 weeks' gestation. There are a number of sonographic values that can be used to determine polyhydramnios, as published by various authors and indicated in Box 7-1. Sonographically, when a fetus has enough room to extend its extremities to their full length, there is too much fluid (Figure 7-1). Quantitatively, polyhydramnios is defined as amniotic fluid exceeding 2000 ml.

Box 7-1.   Interpreting amniotic fluid indices.

Four-quadrant method, normal ranges:

Phelan et al.: 13 cm ± 5 cm

Rutherford et al.: > 5 cm and < 20 cm

Jeng et al.: > 8 cm and < 24 cm

Single deepest pocket (Manning et al.):

< 1 cm = oligohydramnios

1–2 cm = decreased fluid

2–8 cm = normal

> 8 cm = mild polyhydramnios

> 12 cm = moderate polyhydramnios

> 16 cm = severe polyhydramnios

Box 7-2.   Incidence of polyhydramnios.

Idiopathic 34%

Diabetes mellitus 24.6%

Anomalies 20%

Chromosomal 10%–11%

Rh sensitization 11.5%

Multiple gestation 8.4%

Macrosomia 37%

Box 7-3.   Anomalies associated with polyhydramnios.

Neural tube defects

Gastrointestinal

Facial/neck

Skeletal dysplasia

Ovarian cyst (10%)

Unilateral renal disorder (25% with UPJ obstruction)

Hydrops

Polyhydramnios is associated with anomalies, prematurity, PROM, and placental abruption, increasing the risk of morbidity and mortality. It can be associated with conditions that increase urinary or respiratory fluid production (e.g., maternal diabetes, which causes fetal polyuria) and cardiac anomalies that cause high-output failure. Polyhydramnios can also be associated with conditions that

Figure 7-1. A *Severe polyhydramnios demonstrated by the fetus's ability to extend both legs (arrows) with extra room around all sides. AF = amniotic fluid.* **B** *Large single vertical pocket of amniotic fluid indicated by the arrow.*

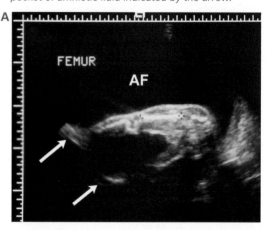

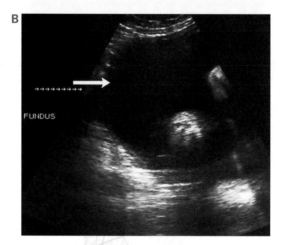

decrease fetal swallowing, such as gastrointestinal abnormalities that cause obstructions, neural tube defects, and muscular abnormalities that affect muscle contractibility. The incidence of such conditions is demonstrated in Box 7-2, and the most commonly associated anomalies are listed in Box 7-3. This chapter addresses those anomalies that can be demonstrated sonographically and are most likely to be encountered in a general practice.

NEURAL TUBE DEFECTS

Neural tube defects (NTDs) are often associated with polyhydramnios because they affect the ability of the fetus to swallow normally. If the amniotic fluid does not circulate through the fetal kidneys as the result of swallowing, the kidneys continue to produce and excrete fluid as fetal urine rather than simply filtering and recirculating the amniotic fluid that has already been produced. This results in an abnormal accumulation of fluid.

The etiology of neural tube defects has been attributed to a folic acid (B vitamin) deficiency. Mothers are encouraged to take supplements during pregnancy and to eat foods rich in folic acid, such as broccoli, green beans, spinach, citrus juices, strawberries, liver, eggs, and yogurt. Doing so decreases the risk of neural tube defects by 40%; continuing this regimen reduces the recurrence rate by 70%. Diabetics, especially those who are insulin-dependent, have a higher incidence of neural tube defects. Drugs—including valproic acid for seizures, aminopterin, and methotrexate—are included as risk factors, as well as hyperthermia. Defects of the central nervous system include those of the brain and spine. These defects are often associated with abnormalities of the face.

Head

Anencephaly

Anencephaly is the most common neural tube defect, affecting approximately 1 in 1000 live births with a 4:1 female to male ratio. It results from a defect in the closure of the anterior neural tube at approximately 6 weeks' gestation, with complete or partial absence of the brain. Folic acid deficiency has been associated with the anomaly. Although anencephaly may be the only abnormal finding, it is not uncommon for anencephalic fetuses also to have cleft defects of the face, spina bifida, clubfoot (talipes equinovarus), and/or abdominal wall defect. The fetus often appears hyperactive as there is extra space for movement due to polyhydramnios, and the amniotic fluid is thought to irritate the exposed brain stem. This condition is not compatible with life, and most live-born fetuses expire shortly after delivery.

Typically, the anencephalic fetus will show well-defined facial bones but no skull or brain. This produces the classic "frog face" appearance of the bulging orbits (Figures 7-2 A and B). Because there is at least a partial brain stem, a small amount of cerebral tissue may be seen as a cap-like structure above the orbits (Figure 7-2C; also see fetal specimen in Figure 7-2D). This anomaly can be isolated but is often associated with spina bifida.

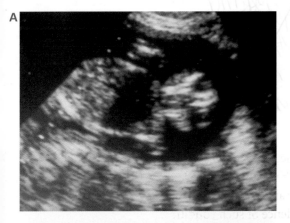

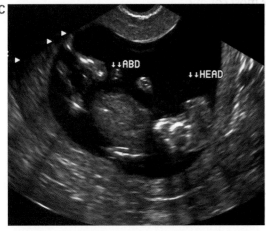

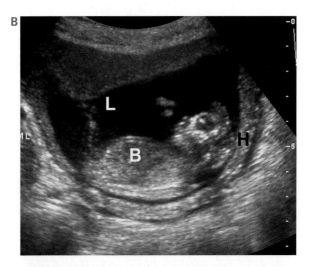

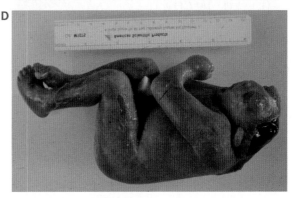

Figure 7-2. A *Classic "frog face" showing the prominent orbits of an anencephalic fetus.* **B** *Long-axis view of an anencephalic fetus. H = head, B = body, L = leg.* **C** *Anencephalic fetus with the "cap-like" remnant of brain tissue.* **D** *Specimen of anencephalic fetus.*

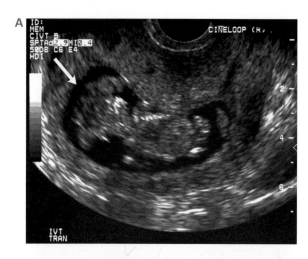

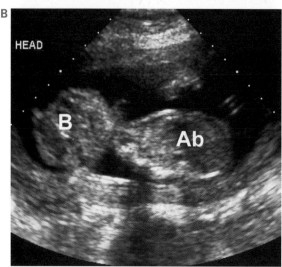

Figure 7-3. A *This fetus with acrania—thought to be a precursor to anencephaly—shows irregularly shaped brain (arrow) with no cranium.* **B** *Long-axis view of fetus with acrania/exencephaly showing no bone around the brain tissue. B = brain, Ab = abdomen.*

Acrania/Exencephaly

Acrania is the absence of the ossified cranium, but the brain is intact and usually well defined. Because there is no skull covering the brain, the cephalic end is often misshapen. **Exencephaly**, in which the cranium is absent and only a partial brain has developed, will ultimately progress to anencephaly because of damage to the exposed brain. Both anencephaly and acrania/exencephaly can be difficult to diagnose with certainty prior to 10 weeks as the skull does not completely ossify until after 10–11 weeks (Figure 7-3).

Microcephaly

Microcephaly is an abnormally small head when compared to the abdomen and femur, measuring less than 3 standard deviations below the norm for age and sex (Figure 7-4). A small head implies a small brain, and the

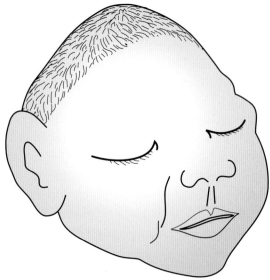

Figure 7-4. *Drawing of very small calvarium of an infant with microcephaly.*

condition is often associated with mental retardation. Various causes include chromosomal abnormalities, exposure to drugs and radiation, intrauterine infections, hemorrhage, and hypoxia. Brain calcifications can be seen, as well as microcephaly, when the insult is due to a TORCH infection.

Encephalocele

Occurring in 1 out of 2000 live births, an **encephalocele** is herniation of brain tissue through a bony defect of the skull. Occasionally, only meninges and fluid herniate out, causing a cystic rather than solid mass outside the fetal skull (Figures 7-5 A and B). This condition may be referred to as a *cranial meningocele*. Most encephaloceles are posterior in location (75%), although they can be frontal (12%) or parietal (13%). Large brain-containing encephaloceles (Figure 7-5C) will cause secondary microcephaly and are most likely to result in severe mental retardation. If the encephalocele is purely cystic, the brain is still confined to the cranium and the head size is not altered significantly. Encephaloceles that are frontal in location have the best prognosis. About 30% of fetuses with an encephalocele also have spina bifida. This anomaly has been associated with hyperthermia, rubella, and cocaine and alcohol abuse.

Hydrocephalus/Ventriculomegaly

Ventriculomegaly is a generalized term for dilated ventricle, while **hydrocephalus** denotes a dilated ventricle specifically caused by increased pressure. The lateral ventricles of the brain contain the echogenic choroid

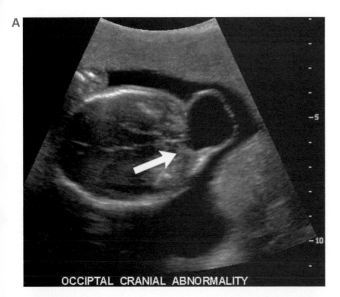

OCCIPTAL CRANIAL ABNORMALITY

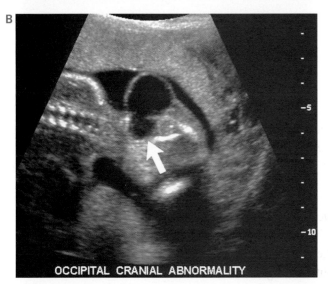

OCCIPITAL CRANIAL ABNORMALITY

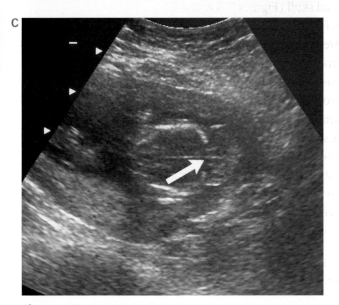

Figure 7-5. A *and* **B** *Cystic occipital encephalocele herniated through a bony defect of the skull (arrow).* **C** *A solid, mostly brain-containing encephalocele. Arrow shows the bony defect.*

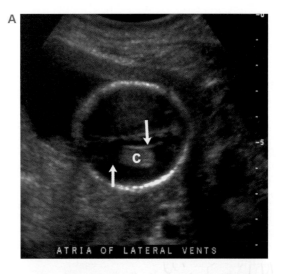

ATRIA OF LATERAL VENTS

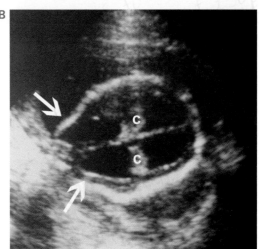

Figure 7-6. A *Normal choroid plexus (C) between the medial and lateral walls of the ventricle (arrows).* **B** *Dangling choroid plexus (C) shown within the dilated ventricles. Note also the lemon sign indicated by the arrows. (Figure continues . . .)*

plexuses, which produce cerebrospinal fluid. The choroid plexus serves as a landmark for identifying the atria of the ventricles, which can be imaged and measured to rule out enlargement and obstruction (Figure 7-6A). Fetal ventricular measurements are consistent throughout pregnancy and should not measure more than 10 mm with the average at 7–8 mm. Mild ventriculomegaly (10–15 mm) can be congenital and of no clinical significance but will most likely result in the patient being referred on for a targeted scan to rule out hydrocephalus. If the lateral ventricle measures more than 10 mm and the choroid does not touch the medial and lateral walls of the ventricles, **hydrocephaly** should be considered. When fluid surrounds the echogenic choroid, it is referred to as the *dangling choroid*—a finding that is specific for hydrocephalus (Figure 7-6B).

C

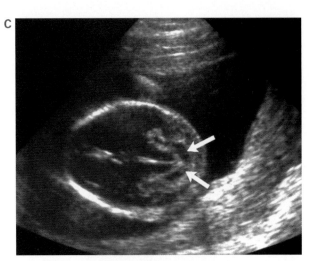

Figure 7-6, continued. C *The banana sign is demonstrated by the flattened cerebellum (arrows) obliterating the region of the cisterna magna.*

Table 7-1. Types of Chiari's malformations.

Type	Description
I	Congenital malformation that is generally asymptomatic. Sometimes the cerebellar tonsils extend into the foramen magnum without involving the brain stem. The most common form of Chiari's malformation.
II	Specifically referred to as Arnold-Chiari malformation. Congenital anomaly almost always associated with spina bifida and hydrocephalus that involves the cerebellum protruding into the cervical spine.
III	The cerebellum and brain stem extend through the foramen magnum and into the spinal cord. The severest form of Chiari's malformation enhancement.
IV	Cerebellar hypoplasia.

There are two types of hydrocephalus, communicating and noncommunicating. In communicating hydrocephalus there is some abnormality in the capacity to absorb fluid from the arachnoid space but no obstruction between the ventricles. Causes include infections, intraventricular hemorrhage, and tumors. Noncommunicating hydrocephalus is caused by an obstruction at some point in the ventricular system, such as aqueductal stenosis or spina bifida. Aqueductal stenosis and the Arnold-Chiari malformation (Chiari's malformation type II) are the most common causes of hydrocephalus. The prognosis is not determined by the ventricular size but instead by the associated anomalies.

Arnold-Chiari Malformation/Spina Bifida

Arnold-Chiari malformation is the term used to describe Chiari's malformation type II, of which there are four specific types defined in Table 7-1. The **Arnold-Chiari malformation** is associated with a neural tube defect. The cranial findings rather than the spinal defect are the most striking. Resulting in **frontal bossing**, the head shape is often referred to as the **lemon sign** as the frontal bones are flattened (Figure 7-6B). This is the result of caudal displacement of the cerebellar tonsils, part of the cerebellum, fourth ventricle, pons, and medulla oblongata through the foramen magnum into the spinal canal. This causes displacement and flattening of the cerebellum, making it look like a banana (the **banana sign**), and obliteration of the cisterna magna (Figure 7-6C). When a fetus demonstrates both the lemon sign and the banana sign together, there is also a 95% chance that there is an

open neural tube defect and hydrocephalus. However, it is important to note that the lemon sign may not be apparent or have value after 24 weeks, as the head shape may return to normal.

Iniencephaly

Iniencephaly—a rare neural tube defect that causes severe retroflexion of the fetal head and serious defects of the spine—can be associated with anencephaly, spina bifida, encephalocele, and hydrocephalus. The fetus has severe lordosis of the cervical spine, which is short, causing hyperextension of the head and neck and putting the fetus in a backward-bending "stargazing" position (Figure 7-7). In addition to severe flexion of the spine, there is usually cervical rachischisis with cervical and often lumbar meningocele. When diagnosed in utero, this rare anomaly is almost always lethal. The male-to-female ratio is 1:10.

Aqueductal Stenosis

Considered one of the most common causes of congenital hydrocephalus, **aqueductal stenosis** is the obstruction of the **aqueduct of Sylvius**, which connects the third and fourth ventricles. The occurrence is 1 in 2000 births with a male-to-female ratio of 2:1. The lateral and third ventricles are enlarged. The fourth ventricle and cerebellum are normal. If the condition is an isolated anomaly, the prognosis is promising, and 50%–80% of these children

Figure 7-7. *The "stargazer" position of a fetus with iniencephaly.*

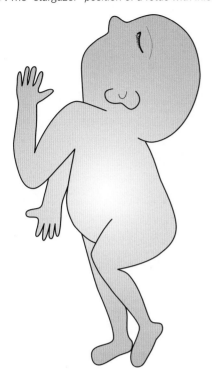

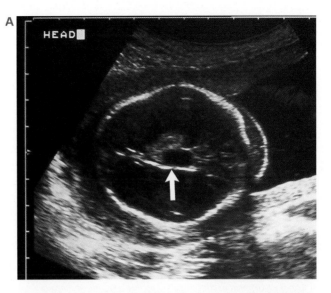

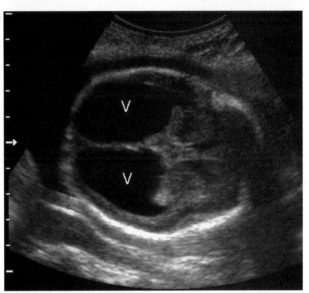

Figure 7-8. A *Hydrocephalus with dilated third ventricle (arrow).* **B** *Dilated ventricles (V).*

will have normal mental function. When there are other associated anomalies, however, the prognosis is poor. Sonographically, the lateral ventricles are enlarged, with the posterior horns measuring larger than the anterior horns. The third ventricle is also dilated, while the cerebellum and fourth ventricle are normal (Figure 7-8).

Agenesis of the Corpus Callosum

The **corpus callosum** is a midline structure that overlies the lateral ventricles and carries nerve that connects the right and left hemispheres of the brain. It is the largest fiber tract within the central nervous system—consisting of 200 to 250 million nerve fibers—and serves a function in learning and memory. Embryologically, the corpus callosum develops later than other CNS structures, usually between 12 and 22 weeks' gestation, making the diagnosis of agenesis of the corpus callosum difficult if not impossible in the first trimester. Developmental failure may be partial or complete, depending on when it occurs. The prognosis depends on associated anomalies, of which there is a high incidence; 85% of these associated anomalies are other CNS abnormalities and 62% are extracranial. Patients may suffer seizures, mental/motor deficits, and psychosis, or they may be asymptomatic. Sonographically, the third ventricle is elevated and the lateral ventricles are displaced laterally, allowing one to see all three structures in the

same plane. The dilated lateral ventricles have a teardrop shape, and the elevated third ventricle may present as an interhemispheric cyst. The cavum septum pellucidum (nerve bundles) that connects the cerebral hemispheres is absent (Figure 7-9).

Dandy-Walker Malformation

Dandy-Walker malformation is the absence (**agenesis**) or, in **Dandy-Walker variant**, incomplete development (**hypoplasia**) of the cerebellar vermis associated with cystic dilatation of the fourth ventricle resulting in a posterior fossa cystic mass. As the fourth ventricle progressively enlarges, the third and lateral ventricles ultimately become dilated as well (Figures 7-10 A and B). There may

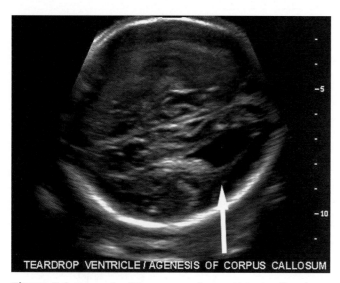

Figure 7-9. *Agenesis of the corpus callosum. Note the dilated teardrop-shaped ventricle (arrow).*

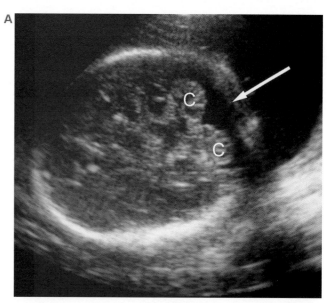

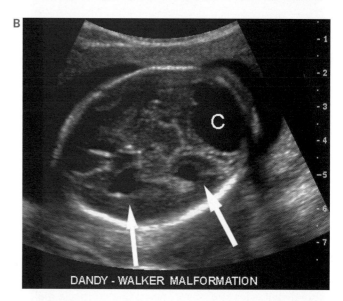

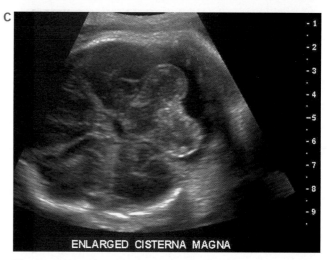

Figure 7-10. A *Enlarged cisterna magna (arrow) with displacement of the cerebellar hemispheres (c).* **B** *Dandy-Walker cyst (c) with dilatation of the lateral ventricle (arrows).* **C** *Prominent or mega cisterna magna.*

also be atresia of the foramen of Magendie (also called the median aperture) and possibly the foramen of Luschka (the lateral aperture of the fourth ventricle). Care should be taken in attempting to make the diagnosis too early as the vermis does not form inferiorly until 18 weeks. The Dandy-Walker malformation occurs in 1 out of 30,000 births, and it is not uncommon for this malformation to be associated with agenesis of the corpus callosum as well as other intra- and extracranial anomalies. The overall postnatal mortality is 35%. Nevertheless, one-third of survivors will have an IQ exceeding 80. This malformation has been associated with congenital infections.

Dandy-Walker malformations are characterized by three findings, including (1) posterior fossa cyst, (2) defect of the cerebellar vermis that results in a communication between the cyst and fourth ventricle, and (3) variable degrees of hydrocephalus. This is a condition that may present with normal levels of amniotic fluid unless associated with chromosomal abnormalities.

Care should be taken not to mistake a mega cisterna magna for a Dandy-Walker malformation. With mega cisterna magna, the cerebellum will be normal with a prominent cisterna magna (Figure 7-10C).

Arachnoid Cysts

The arachnoid is the delicate membrane resembling a spider's web that is interposed between the dura mater and pia mater and, with them, constituting the meninges. **Arachnoid cysts** can develop within the arachnoid and be found anywhere within the brain and spinal cord. Those that develop in the posterior fossa can simulate a

Dandy-Walker malformation. Arachnoid cysts, however, do not communicate with the ventricular system and are not associated with other anomalies; therefore they are usually not associated with polyhydramnios when identified as an isolated anomaly. When an arachnoid cyst is in the posterior fossa, it can be difficult to differentiate from the Dandy-Walker cyst. As the cyst enlarges, the fourth ventricle and the cerebellum are displaced anteriorly. The brain stem may become compressed. Hydrocephalus may develop due to compression caused by the cyst.

Choroid Plexus Cysts

Cysts can develop in the echogenic choroid plexus within the lateral ventricles and are relatively common. **Choroid plexus cysts** can range in size from just a few millimeters to more than 10 mm. They can be single or multiple and unilateral or bilateral, and they usually resolve by 26 weeks. As an isolated finding, choroid plexus cysts are usually of no clinical significance. Nevertheless, demonstration of a choroid plexus cyst warrants a careful fetal survey to rule out any other unusual findings because in several studies these cysts have been associated with trisomies 18 and 21. If choroid plexus cysts measure greater than 10 mm, are multiple, bilateral, and persist after 26 weeks, the likelihood of an associated chromosomal abnormality increases (Figure 7-11).

Vein of Galen Aneurysm

Thought to be due to increased blood flow from an arteriovenous malformation in the fetal head, these rare aneurysms are central and superior in location. **Vein of**

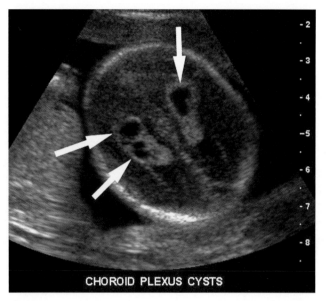

Figure 7-11. *Bilateral choroid plexus cysts (arrows).*

Galen aneurysms may be round or oval and show small branches along the sides of the cyst. Color Doppler will make a definitive diagnosis, revealing flow within the cyst (Figure 7-12). Shunting from the arteriovenous malformation may be severe enough to cause heart failure in utero or in the neonatal period. If hydrops develops in utero, the prognosis is extremely poor. With surgical correction, the mortality rate is about 20%. Survivors tend to progress well, rarely showing symptoms in later life. By itself, the aneurysm should have no effect on the amniotic fluid level; however, hydropic fetuses frequently present with polyhydramnios.

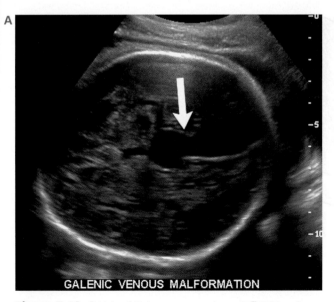
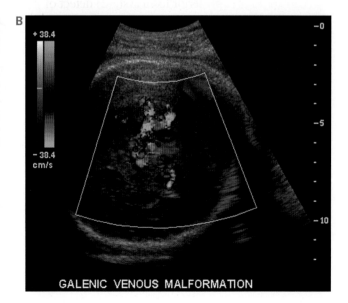

Figure 7-12. A *Vein of Galen aneurysm (arrow).* **B** *With color.*

Holoprosencephaly

Holoprosencephaly, occurring in 1 out of 10,000 births, is thought to result from the abnormal or deficient cleavage of the early forebrain (prosencephalon) at about 5–7 weeks' gestation. This anomaly has been associated with alcohol abuse, TORCH, diabetes mellitus, radiation, excessive vitamin A, and trisomy 13. There are three major varieties of holoprosencephaly—(1) alobar, (2) semilobar, and (3) lobar. The alobar and semilobar types are fatal. Severe cleft defects of the face are also common (Figure 7-13A). With lobar holoprosencephaly, infants may live but are usually severely mentally retarded. Overall, the prognosis for all three is poor.

Alobar Holoprosencephaly In **alobar holoprosencephaly** the lateral ventricles are fused, forming a large **single ventricle** that is horseshoe-shaped. The large ventricle drapes over the fused thalami (Figure 7-13B). There can be variable degrees of falx formation; however, mostly the falx will be absent. Median cleft defects of the face, hypotelorism, cyclopia, single nostril, and proboscis may also be seen (Figures 7-13 C and D). There is a male-to-female ratio of 1:3, and infants usually die at birth or within the first six months of life. This is the severest form of holoprosencephaly. See Box 7-4.

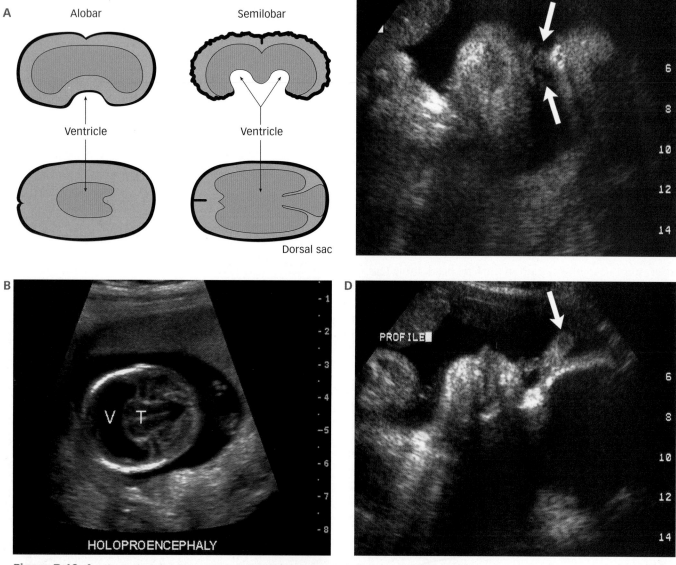

Figure 7-13. A *Schematics of alobar and semilobar holoprosencephaly.* **B** *Horseshoe-shaped ventricle (V) draping over the fused thalami (T).* **C** *Frontal view of fetal face showing severe hypotelorism. The orbits are indicated by arrows.* **D** *Profile of fetal face showing a proboscis (arrow) above the orbit.*

Box 7-4.	**Alobar holoprosencephaly.**

Hypotelorism/proboscis

Monoventricle

Fused thalami

Absent—falx, corpus callosum, third ventricle

Box 7-5.	**Semilobar holoprosencephaly.**

Partial posterior separation of cerebral hemispheres

Monoventricle

No frontal-temporal-occipital horns

Fused thalami

Midline cleft

Semilobar Holoprosencephaly **Semilobar holoprosencephaly** will also show fused thalami and a single monoventricle, but there will be partially developed occipital horns and falx. The cavum septum pellucidum will be absent. There is decreased brain matter, and the prognosis is poor. See Box 7-5.

Lobar Holopresencephaly **Lobar holoprosencephaly** is a little more complex in appearance. It is the mildest form of holoprosencephaly and is not usually detected with sonography. The interhemispheric fissure is well developed anteriorly and posteriorly, but there is still some fusion of the lateral ventricles. The cavum septum pellucidum is absent. These infants are less severely affected and present with varying degrees of mental impairment.

Porencephaly, Hydranencephaly, and Schizencephaly There are several conditions that will destroy brain tissue. These include porencephaly, hydranencephaly, and schizencephaly, rare congenital conditions in which the cerebral tissues are replaced by cerebrospinal fluid. The

prognosis is poor, and the condition may not present until late in the pregnancy. They are among the severest brain anomalies.

Porencephaly **Porencephaly** presents as cystic cavities within the brain matter. The destruction of brain matter may result from severe ischemia or hemorrhage. The fluid-filled cavity or cavities usually communicate with the adjacent ventricles and may even communicate with the subarachnoid space.

Hydranencephaly **Hydranencephaly** is an extreme form of porencephaly and is thought to be the result of early occlusion of the internal carotid arteries. It has been associated with cocaine abuse and congenital infections such as TORCH. The cranium will be filled with fluid. The brain stem and rhombencephalic structures are usually spared. Head size can be normal or microcephalic (Figures 7-14 A and B).

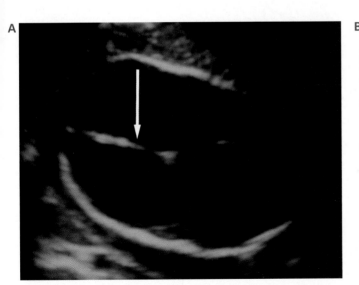
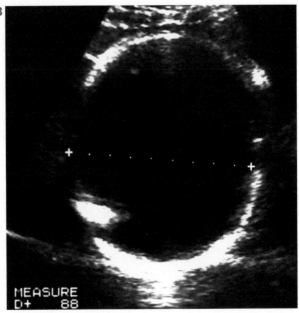

Figure 7-14. A *Hydranencephaly with partial falx (arrow).* **B** *Brain has been completely replaced by fluid, typical of hydranencephaly. (Figure continues . . .)*

C

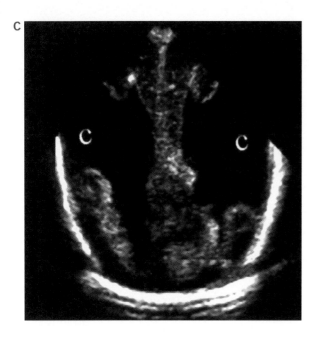

Figure 7-14, continued. *Coronal (**C**) and axial (**D**) images of schizencephaly. Note the clefts (C). **C** and **D** reprinted with permission from De Lange M, Rouse GA: Ob/Gyn Sonography: An Illustrated Review. Pasadena, CA, Davies Publishing, 2004.*

D

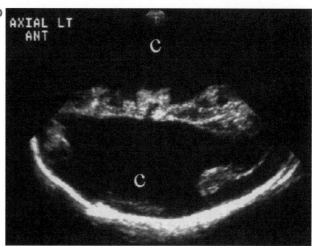

Schizencephaly Thought to result from a destructive vascular insult prior to 20 weeks' gestation, **schizencephaly** is a rare condition in which fluid-filled clefts are seen to extend from the skull through the brain and into the lateral ventricles (Figures 7-14 C and D). Schizencephaly can be unilateral or bilateral.

Spine

Spina Bifida

By six weeks' gestation, the neural tube becomes completely closed at both ends. **Spina bifida** is the failure of this process, resulting in defective closure of a portion of the neural tube and causing nonfusion of the vertebral arches. Although spinal ossification begins at 10 weeks, it is not complete until 20 weeks' gestation. The process of ossification is gradual, but that of the pedicles, lamina, and S1 is sufficient at 18 weeks to assess and rule out spina bifida. Because spinal defects can occur anywhere along the spine, it is important to visualize the entire spine. The most common location for a spina bifida to occur is in the **lumbosacral** region. If fetal position or maternal body habitus precludes adequate visualization of any part of the spine, it should be documented on the clinical data sheet. The higher the location of the defect, the poorer the prognosis.

There are various forms of spina bifida, all of which fall under the classification of **spinal dysraphism**, or neural tube defect. Neural tube defects can be covered by skin (**spina bifida occulta**) or open, exposing the spinal cord (**spina bifida aperta**). Open defects are often associated with a meningocele or myelomeningocele. **Meningoceles** are hernial cysts containing cerebrospinal fluid (CSF), dura, and arachnoid, but no neural tissue. They appear mostly cystic on sonogram. **Myelomeningoceles** are hernial sacs that contain CSF, dura, arachnoid, spinal cord, and/or nerve roots. Sonographically, they appear complex to solid. These sac-like protrusions extend from the spiny defect as a mass along the back of the fetus. **Spina bifida cystica** is a term used to describe both meningoceles and myelomeningoceles (Figures 7-15 A and B). **Rachischisis** is a severe form of spina bifida in which the spine is open throughout the majority of its length.

Patients with spina bifida occulta usually do not have any complications from the spinal defect. However, they may have a dimple or tuft of hair growing over the site of the defect. These patients tend to have a higher sensitivity to latex products.

Spina bifida aperta affects individuals differently depending upon the severity of the defect and whether or not the cord is involved (Figures 7-15 C and D). The most common complications are hydrocephalus, urinary incontinence, and paralysis. There is a 10% risk of mental retardation. Although fetuses with spina bifida may show movement of their extremities in utero, this observation does not preclude paralysis. Paralysis may not become apparent until after delivery.

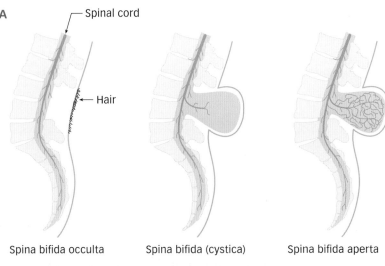

A
- Spinal cord
- Hair

Spina bifida occulta   Spina bifida (cystica)   Spina bifida aperta

Figure 7-15. A *Schematics of spina bifida occulta and aperta.* **B** *Long-axis view of spina bifida with a meningocele (arrow).* **C** *Longitudinal view of the fetal spine showing a defect in the lumbar region.* **D** *Transverse image through the fetal abdomen showing a V-shaped spine (arrows) indicating spina bifida. The arrows are pointing to the posterior ossification centers, which are splayed apart.* **E** *Long-axis view of a fetus with scoliosis. (Figure continues . . .)*

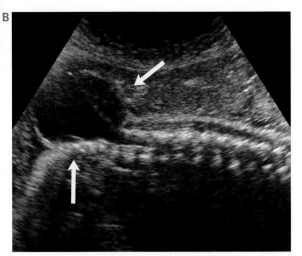

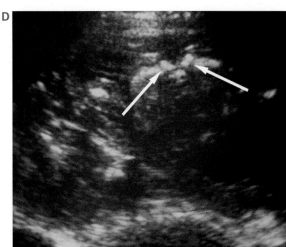

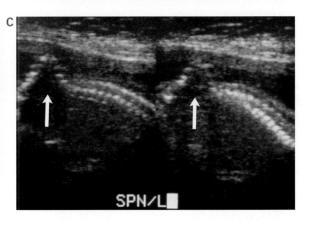

SPN/L

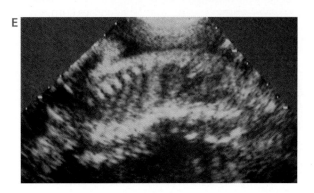

Curvatures of the Spine

Scoliosis is the abnormal lateral curvature of the spine (Figure 7-15E). **Kyphosis** is an exaggerated convex curvature resulting in a humpback. **Lordosis** is an exaggerated anterior curvature of the spine causing severe swayback. These severe curvatures may be associated with spina bifida and abdominal wall defects.

Teratomas

Teratomas in the newborn most often originate from the sacrococcygeal region or the gonads; however, they can occur anywhere near the midline from the brain to the coccyx. These masses are usually complex and may contain calcifications. Teratomas that are predominantly cystic (15%) are most likely to be benign, while those that are mostly solid and mostly inside the fetus are likely to be malignant. Teratomas are considered to be the most common tumors found in newborns, although the occurrence is only 1 in 35,000 births with a 3:1 female-to-male ratio. Based on clinical presentation, four types of **sacrococcygeal teratomas** have been described (Table 7-2). They can displace the rectum and bladder anteriorly and cause compression on the ureters, resulting in hydronephrosis. Arteriovenous shunting can occur within the tumor, potentially leading to cardiac failure in the fetus and ultimately hydrops. Once a teratoma has been diagnosed, serial scans of the pregnancy should be performed to monitor the growth of the tumor and its effect on other fetal structures as well as to watch for developing hydrops. The mother should be monitored for pre-eclampsia. Masses measuring more than 4.5 cm usually require c-section for delivery to avoid dystocia and the risk of hemorrhage at delivery. Rapid tumor growth has also been associated with placentomegaly (due to fetal cardiac failure), fetal distress (hydrops), and preterm labor (Figures 7-15 F–L).

Table 7-2.	Types of sacrococcygeal teratomas.
Type	**Description**
I	Predominantly external (47%)
II	External and internal (34%)
III	Predominantly internal (9%)
IV	Entirely presacral (10%)

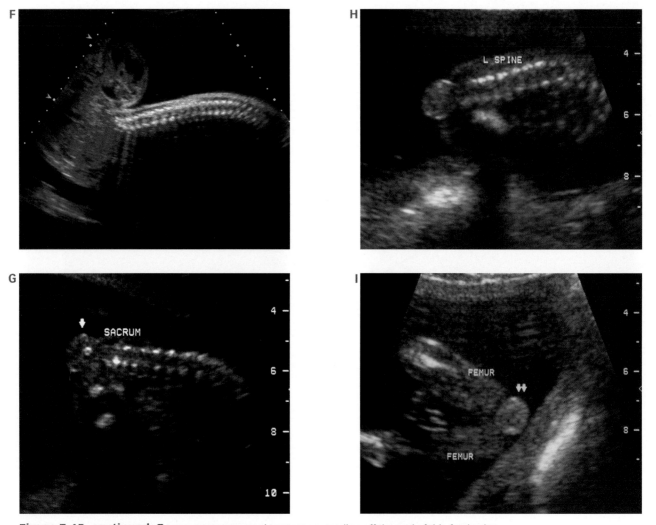

Figure 7-15, continued. F *Large sacrococcygeal teratoma extending off the end of this fetal spine.* **G** *and* **H** *Longitudinal views of the spine showing a smaller teratoma in the lumbosacral region.* **I** *View of the same teratoma shown at the buttock region. Following page:* **J** *and* **K** *This large cystic teratoma extended from the fetal mouth. Following page:* **L** *Cystic mass is seen under the nostrils and upper lip.*

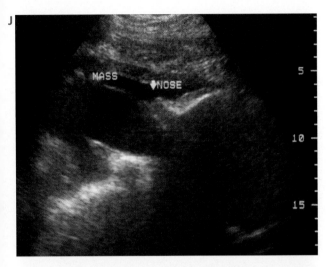

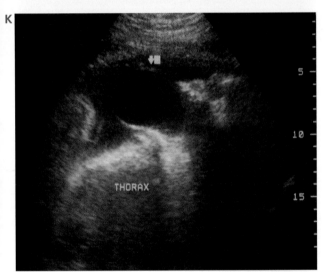

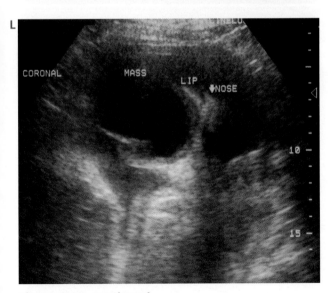

Figure 7-15, continued.

Neck

Neck masses may be anterior or posterior, cystic, solid, or complex, and vascular or avascular. Those that are anterior or anterolateral are less common than the posterior masses. Masses that cause hyperextension of the neck may reduce the fetus's ability to swallow and cause polyhydramnios. Neck masses include goiters, teratomas, hygromas, tracheal atresia, and thyroid cysts. The more common neck masses will be posterior or posterolateral, such as cystic hygromas, occipital encephaloceles, and cervical meningomyeloceles. Although the occipital encephalocele is not a neck mass, cerebrospinal fluid and/or brain tissue protruding from an occipital defect may initially appear to originate from the upper posterior region of the neck. If a posterior neck mass is an isolated anomaly, it would not necessarily be seen in association with polyhydramnios.

Cystic Hygroma

Although cystic hygromas can be anterior in location, most are posterior and lateral. **Cystic hygromas** are the result of a malformation causing obstructed jugular lymph vessels. The obstruction leads to significant enlargement of the lymph sacs, forming cysts. These cysts can be classified as simple or complex. Simple cysts appear without loculations and carry a better prognosis, with 94% of affected fetuses born live. Complex hygromas are more typical and contain multiple loculations. These fetuses have a higher incidence of other anomalies, and only about 12% will be live born. These large multiseptated cystic masses will appear to envelop the fetus (Figures 7-16 A and B).

Cystic hygroma (Figure 7-16) can be an isolated abnormality or associated with a syndrome, the most common of which is Turner syndrome. Hygromas have been associated with alcohol abuse.

In some cases the anomaly resolves in utero as the lymph vessels reconnect with the vascular system. At delivery these infants may show the webbed neck corresponding to the effect of the decompressing hygroma on the neck tissues. A common complication seen with cystic hygromas is the development of hydrops. In the second trimester, there is usually oligohydramnios with a few cases having either a normal amount of amniotic fluid or polyhydramnios. The prognosis typically is poor.

Figure 7-16. A *Long-axis view of a fetus with a large cystic hygroma (arrows) behind the head.* **B** *Cystic hygroma is shown around the fetal skull. Note the multiple septations. AP (**C**) and lateral (**D**) views of a specimen with a cystic hygroma at the posterior neck.*

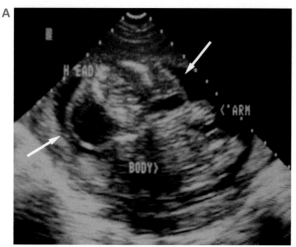

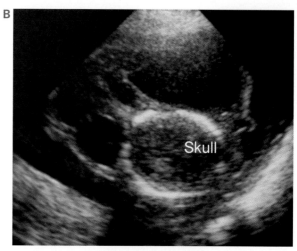

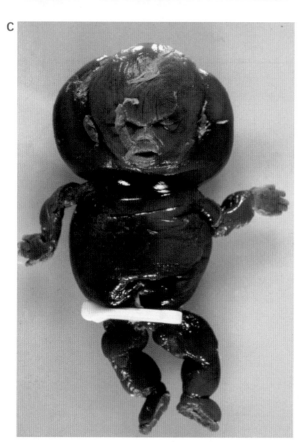

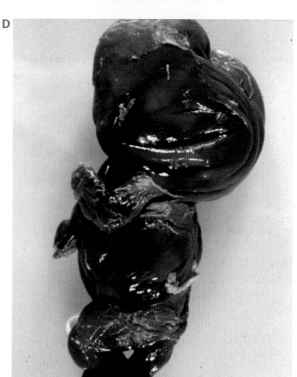

Chest

Pleural Effusion

Pleural effusion, also known as *hydrothorax*, denotes fluid in the chest that conforms to the shape of the thorax, diaphragm, and mediastinal structures. Pleural effusions can be unilateral or bilateral (Figure 7-17) and occur in 1 out of 15,000 pregnancies. Most cases of pleural effu-

sion result from high-output cardiac failure in the fetus, lymphatic dysplasia, or low osmotic pressure within the vascular system. Any cardiovascular or pulmonary abnormality can result in the development of pleural effusions. Pleural effusions may also be primary or secondary to fetal hydrops (hydrops fetalis), the hallmark of which is the abnormal accumulation of fluid in body cavities and soft tissues (e.g., pleural effusion, abdominal ascites, and dermal edema). Fetal hydrops—strictly defined as identification of two or more abnormal fluid collections

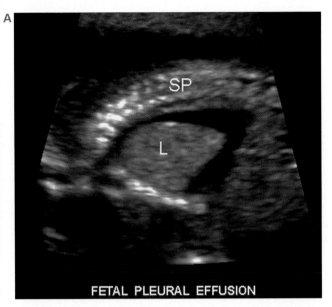

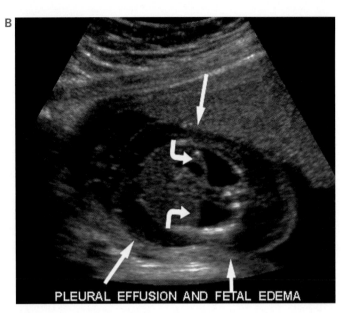

Figure 7-17. A *Longitudinal image of fetal chest demonstrating pleural effusion. SP = spine, L = lung.*
B *Transverse view of fetal thorax demonstrating bilateral pleural effusions (curved arrows) with gross dermal edema (straight arrows) indicating fetal hydrops.*

within body cavities or tissue—is associated with polyhydramnios and thickened placenta in from 30% to 75% of cases. There are two categories of fetal hydrops, immune and nonimmune. **Immune hydrops** results from **Rh isoimmunization** or alloimmune hemolytic disease, in which fetal red blood cells are destroyed by maternal IgG antibodies. **Nonimmune hydrops** (**NIH**) can be the result of about 149 different causes, including fetal, maternal, and placental abnormalities as well as some medications. Nevertheless, anomalies of the fetal heart are the most common cause and chromosomal abnormalities the second most common cause of NIH. See Chapter 10 for more detailed information on immune and nonimmune forms of fetal hydrops.

Congenital Cystic Adenomatoid Malformation

Congenital cystic adenomatoid malformation (**CCAM**) is one of the more common pulmonary masses, constituting 25% of all lung lesions. CCAMs are benign, congenital, hamartomatous lesions. The masses usually involve only one lobe or segment and can be isolated or associated with other anomalies (25%). If found to be an isolated anomaly and the fetus is delivered, resection of the mass is recommended as those left in can develop infection and abscess formation later on. Findings associated with a poor prognosis include mediastinal shift and the development of fetal hydrops.

CCAMs are classified as follows:

- Type I—also referred to as *macrocystic type*—contains defined cysts measuring 2–10 cm in diameter (Figure 7-18). Rarely associated with hydrops, type I lesions carry a 70% survival rate.

- Type II contains medium-sized cysts measuring less than 2 cm and is the type most likely to be associated with other anomalies, such as renal agenesis, diaphragmatic hernia, and other pulmonary malformations.

- Type III—*microcystic type*—contains cysts that are usually too small to resolve sonographically, making the mass appear homogeneously echogenic. There is a 78% mortality rate with this type if it is not detected antenatally.

Pulmonary Sequestration

Pulmonary sequestration is an accessory lobe of lung tissue that is separate from the normal tracheal bronchial tree and that has a systemic arterial blood supply from the aorta. Usually located in the lower posterior basal segments of the lobe, these masses of tissue appear homogeneously echogenic and can resemble microcystic adenomatoid malformation (Figure 7-19). There are two types of pulmonary sequestration, intralobar and extralobar.

Intralobar Sequestration Seventy-five percent of pulmonary sequestrations are of the intralobar type. These share

A

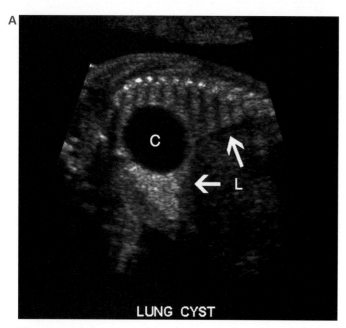

LUNG CYST

B

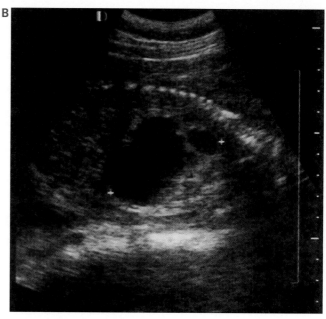

Figure 7-18. A *Long-axis view of fetal chest demonstrating macrocystic adenomatoid malformation in the lung. The arrows are showing the hypoechoic diaphragm. C = cyst, L = liver.* **B** *Macrocystic CCAM. Reprinted with permission from De Lange M, Rouse GA: Ob/Gyn Sonography: An Illustrated Review. Pasadena, CA, Davies Publishing, 2004.*

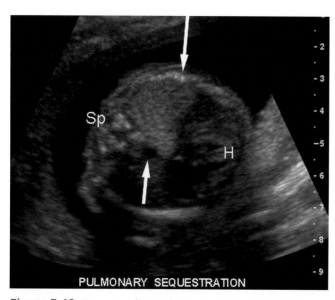

PULMONARY SEQUESTRATION

Figure 7-19. *Transverse image through the fetal chest showing mediastinal shift of the heart by a pulmonary sequestration (arrow). H = heart, Sp = spine.*

a common pleural covering with the main lung lobe and have venous drainage into the pulmonary veins. The arterial supply usually arises from the pulmonary artery. This type is most commonly seen in adults. The right- and left-sidedness is 50/50. Only a small percentage (14%) is associated with other anomalies, most commonly those of the skeleton, foregut, and diaphragm.

Extralobar Sequestration Most commonly seen in fetuses, neonates, and children, extralobar pulmonary sequestration has its own separate pleural covering, and the veins drain into the hemizygous or portal veins. The arterial supply arises directly from the aorta. Although most of these are located in the thorax, a small percentage (5%) may be found below the diaphragm. Most are left-sided (80%), and as many as 60% are associated with other anomalies—most commonly diaphragmatic, pulmonary, or cardiac.

Diaphragmatic Hernia

The diaphragm develops between 6 and 10 weeks' gestation. Incomplete fusion of the diaphragmatic structures results in herniation of the abdominal contents into the fetal chest. This occurs in 1 out of every 3000 births with a male-to-female ratio of 2:1. More than 90% of cases are unilateral and left-sided.

Defects occurring at the foramen of Bochdalek are posterolateral in location. Left-sided defects are easier to identify because the fluid-filled stomach is seen adjacent to and displacing the heart against the chest wall (Figure 7-20). Defects occurring at the right lateral corner allow liver into the chest. The sonographic appearance of liver and lung tissue can be similar, making the defect even more difficult to appreciate. The herniated viscera may

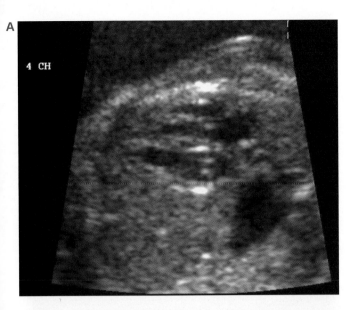

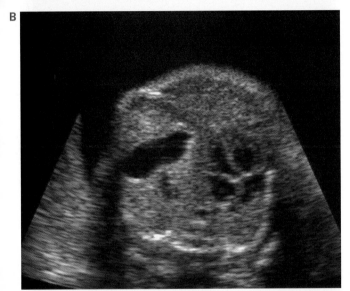

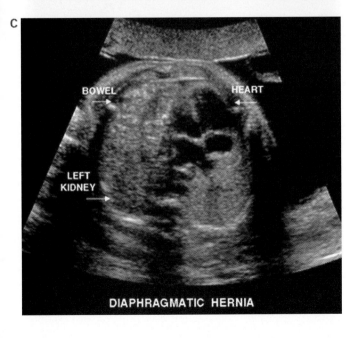

Figure 7-20. A *Transverse image through the fetal chest shows the fluid-filled stomach and heart at the same level. The heart is displaced to the right.* **B** *Four-chamber view of the fetal heart demonstrates the fluid-filled stomach adjacent to and displacing the heart against the chest wall.* **C** *This four-chamber view reveals the left kidney and bowel herniated into the chest, displacing the heart to the right.*

also present as a mass in the chest giving an appearance consistent with CCAM or pulmonary sequestration.

Hernias at the foramina of Morgagni are less common and midline in location. These are more likely to involve other abdominal viscera. With both types of hernias, one should be able to appreciate the diaphragmatic defect. Because **diaphragmatic hernias** are often associated with other anomalies (50%–75%), especially trisomy 18, the prognosis is poor, with a mortality rate exceeding 70% due to pulmonary hypoplasia and anomalies. At least half of the fetuses presenting with associated anomalies are stillborn. The larger the defect/mass and the earlier it is detected (before 25 weeks), the more dismal the outcome. The most common sonographic finding is a mediastinal shift, which often contributes to the development of hydrops.

Heart

Entire textbooks have been written on the fetal heart and congenital heart disease (CHD), and this chapter is not intended to cover the subject extensively. The anomalies mentioned here are the ones that can be detected when imaging the four-chamber view of the heart. Anomalies that cannot be detected with the four-chamber view include very small ventricular septal defects, **tetralogy of Fallot**, **transposition of the great vessels** (**TGV**; also known as **transposition of the great arteries** [**TGA**]), **truncus arteriosus**, and **coarctation of the aorta** (narrowing of part of the aorta). See Box 7-6.

Box 7-6.	Cardiac anomalies easily missed on four-chamber view.
	Tiny VSDs
	Transposition of the great vessels
	Coarctation of the aorta
	Truncus arteriosus
	Tetralogy of Fallot

Box 7-7.	Cardiac anomalies detected with the four-chamber view.

Cardiomyopathy
Ebstein's anomaly
Hypoplastic ventricle
Single ventricle
Aortic/pulmonary stenosis
VSD/ASD
Endocardial cushion defect
Arrhythmias
Masses

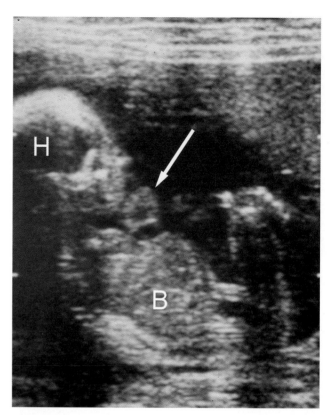

Figure 7-21. *Long-axis view of fetus with ectopia cordis (arrow). H = head, B = body.*

Congenital heart disease constitutes approximately one-third of all congenital malformations and occurs in 1% of live births. Maternal risk factors include but are not limited to diabetes mellitus, collagen vascular disease, TORCH, and Coxsackie virus. Familial factors should also be considered, including genetic syndromes such as Marfan, tuberous sclerosis, Noonan, Holt-Oram, and DiGeorge. Factors indicating a more thorough fetal cardiac examination include a first-degree relative with a congenital heart disease, maternal diabetes mellitus, fetal chromosomal abnormality, an extracardiac anomaly, teratogen exposure, fetal arrhythmia, and fetal hydrops. See Box 7-7.

Ectopia Cordis

Ectopia cordis is very rare, occurring in 1 out of 100,000 births with a male-to-female ratio of 2:1. Although usually associated with other anomalies, it can be an isolated defect that is surgically correctible (Figure 7-21). Most cases of ectopia cordis, however, are associated with limb–body wall abnormalities, early amniotic rupture, or pentalogy of Cantrell, which are usually lethal.

Cardiac Enlargement

An enlarged heart, referred to as **cardiomegaly**, can be due to anything causing cardiac failure or increased cardiac output, such as an arteriovenous (AV) malformation or twin-to-twin transfusion. Other causes include cardiac malformations, cardiac tumors, and **cardiomyopathy**. Fetuses presenting with hypoplastic lungs may give the appearance of cardiomegaly—a common pitfall.

Hypoplastic Ventricle

Although either ventricle can be afflicted with hypoplasia, it most commonly affects the left. The **hypoplastic**

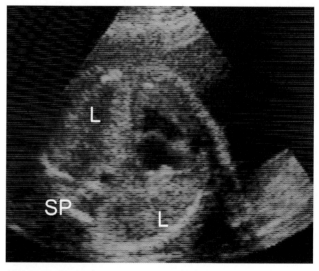

Figure 7-22. *Transverse image through fetal chest showing hypoplastic ventricle. L = lungs, SP = spine.*

left heart syndrome includes a number of structural anomalies associated with a small or absent left ventricle (Figure 7-22). These include aortic atresia, mitral atresia, aortic arch hypoplasia, and coarctation. Fetuses with hypoplastic left ventricle are not usually stressed in utero and do not get into trouble until delivery. There are two procedures that can be performed after delivery. One is the three-stage Norwood procedure, and the second is cardiac transplantation. The Norwood procedure carries a high mortality rate, and many children are unable to progress through all phases of the treatment. While cardiac transplantation has a lower initial operative risk, there is decreased quality of life, and the lack of donors significantly limits the option.

An affected right ventricle may be caused by pulmonary atresia with an intact septum and **tricuspid atresia** (absence or abnormal formation of the tricuspid valve). With **Ebstein's anomaly**, the right atrium enlarges because the tricuspid valve leaflets are incompetent and displaced into the right ventricle. Doppler evaluation reveals very turbulent flow within the right ventricle, which is smaller, but normal flow in the left ventricle. If there is an unbalanced **atrioventricular canal** (**AVC**) defect, double-outlet right ventricle, or single ventricle, either ventricle can be hypoplastic.

Ventricular Septal Defects/Atrial Septal Defects

Ventricular septal defects (**VSDs**) occur in 1 out of 400 births and are among the most common cardiac malformations. They are the result of either (1) a muscular defect due to excessive excavation during ventricular growth or (2) inlet, outlet, or membranous defects due to failure of fusion. VSDs have been associated with exposure to alcohol, valproic acid, and hydantoin. Small defects can be difficult or impossible to identify with sonography and may close spontaneously. Larger defects can usually be surgically repaired. Defects that are identified sonographically are generally larger and more severe (Figure 7-23).

Atrial septal defects (**ASDs**) may be high in the septum (*secundum*) or low at the crux of the heart (*primum*). Primum ASDs are often associated with an inlet VSD. They are very difficult to diagnosis on fetal sonography unless part of the intra-atrial septum is absent. The septum is thin in the area of the foramen ovale and drop-out may occur.

Endocardial Cushion Defect

Endocardial cushion defect is a collection of heart defects consisting of an ASD with VSDs and abnormalities of the atrioventricular valves. This condition is one that has been strongly associated with Down syndrome. In utero heart failure can occur. The prognosis correlates with the severity of the defect. Surgical correction is possible in the majority of cases.

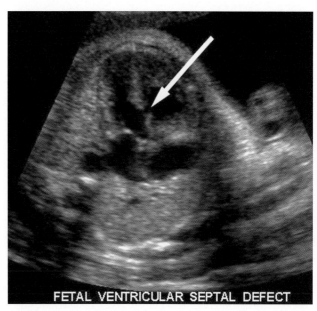

Figure 7-23. *Four-chamber view of the fetal heart demonstrating a ventricular septal defect (arrow).*

Abdomen and Gastrointestinal Tract

Ascites

Fetal abdominal **ascites** is the collection of free intraperitoneal fluid that surrounds the organs and may displace them toward the middle of the abdomen. Intraperitoneal fluid may be related to fetal hydrops, intrauterine infection, perforated bowel obstruction (meconium ileus/peritonitis), and ruptured urinary obstruction (urinary ascites) (Figures 7-24 A and B). One must be careful not to mistake the normally hypoechoic muscle of the abdominal wall for fluid. This is referred to as pseudoascites (Figure 7-24C).

Esophageal Atresia

Occurring in 1 out of 5000 births, esophageal atresia is the congenital lack of continuity of the esophagus where it terminates in a blind-ending pouch. Ninety percent of patients also have a tracheoesophageal fistula (TE), and 50% have other associated anomalies. If esophageal atresia is isolated, functional repair can be performed with a very high success rate. Nevertheless, survival and prognosis depend on the presence and severity of associated anomalies, which can include other gastrointestinal defects (10%), cardiac anomalies (20%), imperforate anus (10%), **VACTERL** (6%), and trisomy 21 (2%–3%). More than 25 other genetic, chromosomal, and sporadic syndromes have also been described with esophageal atresia and tracheoesophageal fistula.

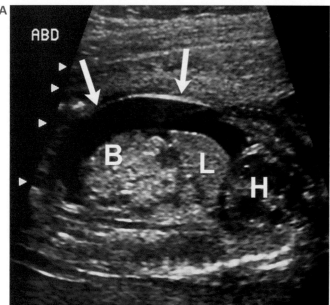

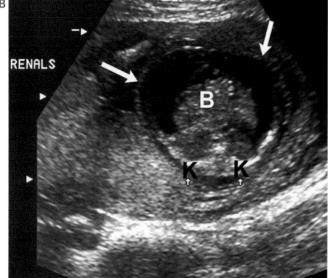

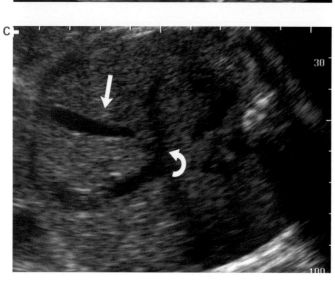

Figure 7-24. *Longitudinal (**A**) and transverse (**B**) views of fetal abdomen demonstrate abdominal ascites (arrows). L = liver, B = bowel, H = heart, K = kidneys. **C** Transverse view through fetal abdomen at the level of the umbilical vein turning into portal (curved arrow) and gallbladder (straight arrow). **D** and **E** Transverse images showing a large fetal gallstone (arrow). The mother had sickle cell anemia. UV = umbilical vein, S = stomach, SP = spine.*

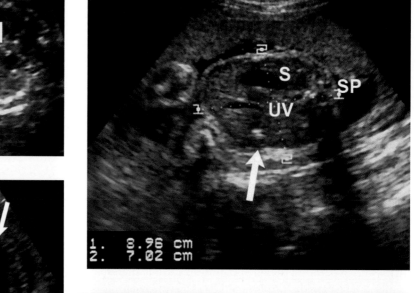

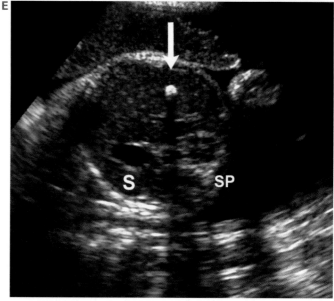

Gallbladder

The fetal gallbladder can be seen after 20 weeks' gestation and is routinely visualized in the third trimester. Absence of the gallbladder may be an indication of **cystic fibrosis**. **Gallstones** in children are not common and even rarer in the fetus. The exception is the patient with **sickle cell anemia**. The presence of fetal gallstones may be an indication for sickle cell anemia. Cystic fibrosis can lead to meconium ileus and peritonitis, and sickle cell anemia is a blood disorder. Both can be associated with polyhydramnios. Since both cystic fibrosis and sickle cell anemia are hereditary, maternal patient history should offer confirmation (Figures 7-24 D–E).

Duodenal Atresia

Considered the most common small bowel obstruction, duodenal atresia occurs in 1 out of 10,000 births. Maternal diabetes, retinoic acid, and alcohol abuse are known teratogens. **Duodenal atresia** results from complete stenosis of the duodenal lumen. It tends to be more common among males and may result from an annular pancreas. One-third of all cases have proven to be associated with trisomy 21. Unless it is associated with other severe anomalies, this condition can be easily corrected, and the prognosis is good. Although duodenal atresia can be detected sonographically as early as 18–20 weeks, it may not be identified until after 24 weeks. The classic sonographic appearance is the double-bubble sign with massive polyhydramnios. The **double bubble** is formed by the normal fluid-filled stomach (first bubble) and the dilated duodenum (second bubble) (Figure 7-25).

Jejunal Atresia

When other parts of the small bowel become obstructed, the cause is usually thought to be ischemic injury from **hypotension** (low blood pressure), vascular accidents/malformations, intussusception, or volvulus. **Jejunal atresia**—absence or closure of the central part of the small intestine—carries a good prognosis if it is an isolated finding. However, 40% of cases have been associated with other anomalies, and more than 15 genetic, chromosomal, and sporadic syndromes have been described with intestinal atresias. The sonographic appearance of a lower intestinal obstruction includes multiple fluid-filled bubbles with some echogenic bowel, dilated loops of bowel, and polyhydramnios. The potential for intestinal rupture is present and will result in **meconium peritonitis**. Most of these cases will resolve in utero with

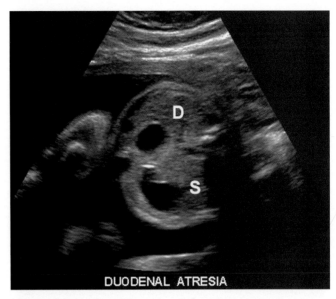

Figure 7-25. *Transverse image of fetal abdomen through the stomach showing the double-bubble sign. S = stomach, D = duodenum.*

normal bowel function. The sonographic appearance of meconium peritonitis includes echogenic ascites, calcifications, and polyhydramnios.

Other Cysts

Cystic masses that may be seen within the fetal abdomen include ovarian, mesenteric, omental, choledochal, gut duplication, sacrococcygeal teratoma, and urachal. These cysts can be challenging if not impossible to differentiate (Figure 7-26). In such situations, it can be helpful to identify fetal sex since, for example, one would not consider an ovarian cyst in a male fetus or a large bladder due to posterior urethral valves in a female fetus. If a cystic mass displaces the bladder anteriorly, one should consider a sacrococcygeal teratoma, anterior meningocele, or either **hydrocolpos**—fluid in the vagina—or **hydrometrocolpos**—fluid in the vagina and uterus (if the fetus is female). **Ovarian cysts** are not uncommon in female fetuses due to maternal and placental hormone stimulation, and these cysts can become quite large, appearing simple or complex. The cysts usually resolve within a few weeks after delivery when hormone stimulation has ceased.

Omental and mesenteric cysts are uncommon with approximately one-third of cases occurring in patients less than 15 years of age. More common than omental cysts, **mesenteric cysts** are lymphatic in origin, benign, and can

Figure 7-26. A *Long-axis view of lower fetal abdomen demonstrates an ovarian cyst. S = stomach, H = heart. Longitudinal (**B**) and transverse (**C**) views of fetal abdomen demonstrate a mesenteric cyst. **D** Meconium cyst from intestinal obstruction.*

A
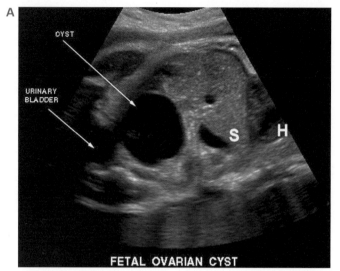

B
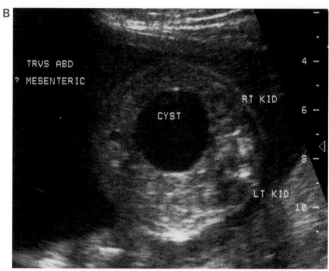

C
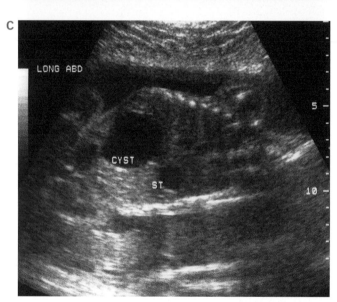

D
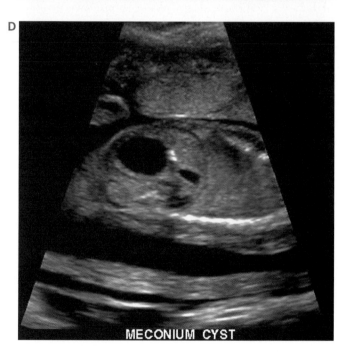

occur anywhere along the gastrointestinal tract from the duodenum to the rectum. They are mostly found within the ileal mesentery of the small bowel or the sigmoid mesentery of the colon. **Omental cysts** are found within the greater and lesser omentum. They may appear as a single simple unilocular cyst or be multiple and complex, ranging in size from a few millimeters to 40 cm. Often they are incidental findings and asymptomatic unless they are hemorrhagic, infected, or torsed, in which case patients could present with abdominal distention and acute abdominal pain. **Gut** or **enteric duplication cysts** are the result of a rare congenital malformation of the intestinal

tract and share at least one common layer with the normal intestine. Most are diagnosed within the first two years of life; the rest are discovered during the newborn period. These are probably best described as diverticula rather than cysts and are identified sonographically by the double wall or "muscular rim" sign, mimicking the gut signature of the intestinal wall. **Sacrococcygeal teratomas** can be mostly cystic, but only rarely, as they contain tissues from all three fetal layers; therefore, they will not be discussed further here. However, the position of an internal teratoma would be deep in the lower abdomen anterior to the lumbar spine, sacrum, or coccyx.

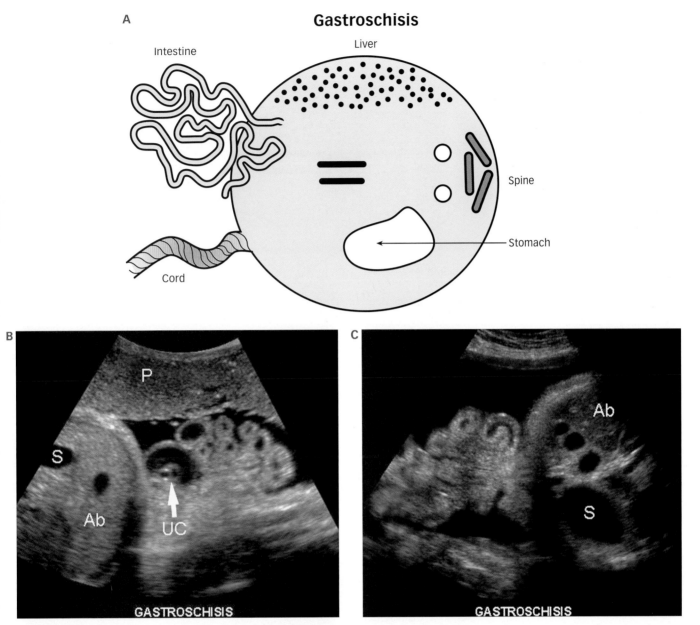

Figure 7-27. A *Schematic of the cord insertion with a gastroschisis.* **B** *and* **C** *Free-floating intestines are seen outside the fetal abdomen. The umbilical cord is seen between the gastroschisis and the abdomen. Ab = abdomen, P = placenta, UC = umbilical cord, S = stomach.*

A **urachal cyst** adjacent to a fluid-filled bladder presents as a double bubble, but these bubbles are anterior and low in the abdomen (caudal to the kidneys), in contrast to the double bubbles of duodenal atresia, which present superior to the kidneys and deep in the abdomen.

Gastroschisis
Gastroschisis is the evisceration of the intestines through a paraumbilical wall defect, occurring in 1 in 4000 births. This condition is rarely associated with other anomalies and does not have an association with chromosomal syndromes or disorders. The bowel loops usually are

seen to the right of the normal umbilical cord insertion (Figure 7-27A). The bowel is free floating, not covered by a membrane. Loops may appear thickened due to irritation from the amniotic fluid. Malrotation of the gut is common, and so the stomach may be inverted and malpositioned as well (Figures 7-27 B and C). Small and large bowel, stomach, and bladder can all be included. Intrauterine growth restriction is a common complication since proteins from the bowel leak into the amniotic fluid. Preterm delivery is also common and warrants close monitoring.

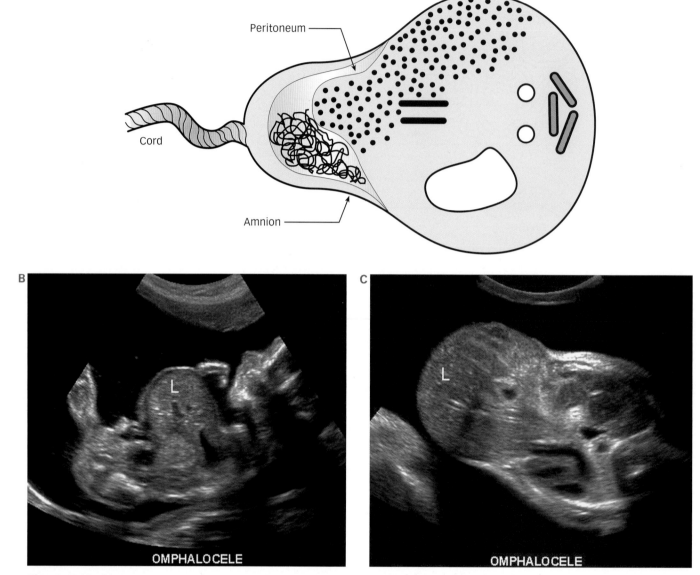

Figure 7-28. A *Schematic of the cord insertion with an omphalocele.* **B** *and* **C** *Longitudinal and transverse images of an extracorporeal liver. L = liver.*

Omphaloceles

The incidence of omphalocele is approximately 1 in 5000 births with a 1:5 male-to-female ratio. An **omphalocele** is an abdominal wall defect that occurs at the base of the umbilical cord. Abdominal viscera herniate into a thin sac composed of peritoneum and amnion, and the umbilical cord inserts into the sac (Figure 7-28A). Omphaloceles are classified as occurring with either intracorporeal or extracorporeal (herniated) liver.

Intracorporeal Liver Omphaloceles with **intracorporeal liver** contain only bowel. These are most commonly associated with chromosomal abnormalities. They can

look similar to a gastroschisis if attention is not paid to the cord insertion site and the surrounding membrane. In some instances, ascitic fluid can build within the sac and cause it to rupture, inhibiting visualization of the surrounding membrane.

Extracorporeal Liver Omphaloceles with **extracorporeal liver** are the most common type (80%), where liver and sometimes bowel herniate into the sac (Figures 7-28 B and C). Any of the other organs can also be involved. The umbilical cord is seen entering the mass and running through the middle of it.

Prognosis The prognosis for omphaloceles depends most on whether there are other associated anomalies and the size of the defect. Very large defects that contain both solid and hollow viscera are more difficult to reduce successfully. Associated anomalies include cardiac (30%–50%), gastrointestinal, and genitourinary.

Cloacal and Bladder Exstrophy

Cloacal exstrophy is an extensive defect in the lower abdomen that involves the bladder and intestinal epithelium while also being associated with an imperforate anus and a wide separation of the anterior pubic arch. **Bladder exstrophy** defect is a failure of the closure of the lower abdomen allowing the bladder to extend outside the abdomen. It is a less common abdominal wall defect, occurring in 1 in 30,000 births with a 3:1 male-to-female ratio. It is not usually associated with other anomalies, and the prognosis is good. Nevertheless, studies have suggested that these patients have a higher risk for developing bladder cancer later in life. The sonographic appearance depends on whether the bladder is urine-filled or not. If not, it will look like a small tissue-like mass with male genitalia seen in a more anterior superior location than usual. If urine-filled, the bladder wall may appear thickened and the bladder will extend out from the anterior abdomen (Figure 7-29). Polyhydramnios is common with cloacal exstrophy but less so with bladder exstrophy.

Limb–Body Wall Complex

Limb–body wall complex (**LBWC**) is the severest form of abdominal wall defect. It is thought to result from adhering amniotic membranes that disrupt normal fetal development. With failure of the amnion and chorion to fuse and an extremely short umbilical cord, the fetus appears to adhere to the placenta. The amnion actually covers over the umbilical cord and extends from the cord all along the abdominal wall. Fetal development is severely disrupted and can include limb defects (95%), malformed organs (95%), scoliosis (77%), and craniofacial defects (56%). In many cases, it is difficult to appreciate any normal anatomy or anything that closely resembles a fetus. Basically what you see are parts of organs and skeletal structures. Other names for this anomaly include **body stalk anomaly**, **cyllosoma**, and **VACTERL** (vertebral, anal, cardiac, tracheoesophageal, renal, and limb) **syndrome**—indicating the severe degree of involvement (Figure 7-30). See Chapter 5 for additional information on limb–body wall complex.

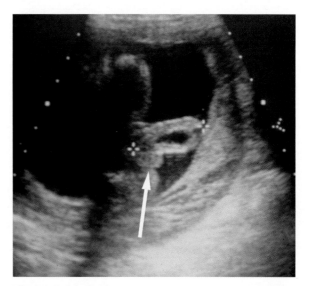

Figure 7-29. *Bladder exstrophy is demonstrated between the calipers. Fluid is seen within the bladder. The scrotum is indicated by the arrow.*

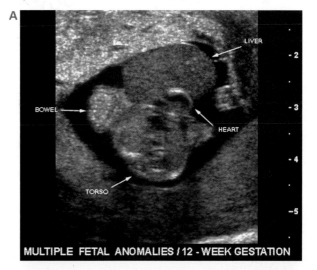

MULTIPLE FETAL ANOMALIES / 12 - WEEK GESTATION

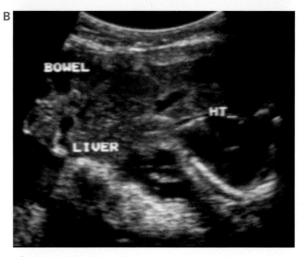

Figure 7-30. A *and* **B** *Fetal organs adherent to placenta and free-floating in a case of limb–body wall complex. (Figure continues . . .)*

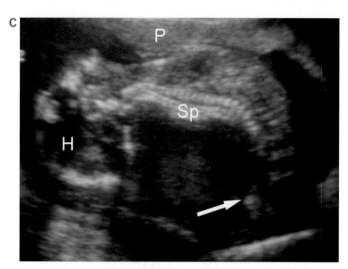

Figure 7-30, continued. C *Fetus is adhering to the placenta (P) with the spine (Sp) in an extreme flexed position causing hyperextension of the head (H), which is typical for arthrogryposis. Note, too, the single flipper-like lower extremity (arrow), suggesting sirenomelia.*

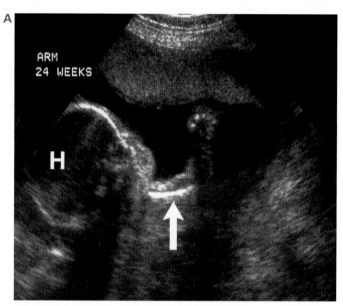

Figure 7-31. A *Image of head (H) and upper arm showing shortened bones in the arm and macrocephaly. The humerus is indicated by the arrow. Following page:* **B** *and* **C** *Lower limbs of dwarf show short length and classic bowing.* **D** *Bones in the forearm as well as the humerus are short in this case of skeletal dysplasia.* **E** *Long-axis view of the chest and abdomen show the classic bell shape.*

Table 7-3.	Bone length anomalies.

Anomaly	Anatomy Affected
Acromelia	Distal segment/terminal part of limb (hand/foot)
Mesomelia	Middle segment
Rhizomelia	Proximal segment
Micromelia	Entire limb

Skeletal Dysplasias

A skeletal dysplasia should be suspected anytime there is a family history or discovery of a shortened femur or decreased echogenicity of the bones during a fetal survey. A short femur length is usually the first indication of skeletal dysplasia and warrants measuring other long bones and foot length to further document the shortening of bones in the extremities, thereby confirming the generalized process. (See Table 7-3.) Fetal foot length is not affected by most skeletal dysplasias. The normal femur length/fetal foot ratio is 1. A FL/FF ratio of less than 0.9 suggests a skeletal dysplasia, while a FL/FF ratio greater than 0.9 is more suggestive of intrauterine growth restriction or genetically small fetus. Other sonographic findings that suggest skeletal dysplasia include a small thorax, abnormal skull and spine, polydactyly, fetal hydrops, and hypomineralization. Volumes have been written on the various types of skeletal dysplasia, but the fact is the disorders are rare. This text focuses only on the ones most likely to be encountered in a general practice.

Achondroplasia

The most common nonlethal skeletal dysplasia is **achondroplasia**. It can be inherited in an autosomal dominant fashion, but most cases are the result of spontaneous mutations. **Homozygous achondroplasia** is lethal and occurs when both parents are affected. In this scenario, the fetus will be stillborn or die shortly after delivery due to respiratory distress.

Typically, achondroplastic dwarfs present with rhizomelia and macrocephaly with hydrocephalus due to a small foramen magnum (Figures 7-31 A–D). A prominent forehead (frontal bossing) and depressed nasal bridge are not uncommon. The trunk length is usually normal but the spine is often lordotic and exhibits a small width. Kyphoscoliosis may be associated. The small thorax causes the abdomen to appear quite protuberant, giving the fetus the classic bell-shaped appearance (Figure 7-31E). Although

Figure 7-31, continued.

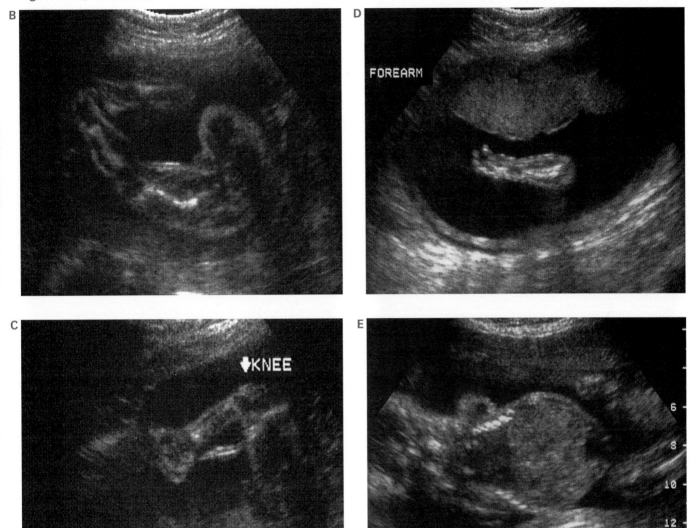

the condition is compatible with life, those affected may have respiratory problems including obstructive sleep apnea because the small chest lacks the ability to expand normally. The small foramen magnum and spinal curvatures contribute to neurologic complications due to compression of the spinal cord. Obesity, later in life, is also common. In most cases this disorder cannot be diagnosed sonographically before 24 weeks, and many findings may not present until the third trimester.

Achondrogenesis

Inherited as an autosomal recessive trait, **achondrogenesis** is lethal. There are several subtypes of which some can be mistaken for thanatophoric dwarfism and osteogenesis imperfecta. Sonographic findings include severely shortened and deformed extremities, poor ossification of the spine and skull with multiple rib fractures, a short trunk and thorax with a bell-shaped abdomen, redundant soft tissue, and severe polyhydramnios. This condition can be detected as early as 13–14 weeks (Figure 7-32).

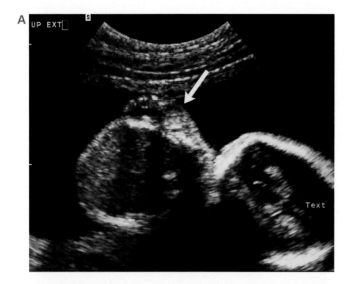

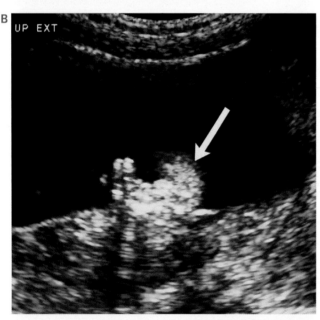

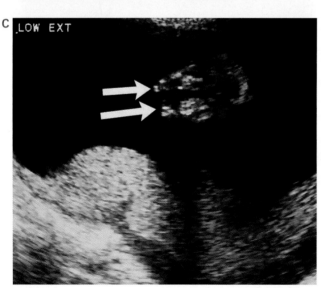

Figure 7-32. *Severely shortened and deformed limbs are indicated by the arrows.*

Thanatophoric Dysplasia

Although rare (1/40,000 live births), **thanatophoric dysplasia** is the most common lethal short-limbed skeletal dysplasia. It is considered a sporadic anomaly probably caused by new dominant mutations. Infants usually die shortly after delivery.

There are two types, 1 and 2. Sonographic findings for both types are the same as for achondrogenesis: The hands are trident-shaped and have short, stubby fingers. The short, bowed femurs have been described as having the appearance of an old telephone receiver. The cloverleaf skull deformity (**kleeblattschädel**), which distinguishes type 2 from type 1, has been described as specific to thanatophoric dwarfs, but in fact it affects only about 14% of them. (See Figures 7-33A and B.)

Osteogenesis Imperfecta

Characterized by hypomineralization of the bone and blue sclera, **osteogenesis imperfecta** is a group of hereditary collagen disorders often referred to as "brittle bone" diseases. There are four types (I–IV). Type IV is the mildest form. In these patients, fractures are uncommon and the blue sclera usually turns white over time. Although the individual may be short in stature, there is no asymmetry or deformation of limbs and they rarely develop deafness. In contrast, type I patients can easily fracture bones with normal activity. They often have scoliosis and the sclera is blue. The skin is thin and bruises easily and the teeth show discolorations. A striking physical finding is the triangular shape of the face. Deafness often occurs at 20–30 years of age. Types I and IV are inherited as an autosomal dominant trait and usually are not diagnosed until after birth.

Type II osteogenesis imperfecta is inherited as autosomal recessive and is lethal, while type III can be inherited as a recessive or dominant trait. Although type III may be compatible with life, it is severe and associated with extreme deformation and handicaps. Death usually occurs in the first or second decade of life due to respiratory complications.

Sonographic findings for types II and III include multiple fractures of long bones and ribs from simple movement in utero. Fractures cause limb shortening and deformation of the bones, including scoliosis of the spine and small thorax. The intracranial anatomy is exaggerated due to demineralization of the skull; pressure over the skull may show indentation of the brain (Figure 7-34).

Figure 7-33. A *Clover-leaf shape of the skull demonstrated in this fetus with type 2 thanatophoric dwarfism. Note the outward bulge in the temporal area (arrows).* **B** *Telephone-receiver shape of the short femur (arrow) in this fetus with type 1 thanatophoric dwarfism.*

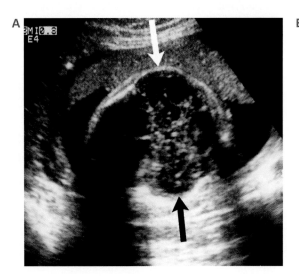
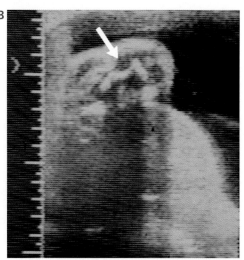

Figure 7-34. A *Osteogenesis imperfecta type II. The skull is not well ossified and flattens with transducer pressure.* **B** *and* **C** *Irregular shape of femurs due to fractures; arrows point to femur.* **D** *Caved-in chest due to broken ribs. The arrows are pointing to the ribs, as seen in transverse cross-section, that are caved in. Sp = spine. Reprinted with permission from De Lange M, Rouse GA: Ob/Gyn Sonography: An Illustrated Review. Pasadena, CA, Davies Publishing, 2004.*

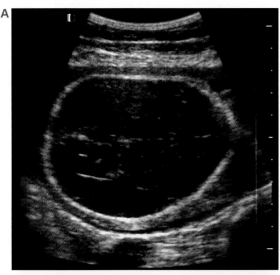
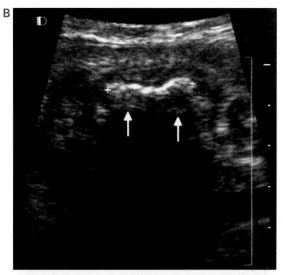
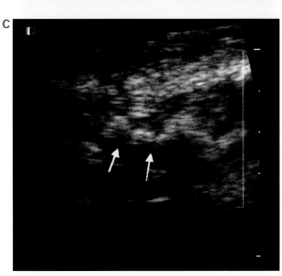
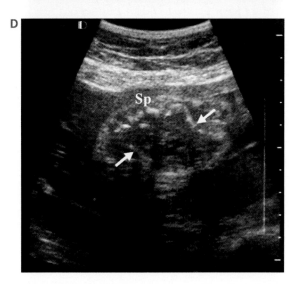

Arthrogryposis

Arthrogryposis is a term used to describe multiple joint contractures and rigidity. It can be caused by anything that inhibits normal fetal movement. Causes can include neurologic disorders such as congenital myotonic dystrophy, congenital myasthenia, and loss of anterior horn cells. Connective tissue disorders might include muscular or articular connective tissue dystrophy or even brain disorders like congenital encephalopathy. Known causative factors include hyperthermia and perinatal infection. There are a number of syndromes associated with arthrogryposis, including autosomal dominant, recessive, and X-linked traits. Joint contractures can also be the result of simple crowding, as seen with oligohydramnios and multiple gestations (Figure 7-35).

Limb Defects

The fetal long bones that make up the limbs are often affected by skeletal dysplasias, and hand and foot deformities are associated with skeletal as well as chromosomal abnormalities. Osteoblasts are cells that arise from the mesoderm and are responsible for the production of bone. Long bones begin as cartilage and convert into bone, whereas flat bones develop directly into bone. With long bones, the shaft or diaphysis (primary ossification center) develops first. At each end of the shaft is a growth center called the metaphysis. The epiphyseal discs are located on either end of the long bone. These secondary ossification centers form during the third trimester and continue after birth. The shaft and epiphysis grow together to form one continuous bone in the adult.

In evaluating fetal limbs, hands, and feet, the mission is to confirm their presence or absence, their shape, and whether there are any fractures. The long bones of the arm include the humerus, radius, and ulna. In the leg we look at the femur, tibia, and fibula. Three epiphyseal centers routinely seen prenatally include those at the distal femur, proximal tibia, and proximal humerus. These may not be identified until after 30 weeks' gestation. The length of long bones of the arms and legs can vary significantly in the normal population, differing from other measurements by as much as 3 weeks while still being normal. In this situation, a repeat scan should be considered to determine if the discrepancy in size is stable or increasing in severity. An increasing discrepancy would indicate a skeletal dysplasia.

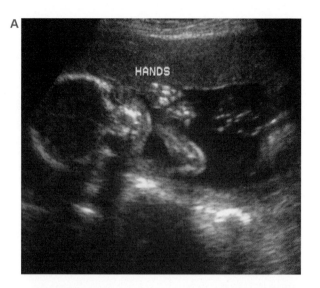

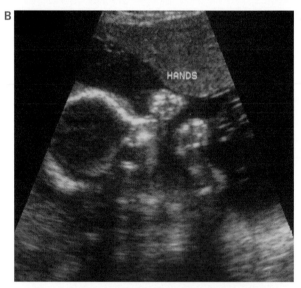

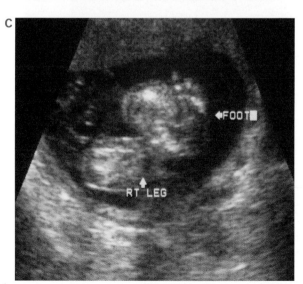

Figure 7-35. A *and* **B** *Fetal hands are fixed in a "praying mantis" position.* **C** *Fetal foot is turned back on the leg in a fixed position.*

When evaluating hands and feet, one should assess presence or absence, number of digits, and posture of the hand or foot. The following is a list of terms denoting various limb abnormalities:

Micromelia—entire limb is short

Hemimelia—missing limb below elbow or knee

Phocomelia—mid portion of limb is absent

Rhizomelia—proximal portion of limb is short (humerus/femur)

Mesomelia—short mid portion (mid phalanx or radius/tibia)

Cubitus varus—elbow deformity; forearm is bent inward (toward midline of body)

Cubitus valgus—elbow deformity; forearm is bent outward (away from midline of body)

Acheiria—absent hand

Apodia—absent foot

Amelia—absent limb

Adactyly—absent digit

Clinodactyly—overlapping digits

Polydactyly—extra digits

Preaxial—located on the radial (thumb) or tibial side

Postaxial—located on the ulnar (pinkie) or fibular side

Syndactyly—fused digits

SCANNING TIPS, GUIDELINES, AND PITFALLS

1. Pseudoascites can be produced when the sound beam is parallel to the abdominal wall muscles. A thin hypoechoic band below the skin and subcutaneous fat simulates fluid. By scanning at different angles, one will recognize the questionable fluid as simply an artifact. Remember, pseudoascites is always parallel to the skin surface (Figure 7-36).

2. Subcutaneous fat and hair may mimic scalp edema. Hair, however, usually shows a more fringe-like appearance (Figure 7-37).

3. Abdominal viscera and fetal heart seen in the same plane can indicate a diaphragmatic hernia or simply that one is scanning in a transverse oblique plane.

Make sure the thorax/abdomen is as round as possible to ensure you are in a true transverse orientation. If so, ribs should not be seen along the periphery.

4. When measuring soft-tissue thickness in the region of the thorax, keep in mind the soft tissues at the level of the scapula are normally thicker than those lower in the thorax. Therefore, soft-tissue thickness of the thorax should always be evaluated at the level of the four-chamber heart.

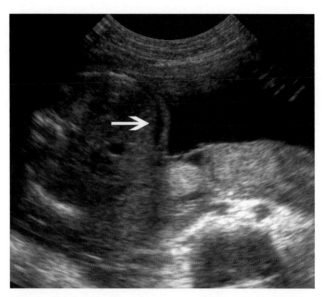

Figure 7-36. *Pseudoascites. The hypoechoic area (arrow) is normal abdominal wall musculature, not fluid.*

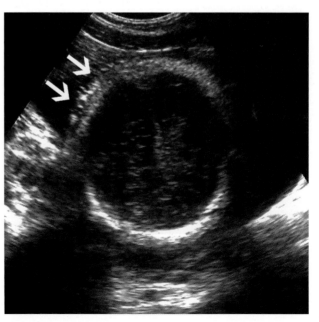

Figure 7-37. *Fetal hair is seen as fringe-like echoes (arrows) around the scalp.*

5. The umbilical cord may be mistaken for a complex cystic mass in the region of the neck when it lies in close proximity or is draped across it. Color Doppler can assist in differentiating the vessels of the cord from a cystic structure.

6. A two-vessel cord can be associated with a number of anomalies and should always warrant a very thorough investigation of the fetus, including the high-risk areas such as face, hands, and feet. Also, a placenta that shows multiple cystic areas (as with molar changes) is frequently an indication of triploidy (Figure 7-38).

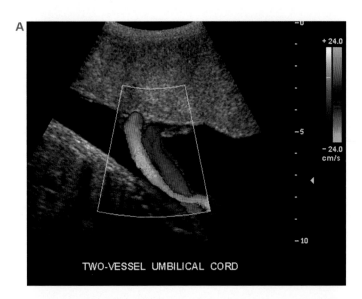

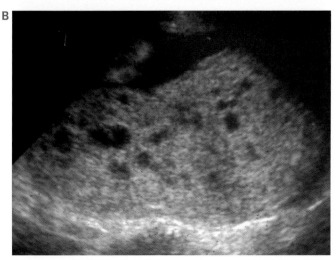

Figure 7-38. A *Two-vessel cord shown with color application.* **B** *Triploidy placenta shows thickening and molar changes.*

REFERENCES

Benacerraf BR: *Ultrasound of Fetal Syndromes*, 2nd Edition. London, Churchill Livingstone, 2007.

Bisset RAL, Khan AN, Thomas NB: *Differential Diagnosis in Obstetric and Gynecologic Ultrasound*, 2nd Edition. Philadelphia, Saunders, 2002.

Callen PW (ed): *Ultrasonography in Obstetrics and Gynecology*, 5th Edition. Philadelphia, Saunders Elsevier, 2008.

DeLange M, Rouse GA: *OB/GYN Sonography: An Illustrated Review*. Pasadena, CA, Davies, 2004.

DuBose T: *Fetal Sonography*. Philadelphia, Saunders, 1996.

Entezami M, Albig M, Gasiorek-Wiens A, et al: *Ultrasound Diagnosis of Fetal Anomalies*. New York, Thieme, 2004.

Hagan-Ansert SL (ed): *Textbook of Diagnostic Ultrasonography*, 7th Edition. St. Louis, Elsevier Mosby, 2012.

Hickey, J: *Essentials of Obstetrics and Gynecology Ultrasound: A Comprehensive Sonographer's Guide*, 2nd Edition. Forney, TX, Pegasus Lectures, 2008.

Hill L: Amniotic fluid index. In Goldberg BB, McGahan JP: *Atlas of Ultrasound Measurements*, 2nd Edition. St. Louis, Mosby/Elsevier, 2006, Chapter 8.

Jeng CJ, Jou TJ, Wang KG, et al: Amniotic fluid index measurement with the four-quadrant technique during pregnancy. J Reprod Med 35:674-677, 1990.

Maizels M, Cuneo B, Sabbagha RE: *Fetal Anomalies: Ultrasound Diagnosis and Postnatal Management*. New York, Wiley-Liss, 2001.

Manning FA, Hill LM, Platt LD: Quantitative amniotic fluid volume determination by ultrasound: antepartum detection of intrauterine growth retardation. Am J Obstet Gynecol 139:254-258, 1981.

McGahan JP, Porto M: *Diagnostic Obstetrical Ultrasound*. Philadelphia, Lippincott, 1994.

Phelan JP, Smith CV, Broussard P, et al: Amniotic fluid volume assessment with the four-quadrant technique at 36-42 weeks' gestation. J Reprod Med 32:540–542, 1987.

Rumack CM, Wilson SR, Charboneau JW (eds): *Diagnostic Ultrasound*, 4th Edition, Volume 2. Philadelphia, Elsevier Mosby, 2011.

Rutherford SE, Phelan JP, Smith CV, et al: The four-quadrant assessment of amniotic fluid volume: an adjunct to antepartum fetal heart rate testing. Obstet Gynecol 70:353, 1987.

Sabbagha RE: Diagnostic accuracy of targeted imaging for fetal anomalies. In Chervenak FA, Isaacson GC, Campbell S (eds): *Ultrasound in Obstetrics and Gynecology*, Volume 2. Boston, Little Brown, 1993.

Sanders RC: *Structural Fetal Abnormalities: The Total Picture*, 2nd Edition. St Louis, Mosby, 2002.

Sauerbrei EE, Nguyen KT, Nolan RL: *A Practical Guide to Ultrasound in Obstetrics and Gynecology*, 2nd Edition. New York, Lippincott Williams and Wilkins, 1998.

SELF-ASSESSMENT EXERCISES

Questions

1. The most common neural tube defect is:

   A. Spina bifida

   B. Hydrocephalus

   C. Anencephaly

   D. Myelomeningocele

   E. Encephalocele

2. Gastroschisis is associated with all of the following *except*:

   A. Chromosomal abnormalities

   B. Preterm delivery

   C. Elevated AFP

   D. Growth restriction

   E. Bowel obstructions

3. Absence of the fetal stomach on sonography would be suggestive of:

   A. Esophageal atresia

   B. Duodenal atresia

   C. Jejunal atresia

   D. Imperforate hymen

   E. Imperforate rectum

4. Of the following, which is a key feature of holoprosencephaly?

   A. Cystic hygroma

   B. Encephalocele

   C. Acrania

   D. Cleft defects

   E. Bowed limbs

5. Nonvisualization of the fetal gallbladder in the third trimester might be indicative of:

   A. Choledochal cyst

   B. Cystic fibrosis

   C. Down syndrome

   D. Bowel atresia

   E. Sickle cell anemia

6. Alobar, semilobar, and lobar are three types of:

   A. Encephalocele

   B. Holoprosencephaly

   C. Congenital cystic adenomatoid malformation

   D. Diaphragmatic hernia

   E. Spina bifida

7. Of the following cardiac anomalies, which is least likely to be seen on the four-chamber view?

   A. VSD

   B. Cardiomyopathy

   C. Endocardial cushion defect

   D. Ebstein's anomaly

   E. Transposition of the great vessels

8. The sonographic appearance of pulmonary sequestration can be similar to that of:

   A. Left-sided diaphragmatic hernia

   B. Right-sided diaphragmatic hernia

   C. Microcystic adenomatoid malformation

   D. Macrocystic adenomatoid malformation

   E. Pericardial effusion

9. Ossification of the lumbosacral region of the fetal spine is sufficient to rule out spina bifida by:

    A. 10 weeks' gestation

    B. 12 weeks' gestation

    C. 14 weeks' gestation

    D. 16 weeks' gestation

    E. 18 weeks' gestation

10. The most common site for a fetal teratoma is the:

    A. Face

    B. Neck

    C. Mediastinum

    D. Axilla

    E. Sacrococcygeal region

11. Which of the following is considered a destructive brain process usually caused by hemorrhage?

    A. Holoprosencephaly

    B. Porencephaly

    C. Hydrocephaly

    D. Anencephaly

    E. Cebocephaly

12. When a fetus is seen to have multiple joint contractures, one should suspect:

    A. Arthrogryposis

    B. Osteogenesis imperfecta

    C. Thanatophoric dwarfism

    D. Achondrogenesis

    E. Cubitus varus

13. Thanatophoric dwarfism has been associated with the:

    A. Cloverleaf-shaped head

    B. Strawberry-shaped head

    C. Lemon-shaped head

    D. Banana-shaped head

    E. Acrania

14 Rhizomelia refers to shortening of the:

    A. Distal end of a limb

    B. Distal segment of a limb

    C. Middle segment of a limb

    D. Proximal segment of a limb

    E. Entire limb

15. A spine that is open for the majority of its length is called:

    A. Scoliosis

    B. Rachischisis

    C. Kyphosis

    D. Lordosis

    E. Platyspondylisis

16. When a limb is missing below the elbow or knee, it is referred to as:

    A. Micromelia

    B. Mesomelia

    C. Phocomelia

    D. Rhizomelia

    E. Hemimelia

17. Of the following, which is considered a nonlethal type of dwarfism?

    A. Osteogenesis imperfecta II

    B. Thanatophoric

    C. Achondroplasia

    D. Achondrogenesis

    E. Camptomelic dysplasia

18. The double-bubble sign is associated with:

    A. Choledochal cyst

    B. Duodenal atresia

    C. Meconium peritonitis

    D. Patent urachus

    E. Bilateral hydroceles

19. This is an image of the fetal head. Additional images also demonstrated cyclopia and a proboscis. This most likely represents:

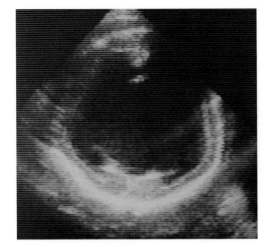

A. Holoprosencephaly

B. Hydranencephaly

C. Hydrocephaly

D. Hypercephaly

E. Encephalomeningocele

20. On a routine obstetric exam, this finding was observed. The patient presented large for gestational age. The most likely diagnosis would be:

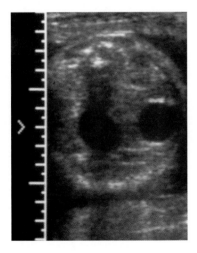

A. Macrosomia

B. Esophageal atresia

C. Duodenal atresia

D. Fetal hydrops

E. Ascites

21. This patient presented with an elevated AFP and was referred for sonographic interrogation. These images show:

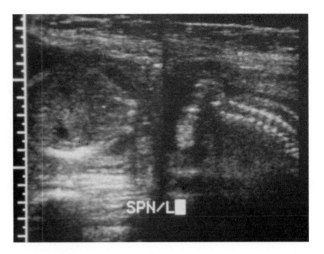

A. Spina bifida occulta

B. Spina bifida with meningocele

C. Spina bifida with myelomeningocele

D. Sacrococcygeal teratoma

E. Rachischisis

22. Based on the following image, which of the following choices would be the most likely diagnosis?

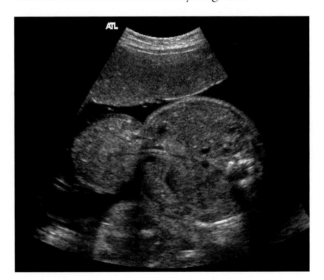

A. Gastroschisis

B. Extralobar sequestration

C. Umbilical hernia

D. Prune belly syndrome

E. Extracorporeal liver

23. This mass was seen extending off the inferior aspect of the fetal spine. A spinal defect could not be observed and no other anomalies were seen. The most likely diagnosis would be:

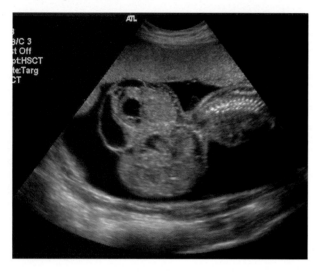

    A. Lumbar myelomeningocele
    B. Sacrococcygeal teratoma
    C. Anal prolapse
    D. Neurofibromatosis
    E. Bladder exstrophy

24. This image of the fetal head (arrows) is demonstrating which shape?

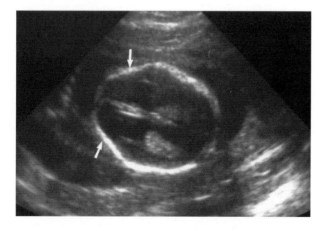

    A. Strawberry
    B. Lemon
    C. Banana
    D. Peanut
    E. Cloverleaf

25. The finding in the image from Question 24 suggests:
    A. Arnold-Chiari malformation
    B. Dandy-Walker malformation
    C. Limb–body wall malformation
    D. Amniotic band syndrome
    E. Congenital cystic adenomatoid malformation

26. The finding in the image from Question 24 is also highly suggestive of:
    A. Fetal alcohol syndrome
    B. Teratomas of the brain
    C. Dwarfism
    D. Spina bifida
    E. Fetal demise

27. What other diagnosis can be made from the image in Question 24?
    A. Mental retardation
    B. Growth retardation
    C. Chromosomal abnormality
    D. Fetal paralysis
    E. Hydrocephaly

Answers

See Appendix F on page 611 for answers and explanations.

Anomalies Associated with Oligohydramnios

Joe Rodriguez, RT, RDMS, and Kathryn A. Gill, MS, RT, RDMS, FSDMS

OBJECTIVES

After completing this chapter you should be able to:

1. Explain the importance and function of amniotic fluid.

2. List the most common causes of oligohydramnios.

3. Discuss the various sonographic indications of intrauterine fetal demise.

4. List and define the Potter syndrome types that can be identified in utero.

5. Explain how fetal urinary tract obstructions can affect amniotic fluid, and describe the sonographic appearances.

6. Explain the difference between symmetric and asymmetric intrauterine growth restriction.

7. List the five parameters evaluated with a fetal biophysical profile.

8. Describe how to perform a fetal biophysical profile.

AMNIOTIC FLUID is a clear, straw-colored sterile liquid that fills the uterus and surrounds the fetus throughout the pregnancy. During the first 12 to 16 weeks of gestation, the amniotic fluid is secreted by various structures such as the placenta, umbilical cord, fetal skin, and amniotic membranes. The fetus then begins a cycle of swallowing fluid and urinating it back into the amniotic cavity. The amniotic fluid thus is mostly fetal urine that is completely recycled through the fetus every few hours. This fluid is composed of several substances, including water, creatinine, urea, bilirubin, proteins, and albumin. The amount of fluid steadily increases until it reaches a peak volume of between 500 and 1000 ml during the third trimester. The amniotic fluid volume begins to decrease after 38 to 40 weeks' gestation. When there is a question of whether the amount of amniotic fluid is normal or not, one can calculate the amniotic fluid index (AFI; see Chapter 4). With experience, however, many sonography practitioners prefer to "eyeball" or qualitatively evaluate fluid levels (Figure 8-1).

Amniotic fluid serves many functions during pregnancy (Box 8-1). It protects the fetus from external trauma and provides a warm environment by helping to conduct and maintain the temperature. The amniotic fluid also allows for regulation of electrolytes and other fluids, and it has some bacteriostatic properties that help protect the fetus from infection. It provides free space for the fetus to move about without tangling the umbilical cord.

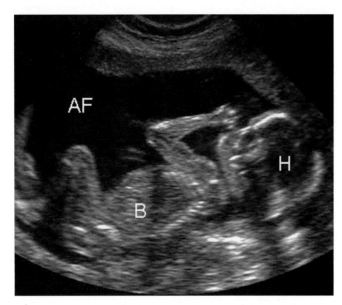

Figure 8-1. *Longitudinal image showing normal amount of amniotic fluid surrounding a second trimester fetus. H = head, B = body, AF = amniotic fluid.*

Adequate fluid is needed to ensure the normal development of the fetal lungs and gastrointestinal tract. As the fetus begins breathing and swallowing, amniotic fluid is washed through the bronchial tree and digestive tract, promoting the healthy development of the fetal lungs and the gastrointestinal tract.

OLIGOHYDRAMNIOS

Oligohydramnios is amniotic fluid volume that falls below normal levels for gestational age. AFI interpretations can vary (see Chapter 4), but it is generally accepted that an AFI of less than 5 cm is conclusive for oligohydramnios. Fluid leakage through the vagina and fetal urinary abnormalities are the most common causes of oligohydramnios. A small tear or rupture of the amniotic membrane may allow fluid to leak out. It can also afford bacteria a means of entering the uterus, creating a high risk of infection for both the mother and fetus. If the fetal kidneys are not functioning properly or if there is distal blockage of the urinary tract, the fetus will not be able to urinate. Fetal urination is vital to maintaining an adequate volume of amniotic fluid. (Both kidneys must be nonfunctioning for oligohydramnios to occur. If one kidney functions, the fluid level will be normal.)

Approximately 8% of pregnancies present with oligohydramnios, and the impact on the fetus is potentially severe: Low fluid volume increases the risk of the fetus

Box 8-1.   Functions of amniotic fluid.

Protection from trauma/infection
Temperature maintenance
Electrolyte regulation
Lung development
Allows fetal movement

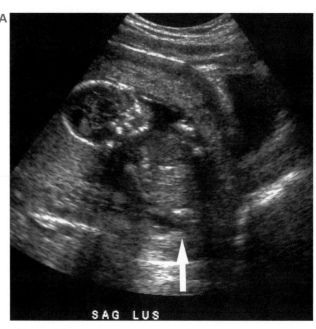

Figure 8-2. A *Longitudinal image of a second trimester fetus in the breech position. Oligohydramnios is causing the fetus to appear in an eccentric position due to its cramped space. Notice how the lower limb appears to be presenting knee first (arrow). Following page: **B** Severe oligohydramnios. The lack of amniotic fluid severely compromises the quality of this second trimester longitudinal scan of the fetal abdomen. The echo textures of the placenta and fetal body are nearly identical, making it difficult to appreciate any subtle abnormality within the fetus. No amniotic fluid pockets can be seen. P = placenta, B = fetal body.*

lying on and compressing the cord, thereby decreasing the blood supply to the fetus. In more extreme cases the cord is compressed completely, blocking the entire blood supply and causing fetal demise. Lack of fluid may also limit the fetus's range of motion within the uterus, creating the possibility of underdeveloped or malformed bones and muscles (Figure 8-2). Box 8-2 lists how oligohydramnios can affect the fetus.

Oligohydramnios is usually diagnosed in the third trimester, although it can occur anytime throughout the pregnancy. Oligohydramnios in the third trimester that is

Box 8-2.   Fetal effects of oligohydramnios.

Facial deformities (Potter facies)
Limb/skeletal deformities
Pulmonary hypoplasia
Cord compression

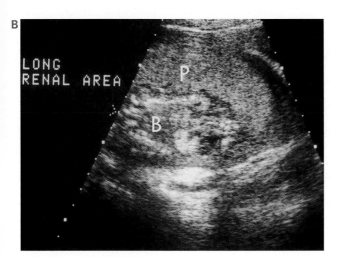

Figure 8-2, continued.

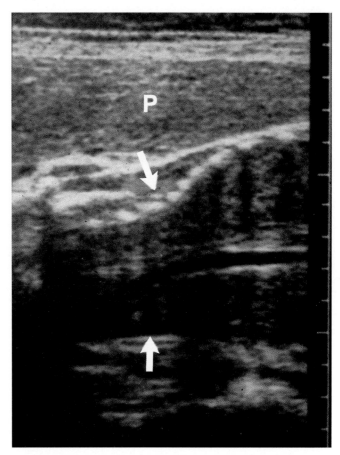

Figure 8-3. *This linear array image through the fetal chest and upper abdomen shows the bell-shaped thorax due to pulmonary hypoplasia (arrows). P = placenta.*

not related to premature rupture of membranes (PROM) or preterm premature rupture of membranes (PPROM) may result in fetal heart decelerations during labor. The outcome is usually favorable with prompt medical care. On the other hand, severe oligohydramnios diagnosed in the second trimester is more ominous due to the high risk of underdeveloped lungs called **pulmonary hypoplasia** (Figure 8-3). Pulmonary hypoplasia is usually lethal, but with proper medical attention the fetus can survive if the process is not too advanced. Under these conditions, fetal well-being is compromised.

One indication of fetal distress is the expulsion of meconium into the amniotic fluid. **Meconium** consists of fetal bowel contents and will give the fluid a green tinge. Small fragments resembling spinach can sometimes be seen floating in the fluid. Meconium-filled amniotic fluid appears quite thick and hazy (Figure 8-4).

Oligohydramnios can develop within 24 hours. The most common clinical signs and symptoms of oligohydramnios are leaking amniotic fluid, fetuses that measure small for gestational age, and decreased fetal movement. Drugs to treat preterm labor, such as ibuprofen and indomethacin,

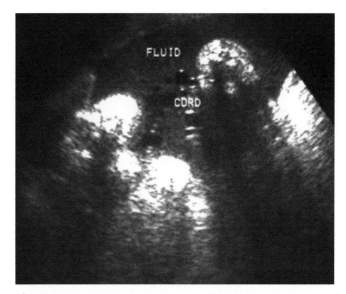

Figure 8-4. *This image shows meconium-filled amniotic fluid. Sonographically, the fluid simulates placental tissue. If one were to measure the deepest AP pocket in this image, it would actually measure approximately 6 cm.*

have been associated with oligohydramnios. These non-steroidal prostaglandin synthetase inhibitors cause the fetal renal blood flow to diminish, which results in decreased urine production and can lead to oligohydramnios. In addition to medications, other iatrogenic causes of oligohydramnios (those resulting from the action of a physician, clinician, or surgeon) include first trimester chorionic villus sampling and second trimester amniocentesis.

ASSOCIATED ANOMALIES: "DRIP"

Box 8-3 lists the conditions associated with oligohydramnios. An easy way to remember these conditions is to use the acronym DRIP, as in "there is just a *drip* of fluid." This mnemonic stands for demise, renal anomalies, iatrogenic causes and intrauterine growth restriction (IUGR), and PROM as well as post dates.

Fetal Demise—The "D" in DRIP

The World Health Organization defines **fetal demise** (death) as "present if the fetus or **neonate** does not breathe or show any other sign of life, such as beating of the heart, pulsation of umbilical cord, or definite movement of voluntary muscles." Fetal demise is usually first suspected when the mother notices a lack of fetal movement, fetal heart tones are inaudible at the office, or there is a decrease in or lack of fundal growth, especially in the first trimester. In contrast to the high fetal mortality rates of the first trimester, the incidence of fetal demise decreases later in pregnancy—to only an estimated 1% after 20 weeks' gestation.

Sonographic Signs
Increased resolution of ultrasound imaging makes the diagnosis of fetal demise easier and more accurate than in the past. Although fetal anatomy is often difficult to image because of problems accompanying fetal demise, the lack

of cardiac activity is indicative of absence of life. Several other signs add supporting evidence. These signs include oligohydramnios due to absorption of the fluid (Figure 8-5A), overlapping of the cranial bones (**Spalding's sign**) (Figure 8-5B), and scalp/trunk edema (**anasarca**) (Figures 8-5 C and D). Intra-abdominal and thoracic gas (**Robert's sign**) can be seen approximately 1–2 days after demise as tissues begin to break down. Thrombus can sometimes be visualized within the fetal heart, but this can be rather difficult to identify. Spalding's, Robert's, and **Deuel's signs** (scalp edema; also called *Deuel's halo sign*) are radiographic findings described decades ago and more

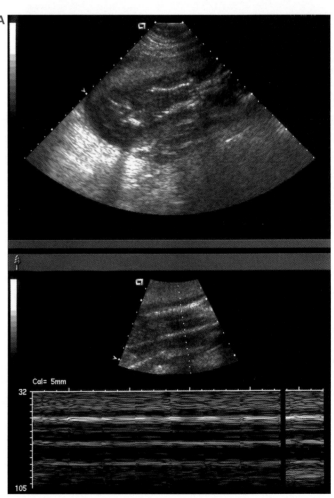

Figure 8-5. A *Longitudinal scan through a fetus showing oligohydramnios and collapse of the chest and abdomen. An M-mode tracing shows no cardiac activity. Following page:* **B** *Image of the fetal head shows collapse and overlapping of the fetal skull (Spalding's sign) and no definition of the brain anatomy or cranial contents.* **C** *Fetal demise. Soft-tissue edema around the fetal head (Deuel's sign).* **D** *Fetal demise. Soft-tissue edema around the fetal abdomen and abdominal ascites indicate gross hydrops.* **E** *General maceration of a fetus shown slumped to the floor of the uterus. The internal fetal anatomy is no longer identifiable. H = head, B = body, P = placenta.*

Box 8-3.	Conditions associated with oligohydramnios.
	D—Demise
	R—Renal anomalies
	I—IUGR/iatrogenic causes
	P—PROM/post dates

recently adopted by sonography practitioners. General **maceration** (degeneration of tissues) usually becomes sonographically apparent 10–14 days after demise (Figure 8-5E). See Box 8-4.

Although it may be detected earlier, normal fetal cardiac activity should be seen transabdominally by 7–8 weeks' gestation with a normal rate of 140 beats per minute ±20. Failure to identify fetal cardiac motion transabdominally by 8 weeks' gestation should automatically warrant the use of the endovaginal scanning technique. Endovaginal ultrasound should be used to evaluate pregnancies earlier than 8 weeks' gestation. Generally speaking, endovaginal technique allows us to see an embryo 1–2 weeks earlier than transabdominal technique. Active cardiac motion should always be identified if the gestational sac measures ≥1.6 cm by endovaginal scanning and ≥2.5 cm by

Box 8-4.	Sonographic signs of fetal demise.

No real-time cardiac motion

Spalding's sign (cranial bones overlapping)

Deuel's sign (scalp edema)

Robert's sign (gas in chest/abdomen)

transabdominal scanning. One should always remember that failure to see a fetal pole by 6 weeks does not necessarily imply a bad outcome. Inaccurate dating of the last menstrual period (LMP) gives the false impression that the fetus is further along than expected. See Chapter 3, Table 3-2.

B

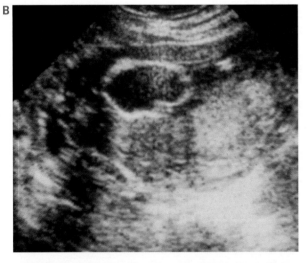

D

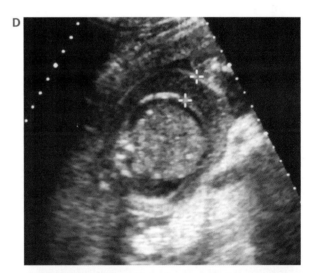

C

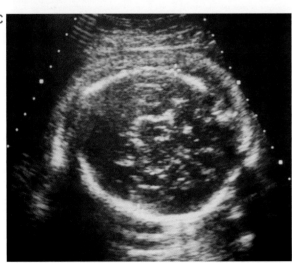

E

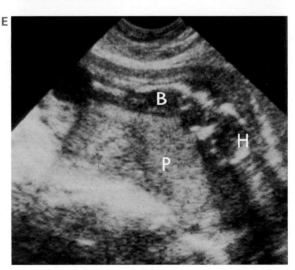

Figure 8-5, continued.

Renal Anomalies—The "R" in DRIP

In the 1940s, pediatrician Edith Potter first described the facial features of newborns delivered with oligohydramnios. They include a flat face with puffy, wide-set eyes, thick epicanthal folds, a parrot-beak nose, recessed chin, and low-set ears. These features were tagged the *Potter facies*. She further described musculoskeletal findings that included spade hands, joint contractures, and foot deformities such as clubbing.

There are five conditions referred to as **Potter sequence** (also known as **Potter syndrome** or **oligohydramnios sequence**):

1. Bilateral renal agenesis (BRA)—classic Potter.

2. Autosomal recessive polycystic kidney disease (ARPKD), formerly termed (and sometimes still called) infantile polycystic kidney disease (IPKD)—Potter type I.

3. Hereditary renal adysplasia (HRA)—Potter type II, including the more common form, unilateral renal adysplasia or agenesis (URA); classic Potter (bilateral renal agenesis) is sometimes considered an extreme form of type II, although here we treat it as a separate category.

4. Autosomal dominant polycystic kidney disease (ADPKD), which is also known as adult polycystic kidney disease (APKD) and is rarely seen in utero—Potter type III.

5. Cystic dysplasia of the kidneys due to long-term obstruction of the fetal kidneys or ureters—Potter type IV.

Because Potter "syndrome" is not a true syndrome (there is not a consistent set of symptoms and signs) but a sequence (a connected series of events), the terms *Potter sequence* and *oligohydramnios sequence* are often used instead of *Potter syndrome*.

Bilateral Renal Agenesis (Classic Potter Syndrome)

Bilateral renal agenesis (**BRA**) is a developmental disorder that occurs in approximately 1 in 3000 to 1 in 10,000 births and usually affects males (70%). It occurs sporadically. Maternal recurrences are rare. Because fetal urination is vital for maintaining the proper volume of amniotic fluid, failure to demonstrate a fetal bladder in the presence of oligohydramnios should always raise the possibility of renal problems. With bilateral renal agenesis, the fetus does not produce urine, resulting in decreased

amniotic fluid levels or severe oligohydramnios (Figure 8-6). Oligohydramnios associated with renal agenesis typically occurs after 18 weeks' gestation, as fetal kidneys are not responsible for the majority of fluid production until after 16 weeks. If fetal kidneys are not identified in their usual location, one should pay careful attention to the lower fetal abdomen to rule out a pelvic kidney (Figure 8-7). Because the fetal structures may be difficult to visualize due to the decreased fluid, the fetal bladder becomes an important landmark for the diagnosis of renal agenesis. The fetal urinary bladder fills and empties approximately every 30–45 minutes; therefore, failure to image the fetal bladder after one hour of scanning makes

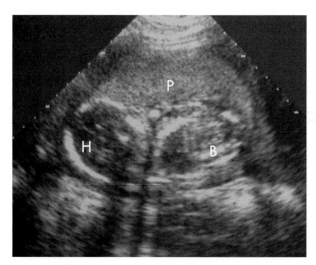

Figure 8-6. *Longitudinal scan demonstrating gross oligohydramnios. The fetus had bilateral renal agenesis. H = head, B = body, P = placenta.*

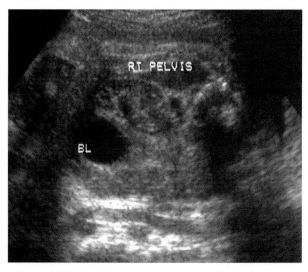

Figure 8-7. *Longitudinal scan shows the fetal kidney just superior and anterior to the fetal bladder (BL).*

the diagnosis of bilateral renal agenesis more likely. If renal agenesis is identified, it is extremely important to determine whether it is unilateral or bilateral. Bilateral agenesis is incompatible with life, with a 40% stillborn birth rate.

Sonographic Signs Bilateral renal outlines should normally be identified in the renal fossae at 15–17 weeks' gestation (Figure 8-8). There are three sonographic signs that make the diagnosis of bilateral renal agenesis convincing: (1) failure to visualize the fetal kidneys (for example, in the absence of kidneys the adrenals will fill the renal fossae and can be mistaken for kidneys; see Figure 8-9), (2) oligohydramnios, and (3) failure to demonstrate the fetal

urinary bladder after one hour of scanning. There is some variation in AFI interpretations depending on which author one reads (see Chapter 4), but it is generally accepted that an AFI of less than 5 cm is diagnostic for oligohydramnios. Visualizing the kidneys can be extremely difficult in the presence of oligohydramnios, particularly during the third trimester. It has been suggested that color Doppler can help to highlight the renal outline and renal arteries to confirm the presence of kidneys (Figure 8-10).

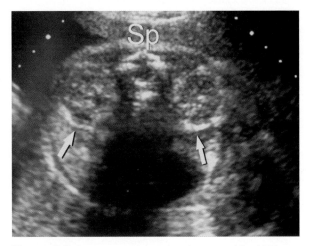

Figure 8-8. *Transverse image showing normal fetal kidneys (arrows) on either side of the spine (Sp).*

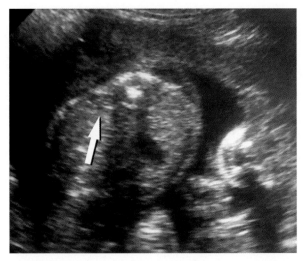

Figure 8-9. *Transverse image at the level of the normal fetal adrenal glands. Note that they look similar to kidneys but are flatter and lie obliquely to the spine (arrow); in the absence of kidneys the adrenals will fill the renal fossae and will look similar.*

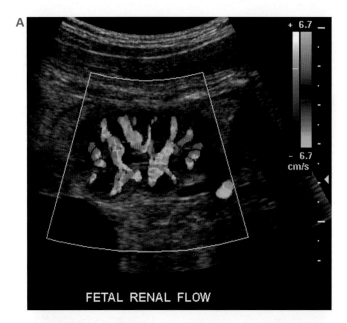

FETAL RENAL FLOW

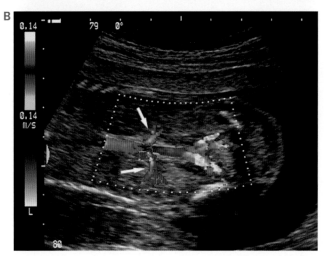

Figure 8-10. A *Color Doppler is used to demonstrate the outline of the kidney. The color settings should be high enough to record as much vasculature as possible without getting flash artifact. This technique is handy when the fetal kidneys are difficult to outline. It should be noted that the kidney will not "light up" if the vascular circulation is compromised or if the color settings are not optimal.* **B** *Color Doppler showing long-axis view of the fetal aorta demonstrating both renal arteries (arrows).*

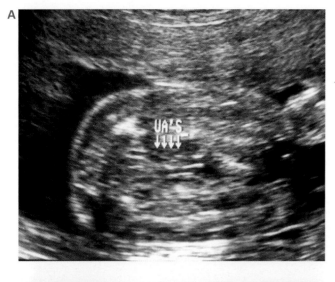

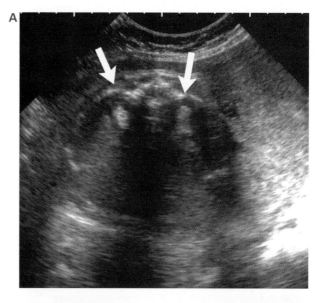

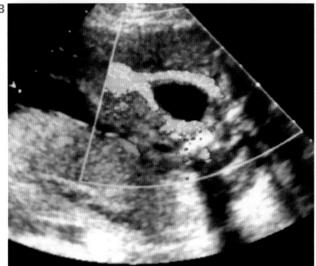

Figure 8-11. A *Scans through the fetal pelvis fail to demonstrate a urinary bladder after an extended period of time. The two umbilical arteries (arrows) are used as landmarks to locate the region of the urinary bladder. It should be seen between the two umbilical arteries.* **B** *A pelvic scan demonstrating a normal distended fetal urinary bladder surrounded by the two umbilical arteries.*

Figure 8-12. A *Transverse image through normal fetal adrenal glands (arrows). Note the reniform architecture.* **B** *This transverse fetal abdomen shows hypoechoic adrenal glands (arrows) filling the renal fossae in a fetus with bilateral renal agenesis.*

The fetal urinary bladder becomes an extremely useful landmark if the fetal kidneys cannot be identified (Figure 8-11). Visualizing a fluid-filled urinary bladder excludes bilateral renal agenesis. A common pitfall is mistaking the adrenal glands for kidneys. Fetal adrenals are large and will fill the renal fossae in the absence of kidneys. The echogenic medulla and hypoechoic cortex of the adrenals mimic the kidneys; however, adrenals are longer and flatter when compared to kidneys (Figure 8-12). Fortunately, the adrenal gland does not have the same color Doppler pattern as the kidney, making it less likely to be mistaken for a kidney when color Doppler is used.

Potter Type I/Autosomal Recessive Polycystic Kidney Disease

Autosomal recessive polycystic kidney disease (**ARPKD**)—also known as **infantile polycystic kidney disease** (**IPKD**)—is an inherited autosomal recessive disorder that results in the formation of multiple tiny renal cysts. The incidence of this disorder is approximately 1 in 40,000 births, and it has a maternal recurrence rate of 25%. The cysts range from microscopic to 2 mm and result from the dilatation of the renal collecting tubules. The numerous interfaces created by these small cysts give the kidney a hyperechoic appearance (Figure 8-13). Although the cysts may disrupt the renal parenchyma and enlarge the

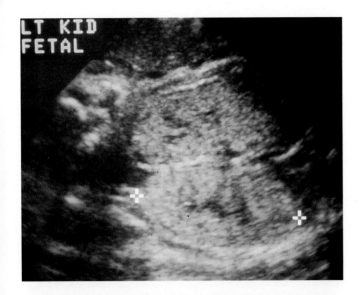

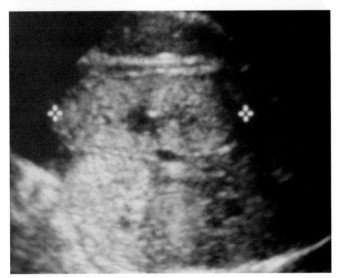

Figure 8-13. *Two images of infantile polycystic kidneys (calipers) filling the abdominal cavity. Note the smooth, hyperechoic pattern.*

kidneys, the basic renal outline is maintained; nevertheless, the kidneys fail to produce an adequate amount of fetal urine. The fetal liver and pancreas may also be affected.

Infantile polycystic kidneys can be diagnosed as early as 16 weeks' gestation. Usually, however, this process is discovered in utero only in severe cases and then only after 24 weeks' gestation. If renal function is compromised, oligohydramnios will be present and the fetal urinary bladder may not be visible. Performing the ultrasound scan shortly after the onset of infantile polycystic disease may result in a normal study. Therefore serial scans may be warranted on mothers who have had previous pregnancies with this condition. Renal function progressively decreases as the disease progresses, and the kidneys may produce a serum-like fluid rather than normal amniotic

fluid. When ARPKD is diagnosed in utero, survivors rarely live past 1 year. The prognosis for these fetuses is poor because of decreased renal function and pulmonary hypoplasia (see Figure 8-3), which results from the severe oligohydramnios. Those born with ARPKD usually are diagnosed after birth; one-third develop end-stage renal disease during childhood, along with hypertension and other conditions that must be managed for life.

Meckel syndrome (also known as **Meckel-Gruber syndrome**) is associated with polycystic kidneys, and the characteristically large echogenic kidneys are usually the most noticeable anomaly associated with the syndrome. These fetuses also have a posterior encephalocele and polydactyly—often missed because the oligohydramnios makes them difficult to visualize.

Potter Type II/Hereditary Renal Adysplasia

Potter type II, hereditary renal adysplasia, most commonly occurs as **unilateral renal adysplasia** or **agenesis** (**URA**), when one fetal kidney is hypoplastic (underdeveloped) and the other is absent (renal agenesis), hypoplastic, or dysplastic (such as multicystic). Potter type II is characterized by severe oligohydramnios and nonvisualization of the fetal kidneys and/or bladder. (Classic Potter, or bilateral renal agenesis, is an extreme form of Potter type II, addressed above as a separate category.)

URA is more common than bilateral renal agenesis, occurring in approximately 1 in 500 to 1 in 1000 births with a male-to-female ratio of 1:1. Since life can be sustained with one-half of one kidney, amniotic fluid levels will be normal in the presence of unilateral renal agenesis, because the remaining kidney will compensate and produce normal amounts of urine. The remaining kidney will also be hypertrophied because it is doing the work of two kidneys. As long as the single kidney is healthy, unilateral renal agenesis is of no clinical significance.

Potter Type III/Autosomal Dominant Polycystic Kidney Disease

Also referred to as **adult polycystic kidney disease** (**APKD**), **autosomal dominant polycystic kidney disease** (**ADPKD**) is linked to mutations in the PKD1 and PKD2 genes, though some cases are sporadic. As with ARPKD, the liver, pancreas, and spleen may also be affected. The incidence of ADPKD is 1 in 800 people, and it usually does not present until adulthood. Although there have been cases reported in fetuses and neonates, they are rare, and it is seldom the cause of oligohydramnios.

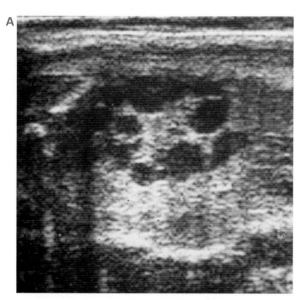

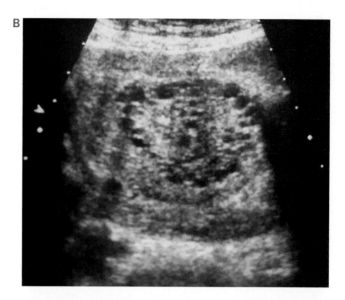

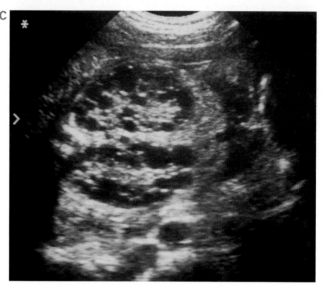

Figure 8-14. A *Longitudinal image through a multicystic fetal kidney. The contour is somewhat irregular due to the variably sized cysts along the cortical periphery. Note the echogenic collecting system sandwiched in the middle with the cysts scattered throughout the renal cortex.* **B** *Longitudinal image through the left fetal kidney in a fetus with bilateral multicystic kidneys.* **C** *Long axis through both multicystic kidneys.*

Potter Type IV

Potter type IV is cystic dysplasia of the kidneys caused by long-term bilateral obstruction of the fetal kidneys or ureters. Genetic predisposition, environmental factors, and chance may result in bilateral renal or ureteral obstruction and subsequent severe cystic dysplasia. These obstructions are relatively common and rarely lead to a dismal fetal outcome.

Multicystic Dysplastic Kidney Disease

Multicystic dysplastic kidney disease (**MCDK** or **MCDKD**) occurs during the embryonic stage of development. It is thought to be the result of complete ureteral obstruction prior to 10 weeks' gestation. The second most common childhood renal disorder, MCDK is characterized by multiple cysts of varying sizes that replace the renal parenchymal tissue. The kidneys are usually enlarged, and the borders may be distorted by cysts along the periphery. Multicystic dysplastic kidneys are usually unilateral and nonfunctioning (Figure 8-14A). Therefore, it is important to examine the contralateral kidney for abnormalities. Approximately 30% of fetuses with unilateral multicystic renal dysplasia present with hydronephrosis or agenesis of the contralateral kidney. Renal agenesis associated with multicystic renal dysplasia is fatal, while hydronephrosis usually has a better outcome. A normal amount of amniotic fluid and the presence of urine in the

fetal bladder are reassurances that the contralateral kidney is functioning properly. The presence of enlarged cystic kidneys and oligohydramnios and the failure to visualize the fetal bladder strongly suggest the diagnosis of bilateral multicystic dysplastic kidneys, which is typically fatal (Figures 8-14 B and C).

Hydronephrosis

Hydronephrosis—Greek for "water in the kidney"—is the dilatation of the renal collecting system caused by obstruction, reflux, or infrequent causes, such as an ectopic ureter. Hydronephrosis is the most common fetal anomaly detected by prenatal ultrasound and is also the most common childhood renal disorder. Figure 8-15A depicts unilateral hydronephrosis of the right kidney in a fetus. Figure 8-15B shows a distended fetal urinary bladder due to a urethral obstruction, which results in

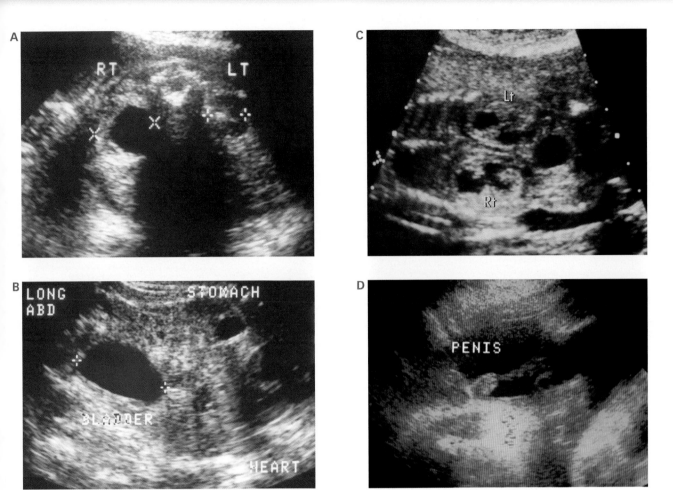

Figure 8-15. A *Transverse scan demonstrates hydronephrosis of the right kidney. The normal left kidney is identified adjacent to the spine in the renal fossa. Careful scanning should be done to avoid mistaking this for a renal cyst.* **B** *Longitudinal scan through the fetal bladder (calipers) shows moderate distention that was due to urethral obstruction.* **C** *Bilateral hydronephrosis. The right (Rt) kidney demonstrates the cystic areas merging together, while the cystic areas on the left (Lt) kidney are demonstrated as two separate renal structures. The two cystic areas in the left kidney are actually dilated calyces; however, the proper angle has not been obtained to visualize them converging into the renal pelvis. A coronal scan gives the best view, showing the calyces merging into the renal pelvis.* **D** *The fetal penis is seen urinating into the amniotic sac. This action confirms the absence of obstruction at the urinary outflow tract.*

bilateral hydronephrosis (Figure 8-15C). Bladder outlet obstructions lead to dilatation of the entire urinary tract. Also note the lack of amniotic fluid in Figures 8-15 B and C. The fetus is unable to urinate due to the obstruction. In contrast, Figure 8-15D shows a male fetus urinating, hence ruling out the presence of an obstruction at the level of the urethra.

Diagnosis Sometimes hydronephrosis is quite apparent, but this is not always so. In the third trimester there is some "normal" dilatation of the fetal renal pelvis that occurs due to **bolus** swallowing of amniotic fluid or a full fetal urinary bladder (Figure 8-16). This "normal" physiologic dilatation spontaneously resolves with fetal urination and time. Hence, the diagnosis of hydronephrosis must always be made with care in order to avoid risky, unnecessary procedures.

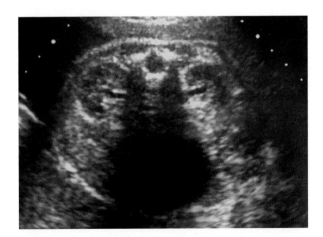

Figure 8-16. *Slight dilatation of the renal collecting system is a common finding in fetuses. This is a transient process that can be affected by how full the fetal bladder is. As the fetus urinates the dilatation can be seen regressing. This transient effect can also be seen as the kidneys collect urine and propel it toward the bladder through peristaltic motion.*

How to Measure for Fetal Hydronephrosis

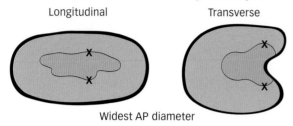

Longitudinal   Transverse

Widest AP diameter

Figure 8-17. *The proper method of measuring a dilated fetal renal pelvis in longitudinal and transverse images.*

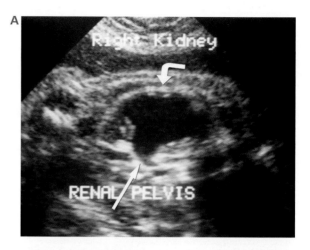

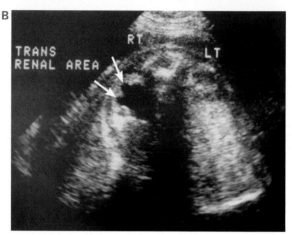

Figure 8-18. A *Longitudinal image of a grossly hydronephrotic right fetal kidney showing severe cortical thinning (curved arrow) and a dilated renal pelvis (straight arrow).* **B** *Transverse image of same fetus comparing the right and left kidneys and showing a dilated renal pelvis with dilated, rounded calyces (arrows) of the right kidney.*

It has been estimated that at least 50% of cases of prenatal hydronephrosis resolve by the time the fetus is born or shortly thereafter. A diagnosis of hydronephrosis can be made if, in the transverse plane (see Figure 8-17), the AP diameter of the renal pelvis is greater than 10 mm and the ratio between the AP diameter of the renal pelvis and the diameter of the kidney is equal to or greater than 50% (Figure 8-18A). Rounded calyces provide further proof of hydronephrosis (Figure 8-18B).

More recent studies have defined hydronephrosis more specifically. Mandel and coworkers have used the following guidelines for renal pelvis measurements: Before 20 weeks' gestation the AP diameter should not be greater than 4 mm; between 20 and 30 weeks' gestation the AP diameter should not be greater than 8 mm; and after 30 weeks' gestation the diameter should not be greater than 10 mm (Table 8-1). As in the adult, dilatation of the fetal renal pelvis can be physiologic rather than pathologic. Therefore, caliectasis is more significant for an obstructive process (Figure 8-19). Finally, anytime hydronephrosis is discovered in the second trimester, an attempt to rule out a chromosomal abnormality—especially trisomy 21—should be made.

Management and Prognosis The outcome of hydronephrosis depends on the severity of the obstruction and at what gestational age the obstruction occurs. It should be

Table 8-1.	Hydronephrosis and renal pelvic diameter.
Gestational Age	**Abnormal AP Diameter**
< 20 weeks	> 4 mm
20–30 weeks	> 8 mm
> 30 weeks	> 10 mm

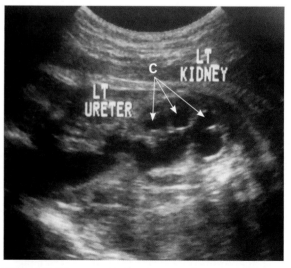

Figure 8-19. *Coronal scan demonstrating left hydronephrosis and hydroureter, which is indicative of an obstruction at the junction of the left ureter and urinary bladder. The right kidney and ureter were normal. C = calyces.*

understood that any chance of fetal survival depends on discovery of the abnormality before the onset of renal failure and pulmonary hypoplasia. Once hydronephrosis is identified, it should be monitored with serial sonographic examinations. As long as renal parenchyma is visible on ultrasound, one can assume that the kidney is still functioning to some degree. As in the adult, thinning of the cortical tissue indicates decreasing renal function.

There have been attempts at therapeutic fetal intervention with varying degrees of success. It has been suggested that if partial obstruction occurs after 20 weeks' gestation the fetus has a good chance of recovering after birth. If partial obstruction occurs before 20 weeks' gestation, when the kidney is still developing, the outcome is less favorable. Referral to a perinatal center for an invasive procedure, such as an in utero **nephrostomy**, can sometimes salvage the kidney by draining its excess fluid.

Fetuses with complete obstruction after 32 weeks' gestation can be delivered early and have a favorable survival rate depending on lung maturity. A wait-and-see approach is usually taken, and prompt postnatal care is available as soon as the fetus is delivered. Late in the third trimester, delivery may be induced early if lung maturity is established.

Ureteropelvic Junction Obstruction

Ureteropelvic junction (UPJ) obstruction is the most common cause of hydronephrosis in fetuses and neonates, with a 4:1 male-to-female ratio. As the name implies, it is caused by an obstruction at the junction of the ureter and the renal pelvis. Causes include a ureteral stricture or kinks, fibrous adhesions, ureteral valves, and an abnormal shape of the **pyelouretral** junction. While cases of incomplete UPJ obstruction may be accompanied by polyhydramnios, cases of bilateral obstruction or a nonfunctional contralateral kidney are often associated with oligohydramnios.

Most cases of fetal UPJ obstruction are unilateral and present with normal amniotic fluid levels and good visualization of the fetal bladder because of the functioning contralateral kidney. With oligohydramnios, carefully evaluate the contralateral kidney to rule out renal agenesis or multicystic dysplasia. MCDK is often associated with a contralateral UPJ obstruction.

In addition, hydronephrosis resulting from a UPJ obstruction must be differentiated from MCDK due to their similar appearances. Hydronephrosis often has a bear claw appearance. The rounded calyces connect with the renal pelvis (Figures 8-20 A and B). On the other hand, MCDK will have multiple, noncommunicating cysts.

A **urinoma**, or urinary ascites—which can result from a ruptured ureter, blown-out calyx, bladder injury, and other causes—may also be seen in the retroperitoneal regions. These will usually be seen posteriorly, adjacent to the fetal spine.

Ureterovesical Junction Obstruction

Any bilateral obstruction—whether it is at the junction with the bladder or at the junction of the renal pelvis—will cause oligohydramnios.

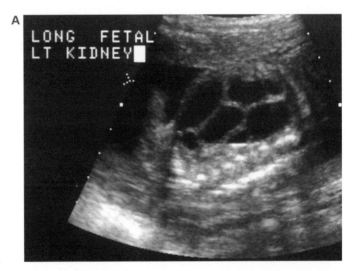

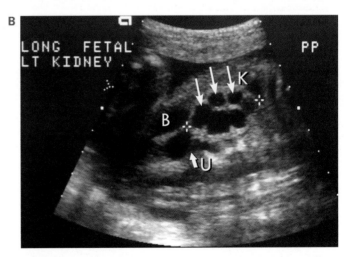

Figure 8-20. A *Longitudinal view of grossly hydronephrotic left kidney simulating multiple cysts. These cysts, however, are all the same size, suggesting hydronephrosis instead. The central cyst is the renal pelvis and the surrounding cysts are the calyces.* **B** *The rounded ends of the calyces (arrows) are identified projecting into the renal cortex, creating the "bear claw" sign. This is characteristic of hydronephrosis and helps to distinguish it from renal cysts. B = bladder, K = kidney, U = ureter.*

Usually associated with primary megaureter, **ureterovesical junction (UVJ) obstruction** is rarely associated with a distal ureteral stricture or valve. Primary megaureter is the result of aperistalsis of the ureter, which is mostly seen in males and can be bilateral in up to 25% of cases. Even when the condition is bilateral, in most cases the prognosis is good. If the ureteral diameter reaches or exceeds 10 mm, however, the outcome is poorer and surgery is usually indicated.

Sonographic findings include a dilated renal pelvis and ureter. A minimally dilated ureter can be mistaken for fluid-filled bowel, and when it is more distended it becomes very serpiginous and may simulate a septated cystic mass. Careful scanning is required to connect the ureter to the kidney and the bladder.

Posterior Urethral Valve

Posterior urethral valve (PUV) is a condition that occurs only in male fetuses, causing obstruction of the entire urinary tract. The male urethra develops tissue projections extending from the back of the posterior urethra into the urethral canal. These projections or valves can partially or completely block the urethra, thereby obstructing the urinary tract. These valves are thought to occur during the early development of the embryo.

PUV will ultimately result in oligohydramnios because the urine cannot get out and circulate. PUVs can present with all or any of the following signs:

- Dilated urinary bladder
- Oligohydramnios
- **Hydroureter** (distention of the ureter caused by obstructed outflow)
- Bilateral hydronephrosis
- Multicystic dysplasia

A grossly distended abdomen, due to the enlarged kidneys and urinary bladder, can inhibit the development of the abdominal wall musculature and obstruct the iliac vessels, resulting in lower limb defects (Figure 8-21A). The urinary bladder typically has a "keyhole" appearance caused by distention of the proximal urethra (Figure 8-21B). The keyhole presentation may not be appreciated when the urinary bladder is grossly distended (prune belly syndrome, also known as Eagle-Barrett syndrome, Figure 8-21C). Other findings include a thick bladder wall. Chronic obstructions can lead to renal cystic dysplasia.

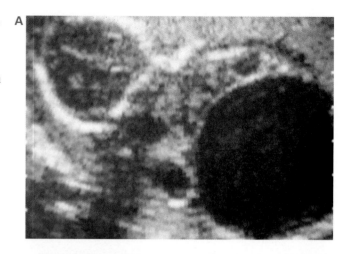

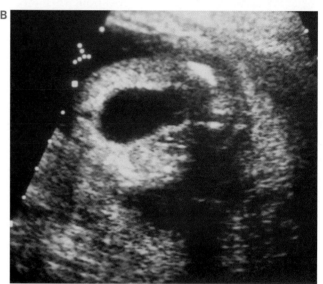

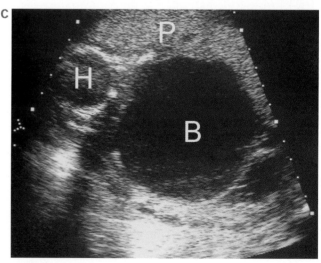

Figure 8-21. A *Longitudinal scan demonstrating a grossly distended urinary bladder in a 28-week fetus. The urinary bladder occupies the entire fetal abdominal cavity and pushes into the chest cavity.* **B** *Fetal urinary bladder with a "keyhole" appearance caused by the distention of the proximal urethra. This is a classic sign for posterior urethral valve (PUV) obstruction.* **C** *Grossly distended bladder in prune belly syndrome. B = bladder, P = placenta, H = head.*

The prognosis depends on when the obstruction occurs and how much fetal lung development has occurred before the onset of oligohydramnios. The overall mortality rate is 50%; 40% of the survivors develop chronic renal failure.

IUGR and Iatrogenesis—The "I" in DRIP

Iatrogenic Causes

Although the "I" in DRIP is usually identified with IUGR, it can also stand for *iatrogenic* associations with oligohydramnios. For example, nonsteroidal prostaglandin synthetase inhibitors can reduce amniotic fluid volume by inhibiting renal vascular flow; when prostaglandin synthetase inhibitors are discontinued, amniotic fluid reaccumulates. Oligohydramnios could also occur following amniocentesis to determine lung maturity, which could cause PROM, or if a practitioner performing a cervical check ruptures membranes. Likewise, oligohydramnios can be a complication of first trimester chorionic villus sampling and second trimester genetic amniocentesis. However, after these procedures, amniotic fluid volume usually returns to normal, and the outcome is generally good.

Intrauterine Growth Restriction (IUGR)

Intrauterine growth restriction (**IUGR**) is usually the result of decreased blood supply to the uterus or to the fetus by way of the placenta. When the placenta is unable to supply adequate blood and nutrients to the fetus, growth is affected, as is fetal renal function. The overall process is complex, but the decrease in fetal renal function due to poor blood supply results in oligohydramnios. Any fetus that does not receive adequate nourishment due to placental insufficiency with not grow as it should.

Fetuses are considered **small for gestational age** (**SGA**) when their weight falls below the 10th percentile for age. When a fetus measures small for dates, IUGR must be ruled out. Many variables must be taken into consideration when trying to establish normal growth. Each year approximately 1 in 100 babies is born SGA by definition, and 10% of those will be normal. Genetics plays a significant role in the latter. Because small people have small babies, it is helpful to ask parents what previous infants weighed at term. Another helpful question to ask is what each parent weighed when he or she was born, as couples tend to have babies close to their own birth weights.

Monitoring fetal growth can be challenging, and to do so accurately requires establishment of the menstrual dates.

This is done utilizing several methods. If the patient is a good historian and has normal regular periods, the best method is by establishing the first day of the last menstrual period (LMP). A fairly accurate estimated date of confinement (EDC) can be predicted from this day. A sonogram performed in the first trimester, ideally at 8–10 weeks, allows us to calculate an EDC that will be accurate within 5–7 days. Other methods include palpation for uterine size upon the first prenatal examination and documentation of first felt fetal movement (**quickening**), usually around 15–20 weeks. To monitor and document growth sonographically, the practitioner must perform serial sonograms at least 2–4 weeks apart. Measurements recorded at shorter intervals may cause errors.

The most common "cause" for a patient to present SGA is incorrect or unreliable dates. This is particularly true of patients with a history of having irregular cycles. In the first trimester, the clinician must rule out fetal demise or missed abortion. During the second and third trimesters, one must consider PROM and oligohydramnios as possible reasons for poor intrauterine growth. Clinical considerations for suspicion of a growth-restricted gestation include predisposing factors, low maternal weight gain, poor fundal height growth (SGA), and history of previous growth-restricted pregnancy. Predisposing factors include chronic maternal disorders such as anemia, hypertension, diabetes, renal disease, and cardiovascular disease. Others include abuses of alcohol, tobacco, and drugs as well as poor nutrition and intrauterine infections. Risk factors for the fetus or infant include **hypothermia** due to lack of subcutaneous fat, **hypoglycemia**, **polycythemia**, and meconium aspiration and asphyxiation, increasing the perinatal mortality rate for IUGR fetuses by a factor of 8.

Symmetric IUGR There are two types of IUGR, symmetric and asymmetric. Of the two, symmetric IUGR is the severest and most difficult to diagnose. Fortunately, symmetric IUGR accounts for only 10% of all cases. Symmetric IUGR fetuses are proportionately small, and growth restriction is caused by an early insult to the pregnancy, prior to 28 weeks' gestation. Associated with serious congenital and chromosomal abnormalities, symmetric IUGR has a poor prognosis. The brain cell size is decreased, and the DNA is usually abnormal. Early insult can result from exposure to radiation, drugs, and infections (TORCH). (See Box 8-5.) Irreversible anomalies associated with symmetric IUGR include trisomies 18 and 21, neural tube defects, and various Potter syndrome types.

Box 8-5.   Causes of symmetric IUGR.

Insult to pregnancy prior to 28 weeks

Radiation

Drugs

Infection

Trisomy

Box 8-6.   Causes of asymmetric IUGR.

Insult to pregnancy after 28 weeks

High altitude

Maternal disease, malnutrition

Placental abnormality

Fibroids

Smoking

Twin-to-twin transfusion

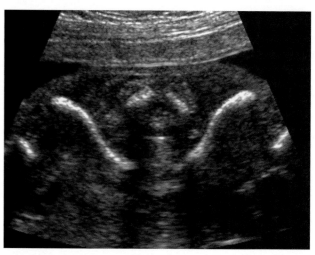

Figure 8-22. *Image taken transverse to the fetus demonstrating the clavicles, which can be measured to estimate gestational age.*

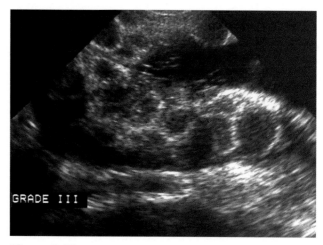

GRADE III

Figure 8-23. *Longitudinal image demonstrating a grade III fundal posterior placenta. The patient was in the early third trimester, too early to be showing a grade III placenta.*

Asymmetric IUGR Asymmetric IUGR is caused by an insult later in the pregnancy, after 28 weeks, and is associated with anything that deflects or interferes with the blood supply to the fetus. Causes include placental masses and abnormalities, fibroids, twin-to-twin transfusion, high altitude, maternal disease, malnutrition, and smoking. (See Box 8-6.) Although these infants also have smaller brain cells, the DNA is normal, allowing for a much better prognosis.

It is easier to identify asymmetric IUGR sonographically, primarily because of the discrepancy in growth between the fetal head and abdomen, which usually does not occur until the third trimester. The fetal brain will grow normally and the head circumference will measure consistently with dates/age. The abdomen, however, will show slowed growth, causing a high **HC/AC ratio** (ratio of head circumference to abdominal circumference). The abdomen measures small because of lack of subcutaneous fat and loss of glycogen stores in the liver. This type of growth is referred to as **head-sparing** due to preferential flowing of blood to the brain at the expense of other organ systems. It is also believed that decreased blood flow to the kidneys affects their function, resulting in oligohydramnios, which is typically associated with asymmetric IUGR. Decreased flow to the placenta causes

premature aging of the placenta and decreased nutrients to the fetus. The fetal long bones are not significantly affected by IUGR, and therefore a high **FL/AC ratio** (the ratio of femur length to abdominal circumference) would also suggest possible IUGR. (See Table 35 in Appendix A.) Studies have shown that the clavicle, specifically, is not altered by IUGR and can be used as a reliable indicator of gestational age when IUGR is suspected (Figure 8-22). Three sonographic findings are typically associated with asymmetric IUGR: (1) oligohydramnios, (2) HC/AC discrepancy, and (3) a premature grade III placenta (Figure 8-23).

Management and Prognosis In cases of suspected IUGR, it is necessary to monitor fetal growth and well-being with the goal of delivering the fetus at the earliest possible time.

Table 8-2. Apgar score.

Heart Rate	Respiration	Tone	Reflex	Color
Absent—0	Absent—0	Flaccid—0	Absent—0	Cyanosis—0
<100 BPM—1	Slow/irregular—1	Slight—1	Slight—1	Acrocyanosis—1
>100 BPM—2	Good cry—2	Active—2	Active—2	Pink—2

Once the fetus is delivered, catch-up growth is common, and the physical and mental status of the infant is usually normal.

Growth-restricted fetuses are at risk for having low Apgar scores at delivery. The **Apgar score** is performed at 1 and 5 minutes after birth. It assesses five parameters of the newborn: (1) heart rate, (2) respiration, (3) muscle tone, (4) reflexes, and (5) skin color. Each parameter is assigned a number value of 0–2; the maximum total score is 10. (See Table 8-2.) This score is helpful in predicting neonatal difficulties. For example, of infants with a score of 2 or less at birth, 78% will not survive the neonatal period. Of those with scores of 8 or higher, only 1% will die in the first 28 days of life.

As noted above, asymmetric IUGR fetuses have abdomens that measure disproportionately small, while the head and limb measurements correspond with the expected gestational age. This abnormality occurs in the third trimester and accounts for the majority of IUGR pregnancies. Factors associated with asymmetric IUGR include placental insufficiency, fetal hypoxia, gestational diabetes, maternal pre-eclampsia, and chronic hypertension. Other causes include high-risk maternal lifestyles that involve tobacco, drug, or alcohol abuse. If caught in time, these high-risk maternal factors can be eliminated, enhancing the fetus's chance of a normal life. It is important to remember, however, that measurement discrepancies and abnormal ratios can indicate problems other than IUGR, as indicated in Box 8-7.

PROM and Post Dates—The "P" in DRIP

Although the "P" in our DRIP list of anomalies associated with oligohydramnios is usually connected with premature rupture of membranes (PROM), it can also stand for post dates. Both conditions are associated with low amniotic fluid levels.

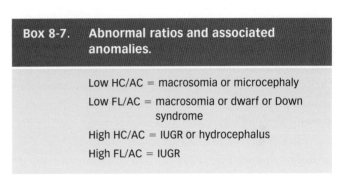

Box 8-7.   Abnormal ratios and associated anomalies.

Low HC/AC = macrosomia or microcephaly

Low FL/AC = macrosomia or dwarf or Down syndrome

High HC/AC = IUGR or hydrocephalus

High FL/AC = IUGR

Post-Term Pregnancies

Post-term pregnancies are defined as pregnancies that go beyond 42 weeks' gestation and occur in approximately 5%–10% of all pregnancies, most of which will be first-time pregnancies. The incidence of fetal morbidity and mortality increases as the pregnancy goes beyond 42 weeks' gestation, making the proper diagnosis and dating more critical.

A relationship between post-term pregnancies, oligohydramnios, and diminished placental function was recognized more than 40 years ago, and animal studies have confirmed that fetal hypoxemia significantly affects urine production. Placental function begins to decrease after 38 weeks' gestation, and this compromises fetal well-being if birth is delayed beyond 42 weeks. We expect amniotic fluid levels to decrease as a pregnancy progresses to term. At 42 weeks, however, the amniotic fluid level the patient had at 40 weeks will be diminished by half. It has been reported that oligohydramnios can develop within a 24-hour period. Therefore, the postmature pregnancy must be monitored carefully.

Postmature fetuses have an increased risk for other problems. These problems include decreased placental function, which denies the fetus enough nourishment, a difficult delivery due to size, and the possibility that the fetus may aspirate meconium (baby stool), causing lung damage. Meconium aspiration may also occur just before delivery or anytime the fetus is distressed.

The pregnancy may present with oligohydramnios, and there may be **macrosomia** (increased body size). Because of lack of fluid, the entire exam may be extremely difficult to image. Meconium may be seen within the amniotic fluid, indicating fetal distress. Fetal breathing motions are often exaggerated due to labored breathing, and the placenta often shows an advanced grade III stage.

PROM and PPROM

The "P" in DRIP is also associated with **premature rupture of membranes (PROM)**. As the pregnancy reaches maturity and the onset of labor begins, the cervical membranes spontaneously rupture, resulting in the expulsion of amniotic fluid. PROM occurs when there is spontaneous rupture of membranes after 37 weeks' gestation but before the onset of labor. PROM is the most common cause of oligohydramnios. Premature rupture of membranes prior to 38 weeks' gestation is classified as **preterm premature rupture of membranes (PPROM)** and is associated with a high incidence of premature births and stillbirths. The diagnosis of premature rupture of membranes can easily be made clinically. In some instances, however, the leaking fluid may be chronic, slow, and therefore not as noticeable. A common symptom of both PROM and PPROM is uncontrollable leaking of fluid from the vagina and soaking of undergarments and bedding.

PROM and PPROM occur in approximately 5% of all pregnancies and are associated with a 10% premature birthrate. There is a recurrence rate of about 32% in subsequent pregnancies. There is a high risk of maternal and fetal infections (especially Group B streptococcus) associated with this process because the open cervical canal allows micro-organisms to enter. Premature rupture of membranes prior to 26 weeks' gestation has a higher incidence of developmental abnormalities and fetal death, accounting for 20% of perinatal deaths. Persistent leaking and second trimester oligohydramnios usually have a bad outcome for the fetus, with a survival rate of only 10%.

Summary of Sonographic Signs

Lack of amniotic fluid will be obvious. A low amniotic fluid index (AFI) is considered a sign of oligohydramnios. In most cases, however, the uterine wall will be in close contact with and wrapping around the fetus. If the fluid volume is borderline, which may be the case with chronic

leakage, serial scans may be necessary to see if the fluid does regenerate itself. It has been documented that low volumes of amniotic fluid have regenerated and presented as normal volume on subsequent studies. Again, amniotic fluid volumes can vary significantly from day to day, and maternal hydration may assist in increasing amniotic fluid.

ADDENDUM: THE FETAL BIOPHYSICAL PROFILE

Purpose and Indications

The fetal **biophysical profile (BPP)**—which includes a nonstress test (NST) and four ultrasound examinations—is one method of performing antepartum surveillance to evaluate fetal well-being. Other methods of antepartum surveillance include the nonstress test, contraction stress test (CST), and Doppler flow studies. Although all of these screening tests can yield high false-positive and false-negative results, they can add useful information in the at-risk pregnancy. If the test performed is favorable, it is very reassuring to both clinician and patient. Although a positive test result—not reassuring to the parents—may have a high probability of being falsely positive, it will prompt further investigation; thus the outcome is not reliant on one test.

Although the BPP is performed for a host of reasons that extend beyond oligohydramnios, it is particularly germane to conditions related to amniotic fluid volume, including those associated with oligohydramnios and polyhydramnios. It is also used to assess the health of the fetus if the mother has hyperthyroidism, bleeding problems, lupus, chronic kidney disease, diabetes, hypertension, pre-eclampsia, multiple gestations, a history of stillbirths, PROM, and a post-term pregnancy (Box 8-8). Therefore it is particularly useful when assessing several conditions related to DRIP.

The biophysical profile can be easily performed during a routine obstetric exam and should be considered anytime oligohydramnios or IUGR is suspected. Four sonographic criteria for IUGR are:

1. HC/AC discrepancy
2. Oligohydramnios
3. Estimated fetal weight of less than 2700 grams
4. Grade III placenta

These findings warrant close clinical follow-up.

Box 8-8.	Indications for performing fetal biophysical profile.

Suspected IUGR

Post dates

Maternal hypertension

Diabetes mellitus

Multiple gestations

PROM

History of stillbirths

Oligohydramnios

Assessment Technique

The fetal BPP evaluates five parameters (Box 8-9): (1) fetal heart rate (by means of the NST, using cardiotocography) and ultrasound evaluation for (2) gross fetal body movements, (3) fetal breathing motion, (4) amniotic fluid level, and (5) fetal tone. If the criteria are met for each parameter, the number 2 is assigned to that parameter. If not, a 0 is assigned. Upon completion, the number values are added for a BPP score. Scores are rated as follows:

(1) Nonstress Test

Nonstress test   (2) reactive = 2 or more fetal heart accelerations of 15 bpm for 30 seconds' duration during a 20-minute period

(0) nonreactive = 1 or fewer fetal heart accelerations of 15 bpm for 30 seconds' duration during a 45-minute period

Fetal heart accelerations generally relate to normal fetal movements. Nonstress tests (and fetal breathing movements) will be depressed when the fetal umbilical vein pH falls below 7.2. If it falls below 7.1, fetal movements and tone will be absent. The NST is most reliable from 32 weeks to term.

(2) Gross Fetal Body Movements

Fetal motion   (2) 3 or more gross body movements

(0) fewer than 3 movements

These movements may include limbs and/or the torso. In terms of embryology, those variables that develop first are the most resistant to anoxia. Fetal movement and tone develop between 7.5 and 9 weeks.

Box 8-9.	Parameters measured by the fetal biophysical profile.

Heart rate

Body movement

Respiration

Amniotic fluid volume

Tone

(3) Fetal Breathing Motion

Fetal breathing   (2) 1 episode

(0) no episode

Fetal breathing can be detected by 17–18 weeks' gestation and can include hiccups. A fetus that is sleeping will not show breathing motions. Because this can be misinterpreted, fetal state is also an important factor to consider when interpreting the BPP. Fetal state is defined as 1F (quiet sleep), 2F (rapid eye movement sleep), or 4F (active state). Fetal state will dictate the amount of time required to identify fetal breathing. During quiet sleep (1F), the average time to obtain a normal BPP is 26.3 minutes as opposed to 3–5 minutes when the fetus is in rapid eye movement sleep (2F) or an active state (4F). Fetal breathing motion of any kind, regardless of duration, is now considered normal for the BPP. Of note, fetal breathing can be stimulated by caffeine and hyperglycemia, while breathing movements may be inhibited by hypoglycemia, supine hypotensive syndrome, cigarette smoking, alcohol, diazepam, and meperidine.

(4) Amniotic Fluid Level

Amniotic fluid   (2) single 2 × 2 cm pocket

(0) < 2 × 2 cm pocket

A decrease in amniotic fluid leading to oligohydramnios is a major sign of chronic fetal compromise. **Hypoxia** results in cardiac compromise, which leads to a decrease in perfusion of major organs such as the kidneys. Decreased blood flow to the kidneys results in decreased urine production and subsequent oligohydramnios. Fetal acidosis can result in a reduction of amniotic fluid by 17.5 weeks. Intrauterine death is often caused by cord compression.

Many texts suggest that at least one pocket of at least 2 cm (vertical dimension) is considered (2) for BPP purposes. One study has even suggested that the AFI calculation may overcall oligohydramnios. A study performed by

Chauhan et al. in 2004 actually concluded there was no advantage to performing the AFI for reasons of a biophysical profile. Therefore, the 2 cm deepest single pocket rule is considered more accurate when performing the fetal biophysical profile. There is much controversy over what value should indicate oligohydramnios. A single criterion should be established and used consistently in each lab.

(5) Fetal Tone

Fetal tone   (2) 1 episode of extension and flexion

                     (0) constant full or partial extension without return

Fetal tone, which measures the extension and flexion of the limbs, can be very difficult to evaluate when there is crowding due to oligohydramnios. On the other hand, gross body movements rarely occur without tone.

Dynamic fetal biophysical activity is cyclical, occurring every 20–40 minutes. A 30-minute time frame allows for tone, movement, and breathing to be observed as they would occur naturally when the fetus is awake.

Modified Assessment Technique

If the nonstress test is not available or has not been done, a modified biophysical profile (minus the NST) can be performed. Manning reported in 1987 that the NST would add no additional predictive value in a patient with a modified BPP of 8/8. On its own merits, the BPP has fewer false-positive results in comparison with the NST. If one or more of the ultrasound parameters are abnormal, however, the NST should be obtained. BPP scores with the NST are to be interpreted as follows:

8–10   No indication for intervention. Recommend repeat BPP in 1 week (twice weekly for post dates or insulin-dependent diabetics). If the mother's condition is not deteriorated, a fetus should not die or become severely compromised within half a week.

4–6   Deliver if cervix is favorable and fetal lungs are mature; otherwise repeat in 12–24 hours.

0–2   Deliver immediately. If lungs are immature, administer steroids and deliver in 48 hours.

Overall, confirmation of fetal breathing, determination of amniotic fluid volume, and results of the NST appear to be the most important variables of the BPP. It is doubtful that additional parameters will be added to the BPP. However, by incorporating the fetal state and Doppler flow studies of the umbilical and middle cerebral arteries as well as the ductus venosus, the examiner can make a more complete assessment of the fetal condition.

SCANNING TIPS, GUIDELINES, AND PITFALLS

1. Regarding the amniotic fluid index (AFI), measurements have been introduced to quantify the amniotic fluid within the pregnant uterus. This technique is accomplished by dividing the pregnant uterus into four quadrants and taking a vertical measurement of the deepest pocket of fluid in each quadrant. The quadrants measured must be free of fetal parts and the umbilical cord. (It is helpful to turn on the color Doppler when a pocket is found to make sure the umbilical cord is not in the way.) The sum of the four measurements equals the amniotic fluid index (AFI). It is generally accepted that a normal AFI in the third trimester is between 8 and 20 cm and that a measurement of less than 5 cm is classified as severe oligohydramnios. For more information on AFIs, see Chapter 4.

2. Multicystic renal dysplasia can be easily mistaken for hydronephrosis. Multicystic renal dysplasia presents as rounded cystic structures that do not communicate with each other. If no communications between the cystic structures can be identified and if those structures do not converge at the renal pelvis, hydronephrosis can safely be excluded. Urinary ascites may be present with massive obstruction due to leaking or rupture of the urinary tract.

3. Always check the fetal pelvis when the kidneys cannot be located in their normal position. Pelvic kidneys can fool us in an adult, so why not in the fetus? Always look closely at the area around the bladder before diagnosing renal agenesis (Figure 8-24). Color Doppler should also be used to identify renal vascularity.

4. Oligohydramnios can be a cause of dolichocephaly. When the fetal head is too long and narrow, the shape will affect the biparietal diameter measurement, making it smaller than the other measurements. When the cephalic index indicates dolichocephaly, one must delete the BPD measurements and average only HC, FL, and AC for average gestational age. The head circumference can still be used as it is not affected by head shape.

5. Meconium-containing amniotic fluid can make one think there is oligohydramnios because of the

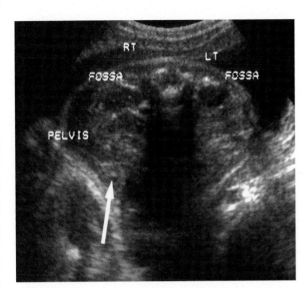

Figure 8-24. *Transverse image showing fetal renal fossae, with the kidney sitting below the normal position (arrow).*

low-level echoes that blend in with fetal surfaces, placenta, and uterine wall. Even though the fluid is not normal in echo appearance and the findings suggest fetal distress, there is fluid all the same. Oligohydramnios should not be reported.

6. Fetuses with renal agenesis demonstrate slightly prominent adrenal glands adjacent to the fetal spine. Care should be taken not to mistake these glands for hypoplastic kidneys. A normal kidney will have a more echogenic central echo complex, and the renal outline can be appreciated with color Doppler.

7. A fetal biophysical profile is indicated whenever oligohydramnios or its complications are suspected.

Acknowledgements: I would like to thank David Heflin BS, RDMS, of the Murray Women's Clinic in Murray, Kentucky, for his support and gracious permission to use some of his scans. I would also like to thank Shonda Bathe, RDMS, of Southeast Missouri Hospital for her valuable input on this project. And a big thanks to my great ultrasound staff at Southeast Missouri Hospital for putting up with me during the time it took to put this chapter together and for always being on the lookout for interesting cases for this chapter. Finally, I would like to express my appreciation to a dear friend, Bill Conklin, MD, who always believed in me and encouraged me to be the best. —Joe Rodriguez, RT, RDMS

REFERENCES

Anderhub B: *General Sonography: A Clinical Guide.* St. Louis, Mosby-Year Book, 1995.

Babcook CJ, Silvera M, Drake C, et al: Effect of maternal hydration on mild fetal pyelectasis. J Ultrasound Med 17:539–544, 1998.

Beck WW: *Obstetrics and Gynecology: A National Medical Series for Independent Study.* Philadelphia, Harwal, 1993.

Callen PW (ed): *Ultrasonography in Obstetrics and Gynecology,* 5th Edition. Philadelphia, Saunders Elsevier, 2008.

Chamberlain PF, Manning FA, Morrison I, et al: Ultrasound evaluation of amniotic fluid volume I: the relationship of marginal and decreased amniotic fluid volume to perinatal outcome. Am J Obstet Gynecol 150:245–249, 1984.

Chauhan SP, Doherty DD, Magann EF, et al: Amniotic fluid index vs. single deepest pocket technique during modified biophysical profile: a randomized clinical trial. Am J Obstet Gynecol 191:661–668, 2004.

Cox S, Williams ML, Levino, KJ: The natural history of preterm ruptured membranes: what to expect of expectant management. Obstet Gynecol 71:558–562, 1988.

Davidson AJ, Hartman DS: *Radiology of the Kidney and Urinary Tract,* 2nd Edition. Philadelphia, Saunders, 1994.

Feldman DM, DeCambre M, King E, et al: Evaluation and follow-up of fetal hydronephrosis. J Ultrasound Med 20:1065–1069, 2001.

Hagen-Ansert SL (ed): *Textbook of Diagnostic Sonography,* Volume 2, 7th Edition. St. Louis, Elsevier Mosby, 2012.

Hill LM, Lazebnik N, Many A: Effect of indomethacin on individual amniotic fluid indices in multiple gestations. J Ultrasound Med 15: 395–399, 1996.

Hill LM, Macpherson T, Romano L, et al: Prenatal sonographic findings of fetal megacalycosis. J Ultrasound Med 21:1179–1181, 2002.

Maizels M, Cuneo BF, Sabbagha RE: *Fetal Anomalies Ultrasound Diagnosis and Postnatal Management.* New York, Wiley-Liss, 2002.

Manning FA, Morrison I, Lange IR, et al: Fetal biophysical profile scoring: selective use of the non-stress test. Am J Obstet Gynecol 156:709, 1987.

McGahan JP, Porto M: *Diagnostic Obstetrical Ultrasound.* Philadelphia, Lippincott, 1994.

Pillai M, Jems D: The importance of the behavioral state in biophysical profile assessment of the term human fetus. Br J Obstet Gynecol 97:1130–1134, 1990.

Rumack CM, Wilson SR, Charboneau JW (eds): *Diagnostic Ultrasound*, 4th Edition. Philadelphia, Elsevier Mosby, 2011.

Sauerbrei EE, Nguyen KT, Nolan RL: *A Practical Guide to Ultrasound in Obstetrics and Gynecology*, 2nd Edition. New York, Lippincott Williams & Wilkins, 1998.

Shipp TD, Bromley B, Pauker S, et al: Outcomes of singleton pregnancies with severe oligohydramnios in the second and third trimester. Ultrasound Obstet Gynecol 7:108–113, 1996.

Vintzileos AM, Gaffney SE, Sallingen LM, et al: The relationship between fetal biophysical profile and cord pH in patients undergoing cesarean section before the onset of labor. Obstet Gynecol 70:196–201, 1987.

SELF-ASSESSMENT EXERCISES

Questions

1. All of the following are considered to be functions of amniotic fluid *except*:

   A. Allows for fetal movement

   B. Critical to fetal lung development

   C. Helps regulate fetal blood flow

   D. Provides protection for the fetus

   E. Helps maintain temperature

2. Which statement is true of the amniotic fluid index?

   A. It is a qualitative means of calculating amniotic fluid.

   B. It is a quantitative means of calculating amniotic fluid.

   C. It is a method for performing an amniocentesis.

   D. It is not a reliable method for evaluating amniotic fluid levels.

   E. It is part of the basic guidelines for performing obstetric sonograms.

3. Which of the following statements is true for fetal demise?

   A. Lack of cardiac activity demonstrated during real-time examination is the most accurate means of diagnosing fetal demise.

   B. Spalding's sign refers to scalp edema and is always associated with fetal demise.

   C. Anasarca refers to collapse and overlapping of the cranial bones, which is always associated with fetal demise.

   D. Fetal demise cannot be verified with ultrasound prior to 12 weeks' gestational age.

   E. Deuel's sign is specific for fetal demise.

4. A fetal pole with cardiac motion should always be identifiable by the time a gestational sac measures:

   A. 2 mm

   B. 2.5 cm

   C. 2 cm

   D. 3.5 mm

   E. All of the above

5. Which of these findings would not lead you to suspect fetal demise?

   A. Lack of fetal motion

   B. Increased fundal height

   C. Negative fetal heart tones in office

   D. Decreased fundal height

   E. Identification of Spalding's sign

6. Which of the following statements about bilateral renal agenesis is incorrect?

   A. There is an increase in amniotic fluid volume.

   B. There is a decrease in amniotic fluid volume.

   C. Fetal urinary bladder will not be identified.

   D. Adrenal glands may enlarge and mimic fetal kidneys.

   E. The condition is terminal.

7. Infantile polycystic kidneys will give the kidney a:

   A. Hypoechoic appearance

   B. Hyperechoic appearance

   C. Irregular and distorted appearance

   D. Abnormally small appearance

   E. The appearance of absent kidneys

8. Multicystic dysplastic kidneys are usually:

    A. Bilateral but functional

    B. Bilateral and nonfunctional

    C. Unilateral but functional

    D. Unilateral and nonfunctional

    E. Pelvic in location

9. Bilateral fetal hydronephrosis usually means:

    A. There is an obstruction at the ureteropelvic junction.

    B. There is an obstruction at the urethral outflow tract.

    C. There is an obstruction along one of the ureters.

    D. The prognosis is fatal.

    E. There is polyhydramnios.

10. Which statement is *not* true regarding fetal hydronephrosis?

    A. The ratio of the renal pelvis AP diameter to the kidney diameter should be less than 50%.

    B. This process affects males more than females.

    C. The AP diameter of the renal pelvis should be greater than 10 mm in the third trimester.

    D. The ends of the calyces will be rounded as they enter the kidney.

    E. It is the most common fetal renal abnormality.

11. If one fetal kidney shows dilation of the fetal renal pelvis and calyces but there is no evidence of a dilated ureter or bladder, the most likely diagnosis would be:

    A. Obstruction at the ureteropelvic junction (UPJ)

    B. Obstruction at the ureterovesical junction (UVJ)

    C. Posterior urethral valves (PUVs)

    D. Obstruction at the mid-ureteral junction (MUJ)

    E. Renal hypoplasia

12. Of the following statements, which is not true of PUV?

    A. It causes bilateral hydronephrosis.

    B. It causes dilation of the entire urinary tract.

    C. It causes unilateral hydronephrosis.

    D. It is often fatal.

    E. It is associated with oligohydramnios.

13. Asymmetric growth restriction is not usually associated with:

    A. Oligohydramnios

    B. Low fetal weight

    C. SGA

    D. Anomalies

    E. Decreased mental capacity

14. The most common cause for a patient presenting SGA is:

    A. Incorrect dates

    B. Genetic

    C. Intrauterine infection

    D. Cigarette smoking

    E. Radiation exposure

15. These images demonstrate fetal kidneys. The most likely diagnosis would be:

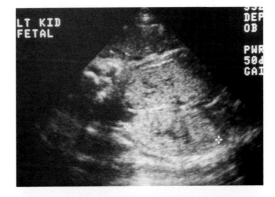

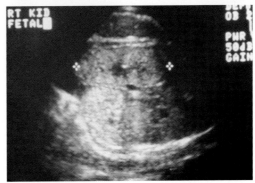

    A. Normal kidneys

    B. Multicystic kidneys

    C. Polycystic kidneys

    D. Hydonephrotic kidneys

    E. Hypoplastic kidneys

16. This transverse image through the fetal abdomen demonstrates:

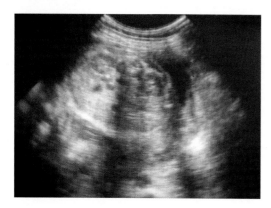

A. Normal kidneys

B. Enlarged kidneys

C. Hydronephrosis

D. Renal agenesis

E. Hypoplastic kidneys

17. Infantile polycystic kidneys are:

A. Not hereditary

B. Autosomal dominant

C. Autosomal recessive

D. Compatible with life

E. Associated with mental retardation

18. How long after demise does general fetal maceration usually become sonographically apparent?

A. 12 hours

B. 24 hours

C. 4 days

D. 10–14 days

E. 1 month

19. After fetal demise, gas can sometimes be seen in the fetal chest and/or abdomen due to breakdown of fetal tissues. This is called:

A. Spalding's sign

B. Robert's sign

C. Haley's sign

D. Murphy's sign

E. Deuel's sign

20. Premature rupture of membranes (PROM) is described as:

A. Rupture of membranes after 37 weeks' gestation but before onset of labor

B. Rupture of membranes before 37 weeks' gestation regardless of the onset of labor

C. Rupture of membranes prior to 37 weeks' gestation

D. Not important to the outcome of the fetus

E. A routine event

Answers

See Appendix F on page 612 for answers and explanations.

Multiple Gestations and Their Complications

Kathryn A. Gill, MS, RT, RDMS, FSDMS

OBJECTIVES

After completing this chapter you should be able to:

1. List the risk factors—both fetal and maternal—for multiple gestations.

2. Describe the roles of zygosity, chorionicity, and amnionicity and how they can be determined sonographically.

3. Explain the importance of documenting fetal presentation, growth disturbances, and demise in multiple gestations.

4. List and define the complications and anomalies specifically associated with the monozygotic gestation.

5. Explain the role of ultrasound in managing patients pregnant with multiple fetuses.

6. Recite the key tips for scanning the patient with multiple gestations.

MULTIPLE GESTATIONS, TWINS SPECIFICALLY, ACCOUNT for approximately 1 of every 40–45 births, and the incidence for triplet births is 1 in 1300. The incidence of naturally conceived quadruplets in the United States is extremely low, estimated to be 1 in 13 million. Although this is a relatively small proportion of births, multiple gestations represent 10%–14% of all perinatal deaths. A number of complications—some of which are unique to twins—can arise in multiple gestations. This chapter reviews multiple gestations and their complications and discusses the clinical usefulness of monitoring these pregnancies with ultrasound techniques. Although the chapter focuses on twins (the most common multiple gestation), the principles hold for other multiples as well.

RISK FACTORS

Several factors may predispose a woman to producing multiple gestations (Box 9-1), including hormonal fluctuations that come with advanced maternal age, history of multiple gestations or multiparity, race/ethnicity

Box 9-1.	Factors predisposing a woman to multiple gestations.
	Advanced maternal age (AMA)
	Maternal family history
	Previous multiple gestation/multiparity
	African American ethnicity
	Multigravida (>7) status

Box 9-2.	Risks posed to mother by multiple gestations.

Anemia

Pregnancy-induced hypertension

Hyperemesis gravidarum

Pyelonephritis

Postpartum hemorrhage

Placenta previa

Placental abruption

Box 9-3.	Risks posed to fetus by multiple gestations.

Preterm labor and delivery

Intrauterine growth restriction

Anomalies

Increased morbidity/mortality

(twins are more prevalent among African Americans than Caucasians), multigravida (>7), and maternal family history. Paternal family history is not considered a significant risk factor because twinning depends on the number of eggs that are fertilized, not the genetic characteristics of the sperm.

Although much of this discussion focuses on the fetal risks of multiple gestations, there are also maternal risks to consider. Maternal risks include anemia, hyperemesis gravidarum, pregnancy-induced hypertension (PIH), pyelonephritis, and postpartum hemorrhage, as well as placenta previa and placental abruptions (Box 9-2).

Once the sonographer identifies an intrauterine pregnancy with more than one fetus, the patient is automatically considered at high risk. Compared to singletons, multiples are at increased risk for morbidity and mortality by a factor of 5 to 10. These risks increase if the fetuses are the same sex. Premature delivery and associated cerebral hemorrhage are common; many multiples are born prior to 37 weeks. Mortality associated with preterm delivery has been estimated at 20%. Intrauterine growth restriction and growth discrepancies are also more frequent among multiple gestations. Today prematurity and low birth weight are considered the most common causes of perinatal death among multiple gestations. Finally, there is an increased incidence of structural fetal anomalies among twins and other multiple gestations (Box 9-3).

Sonographically, there are three things that one should attempt to define:

- Zygosity
- Chorionicity
- Amnionicity

Zygosity is the most difficult to define and can be accomplished only if the sexes of the two fetuses can be differentiated sonographically (i.e., one male and one female) or when fetal blood sampling reveals that the blood types of the fetuses differ. Chorionicity and amnionicity, on the other hand, can be determined sonographically with a high degree of accuracy during the first trimester.

ZYGOSITY

Zygosity denotes the number of eggs fertilized. Twins may be monozygotic or dizygotic. **Monozygotic (identical) twins** are the result of the fertilization of a single egg (ovum) that subsequently splits into what will become two chromosomally identical individuals. **Dizygotic (fraternal) twins** result from the fertilization of two separate eggs. Using diagnostic ultrasound, the examiner can determine zygosity only when a difference in sexes can be appreciated. Percutaneous fetal blood sampling performed under ultrasound guidance can help determine zygosity if there is a clinical need to do so. If the fetuses have different blood types, they must be fraternal.

Dizygotic twins are the most common type of twins in the United States. Because dizygotic twins develop from separate eggs fertilized by different sperm, the twins are genetically distinct and may have different sexes and blood groups. Only one-third of dizygotic twins are the same sex.

Monozygotic twins are natural clones who share 100% of their genes. They constitute only about one-third of all twin pregnancies in the United States. About one-quarter of identical twins are **mirror-image twins**, characterized by opposite or reversed features. For example, one twin will be right-handed while the other is left-handed. They may show other mirror-image reversals as well, such as opposite hair whorls and moles on opposite sides of the face or body. Mirror-image twinning is common among conjoined twins and thought to be the result of late splitting of the fertilized egg.

Polar body twinning or half-identical twins are currently being studied, and the results may explain why some fraternal twins look almost identical. This phenomenon occurs when the egg splits before fertilization. Each half is then fertilized by different sperm.

Monozygotic twins are at risk for many complications, some of which are unique to this type of twinning (see the section headed "Complications Specific to Monozygotic/Monochorionic Twins" below). There is an increased incidence of anomalies among monozygotic twins, such as anencephaly, holoprosencephaly, hydrocephaly, sacrococcygeal teratomas, and sirenomelia (mermaid syndrome). Even though these twins develop from the same egg, the anomalies tend to be discordant (i.e., present in one twin but not in the other).

CHORIONICITY AND AMNIONICITY

Sonographically, twin pregnancies and other multiple gestations are classified by the number of **amnions** (sacs or dividing membranes) and **chorions** (placentas). Development of the amnion/chorion depends on the type and timing of twinning, and it is important to realize that

Table 9-1.	Amnionicity and chorionicity by type of twin.
Type of Twin	**Amnionicity/Chorionicity**
Dizygotic	100% diamniotic/dichorionic
Monozygotic	30% diamniotic/dichorionic
	60% diamniotic/monochorionic
	10% monoamniotic/monochorionic

the development of the chorion precedes that of the amnion. Therefore a separating membrane between fetuses can be difficult to appreciate early in the first trimester.

All dizygotic and most monozygotic twins are **diamniotic**, and all dizygotic twins are **dichorionic** (Table 9-1). Chorionicity as well as amnionicity of monozygotic twins is determined by when the zygote divides (Figure 9-1A):

- Very early division—4 days or sooner after fertilization—results in diamniotic/dichorionic monozygotic twins, just like dizygotic twins. This occurs in about 30% of these cases (Figure 9-1B).

A

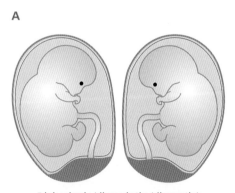

Dichorionic/diamniotic (dizygotic)

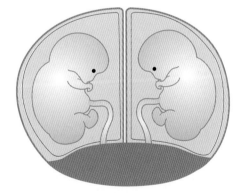

Dichorionic/diamniotic (monozygotic with fusion of two placentas)

Figure 9-1. A *The various types of twin amnionicity and chorionicity. (Figure continues . . .)*

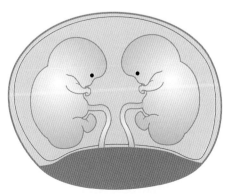

Monochorionic/monoamniotic

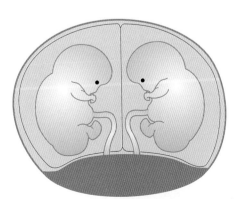

Monochorionic/diamniotic

Figure 9-1, continued. B *Longitudinal image of a first trimester twin pregnancy showing both placentas along the posterior uterine wall (arrows).* **C** *Early second trimester image of twins sharing a single amniotic sac. There is no separating membrane between them.* **D** *First trimester monoamniotic twins.*

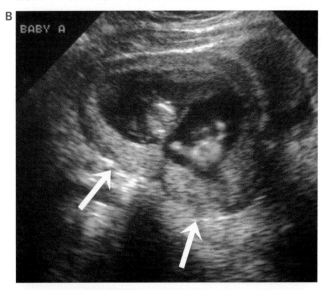

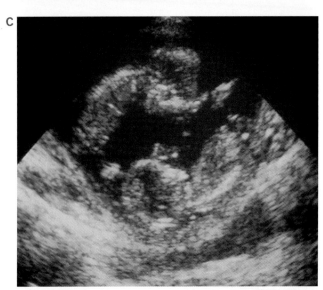

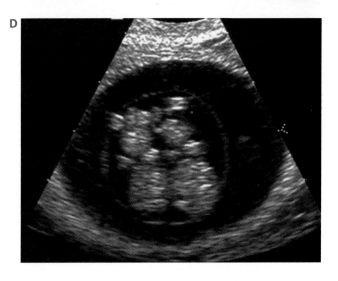

- When division occurs 4–7 days after fertilization, the monozygotic twins are diamniotic/**monochorionic**, which is the most common result (60%).

- Delayed division (7–13 days) occurs in only 10% of cases, resulting in a monochorionic/**monoamniotic** gestation. These twins have the poorest prognosis because cord entanglement causes demise in about 50% (Figure 9-1C). Sonographic identification of the separating membranes is important because it demonstrates that the fetuses are in separate sacs and therefore unable to become intertwined (Figure 9-1D).

- When division of the single zygote occurs after 13 days, the result is conjoined twins.

Sonographically, one can best identify chorionicity and amnionicity in the first trimester. A very thick separating membrane (two layers of amnion and two layers of chorion) would be indicative of a dichorionic/diamniotic gestation (Figure 9-2A). Identification of double yolk sacs implies diamnionicity, although one must be cautious since the separating membrane of a monochorionic/diamniotic pregnancy (two layers of amnion and one layer of chorion) is sometimes difficult to appreciate early in the pregnancy. Therefore identification of yolk sacs can be

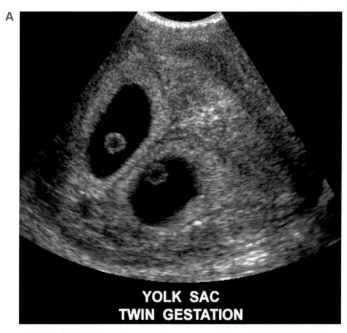

YOLK SAC
TWIN GESTATION

Figure 9-2. A *Transvaginal image showing a thick separating structure corresponding to two layers of amnion and two layers of chorion (diamniotic/dichorionic). Following page:* **B** *and* **C** *In these images, identification of two yolk sacs indicates the gestation will be diamniotic. However, viability cannot be verified until embryos and heartbeats can be seen.*

used to determine the number of amniotic sacs prior to visualization of the embryos (Figures 9-2 B and C). A twin gestation should not be ruled out until defined embryos can be identified at 6–7 menstrual weeks (Figure 9-3).

As pregnancy progresses into the second and third trimesters, identifying the number of placentas can become challenging because two placentas can appear as one if they abut each other or are fused (see Figure 9-1B). Again, the separating membrane can be evaluated for thickness. A membrane measuring more than 2 mm would suggest dichorionicity, and one that is thin and wispy (<2 mm) would indicate a single placenta (Figure 9-4). This rule may lose its accuracy later in pregnancy as crowding and

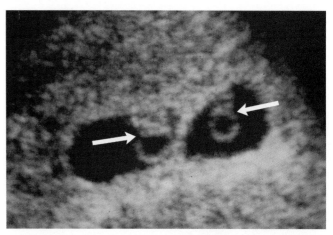

Figure 9-3. *In this magnified image, early twin embryonic disks (arrows) are seen between the yolk sac and the smaller amnion.*

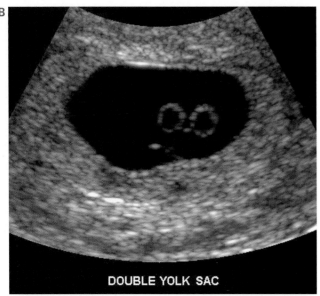

DOUBLE YOLK SAC

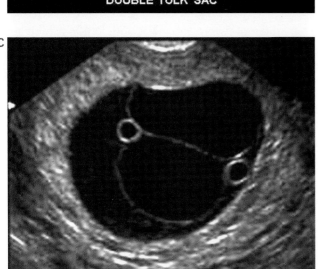

Figure 9-2, continued.

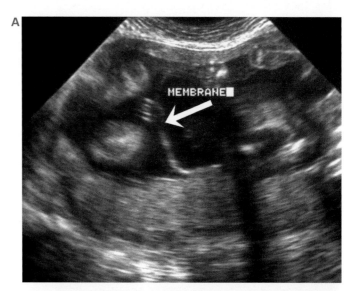

MEMBRANE

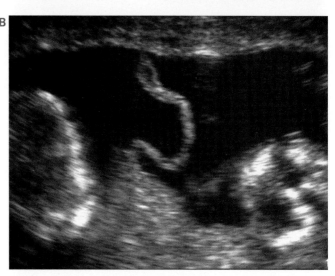

Figure 9-4. A *In this longitudinal image, the placenta appears to be a single posterior placenta, but the thick separating membrane suggests otherwise (arrow).* **B** *A more magnified view shows a thick membrane.*

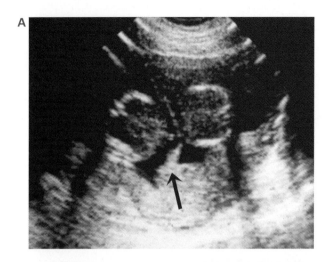

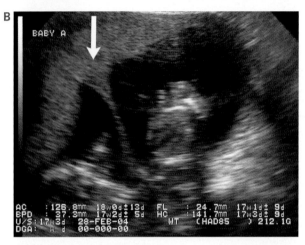

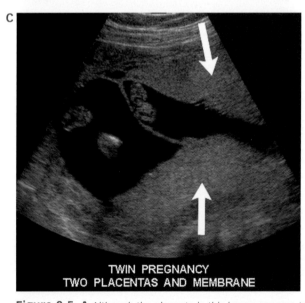

Figure 9-5. A *Although the placenta in this image appears to be single and posterior, the arrow is showing proliferation of the chorionic villi between the membranes, known as the "twin peak sign." This indicates there are two placentas—dichorionic.* **B** *Note the peak indicated by the arrow. Also, the separating membrane is thick. Both signs confirm a dichorionic gestation.* **C** *In this image, there are clearly two placentas (arrows), one anterior and one posterior. The separating membrane appears thin because of the increasing amniotic fluid within each sac, which causes thinning.*

increased amniotic fluid cause ill definition and thinning of the visible membrane. The **twin peak sign** (also known as the lambda or chorionic peak sign) can also suggest dichorionicity, but it is not 100% reliable. This sign refers to chorionic villi that grow into the potential interchorionic space for a short distance beyond where the membranes meet (Figure 9-5). There is no potential space if there is only one chorion/placenta.

Identifying the number of placentas and amniotic sacs is critical to the management of any multiple pregnancy. For twins and other multiples who have their own individual placentas and sacs, the risk of morbidity and mortality is much less than that for twins who share a single placenta and/or sac; most complications are related to twins that share a placenta. Therefore monozygotic twins are at increased risk for many complications, some of which are specific to monochorionicity.

FETAL PRESENTATIONS

It is important to document fetal position, especially near term. With twins and other multiple gestations the position of each fetus is relevant, and labeling the fetuses correctly is imperative. Fetal position may dictate the method of delivery. The presenting fetus is labeled Fetus (or Twin) A. The remaining fetus(es) are labeled sequentially and alphabetically (Figure 9-6). Some practitioners identify the fetuses numerically (Twin 1, Twin 2; Figure 9-12A). In almost 50% of twin pregnancies both twins are cephalic near term; about 37% are cephalic/breech. In a small percentage of twin pregnancies both twins are breech. In the remainder of twin pregnancies both fetuses exhibit a **transverse lie**, positioned horizontally across the mother's abdomen presenting shoulder-first. Malpresentation is diagnosed if one or both twins are in a position other than cephalic. Monoamniotic and malpresented twins usually require delivery by cesarean section, which in both cases reduces trauma and the risk of cord prolapse.

GROWTH DISTURBANCES

One of the primary reasons for closely monitoring a multiple gestation is to watch for growth discordancy. Intrauterine growth restriction (IUGR) can occur regardless of the type of twinning or other multiple gestation, and the growth differences can carry into adulthood, affecting height, weight, and even IQ. This is an area where zygosity plays an important role. Dizygotic twins

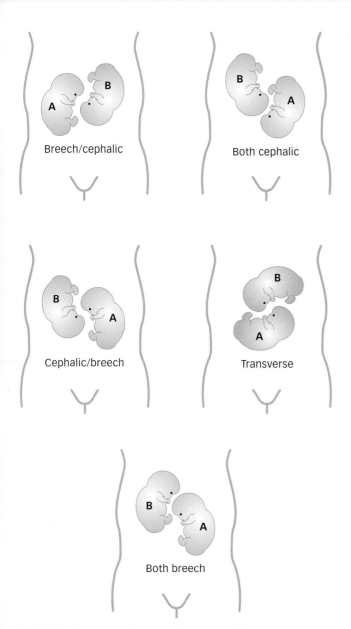

Figure 9-6. *Drawing demonstrating twin positions.*

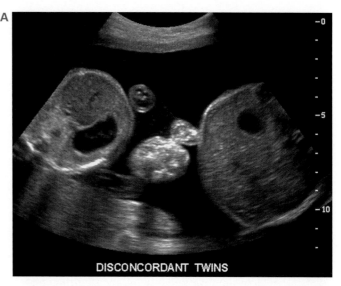

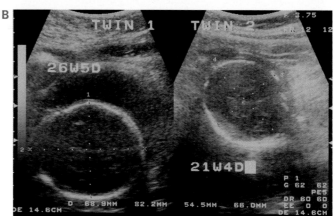

Figure 9-7. **A** *This image of transverse fetal abdomens clearly shows a difference in size between the twins.* **B** *There is an obvious difference in the size of the fetal skulls as well.*

may vary in size since they develop from separate eggs fertilized by different sperm and are genetically different. This is especially true if one fetus is male and the other is female (Figure 9-7). Low birth weights, defined as <2500 grams at birth, are more common (10×) in twins when compared to singletons, and this probability should be factored in when monitoring growth. Singleton charts can be used with twins up to 30 weeks of age. After that, multiple gestation charts are available and should be used since there is slower fetal growth with twins when compared to singletons. For gestations of higher numbers (triplets, quads, and so forth), fetal growth slows after 20 weeks. See Tables 36–43 in Appendix A.

With monozygotic twins, however, fetal size should remain the same throughout pregnancy since the fetuses are genetically identical. Any growth discordancy between monozygotic twins suggests a problem with the circulatory system between fetuses and placenta and may be associated with twin-to-twin transfusion syndrome (TTTS). TTTS happens when the twins are monochorionic and is much severer than simple IUGR. **Discordancy** is defined as a weight difference between fetuses of more than 500 grams (20%–25%). Other parameters suggesting growth discordancy include biparietal diameter (BPD) differences of more than 5 mm, abdominal circumference (AC) differences of more than 20 mm, and head circumference (HC) differences of more than 5% (Box 9-4).

> **Box 9-4.   Hallmarks of discordant growth.**
>
> Weight differences >20%–25% (500 g)
> Biparietal diameter differences >5 mm
> Head circumference differences >5%
> Abdominal circumference differences >20 mm

VANISHING TWIN

The **vanishing twin** phenomenon is not uncommon. Various studies have estimated that it occurs between 10% and 50% of the time when twins are identified before 10 weeks. Prior to visualization of an embryo, when one twin dies an empty sac can be seen; subsequently it is resorbed and disappears. The same is usually true if there is an identifiable embryonic or fetal pole absent a heartbeat (6–13 weeks; see Figure 9-8). Occasionally, however, the co-twin becomes incorporated into the developing twin. This is referred to as a **fetus in fetu**. On radiographs or ultrasound, a well-defined axial skeleton may be seen in the retroperitoneum, usually close to the umbilical circulation. For the surviving twin there is usually minimal or insignificant risk.

FETAL DEMISE

Demise of a twin in the second or third trimester carries varying risks depending on the chorionicity of the pregnancy. Risks are usually minimal in the dichorionic/diamniotic gestations and increase significantly if the twins share a single placenta. If demise occurs in the third trimester there is an increased risk for preterm labor and delivery as well as obstruction of the birth canal by the dead twin. When a dead, macerated fetus is still visible, it is referred to as a **fetus papyraceous**, a paper-thin or mummified fetus. In rare instances a fetus may die and calcify, becoming a **lithopedion**.

CONGENITAL ANOMALIES

There are three categories of anomalies associated with multiple gestations:

- *Deformation*, such as clubbing of the foot due to physical constraints.
- *Disruption*, due to intrauterine events such as IUGR.
- *Malformations*, such as the conjoined twin.

Compared to singletons, multiple gestations are twice as likely to present with congenital anomalies, and the risks increase if the twins are monozygotic. Although both

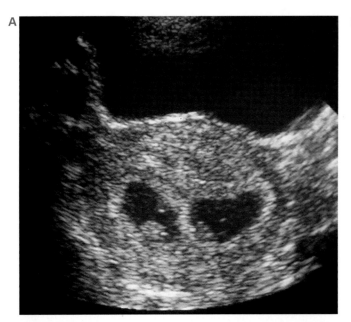
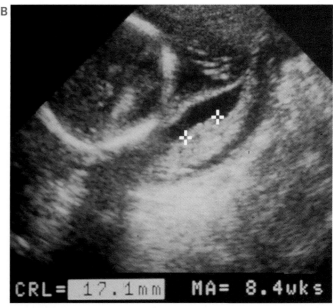

Figure 9-8. A *Transverse image of a twin pregnancy at 8½ weeks. Patient presented as a threatened aborter. Both fetuses were viable and bed rest was ordered until bleeding stopped.* **B** *Upon return for follow-up growth, a single fetus was identified. Adjacent to the fetal head, a collapsed sac was seen. Apparently, one twin died shortly after the first sonogram and had not completely reabsorbed (vanishing twin indicated by calipers).*

twins can be affected, anomalies are usually discordant regardless of type of twinning. Concordant anomalies are most likely to occur in the monozygotic pregnancy. The most common anomalies are those that affect the central nervous, musculoskeletal, cardiovascular, and gastrointestinal systems. Structural musculoskeletal anomalies such as clubbing of the feet may be caused by crowding. Sirenomelia (mermaid syndrome), although rare, is 100 times more commonly seen in twins, with a higher incidence among monozygotic twins (Figure 9-9).

COMPLICATIONS SPECIFIC TO MONOZYGOTIC/MONOCHORIONIC TWINS

It is well documented and has been demonstrated by pathologists that artery-to-artery, vein-to-vein, and artery-to-vein **anastomoses** (pathologic connections, openings, or communications between blood vessels) occur in monochorionic twin pregnancies. Superficially, arteries

anastomose with arteries and veins with veins. Deep in the placenta, arteries anastomose with veins. Usually these anastomoses do not interfere with the normal growth of the fetuses, allowing for a balanced flow of blood to each. Nevertheless, these communications within the placenta can result in complications such as twin-to-twin transfusion and twin embolization syndromes (Box 9-5).

Twin-to-Twin Transfusion Syndrome

Occurring in approximately 15%–30% of monochorionic gestations, **twin-to-twin transfusion syndrome (TTTS)** is a very serious complication in which unbalanced arterial venous shunting causes growth restriction of one twin and overgrowth or hydrops in the other (Figure 9-10). Also referred to as **fetal parabiotic syndrome**, the artery-to-vein **anastomosis** within the shared placenta causes a mixing of fetal blood, shunting too much to the recipient twin and not enough to the donor twin (Figure 9-11). The recipient twin will be large for gestational age (LGA) and the donor twin will be small for gestational age (SGA). The extreme of this

Box 9-5.	Complications associated with monozygosity.

Twin-to-twin transfusion syndrome (TTTS)

Twin embolization syndrome (TES)

Twin reversed arterial perfusion (TRAP) sequence

Conjoined twins

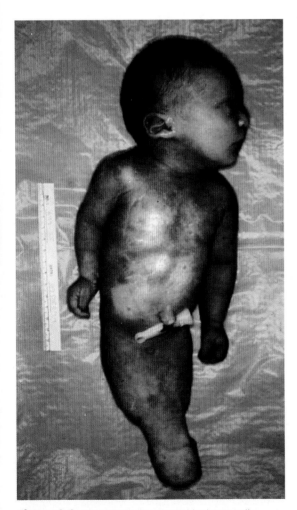

Figure 9-9. *Specimen of a fetus with sirenomelia (mermaid syndrome).*

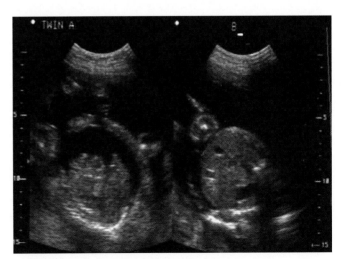

Figure 9-10. *Twin abdomens showing gross discordancy with the larger twin exhibiting abdominal ascites.*

Figure 9-11. *Drawing showing vascular anastomosis within a shared placenta.*

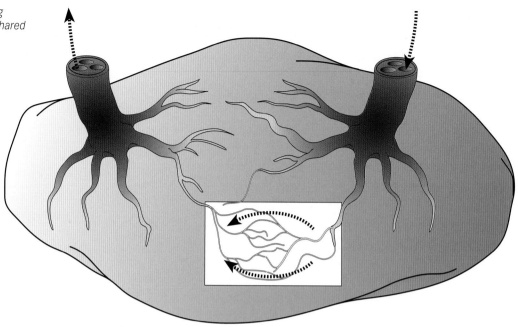

complication is called the **stuck twin syndrome**, a term referring to a severely growth-restricted (donor) twin. In this syndrome, the "stuck" donor twin not only is SGA but also is contained within a severely oligohydramniotic sac. The LGA twin has polyhydramnios, which pushes the small twin's sac against the uterine wall, creating the appearance that the donor twin is stuck to the uterus (Figure 9-12A). Stuck twin syndrome has also been termed **twin oligohydramnios/polyhydramnios sequence** (**TOPS**). The severe oligohydramnios often makes it impossible to visualize the separating membranes. The recipient twin will be further compromised if cardiac overload results in the development of fetal hydrops (Figure 9-12B).

The most striking sonographic findings in TTTS relate to the significant **discordance** in both size and growth of the fetuses and the amount of amniotic fluid noted in each sac. If such a discordance is seen in the second trimester, it is most likely due to TTTS or associated with other, unrelated anomalies. It is important to differentiate TTTS from simple IUGR because TTTS carries a poorer prognosis. Although the "stuck twin" does not necessarily indicate TTTS, it is most commonly seen with this syndrome, as is hydrops in the larger twin. Hydrops is not usually seen with simple IUGR. Severe polyhydramnios and hydrops of the other twin are indicative of TTTS. With simple IUGR of one twin, the other twin is normal while the growth-restricted twin may appear to be a stuck twin because of the oligohydramnios in its sac.

Twin Embolization Syndrome

Demise of one twin, when twins share a single placenta, puts the surviving twin at increased risk for morbidity and mortality because of the shared circulation of vessels within the common placenta. When one fetus dies, its tissues necrose. As the tissues break down, clots and debris can be transmitted to the surviving twin, causing obstructions to blood flow and/or organ infarction—the **twin embolization syndrome** (**TES**), sometimes known as thrombotic emboli syndrome. TES occurs in 1%–7% of twin pregnancies. These events can occur as early as seven days after demise but usually occur two weeks after the death of one fetus. Organ systems most likely to be affected include the central nervous system and the gastrointestinal/genitourinary (GI/GU) tracts. If demise occurs early in the pregnancy, the effect may include atresia of organ systems such as bowel obstructions or limb reductions. Late fetal death causes more destructive effects in critical organs such as the brain and kidneys. Ventriculomegaly, cortical atrophy, porencephaly, hydranencephaly, microcephaly, and renal defects are among the more common findings associated with TES (Figure 9-12C).

Twin Reversed Arterial Perfusion Sequence

Twin reversed arterial perfusion (**TRAP**) **sequence**, also called **acardiac parabiotic twinning**, is a rare complication of monozygotic gestations involving 1 in 30,000 births. The most popular theory for this occurrence is

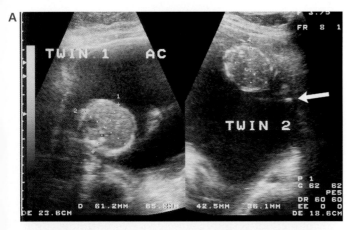

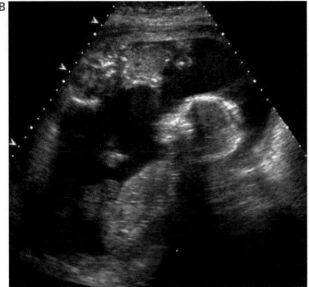

that reversal of blood flow through a large artery-to-artery, vein-to-vein anastomosis creates a single circulation of blood between the two fetuses. Consequently, one twin has reversed flow, causing serious malformations, including disruption of the development of the heart. The normal twin (*pump twin*) will have normal circulation but also has to provide circulation for the other twin (*perfused twin*). The blood pumped to the perfused twin is reversed through the umbilical arteries and the arterial anastomoses in the placenta. The arterial pressure in the normal twin exceeds that of the other twin, causing the reversal of blood flow in the abnormal twin. This results in a deficiency of blood supply to the upper body and leads to atrophy of the heart and upper body organs. This mismatch creates a huge single circulation of blood flow between the normal and abnormal fetuses. The increased cardiac load on the normal fetus often results in cardiac failure and hydrops of that twin.

Hemodynamic forces are critical to cardiac development, and the alteration in flow in TRAP causes severe anomalies, including absent heart or incomplete heart development. **Acardia** in twins is classified by degree of development. Classifications include **acardius acephalus** (60%–70%; Figure 9-13), **acardius anceps** (rare; Figure 9-14), **acardius acormus** (rare), and **acardius amorphus** (Figure 9-15A). Acardius amorphus and acardius acephalus are the most common.

Figure 9-12. A *These twin abdomens show slight discordant growth, but Twin 2 appears to be stuck to the anterior uterine wall. The arrow is pointing to the intertwine membrane showing Twin 2 has a small oligohydramniotic sac. The polyhydramnios in Twin 1's sac is pushing the smaller twin against the anterior uterus, making it look stuck to the uterine wall.* **B** *The smaller twin is stuck to the anterior uterine wall while the larger one sits on the posterior aspect of the uterus. The separating membrane cannot be appreciated.* **C** *Images show gross brain destruction (hydranencephaly) from TES.*

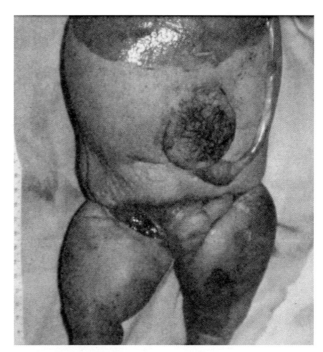

Figure 9-13. *Specimen of an acardiac twin with lower body formation—acardius acephalus.*

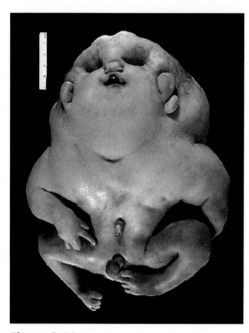

Figure 9-14. *Specimen of acardius anceps.*

Sonographically, the pump twin is usually normal but, as mentioned above, may become hydropic because of cardiac overload from supporting circulation for both itself and the perfused co-twin. The mortality rate for the pump twin is 50% and may be related to the size of the co-twin and patency of circulation. The hydropic fetus may have a polyhydramniotic sac, while the acardiac twin frequently is associated with oligohydramnios. Sonographic findings related to the acardiac twin include gross skin edema and cystic hygromas. Typically, the acardiac twin shows some lower abdomen and limb development or is simply present as an amorphous lump of tissue (Figures 9-15 B and C). Upper body and head development is rare. The umbilical cord of the acardiac twin frequently (50% of the time) shows only two vessels, and Doppler interrogation can demonstrate the reversal of blood flow. Table 9-2 correlates type of acardia with fetal development.

Figure 9-15. A *Specimen of acardius amorphus.* **B** *and* **C** *Sonographic images of acardiac twins of the amorphus type. Each shows gross skin edema and partial spine/rib development.*

A

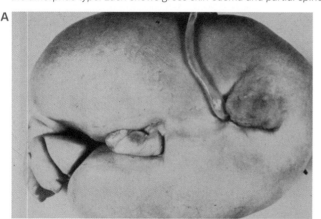

C

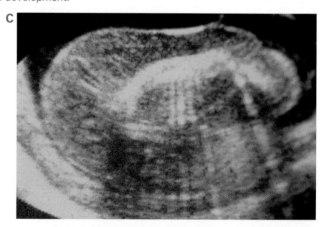

B

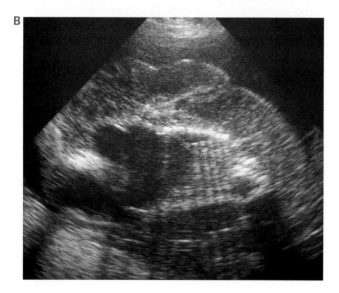

Table 9-2.	Types of acardia associated with degree of fetal development.
Type	**Degree of Fetal Development**
Acardius anceps	Head + body + extremities without heart
Acardius acormus	Head only
Acardius acephalus	Lower body + lower extremities
Acardius amorphus	Teratomatous tissue

Sonographic management involves monitoring the normal twin for evidence of hydrops. Polyhydramnios associated with fetal hydrops can cause discomfort for the mother, and placental edema may be seen. The acardiac twin growth should also be monitored because the size of the perfused twin affects the prognosis for the pump twin. The larger the perfused twin, the worse the prognosis for the pump twin. Preterm delivery is a complication and necessitates close clinical follow-up.

Conjoined Twins

Chang and Eng Bunker were conjoined twins from Siam (modern Thailand) who made their fortunes with the Barnum and Bailey circus—hence the term *Siamese*

twins. They were connected by a fibrous band of tissue that attached their lower chests. Two theories have been proposed to explain this phenomenon, today known as **conjoined twins**. One is that they result from the late division or *fission* (13 days after fertilization) of a single fertilized egg. Another theory emanating from a more recent study suggests that conjoined twins result from the secondary *fusion* of two separate monozygotic discs. Regardless of the cause, this is a rare anomaly of monozygotic twinning. It occurs sporadically (1 in 50,000 births), and most conjoined twins tend to be female. Conjoined twins are classified according to the site of fusion (Figure 9-16A).

A

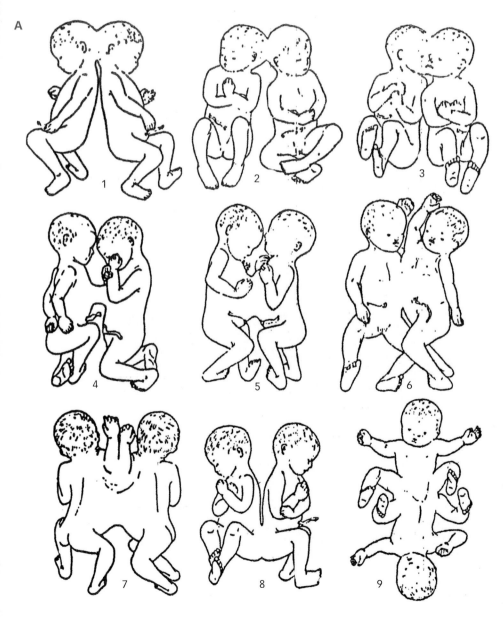

Figure 9-16. A *Various forms of twin attachments. Reprinted with permission from Patten BM:* Human Embryology. *New York, McGraw-Hill, 1968.* **1–3** *Craniopagus.* **4–7** *Thoracopagus.* **8–9** *Pygopagus. (Figure continues . . .)*

Conjoined twins are most commonly fused at the thorax with or without fusion of the upper abdomen. The fetuses are face-to-face, often causing hyperextension of the necks. Thoracic fusion of conjoined twins is termed **thoracopagus**. (*Pagus* is Greek for *fastened*.) The majority of these twins will exhibit conjoined hearts and half will share portions of their intestinal tracts. **Craniopagus** is head-to-head fusion, **omphalopagus** is abdomen-to-abdomen fusion (Figures 9-16 B–E), and **xiphopagus** is fusion of the anterior abdominal wall to the umbilicus and can be considered a subgroup of thoracopagus with a less complicated union. Although the twins usually share a liver, their upper intestinal tracts typically are separate. Omphalopagus twins, however, will show a communication of peritoneum. It is not uncommon for them to have multiple (up to seven) umbilical vessels

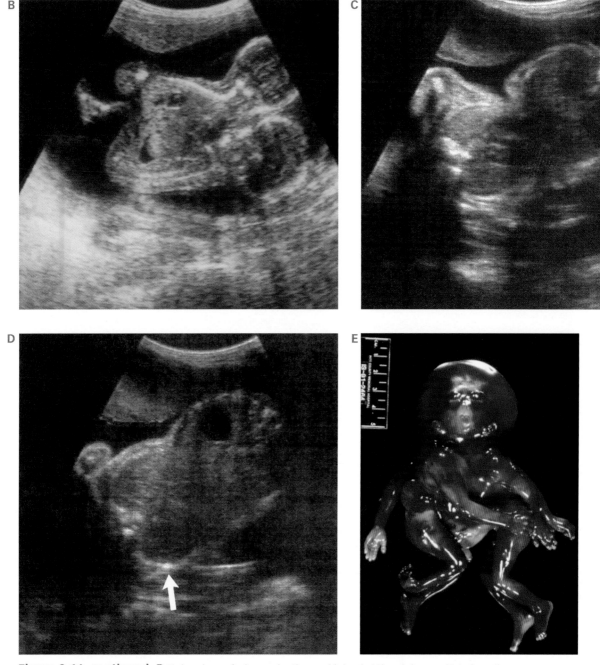

Figure 9-16, continued. B *Twins shown facing each other and joined at the abdomen. Note how the anterior twin has a hyperextended head/neck.* **C** *Transverse image of fetal abdomens showing they are joined at the liver.* **D** *This transverse image suggests the fusion extends to the lower chest region, as we see the heart (arrow) of the twin on the right.* **E** *Specimen of a craniothoracopagus twin.*

in the cord and exhibit an omphalocele. **Pygopagus** twins are joined dorsally at the buttocks and sacrum and face away from each other. The lower genital tract and external genitalia are fused and these twins often exhibit a single rectum and anus. **Ischiopagus** twins, constituting only about 5% of conjoined twins, share a common ischium and sacrum. Their intestinal tracts usually are joined at the ileum and empty into a single colon. This classification can be further divided into *ischiopagus tetrapus* twins (with four normal legs attached to the pelvis) and *ischiopagus tripus* twins (with two of four legs fused into a deformed limb). Of the two, ischiopagus tripus twins are most common. Joining at the head is the least common attachment and shows fusion of the skulls, often with shared sinuses and vascularity. The skulls may

fuse at the brow, vertex, or parietal bones and may fall under one of two subgroups, the *partial* or *total* form. With the partial form, the brains are separated by bone or dura, allowing for easier postnatal surgical separation. With the total form, the brains are connected or separated only by the arachnoid. Among the rarest forms of fusion is the **dicephalus**, two heads on a single body (Figure 9-17).

The prognosis for separation of conjoined twins depends on the degree of fusion and the organs shared. A large proportion of conjoined twins are stillborn or die shortly after delivery (40%–60%), usually because of associated congenital anomalies, including congenital heart disease and GI/GU abnormalities. Sonography can play a critical role in making this determination. (See Table 9-3.)

Figure 9-17. A *Specimen of a dicephalus twin.* **B** *and* **C** *These transverse images show two fetal heads facing each other.*

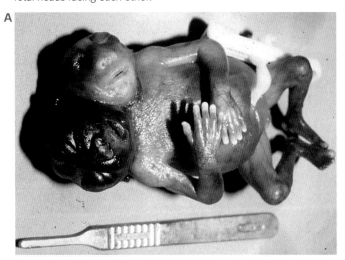
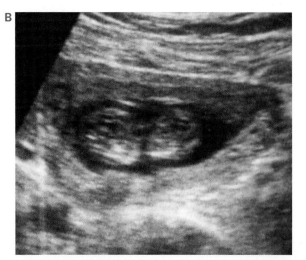
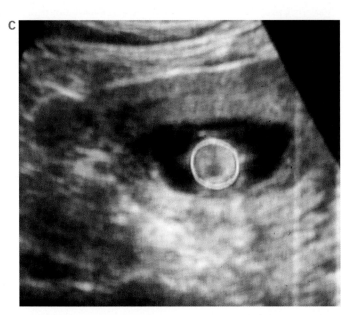

Table 9-3.	Frequency of conjoined (Siamese) twins by site of fusion.

Type (Site) of Fusion	Frequency
Thoracopagus	30%
Omphalopagus	25%
Pygopagus	20%
Craniopagus	15%
Ischiopagus	5%

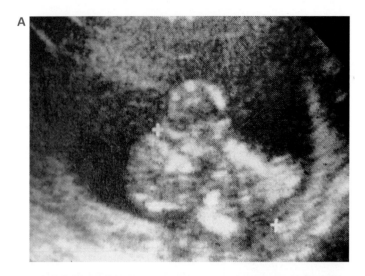

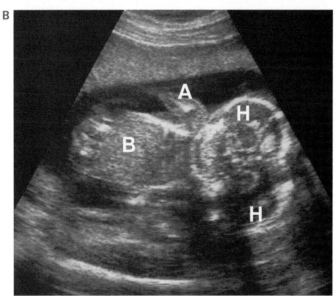

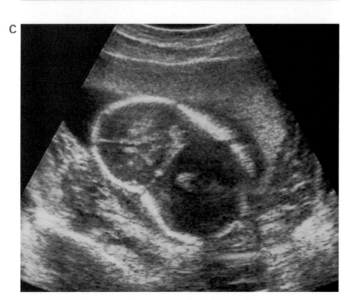

Figure 9-18. A *Very early twins showing close face-to-face orientation.* **B** *Craniopagus twins showing long axis through heads and body. H = head, B = body, A = arm.* **C** *Transverse through both heads.*

Sonographic findings associated with conjoined twins include the inability to identify a separating membrane, as these twins are monochorionic/monoamniotic. It is not uncommon for one or both to develop hydrops and polyhydramnios. Conjoined twins are positioned close to each other (Figure 9-18) and often assume an eccentric position in the uterus. Often, heads, spines, and/or extremities will be in extended or unusual positions. The sonographer should be suspicious if he or she finds no change in fetal positions upon follow-up examination. The umbilical cord contains more than three vessels; color Doppler can assist in verification.

SONOGRAPHIC MANAGEMENT

Multiple gestation should be identifiable on transvaginal sonography by 6 weeks' menstrual age, and monoamniotic twins should be recognized by 7–8 weeks. Visualization of the dividing membrane helps determine chorionicity by evaluating the thickness: A membrane measuring 2 mm or more in the first and early second trimesters suggests a dichorionic/diamniotic pregnancy.

Multiple gestations should be monitored regularly for growth, position, and fetal well-being at four-week intervals after 20 weeks' menstrual age. Fetal biophysical profiles and Doppler evaluations can help monitor fetal well-being. Two-week intervals are recommended in complicated cases. Although Doppler can be helpful in monitoring twins, most clinicians find that monitoring weights among and between the fetuses is most helpful. Other reasons for monitoring the multiple gestation include evaluating patients who are prescribed tocolytic agents for preterm labor, measuring the cervical length, and observing the status of a cerclage. (See Table 9-4.)

Performing amniotic fluid indices on individual sacs has not proven to be useful or reliable. Therefore amniotic fluid levels are subjectively monitored with close attention to rule out a stuck twin scenario. One can qualitatively check the hydrostatic pressures by observing the separating membrane. If the pressures are equal on both sides, the membrane will be flaccid. If the stuck twin scenario is suspected, the membrane will bulge from the polyhydramniotic side toward the smaller oligohydramniotic sac.

Finally, once an additional fetus has been identified, the practitioner must be sure to scan the entire uterine cavity so as not to miss anyone else. Triplets and quadruplets

Table 9-4.	The maternal and fetal risks posed by twinning and other multiple gestation.

Maternal Risks	Fetal Risks
Anemia	Preterm labor and delivery
Pregnancy-induced hypertension	Intrauterine growth restriction
Hyperemesis gravidarum	Increased morbidity/mortality
Pyelonephritis/urinary tract infection	Discordant growth/anomalies
Placenta previa/abruption	Vanishing twin/demise

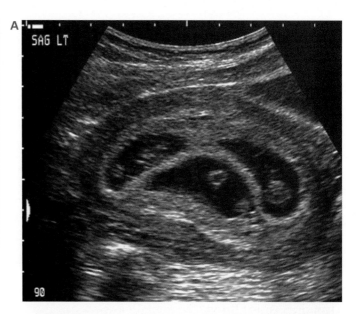

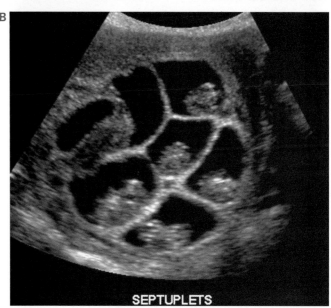

Figure 9-19. **A** *Image demonstrating gestation of triplets all separated by thick membranes.* **B** *Image of septuplets.*

are not as uncommon as they once were, particularly in those patients who have undergone fertility assistance. The incidence of *super twins* (three or more fetuses) increased 178% between 1984 and 1994 (Figure 9-19). It has been estimated that 60% of triplets, 90% of quadruplets, and 99% of quintuplets born in the United States today are the result of fertility treatments. Never in recorded history have sextuplets been naturally conceived—and there is a reason. The human uterus is not designed to accommodate large numbers of fetuses, and more fetuses die than live in large multiple births. For this reason, patients who undergo fertility-assisted procedures may be given the option of selective feticide in cases where more than four viable fetuses are identified after 10 weeks. Sonography practitioners may be asked to assist by localizing the fetuses and guiding the injection of potassium chloride or air into the chest until asystole is documented.

SCANNING TIPS, GUIDELINES, AND PITFALLS

Multiple gestations can be quite challenging in the second and third trimesters, as fetal movement and crowding add to the difficulty of separating body parts. Scan one fetus at a time, thoroughly, documenting all anatomic structures and measurements before going on to the next fetus. Bouncing back and forth between babies only confuses the examiner. Remember to establish the lie of each fetus before imaging anything. Once you know the fetal lie, you can start at the head and systematically work your way down the body, imaging as you go.

Breech fetuses have a higher incidence of **dolichocephaly** (having a cranial length greater than the cranial width, or

a cephalic index less than 76), and this is particularly true among twins that are breech. The cephalic index should always be checked before one determines growth discrepancies based on BPD differences > 5 mm. Dolichocephaly can be the result of crowding. When determining the differences in abdomen sizes, pay close attention to whether the size difference has to do with hydrops of one twin as opposed to IUGR. The prognosis for the twin with hydrops is much poorer than that for a twin with simple IUGR.

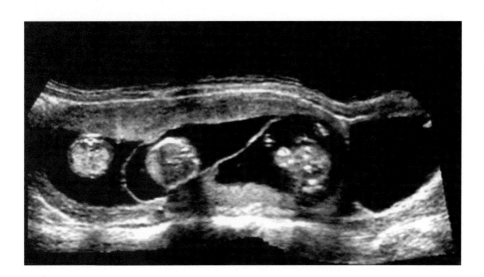

Figure 9-20. *The extended view option, such as with SonoCT, allows one to demonstrate multiple fetuses on one image.*

Tips and Guidelines

1. Establish the lie of each fetus before imaging anything. Start at the head of one fetus and systematically work your way down the body, imaging as you go.

2. Scan one fetus at a time, thoroughly, documenting all anatomic structures and measurements before moving to the next fetus.

3. Document the total number of fetuses in a single image (Figure 9-20).

4. Ascertain that each fetus has all of its parts.

5. Always check the cephalic index before determining growth discrepancies based on BPD differences > 5 mm.

6. Be sure to determine whether abdominal size differences are the result of IUGR rather than hydrops in one fetus.

7. Allow yourself plenty of time. When scheduling follow-up examinations on twins, allow two appointment slots, for triplets allow three, and so on. Appropriate scheduling will minimize stress on you and make your day run more smoothly.

Pitfalls

8. A subchorionic hemorrhage (implantation bleed) adjacent to an intrauterine sac can be mistaken for a second sac or vanishing twin.

9. A placental cyst could simulate or be mistaken for a saclike structure.

10. An intrauterine pregnancy within a bicornuate/septate uterus with fluid in the opposite side surrounded by decidualized endometrium could trick one into thinking there is a gestational sac in each horn or side of the uterus (Figure 9-21).

11. Identification of the extracoelomic space, which may be seen with a single gestation up to 8 weeks, can be mistaken for another saclike structure.

See Appendix C for an example of a clinical data sheet designed for twin obstetric ultrasound.

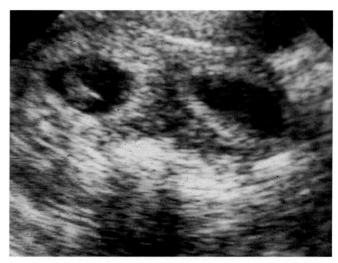

Figure 9-21. *Transverse image of a bicornuate uterus with an intrauterine gestational sac in the right horn.*

REFERENCES

Benacerraf BR: *Ultrasound of Fetal Syndromes*. New York, Churchill Livingstone, 1998, pp 431–448.

Benacerraf BR: *Ultrasound of Fetal Syndromes*, 2nd Edition. New York, Churchill Livingstone, 2007.

Benson CB, Doubilet PM: Twin pregnancy. In McGahan JP, Porto M: *Diagnostic Obstetrical Ultrasound*. Philadelphia, Lippincott, 1994, pp 434–448.

Burn J: Twins and twinning. In Chervenak FA, Isaacson GC, Campbell S: *Ultrasound in Obstetrics and Gynecology*. Boston, Little Brown, 1993, pp 783–793.

Carr-Hoeffer C: Twin reversed arterial perfusion sequence. In *OB-GYN Ultrasound Today*, Lesson 5, Volume 5. Hattiesburg, MS, Chrestomathic Press, 2000.

Cullinan JA: Sonography of multiple gestations. In Fleischer AC, Manning FA, Jeanty P, et al: *Sonography in Obstetrics and Gynecology, Principles and Practice*, 5th Edition. New York, McGraw-Hill Medical, 1996, pp 547–562.

Egan JFX, Borgida AF: Ultrasound evaluation of multiple pregnancies. In Callen PW (ed): *Ultrasonography in Obstetrics and Gynecology*, 5th Edition. Philadelphia, Saunders Elsevier, 2008, pp 266–296.

Jaffe R, Abramowicz, JS: *Manual of Obstetric and Gynecologic Ultrasound*. Philadelphia, Lippincott-Raven, 1997.

Jeanty P: Sonography in multiple gestation. In Fleischer AC, Toy EC, Lee W, et al: *Sonography in Obstetrics and Gynecology, Principles and Practice*, 7th Edition. New York, McGraw-Hill Medical, 2011.

Kurtz AB, Middleton WD: *Twin (Multiple) Gestations in Ultrasound: The Requisites*. St. Louis, Mosby, 1999, pp 341–355.

Mehta TS: Multifetal pregnancy. In Rumack CM, Wilson SR, Charboneau JW, et al: *Diagnostic Ultrasound*, 4th Edition. St. Louis, Elsevier Mosby, 2005, pp 1145–1165.

Mitchell C, Trampe B: Sonography and high-risk pregnancy. In Hagen-Ansert SL (ed): *Textbook of Diagnostic Sonography*, 7th Edition. St. Louis, Elsevier, 2012, pp 1181–1188.

Nolan RL: Multiple gestation. In Sauerbrei EE, Nguyen KT, Nolan RL: *A Practical Guide to Ultrasound in Obstetrics and Gynecology*, 2nd Edition. Philadelphia, Lippincott-Raven, 1998, pp 417–433.

Sanders RC, Blackmon LR, Hogge WA, et al: *Structural Fetal Abnormalities: The Total Picture*. St. Louis, Mosby, 1996, pp 221–234.

Sanders RC, Blackmon LR, Hogge WA, et al: *Structural Fetal Abnormalities: The Total Picture*, 2nd Edition. St. Louis, Mosby, 2002.

Spencer R: *Conjoined Twins: Developmental Malformations and Clinical Implications*. Baltimore, Johns Hopkins University Press, 2003.

Spitz L: Conjoined twins: a review. Prenatal Diagn 25:814–819, 2005.

SELF-ASSESSMENT EXERCISES

Questions

1. Amnionicity refers to the number of:
   A. Placentas
   B. Sacs
   C. Ova
   D. Cords
   E. Fetuses

2. Which of the following is *not* a maternal complication of twinning?
   A. Trophoblastic disease
   B. Pregnancy-induced hypertension (PIH)
   C. Anemia
   D. Hyperemesis gravidarum
   E. Postpartum hemorrhage

3. The stuck twin syndrome is associated with:
   A. Conjoined twins
   B. Twin reversed arterial perfusion (TRAP)
   C. Vanishing twin
   D. Twin peak
   E. Twin-to-twin transfusion syndrome (TTTS)

4. The membrane separating these twins indicates what about this pregnancy?

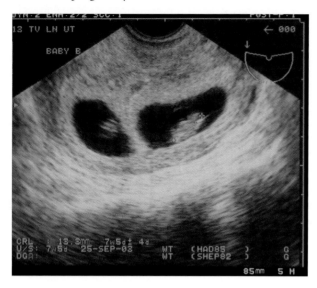

A. Diamniotic/dichorionic

B. Diamniotic/monochorionic

C. Monoamniotic/dichorionic

D. Monoamniotic/monochorionic

E. Amniotic band syndrome

5. A complication that can occur when one twin dies in utero and shares a common placenta with the surviving twin is called:

A. Twin-to-twin transfusion syndrome (TTTS)

B. Acardiac parabiotic twinning

C. Twin embolization syndrome (TES)

D. Twin reversed arterial perfusion (TRAP) sequence

E. Dizygotic twin syndrome

6. The most common form of conjoined twinning is called:

A. Craniopagus

B. Pygopagus

C. Ischiopagus

D. Thoracopagus

E. Omphalopagus

7. For how many weeks can a singleton gestational age chart be used for twins before their growth rates slow and a multiple gestation chart should be used?

A. 20

B. 25

C. 30

D. 35

E. 40

8. This image suggests the pregnancy is:

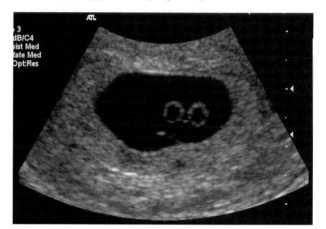

A. Dizygotic

B. Monozygotic

C. Diamniotic

D. Monoamniotic

E. Dichorionic/diamniotic

9. Which of the following characteristics of multiple gestations is the most difficult to define sonographically?

A. Zygosity

B. Amnionicity

C. Chorionicity

D. Gender

E. Twin presentation

10. Which of the following statements is *not* true of dizygotic twins?

A. They are chromosomally different.

B. They are always diamniotic.

C. They are always dichorionic.

D. They are considered identical twins.

E. They are the most common type of twin.

11. Twins that are connected at the pelvic region would be termed:

    A. Craniopagus

    B. Thoracopagus

    C. Pygopagus

    D. Omphalopagus

    E. Xiphopagus

12. Twins' growth is considered discordant if:

    A. Their BPDs differ by 2 mm.

    B. Their abdominal circumferences differ by 5 mm.

    C. Their cephalic indices are different.

    D. One amniotic sac has polyhydramnios.

    E. Their weights differ by more than 500 grams.

13. A cesarean section will be required if:

    A. The twins are monochorionic.

    B. The twins are diamniotic.

    C. The presenting twin is breech.

    D. The twins are discordant in growth.

    E. The twins are monozygotic.

14. Which of the following conditions causes acardia?

    A. Twin-to-twin transfusion syndrome (TTTS)

    B. Stuck twin syndrome

    C. Conjoined twins

    D. Twin embolization syndrome (TES)

    E. Twin reversed arterial perfusion (TRAP) sequence

15. You are scanning a twin gestation and one twin has fetal hydrops while the other is small for gestational age. You suspect:

    A. Intrauterine growth restriction (IUGR)

    B. Twin embolization syndrome (TES)

    C. Twin reversed arterial perfusion (TRAP) sequence

    D. Twin-to-twin transfusion syndrome (TTTS)

    E. Acardiac parabiotic twinning

16. Which of the following is not thought to be a predisposing factor for having twins?

    A. Maternal family history

    B. Paternal family history

    C. Mother of advanced maternal age

    D. Multigravida > 7

    E. Race/ethnicity

17. A diamniotic/monochorionic pregnancy is suggested by a separating membrane that measures:

    A. < 2 mm

    B. > 2 mm

    C. < 4 mm

    D. > 4 mm

    E. 1 cm

18. Of the following statements, which describes this image most accurately?

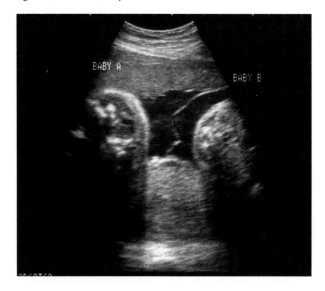

    A. The twins are identical.

    B. The twins are diamniotic/monochorionic.

    C. The twins are conjoined.

    D. The twins are growth discordant.

    E. The twins are diamniotic/dichorionic.

19. Which of the following statements is true for twins?

    A. 100% of monozygotic twins are diamniotic/mono-chorionic.

    B. Most complications relate to chorionicity.

    C. Twin-to-twin transfusion syndrome (TTTS) is specific to dizygotic twins.

    D. Zygosity refers to the gender of the fetus.

    E. Twin embolization syndrome (TES) frequently occurs when one twin dies in utero.

20. All of the following statements concerning dizygotic twinning are true *except*:

    A. Dizygotic twins are considered fraternal.

    B. Women over the age of 40 have a higher incidence.

    C. Conjoined twins are usually dizygotic.

    D. Dizygotic twinning is more common among African Americans than among Caucasians.

    E. 100% of dizygotic twins are diamniotic/dichorionic.

Answers

See Appendix F on page 614 for answers and explanations.

Maternal Disorders and Pregnancy

Kathryn A. Gill, MS, RT, RDMS, FSDMS

OBJECTIVES

After completing this chapter you should be able to:

1. List the maternal and fetal complications associated with hypertension during pregnancy.

2. Explain how diabetes can affect pregnancies.

3. Define the difference between immune and nonimmune fetal hydrops and explain how hydrops presents sonographically.

4. Discuss causes of abdominal pain during pregnancy.

5. Explain the significance of a pelvic mass during pregnancy and discuss how sonography can assist with monitoring and treatment.

ALTHOUGH MOST OBSTETRIC ULTRASOUND examinations focus on the fetus, the sonographer must be knowledgeable about maternal complaints and disorders that may affect the pregnancy. Some conditions may be unique

to pregnancy, while others may be chronic and occur in nonpregnant patients as well. This chapter discusses common maternal complaints and disorders, their impact on the fetus, and how the sonographer should monitor these patients.

SUPINE HYPOTENSIVE SYNDROME

Supine hypotensive syndrome is a common condition resulting from the fetus pressing on the maternal inferior vena cava (IVC). This usually occurs in the third trimester when the patient is supine. The weight of the pregnant uterus obstructs the blood flow within the IVC, causing the patient to begin to feel faint, clammy, and nauseated. The problem can be remedied by simply rolling the patient onto her left side (i.e., into a left lateral decubitus position) and instructing her to take in slow, deep breaths.

HYPEREMESIS GRAVIDARUM

Hyperemesis gravidarum is nausea and vomiting to the point of dehydration and sometimes requires hospitalization. It is usually the result of excess circulating hormones such as estrogen and progesterone. This condition can be associated with multiple gestations or trophoblastic disease. If trophoblastic disease is ruled out, the pregnancy should be monitored for growth restriction until the condition subsides, as the mother may not be able to keep food down, possibly depriving the fetus of nourishment. When the pregnant patient presents with nausea and vomiting, other conditions to be ruled out include maternal gallstones and peptic ulcer disease.

PREGNANCY-INDUCED HYPERTENSION

Pregnancy-induced hypertension (**PIH**) is caused by prostaglandin abnormalities and affects approximately 10% of all pregnancies, usually first pregnancies. The condition is most prevalent in patients younger than 18 and older than 35 years. **Prostaglandins** are hormone-like lipid compounds found in many tissues and affect the contractility of the uterus and other smooth muscle. They have the ability to lower blood pressure and regulate body heat.

PIH usually presents after the 20th week of gestation and can be life-threatening. Typically, patients present with high blood pressure, **proteinuria**, generalized edema (including **pitting edema**), and weight gain (Figure 10-1). Maternal blood pressure is considered elevated at 140/90 mmHg or higher. Excessive maternal weight gain would be 2 pounds or more per week. These clinical findings are referred to as **pre-eclampsia**, and the patient should be monitored for intrauterine growth restriction as the placenta becomes edematous, restricting blood flow (Box 10-1).

Further progression results in **eclampsia**, sometimes referred to as the *convulsive stage*, with the patient presenting with severely high blood pressure (160/110 mmHg × 2 taken six hours apart), headaches, blurred vision, and/or abdominal pain (Box 10-2). These are severe signs and carry a 17% maternal mortality rate due to stroke and 37% fetal mortality rate due to demise and/or placental abruption. Other maternal risks include seizures, coma, and renal, liver, and heart failure. Sonographic find-

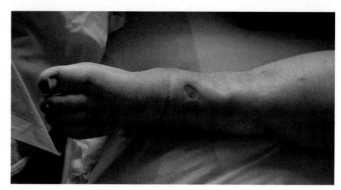

Figure 10-1. *Pitting edema demonstrated at the ankle and lower calf region.*

Box 10-1.	Pre-eclampsia.
	Hypertension
	Proteinuria
	Edema
	Weight gain

Box 10-2.	Eclampsia.
	Severe hypertension
	Headaches
	Blurred vision
	Abdominal pain

ings include a small placenta that may have an advanced grade. **Oligohydramnios**, a deficiency of amniotic fluid (see Chapter 8), is also common and associated with the resultant growth restriction of the pregnancy. In severe cases, the mother may develop maternal ascites, pleural effusions (Figure 10-2), and risk of placental abruption.

PIH can affect maternal kidneys, brain, and liver. A variant of severe eclampsia, recognized in 1982, is characterized by pain in the right upper quadrant due to liver enlargement, along with nausea, vomiting, and abnormal liver enzymes. The condition is referred to as **HELLP syndrome**, an acronym for hemolysis, elevated liver enzymes, and low platelets. It occurs in 2%–12% of pre-eclamptic patients. Maternal risk factors include young age, African

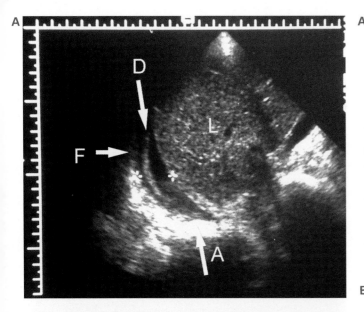

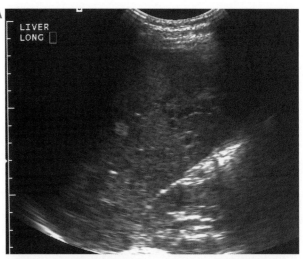

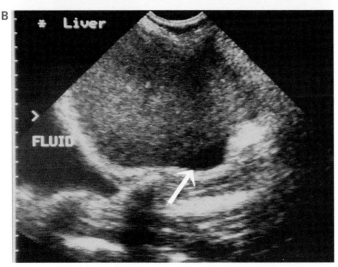

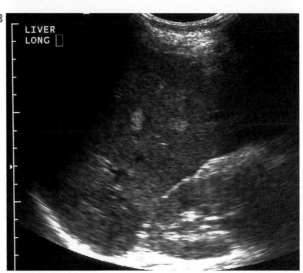

Figure 10-2. A *Longitudinal image of the maternal liver, which is enlarged. There is pleural effusion and a small amount of ascites. L = liver, F = pleural effusion, A = ascites, D = diaphragm.* **B** *Longitudinal image through the right upper quadrant showing maternal abdominal ascites (arrow).*

American ethnicity, familial predisposition, and other underlying factors, such as hypertension, diabetes, and renal disease. In severe cases the liver may rupture and show a subcapsular hematoma with a 3.5% maternal mortality rate. Since symptoms for this disorder may mimic other conditions, it is critical to make the diagnosis early. Sonographic findings include altered liver and kidney echo patterns with patchy increased echoes throughout (Figure 10-3). The liver and kidneys may enlarge, and fluid may be seen around them.

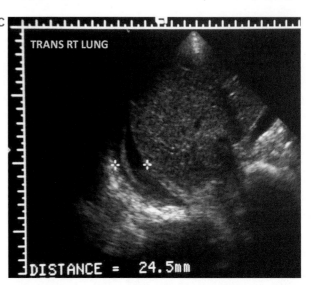

Figure 10-3. A *and* **B** *Patient with HELLP syndrome. Liver shows mottled appearance and decreased visualization of vasculature due to enlarged liver.* **C** *Subcapsular fluid and pleural effusion in patient with HELLP syndrome.*

CHRONIC HYPERTENSION

Chronic hypertensives constitute only about 2% of all pregnancies. These patients usually present with obesity and have a blood pressure exceeding 140/90 before pregnancy. Mothers and fetuses are monitored the same as those with PIH.

HYDROPS

Edith Potter—best known for describing abnormal facial findings in fetuses and infants with renal abnormalities—first spoke of hydrops in 1943. **Hydrops** is defined as two or more abnormal serous fluid collections, and these usually include pleural effusions (Figure 10-4), abdominal ascites, and anasarca. In some cases, cardiomegaly may be present, and it has been suggested that **hydroceles** (Figure 10-5) in male fetuses may be an early indication of the development of abdominal ascites. Placental edema may also be present, causing pre-eclampsia. There can be many causes for the development of **fetal hydrops** (**hydrops fetalis**), but, regardless of the cause, once fetal hydrops develops the prognosis is poor, even at term, with a survival rate of only 25%. Any time fetal hydrops is identified, one should rule out a maternal immune cause first. Most cases are accompanied by viral infections that cause mild maternal symptoms, such as a cold, fever, and/or swollen lymph nodes. Fetal hydrops can be seen 10–14 days after onset of symptoms.

Nonimmune Hydrops

Hydrops usually stems from fetal anemia, which requires the heart to pump a much greater volume of blood to deliver the same amount of oxygen. This anemia can have either an immune or a nonimmune cause. **Nonimmune hydrops** (**NIH**) can also be unrelated to anemia, as, for example, when a tumor or congenital cystic adenomatoid malformation increases the demand for blood flow.

There are approximately 150 causes of nonimmune hydrops, and all carry a 50%–98% mortality rate. Causes include **TORCH infections** (toxoplasmosis, other [syphilis, varicella-zoster, parvovirus B19], rubella, cytomegalovirus, and herpes), blood disorders, cardiac abnormalities, abdominal and pulmonary masses, diabetes, PIH, and renal and chromosomal abnormalities, among many others.

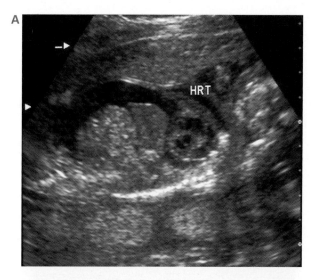

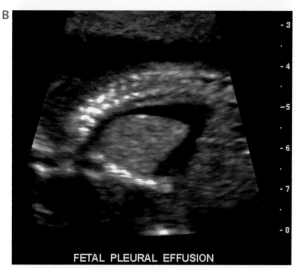

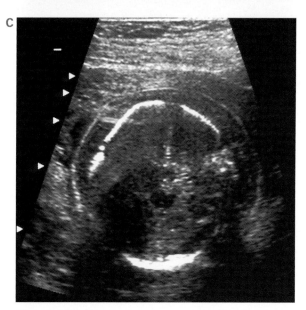

Figure 10-4. A Longitudinal scan through a fetal chest and abdomen showing abdominal ascites and pleural effusion. **B** Fetal lung surrounded by pleural effusion. **C** Fetal head showing a thick halo associated with gross scalp edema.

Figure 10-5. A *Transverse image through fetal chest showing an enlarged heart surrounded by pericardial fluid (arrows). Skin edema is also seen.* **B** *Fetal scrotum demonstrating a hydrocele.* **C** *The four Rh combinations and the outcome for the offspring.*

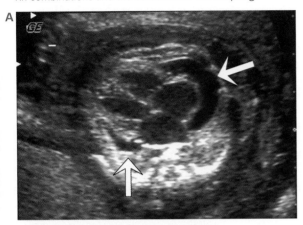

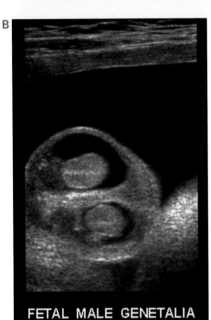

FETAL MALE GENETALIA

Alpha thalassemia is a rare, lethal type of fetal nonimmune hydrops seen in patients of Asian or Mediterranean descent (Box 10-3).

Causes that are considered treatable include fetal anemia associated with **parvovirus**, fetal cardiac arrhythmias associated with tachycardia and heart block, high-pressure fluid seen with pleural and pericardial effusions, and hydrops associated with twin-to-twin transfusion syndrome (TTTS). Several mild childhood diseases that present with a rash can be contracted during pregnancy and cause the fetus to develop hydrops. These viruses were numbered by a French physician in 1905. The more common include first disease (German measles), third disease (scarlet fever), fifth disease (erythema infectiosum, caused by a

Box 10-3.	Conditions associated with nonimmune hydrops.

Cardiovascular and pulmonary abnormalities
Skeletal dysplasias
Chromosomal abnormalities
Blood disorders
Twin-to-twin transfusion syndrome
Diaphragmatic hernia and GI tract obstructions
TORCH infections
Sacrococcygeal teratomas
Placenta/cord anomalies
Fetal liver disease
Maternal disease
Medications

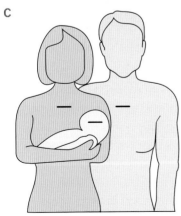

The Rh type of a child born of parents who are both Rh− can only be negative.

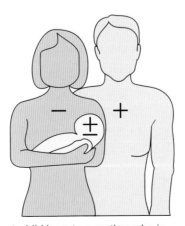

A child born to a mother who is Rh− and a father who is Rh+ can be either Rh− or Rh+. About 60% of the time, the children of these parents are Rh+.

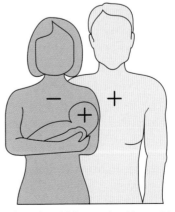

When the child conceived by an Rh− woman is Rh+, difficulties may occur for that child or for the mother's future children. The greatest problem is a condition called hemolytic disease of the newborn.

parvovirus), and sixth disease (roseola). All are contracted nasopharyngeally and cause symptoms similar to those of mononucleosis.

Untreatable causes include viral sources seen with TORCH, lymphatic sources, and those associated with cardiomyopathy. Cytomegalovirus (CMV) and toxoplasmosis are among the most common viral sources, while a cystic hygroma, a lymphatic lesion typically found in the head and neck area, is the most common lymphatic source. Valvular disease is most responsible for cardiomyopathy and hydrops associated with heart abnormalities.

Immune Hydrops

Mothers can develop antibodies to about 100 red blood cell surface antigens, and approximately one-third of these antibodies can result in fetal anemia. Most of these, however, are caused by blood group incompatibilities such as ABO incompatibility and rhesus (Rh) isoimmunization, whereby the mother's immune system recognizes the fetus as a foreign substance and attacks it.

Rh blood group antibodies have only one function, and that is to destroy Rh+ cells. If both parents are Rh−, there is no need for concern, because the fetus will be Rh− as well. However, mothers who are Rh− must be monitored for the development of fetal hydrops if the father is Rh+. During the last month of pregnancy the fetus acquires antibodies from the mother, and during birth fetal blood cells are allowed to enter the mother's bloodstream, where they persist. If the fetal blood factor differs from the mother's, the mother becomes immunized to the fetal foreign antigen. With subsequent pregnancies, **hemolysis** (destruction of red blood cells) can occur when the maternal immune system attacks the fetus. Severe fetal anemia causes **erythroblastosis fetalis (EBF)**, which is associated with fetal hydrops, congestive heart failure, and ultimate demise. For patients who have had a previous stillborn or hydropic infant due to the Rh factor, there is a 90% chance that the next Rh+ infant will be stillborn if untreated (Figure 10-5C).

When fetal red blood cells are destroyed, more are made by the bone marrow. If production is inadequate, the liver and spleen produce red blood cells. When the liver and spleen production proves to be inadequate, severe fetal anemia and hydrops occur. Fetal hydrops associated with the Rh− mother is called **immune hydrops**.

Other causes of immune hydrops include ABO incompatibility and irregular blood group incompatibilities. A fetal hematocrit of 15% or less results in hydrops. Ultrasound-guided percutaneous umbilical blood sampling (PUBS)—also known as **cordocentesis** or fetal blood sampling—can be very helpful in getting a fast diagnosis. For additional information on immune hydrops or Rh isoimmunization, see Chapters 7 and 12.

Role of the Sonographer

The role of the sonographer in monitoring the Rh− patient is to perform an early ultrasound examination to confirm gestational age and then to perform serial sonograms to monitor for erythroblastosis fetalis. Monitoring usually begins at about 20 weeks' gestation, and sonograms are performed at four-week intervals until delivery. Sonographic findings might include an enlarged umbilical vein, enlarged heart, cardiac arrhythmia, enlarged thoracic circumference due to cardiomegaly, pleural effusions, polyhydramnios, and thick placenta. Sonography can also assist in performing amniocenteses to check for bilirubin in the amniotic fluid, indicating an abnormal amount of fetal red blood cell destruction, and to guide physicians during intrauterine transfusions. These transfusions may begin at 26 weeks. Although blood flow within the uterine and umbilical arteries in the isoimmunized pregnancy will be normal, fetal anemia is associated with increased cardiac output. The increase in cardiac output causes increased blood flow in the umbilical vein and increased velocity in the IVC, descending thoracic aorta, common carotid arteries, and middle cerebral arteries. Doppler ultrasound may be helpful in monitoring fetal well-being and in determining the best time to intervene.

In Utero Blood Transfusion

Intervention usually involves in utero blood transfusion. It is important to check the fetus for anemia prior to performing transfusion. A needle is placed within the umbilical vein at the site where the cord inserts into the placenta. This is where it will be stablest. Once the needle is in the vein, blood can be aspirated and tested by means of cordocentesis. The needle can be left in place while laboratory tests are performed to determine the feasibility of transfusion. If the situation is favorable, packed red blood cells are introduced into the umbilical vein. The fetal heart must be monitored to check for cardiac overload. An increase in fetal heart rate during transfusion usually indicates a favorable prognosis. Bradycardia, or slowing of heart rate, is worrisome. Demise occurring within 24 hours of transfusion is usually the result of the procedure itself. Demise occurring more than 24 hours after the procedure is usually due to the condition.

DIABETES MELLITUS AND PREGNANCY

An association between diabetes mellitus and congenital malformations has been suspected since the early 19th century. Since the early 1990s, we have seen significant improvements in the medical, obstetric, and neonatal care of diabetic pregnancies, and this has resulted in a decrease in fetal and neonatal morbidity and mortality. Still, the incidence of malformations in these pregnancies has not significantly changed; the estimated frequency among diabetic mothers is 3%–6%. Diabetes is considered the leading cause of fetal malformations and is responsible for 40% of all perinatal deaths. For this reason, the diabetic patient is categorized as "high risk," and the sonographer must be knowledgeable about the complications that can occur during pregnancy.

Definition of Diabetes

Diabetes mellitus is the most common endocrine disorder and is estimated to occur in one of every 324–350 pregnancies in the United States. It belongs to a family of chronic diseases that affect many functions and body systems, primarily those of carbohydrate metabolism related to insulin deficiency. **Endocrine glands** produce hormones that are delivered directly to the bloodstream. The culprit causing diabetes is the pancreas, which produces insulin. Insulin acts as a regulator for the passage of **glucose** (simple sugar) from the bloodstream into fat and muscle cells. Glucose, not needed immediately by the body, is stored in the liver as **glycogen** and converted back to glucose when needed. Most of the glucose is used by the brain and red blood cells, and the remainder is metabolized by muscle and fat tissue. The pancreas is sensitive to any rise in glucose and responds by excreting insulin. This allows for storage of glycogen in the liver to be enhanced and hoarded until the amount circulating in the blood is utilized. When there is a lack of insulin or when the body is unable to use insulin effectively, there is an increase in the blood glucose levels (**hyperglycemia**), and these blood levels can vary widely.

Types and Classifications of Diabetes

Diabetes mellitus falls under three types and several classifications. The types include type 1, type 2, and gestational diabetes. These can be further classified alphabetically in a system referred to as **White's classification**. The causes of the different types are unknown. Nevertheless, each is associated with several identifiable clinical characteristics (see Table 10-1).

Type 1 Diabetes

Type 1 and type 2 diabetes share the presence of a diabetic family history, but they differ in the sources of their remaining causes. **Type 1 diabetes** may be due to a fault in the immune system that causes the pancreas to cease insulin production. These patients experience juvenile onset of diabetes and are insulin-dependent; therefore, they require continued regular injections of exogenous insulin for survival. Of all diabetics, 10% are type 1 and, for the pregnant patient, type 1 is considered more serious, putting the patient at a high risk for complications. Type 1 can be further classified, using White's classification, as types C–T.

Type 2 Diabetes

Most **type 2**, or **class B**, **diabetics** are considered non–insulin-dependent. With type 2, the pancreas produces insufficient amounts of insulin. The reason for this phenomenon is unknown, but 85% of all diabetics fall under the category of type 2. Typically, they are overweight and

Table 10-1.	White's diabetes classification.
Class A	Highest probability of fetal survival. No insulin; minor dietary regulation.
Class B	Onset at age 20 or later. Less than 10 years' duration before pregnancy.
Class C	Onset or duration between 10 and 19 years. Minimal vascular disease.
Class D	Onset before age 20 with 20+ years' duration. Moderate to advanced vascular disease.
Class E	Same as Class D + calcification of pelvic vessels.
Class F	Same as Class D + nephritis.
Class G	Many organ failures.
Class H	Cardiomyopathy.
Class R	Active retinitis.
Class T	Renal transplant.

Reprinted with permission from Gill K: Diabetes mellitus and pregnancy. Ob-Gyn US Today, 3(10):158, 1998.

middle-aged or older. Obesity is suggested to be a major factor, because the more fat content there is in the body, the higher the body's resistance to insulin. Type 2 diabetes can be managed with diet and weight reduction in most cases.

Gestational Diabetes

The occurrence of **gestational**, or **class A**, **diabetes** is more prevalent in individuals with a family history of diabetes, a history of sugar in the urine, obesity, and a history of glucose intolerance. For the gestational diabetic, insulin insufficiency usually occurs during the second trimester and disappears shortly after delivery. Gestational diabetes is similar to type 2 diabetes since both occur during the adult years and are associated with obesity. Although gestational diabetics are considered non-insulin-dependent, they are at risk for developing diabetes later in life. Gestational diabetes affects approximately 25 of every 1000 pregnant women and is the most common type in this population. Risk factors for gestational diabetes include a family history of diabetes, being a borderline diabetic, having had a stillbirth or macrosomic infant, having had a child with a congenital anomaly, advanced maternal age (35 years or older), or weighing 170 pounds or more before pregnancy (Box 10-4).

Maternal Complications of Diabetes

It is important for the obstetric sonographer to have knowledge of the effects of diabetes on a pregnancy so that he or she can perform a thorough evaluation of the fetus and be aware of the maternal complications as well. Diabetic mothers experience an increased incidence of urinary tract infections, vaginal infections, PIH, and polyhydramnios as well as hypoinsulinism, hyperglycemia, and postpartum hemorrhage (Box 10-5).

Fetal Complications of Diabetes

Glucose is the primary fuel for fetal growth. The fetus of the diabetic mother is exposed to high levels of glucose, producing excess levels of insulin that cause growth discrepancies in fetal body parts. These fetuses may be macrosomic or growth-restricted, and they can also exhibit a wide range of anomalies and malformations. (See Box 10-6 for a summary of fetal complications from diabetes.)

Large for Gestational Age and Macrosomia

Patients classified as class A or B will most likely produce fetuses that are **large for gestational age** (**LGA**). Usually, the head and brain will grow normally; however,

the trunk and abdominal organs will have an increased growth rate, producing asymmetrical growth seen at 28–32 weeks of gestational age. Between 25% and 42% of fetuses born to diabetic mothers are LGA, and between 10% and 50% show **asymmetrical macrosomia**, weighing more than 4500 grams at birth. LGA and macrosomia put a fetus at increased risk for perinatal morbidity and mortality.

Complications that result from trauma during delivery include shoulder dystocia, fractures, **facial/brachial plexus palsies**, perinatal asphyxia, meconium aspiration, and

---

Box 10-4.   Risk factors for gestational diabetes.

Borderline diabetic
170+ lbs pre-pregnant
> 35 years of age
Previous infant > 9 lbs at birth

Box 10-5.   Diabetes and maternal complications.

Endocrine imbalance
Increased urinary tract and vaginal infections
Pregnancy-induced hypertension (4×)
Polyhydramnios (10×)
Hypoinsulinism
Hyperglycemia
Postpartum hemorrhage

Box 10-6.   Diabetes and fetal complications.

Large for gestational age/macrosomia
Growth restriction
Central nervous system anomalies
Cardiac anomalies
Gastrointestinal anomalies
Genitourinary anomalies
Postnatal hypoglycemia/hyperinsulinism
Hydrops
Respiratory distress
Demise (2×)

neonatal metabolic complications. Fetal size and weight in the diabetic patient can be quite misleading, based on ultrasound measurements alone, and at delivery infants may present with **infant respiratory distress syndrome** (also known as **hyaline membrane disease**) because their lungs have matured more slowly. The timing and management of delivery of the infants of diabetic patients depend on good gestational dating and fetal weight estimations. When interpreting a **lecithin-to-sphingomyelin (L/S) ratio** for fetal lung maturity in nondiabetic patients, physicians would consider fetal lungs mature if the ratio is 2:1. However, in the diabetic patient, the L/S ratio must be 3–3.5:1 before delivery should be attempted. Therefore, it is wise to perform amniocentesis on these patients before labor is induced or cesarean section is performed.

Fetuses with **symmetrical macrosomia**, where all fetal measurements are symmetrically large, are thought to be the product of genetics rather than diabetes. Mothers of these fetuses typically have delivered large babies in the past, and often both parents will indicate that, at delivery, they were large babies themselves.

Polyhydramnios

Another cause of LGA is **polyhydramnios**, or excess amniotic fluid, not uncommon in the diabetic pregnancy, especially gestational diabetes (Figure 10-6). The etiology of this condition is unknown. Many studies have been performed to determine if fetal polyuria due to fetal hyperglycemia in the diabetic patient could explain the increase in amniotic fluid, but none has proven this assumption to be true. Other theories of the cause include increased amniotic fluid osmolality due to increased glucose and/or decreased fetal swallowing. In most cases, polyhydramnios does not present until the third trimester. Most seasoned sonographers perform a qualitative means of evaluating amniotic fluid levels by simply eyeballing the overall appearance of the fluid. A quantitative means is available by calculating the amniotic fluid index (AFI). When using the AFI, make sure that you and the referring clinician agree upon the numeric value for normal and abnormal findings, because there are three published ranges for normal values. (See Chapter 4 for more on the AFI.)

Placental and Umbilical Cord Anomalies

The placenta in patients with classes A–C diabetes is usually larger than normal because of villous edema. A normal placenta should not measure more than 4–5 cm at term and should not measure more than 3 cm at 20

weeks. To measure the placenta, calipers are placed at the widest anterior/posterior (AP) dimension of the placenta, excluding the vascular retroplacental space (Figure 10-7A). Septal cysts may be seen because of the obstruction of septal venous drainage. In classes D–H, one should expect the placenta to be thinner than normal because of vascular insufficiency and atrophy.

If the placenta is enlarged, it is not uncommon for the umbilical cord also to be large; the incidence of enlarged umbilical cords is five times greater in diabetics. Single umbilical arteries can be associated with this condition, having been found in 6.4% of diabetic pregnancies (Figures 10-7 B and C). Single umbilical arteries or two-vessel cords are also associated with malformations such as inguinal hernias, clubfoot, polydactyly, pulmonary hypoplasia, and vertebral and genitourinary anomalies.

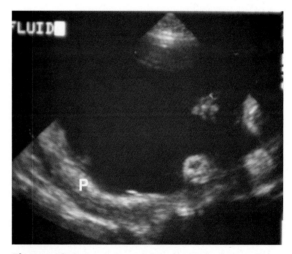

Figure 10-6. *Gross polyhydramnios is causing placental compression posteriorly. P = placenta.*

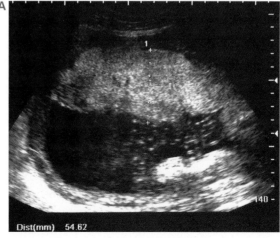

Figure 10-7. A *An edematous placenta measuring 5.5 cm. (Figure continues . . .)*

B

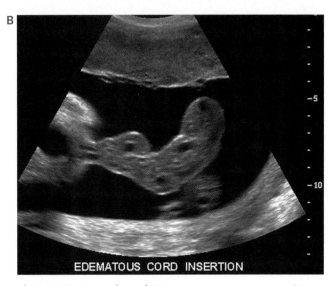

EDEMATOUS CORD INSERTION

C

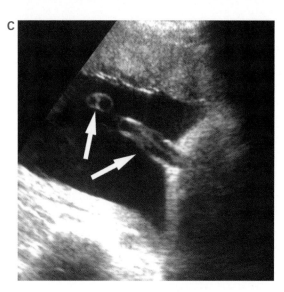

Figure 10-7, continued. B *Edematous umbilical cord.* **C** *Cord insert into the fetal abdomen showing only two vessels (arrows).*

Intrauterine Growth Restriction

Intrauterine growth restriction (**IUGR**), which refers to the poor or restricted growth of the fetus in utero, is a complication among class C diabetics, as well as patients in classes D–H, who are at risk for the most unfavorable outcomes, such as fetal anomalies, hydrops, and demise. Insulin-dependent diabetics frequently experience circulatory problems. During pregnancy, poor circulation can lead to uteroplacental vascular insufficiency, causing a decrease in nutrients received by the fetus. Fetal anomalies are produced by the teratogenic effect of hyperglycemia; many studies have proven that hyperglycemia disrupts organogenesis. The fetus of a diabetic patient who is in poor glycemic control or experiences a change in glycemic control during the fifth to eighth weeks of gestation is at considerable risk for serious congenital abnormalities, including those of the central nervous system, heart, gastrointestinal tract, and genitourinary system.

Central Nervous System Anomalies

Central nervous system (CNS) anomalies in the fetuses of diabetic patients can include **neural tube defects** (**NTDs**), openings or other defects in the brain or spinal cord. The most common neural tube defects seen in diabetic patients are anencephaly, encephalocele, holoprosencephaly, spina bifida, and meningomyelocele. Careful evaluation of the fetal skull, brain, and spine is necessary to rule out these abnormalities. Anencephaly, absence of the cranium and brain, occurs three times more frequently in the fetuses of diabetic patients (Figure 10-8). Posterior

A

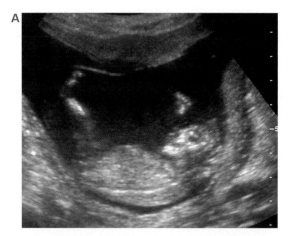

B

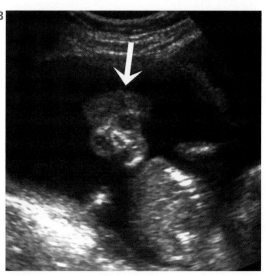

Figure 10-8. A *Anencephalic fetus shown with leg extended and hand above the face.* **B** *Frontal view of face of anencephalic fetus. Minimal brain tissue is present with no bony covering (arrow).*

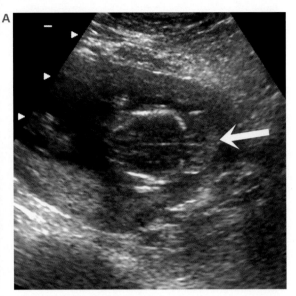

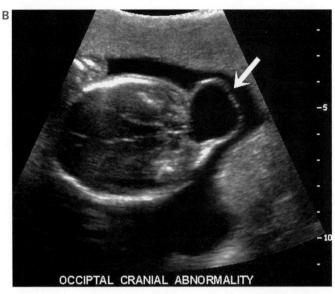

OCCIPTAL CRANIAL ABNORMALITY

Figure 10-9. A *A posterior encephalocele (arrow). Note the bony defect through which the brain tissue protrudes.* **B** *Posterior cystic encephalocele (arrow).*

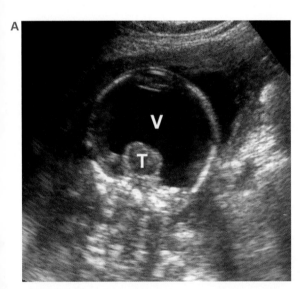

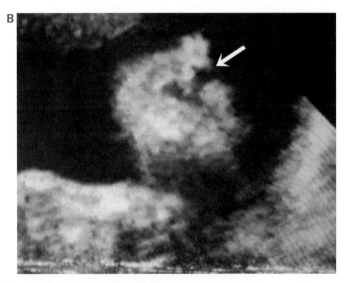

Figure 10-10. A *Fetal head showing a large horseshoe-shaped ventricle and fused thalami associated with alobar holoprosencephaly. V = ventricle, T = thalami.* **B** *Frontal view of fetal nose and mouth showing a cleft defect of the lip (arrow).*

encephaloceles with protrusion of the cerebellum into a subcutaneous sac are uncommon in the fetuses of nondiabetics (Figure 10-9). There are varying forms of holoprosencephaly, all carrying a poor prognosis. The severest form is the alobar type, resulting in one large, single, horseshoe-shaped ventricle draping over fused thalami. This anomaly is often associated with a cleft defect of the face (Figure 10-10). Holoprosencephaly is 40 times more common among diabetic pregnancies.

The lumbosacral region of the spine is of particular interest because most spinal defects occur in this area (Figure 10-11A). However, it is also important to screen for **caudal regression syndrome**, the complete or partial congenital absence of the lower spine and/or sacrum, which is often associated with genitourinary abnormalities such as renal agenesis, hypoplastic femurs, clubfeet, and muscular atrophy below the level of the spinal termination (Figures 10-11 B and C). Additionally, some

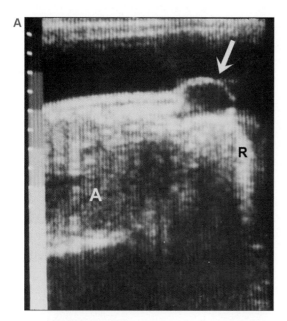

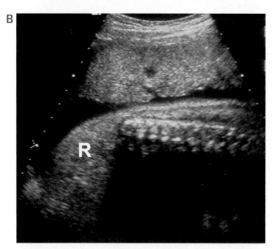

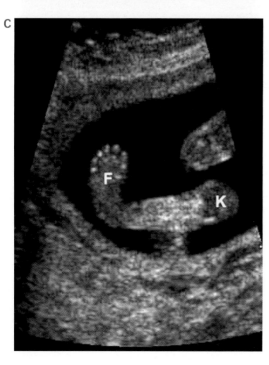

Figure 10-11. A *Longitudinal image of a fetal spine showing a meningocele (arrow). A = abdomen, R = rump.* **B** *Longitudinal image of spine showing how it abruptly ends before reaching the rump end. R = rump.* **C** *Image showing the lower leg and foot of a fetus with clubfoot. Note how the foot is turned inward. K = knee, F = foot.*

fetuses present with lower limb fusion, called **sirenomelia**, or **mermaid syndrome** (Figure 10-12). This condition is often thought to be the most specific abnormality associated with maternal diabetes, occurring 200–600 times more often in the diabetic than in the nondiabetic. The incidence among diabetic mothers is 0.2%–0.5%. See Chapter 11 for additional information on sirenomelia, or mermaid syndrome.

Another syndrome that has been associated with diabetic pregnancies is **femoral hypoplasia–unusual facies syndrome**. This involves hypoplasia of the femur and/or humerus and may include absence of the fibula. These findings can be identified sonographically if the limbs are thoroughly evaluated. The facial characteristics, however, are usually too mild to detect with ultrasound.

Cardiac Anomalies

Probably the most common anomaly seen in diabetic pregnancies, congenital heart disease is four times more common in the fetuses of diabetic patients than in those of nondiabetic patients. Of the major cardiac defects, ventricular septal defects (VSDs) are the most common (Figure 10-13). Others include atrial septal defects (ASDs), tricuspid atresia, hypoplastic left ventricle, and situs inversus (also known as situs transversus). Abnormalities of the great vessels may also be encountered, such as coarctation of the aorta, transposition of the great vessels, truncus arteriosus, and pulmonary artery atresia.

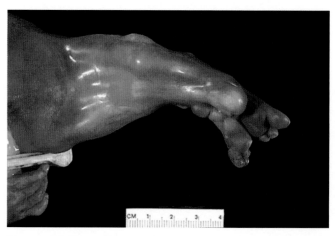

Figure 10-12. *Specimen of sirenomelia, or mermaid syndrome.*

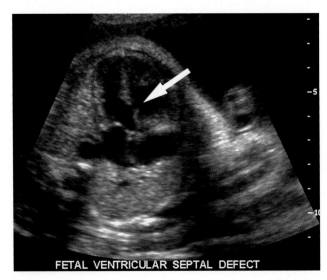

Figure 10-13. *Four-chamber view of heart shows a rather large ventricular septal defect (arrow).*

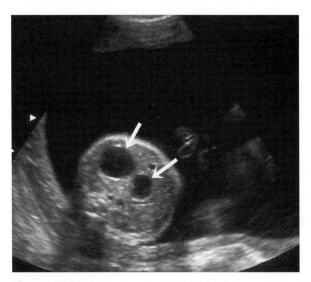

Figure 10-14. *Transverse image of a fetal abdomen demonstrating duodenal atresia. Note the classic "double bubble" (arrows) and polyhydramnios.*

Gastrointestinal Anomalies

Situs inversus, duodenal atresia, and imperforate anus are among the gastrointestinal (GI) abnormalities most frequently seen in fetuses of diabetics. The fetal stomach takes on an adult shape and position at around the 9th or 10th week of gestation. The colon is first identified toward the end of the second trimester and can easily be identified in most fetuses by 28 weeks. Dilation of any part of the fetal GI tract can usually be easily identified with sonography. Duodenal atresia will present with the classic "double bubble sign" and is readily identifiable but usually not until after 24 weeks of gestation (Figure 10-14). Other GI abnormalities that can occur in infants of diabetic mothers include small left colon syndrome and inguinal hernias; however, these are not routinely identified with ultrasound prenatally.

Genitourinary Anomalies

In the fetus of a diabetic mother the kidneys and bladder should be evaluated for function and size. The genitourinary anomalies seen in these patients include hydronephrosis (Figure 10-15A), agenesis, ureteral duplication, and multicystic dysplasia (Figure 10-15B) of the kidneys.

Fetal kidneys may not be routinely identified until 15–17 weeks of gestation, but the fetal bladder can be seen much earlier, at around 10–12 weeks. If the fetal bladder is identified, we can assume there is at least one kidney present and functioning. Kidney size can be ascertained by measuring the abdomen at the level of the kidneys in

A
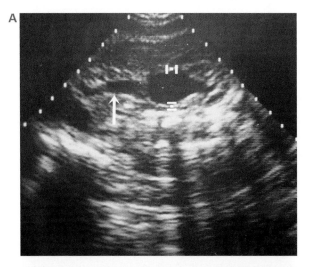

B
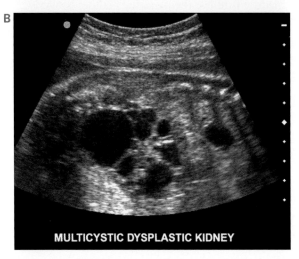

MULTICYSTIC DYSPLASTIC KIDNEY

Figure 10-15. A *Longitudinal view through a fetal kidney showing hydronephrosis (calipers) and a dilated ureter (arrow).* **B** *Long-axis view through a fetal kidney showing multicystic dysplasia. (Figure continues . . .)*

C

D

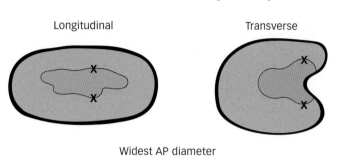

How to Measure for Fetal Hydronephrosis

Longitudinal   Transverse

Widest AP diameter

Figure 10-15, continued. C *How to measure AP or transverse fetal kidney and compare to AP or transverse measurement of the fetal abdomen. The ratio of kidney to abdomen should be 1:3.* **D** *How to measure the dilated fetal renal pelvis.*

either a transverse or AP diameter and comparing the same measurement (transverse or AP) of the kidney. The normal ratio between the two should be 1:3 (Figure 10-15C). Because the fetal kidneys are responsible for amniotic fluid production, lack of renal function causes **oligohydramnios**, a deficiency of amniotic fluid. Normal fetal bladder filling and emptying should occur every 30–60 minutes. Remember, though, that renal abnormalities affecting function must be bilateral before oligohydramnios will result.

Fetal **hydronephrosis** is determined by visualization of a dilated renal pelvis and collecting system. This can be misleading, because mild dilatation can be physiologic if the fetal bladder is full or the maternal bladder is overly distended. By measuring the AP diameter of the renal pelvis, one can differentiate physiologic from pathologic dilatation (Figure 10-15D). A fetal renal pelvis measuring more than 10 mm is considered pathologic. A 5–6 mm renal pelvis is most likely due to a physiologic cause but still warrants follow-up. Measurements of 6–8 mm would require careful follow-up to monitor for continued enlargement and possible intervention.

Patient Workup and Management

Upon the diabetic patient's first prenatal visit, a thorough medical history should be taken as well as a baseline blood workup to include the HgBA1C (glycosylated hemoglobin) test and urinalysis. At this time, an attempt

to classify the patient accurately is important in proper management. The following information should be documented:

- Progress and outcome of any/all previous pregnancies
- Baseline blood pressure
- Urinalysis and culture results
- Baseline glycosylated hemoglobin measurement (normal value < 6.5%)
- Thorough instructions on insulin dosage, diet to be followed, and home glucose monitoring

If maternal glucose levels (and therefore HgBA1C) are controlled, the perinatal outcome is good. If fluctuations in blood sugar or hyperglycemia occur in the mother, these changes will also occur in the fetus. A correlation between the mother's glucose levels and adiposity in the infant has been observed. **Ketoacidosis**, the accumulation in the blood of fat by-products called **ketones**, can occur at any time during the pregnancy and cause coma or death in utero (Table 10-2).

It is now recommended that all obstetric patients have a diabetic evaluation at no later than 24–28 weeks' gestation. The patient is given a 50-gram glucose load and the plasma glucose levels are measured one hour later. If these are abnormal, an oral **glucose tolerance test** is given. Patients showing an abnormal oral glucose tolerance test but normal fasting blood sugar levels are classified as class A diabetics. Their incidence of intrauterine fetal demise is

Table 10-2.	HgBA1C levels and malformation rates.
< 7% normal	1%
7% < 8.5%	5%
8.5% ≤ 10%	10%
> 10%	20%

no greater than that seen in nondiabetic patients and they are managed no differently, with the exception that fasting and postprandial glucose levels are measured weekly. If normal levels are exceeded, the patient is placed on human insulin and the baby will be surveyed as insulin-dependent.

Classes B–R are considered insulin-dependent. In these patients, who are at higher risk for complications, the following measures should be taken:

- Instructions to regulate diet and insulin
- Sonogram to date pregnancy and search for anomalies
- Education about pregnancy and diabetes
- Ophthalmologic evaluation

During the second trimester, a careful search for malformations is performed by obtaining a **maternal serum alpha-fetoprotein** (**MSAFP**) sample with a **maternal serum quad screen** around 16 weeks' gestation, and an ultrasound and fetal echocardiography at 18–20 weeks' gestation is recommended to rule out cardiac malformations. Other considerations to be monitored are fundal height and uterine growth, incidence of urinary tract infections, and early signs of pre-eclampsia.

Role of Sonography

Ideally, we would like to evaluate the diabetic patient at least three times during the course of the pregnancy. During the first trimester, we want to establish good dates for monitoring growth. If an early growth delay is observed, there is a 27% chance of a fetal anomaly. The second trimester sonogram is done to screen for anomalies and perform a fetal echocardiogram. Amniocentesis is reserved for suggestive ultrasound findings. The third trimester sonogram allows us to estimate fetal weight and perform a fetal biophysical profile for fetal well-being.

The basic guidelines for performing an obstetric examination should allow us to identify most of the abnormalities and complications recognizable by sonography. These require us to establish fetal lie, number, and viability; placental location and appearance; and amniotic fluid level. Observing these structures will allow us to rule out polyhydramnios, abnormal placental thickness, and fetal demise. The basic guidelines require us to image the fetal brain, heart, stomach, kidneys, bladder, and spine, all of which can be affected by maternal diabetes. The four-chamber view of the heart will rule out 50%–70% of structural cardiac abnormalities. The four basic measurements that we evaluate—biparietal diameter (BPD), head circumference (HC), abdominal circumference (AC), and FL (femur length)—will assist in determining if the fetus is growing at a normal rate, and ratios can help in determining macrosomia, growth restriction, and skeletal abnormalities such as femoral hypoplasia. Combining the various fetal measurements assists in weight estimations, which may be important in determining the course of delivery even though sonographic weight estimations tend to underestimate the LGA fetus and overestimate the small-for-gestational-age (SGA) fetus. One rule of thumb is the growth rate for AC. If the AC measurements show more than 12 mm of growth per week, one should suspect LGA. Other measurements might include humeral and femoral soft-tissue thickness to check for macrosomia. If one subtracts the BPD measurement from that of the chest diameter and the result is equal to or greater than 14 mm, LGA/macrosomia should be suspected. These fetuses will have a 3%–13% risk for shoulder dystocia.

Doppler Evaluation

Fetal Doppler sonography is beginning to play a valuable role in evaluating the high-risk or compromised pregnancy. This is particularly true in the evaluation of the fetal heart and the placenta. Color Doppler applications have assisted in detecting subtle cardiac anomalies in utero. Transvaginal color Doppler provides more detailed information about intracardiac flow. The ideal time to evaluate the fetal heart, transvaginally, is at 13–16 weeks' gestation. Utilizing color Doppler in conjunction with fetal echocardiography aids the sonographer/sonologist in making a final diagnosis relative to cardiac anomalies.

Doppler waveform analysis of fetoplacental or uteroplacental circulation is still in its infancy; however, it provides clinically useful physiologic information in managing a high-risk pregnancy. Still, fetal Doppler applications are far from conclusive. Doppler information alone should not be relied upon but should be correlated with other sonographic findings, laboratory values, and clinical information.

See Chapter 12 for more information about the clinical applications of Doppler sonography in obstetrics and gynecology.

THYROID DISEASE

After diabetes, maternal thyroid disease is the second most common endocrine disorder seen in pregnancy. **Hyperthyroidism**, or **Graves' disease**, is associated with a diffuse toxic goiter. If untreated, pregnant patients with this condition experience a stillbirth rate of 8%–15% and 25% premature deliveries. **Hypothyroidism** is associated with similar unfavorable perinatal outcomes. Untreated hypothyroidism may cause intellectual impairment of the newborn and goiter (Figure 10-16).

ADNEXAL MASSES

Adnexal masses may cause a patient to present as LGA on physical examination. The most common ovarian masses encountered during pregnancy are the **corpus luteum** and **theca-lutein cysts**, both of which are hormonally stimulated (Figure 10-17A). Ovarian masses that enlarge with pregnancy are often found behind the cervix. The corpus luteum cyst should subside by 12–16 weeks. Because they usually do not cause pain or other symptoms, **cystadenomas** and **dermoids** may be discovered incidentally and a **pedunculated fibroid** may mimic an ovarian mass (Figures 10-17 B and C). The decision to intervene surgically will depend on the

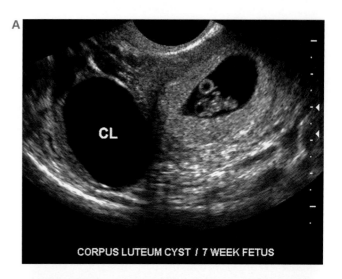

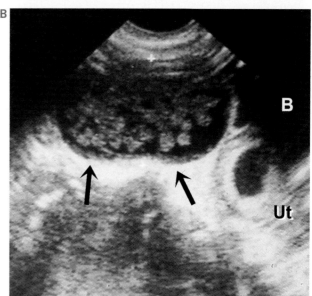

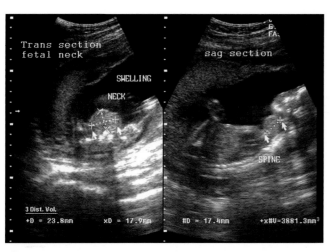

Figure 10-16. *Fetal goiter in a mother with hypothyroidism.*

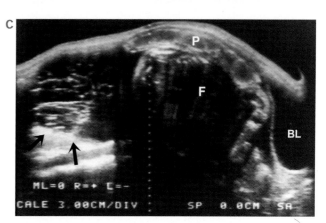

Figure 10-17. A *Image demonstrates an early intrauterine pregnancy with a normal corpus luteum cyst in the adnexa. CL = corpus luteum.* **B** *Longitudinal image through a uterus containing a first trimester pregnancy. Superior to the uterus is a large complex mass that proved to be a benign dermoid (arrows). B = bladder, Ut = uterus.* **C** *Longitudinal articulated arm scan demonstrates a late third trimester pregnancy. Note the grade III placenta anterior. Superior to the uterine fundus is a multiseptated cystadenoma (arrows). P = placenta, F = fetus, BL = maternal bladder.*

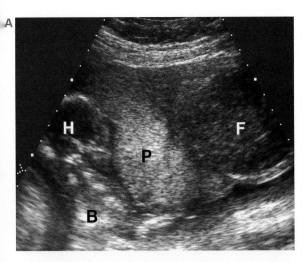

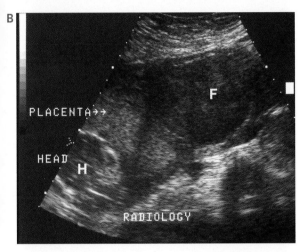

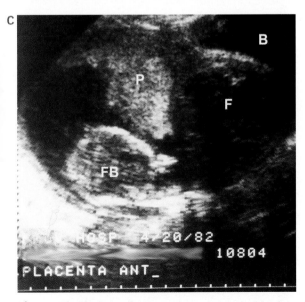

sonographic characteristics of the mass, the likelihood of torsion, symptoms, and the stage of pregnancy. Ovarian masses that have thick, irregular walls and/or septations, defined mural nodules, solid components, and ascites are worrisome for malignancy.

Adnexal masses will be displaced as the uterus enlarges with progression of the pregnancy, which may lead to torsion and thus severe pain. **Ovarian torsion** is cause for immediate surgery, because rupture can be life-threatening. Otherwise, if surgery must be considered, it is best to wait until the second trimester. The risk for spontaneous abortion is greatest in the first trimester, and surgeries performed in the third trimester may induce preterm labor.

Masses such as uterine **fibroids** may compete with the uterus for blood supply, and this can result in growth restriction of the fetus or abruption of the placenta (Figure 10-18). Generally, fibroids do not interfere with pregnancy. However, large fibroids located in the lower uterine segment may obstruct the vaginal canal and necessitate

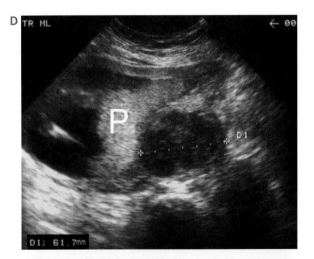

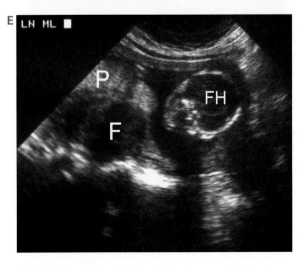

Figure 10-18. A *and* **B** *Intrauterine pregnancy with a large fibroid adjacent to the placenta. F = fibroid, P = placenta, H = fetal head, B = fetal body.* **C** *Longitudinal image through the lower uterine segment of a second trimester pregnancy. A large fibroid is seen in the cervical region. B = bladder, P = placenta, F = fibroid, FB = fetal body.* **D** *Fibroid (calipers) immediately posterior to the placenta. P = placenta.* **E** *Longitudinal view of same. P = placenta, F = fibroid, FH = fetal head.*

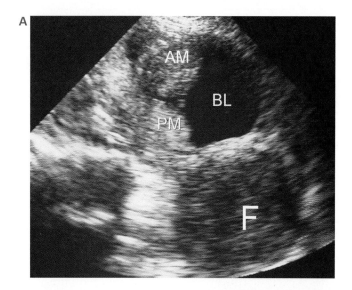

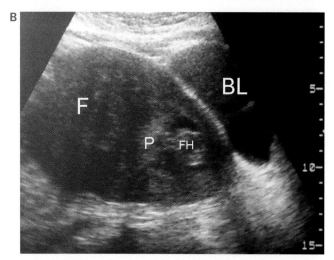

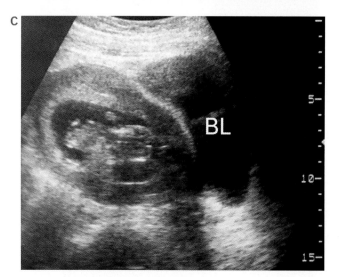

Figure 10-19. A *Large fibroid in the cervical region. Note the contracted anterior and posterior myometrium. F = fibroid, AM = anterior myometrium, PM = posterior myometrium, BL = bladder.* **B** *Longitudinal image of an early gestation crowded by multiple fibroids. F = fibroid, BL = bladder, P = placenta, FH = fetal head.* **C** *Longitudinal image shows more of the gestational sac with the fetus inside, BL = bladder.*

cesarean section for delivery (Figure 10-19A). Fibroids have been associated with first trimester spontaneous abortions and infertility as well (Figures 10-19 B and C). Since fibroid growth is influenced by estrogen, these masses have a tendency to enlarge during pregnancy. Rapid growth may result in cystic degeneration, which can also be a source of pain during pregnancy.

If a patient presents with acute abdominal pain during pregnancy, the sonographer should first rule out a hemorrhagic corpus luteum cyst, a degenerating fibroid, ovarian torsion, and, although rare, coexisting ectopic pregnancy. Maternal causes of acute abdominal pain might include urinary tract infections or obstruction, **cholecystitis**, or intestinal obstruction.

OTHER DISORDERS

During pregnancy, miscellaneous problems can arise. The association of gallstone formation and estrogen is well known and gallstones are not uncommon during pregnancy. Progesterone during pregnancy may affect the contractility of the gallbladder, causing gallbladder stasis and increasing the risk for stone formation. If a patient presents with right upper quadrant pain with or without nausea and vomiting, the gallbladder should be evaluated (Figure 10-20).

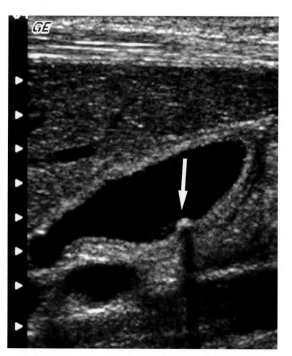

Figure 10-20. *This longitudinal image through a maternal gallbladder shows some wall thickening consistent with cholecystitis and a gallstone (arrow).*

Urinary tract disorders are also common during pregnancy. Flank pain may indicate an obstruction or infection (**pyelonephritis**). Hydronephrosis is common, occurring in approximately 80% of cases, and can begin as early as 11–15 weeks' gestation. Obstruction is the result of hormonal stimulation (progesterone) and mechanical compression of the ureters by the enlarged uterus. Progesterone has a relaxing effect on the smooth muscle of the ureters, which allows for dilation. Hydronephrosis is seen more on the right side, with a 3:1 predominance, as the uterus tends to dextrorotate against the right pelvic brim (Figure 10-21). Patients are advised to assume a left lateral

decubitus position to help relieve the compression. If the pain is severe, a ureteral stent or nephrostomy tube can provide temporary relief until the fetus can be delivered. Chronic renal disease in the mother can cause growth restriction, preterm delivery, and stillbirth.

Hyperthermia/pyrexia may cause neural tube defects, intrauterine death, abortion, or preterm labor. The **TORCH infections** can cause demise and abortion in the first trimester and growth restriction, hydrops, and fetal death in the second and third trimesters. The fetal brain may show evidence of hydrocephalus, calcification, and microcephaly. Infants who are live-born may suffer mental retardation. Parvovirus B19 and human immunodeficiency virus (HIV) can be added to the list of infections that can induce these anomalies. In mothers with HIV infection, treatment with azidothymidine (AZT) starting at 14 weeks' gestation, continuing throughout the pregnancy, and then given intravenously during labor, followed by treating the neonate for the first six weeks of life, has been documented to decrease the rate of vertical transmission from 25% to 8%.

Mothers who have epilepsy have twice the risk of having children with fetal anomalies and offspring who inherit the disorder. Women with the genetic disorder phenylketonuria (PKU) are at increased risk for spontaneous abortion and of having children with microcephaly and mental retardation. PKU is a recessive inherited metabolic disorder. Patients are usually blonde and blue-eyed with defective pigmentation. They have a hypersensitivity to light and are prone to eczema. If untreated, patients develop mental retardation, tremors, poor muscle coordination, excessive sweating, and sometimes convulsions.

SCANNING TIPS, GUIDELINES, AND PITFALLS

1. When a patient is in her third trimester of pregnancy, it can be difficult to evaluate the upper abdomen while she is lying supine. The enlarged uterus pushes everything superiorly, including bowel. If one needs to evaluate the gallbladder and pancreatic head region, it is sometimes helpful to scan these patients in the upright position. All the organs will drop slightly when the patient is standing, making sonographic access somewhat easier.

2. Elevating the patient's head will help take some pressure off the IVC and inhibit the onset of supine hypotensive syndrome.

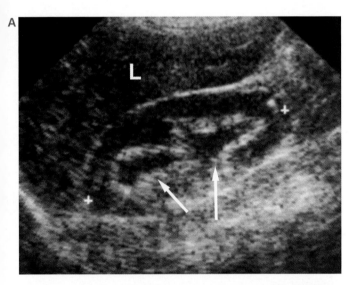

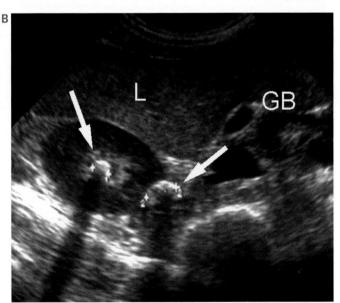

Figure 10-21. A *This longitudinal right kidney (calipers) shows hydronephrosis (arrows). L = liver.* **B** *Transverse maternal kidney in a patient with renal stones. One is shown in the renal pelvis region and another at the ureteropelvic junction (arrows). L = liver, GB = gallbladder.*

3. If a patient cannot lie on her back because of supine hypotensive syndrome, it is possible to perform some imaging with the patient in the decubitus position.

4. Patient body habitus and fetal position can affect one's ability to demonstrate fetal anatomy. If certain fetal parts/organs are not readily seen, make a technical note that the anatomy was not well demonstrated. When available, harmonics can assist in better visualization.

5. If a patient has a chronic maternal disorder, it is important to check medications that the patient might have taken or may be taking during pregnancy, because some are known to cause fetal anomalies. See Table 44 in Appendix A.

6. Abdominal or pelvic pain during the first trimester is often related to round ligament pain. As the uterus expands, it pulls on the ligament, causing a sharp or dull crampy sensation. These patients may present clinically as possibly having ectopic pregnancy or torsed ovary, both of which are considered surgical emergencies. Other causes of pain include a degenerating fibroid or a hemorrhagic corpus luteum cyst.

REFERENCES

Alvarez M, Chitkara U, Wein R, et al: Ultrasonic evaluation of the fetal heart in diabetic pregnancy. J Ultrasound Medicine S218, 1988.

Callen PW (ed): *Ultrasonography in Obstetrics and Gynecology*, 5th Edition. Philadelphia, Saunders Elsevier, 2008.

Carroll B: Duplex Doppler in obstetrical ultrasound. The Radiological Clinics of North America 25:15–20, 1990.

Chervenak FA, Isaacson GC, Campbell S: *Ultrasound in Obstetrics and Gynecology*, Volumes 1 and 2. Boston, Little Brown, 1993.

Ciccone V, Rouse G, De Lange M: Sonographic evaluation of fetal structural anomalies associated with maternal diabetes mellitus. JDMS 1:15–20, 1992.

DiSalvo DN: Sonographic imaging of maternal complications of pregnancy. J Ultrasound Med 22:69–89, 2003.

Doubilet PM, Benson CB: Fetal growth disturbances. In Miller WT (ed): *Seminars in Roentgenology*. Philadelphia, Saunders, 1990, pp 313–315.

Gabbe SG: Diabetes mellitus: ways of individualizing care. Contemporary OB/GYN, 1990, pp 68–77.

Levine D: Fetal hydrops. In Rumack CM, Wilson SR, Charboneau JW, et al (eds): *Diagnostic Ultrasound*, 4th Edition. St. Louis, Elsevier Mosby, 2011, pp 1424–1454.

McGahan JP, Porto M: *Diagnostic Obstetrical Ultrasound*. Philadelphia, Lippincott, 1994.

Merlob P, Reisner SH: Fetal effects from maternal diabetes. In Buyse M (ed): *Birth Defects Encyclopedia*. Cambridge, Blackwell, 1990, pp 700–702.

Mitchell C, Trampe B: Sonography and high-risk pregnancy. In Hagen-Ansert SL (ed): *Textbook of Diagnostic Sonography*, 7th Edition. St. Louis, Elsevier, 2012, pp 1176–1179.

Nyberg DA: Intra-abdominal abnormalities. In Nyberg DA, Mahony BS, Pretorius DH (eds): *Diagnostic Ultrasound of Fetal Anomalies: Text and Atlas*. Chicago, Year Book, 1990, pp 342–394.

Todros T, Merrigi E, Catella G: Growth of fetuses of diabetic mothers. J Clin Ultrasound 17:333, 1989.

SELF-ASSESSMENT EXERCISES

Questions

1. Diabetes primarily affects the metabolism of:
   A. Bilirubin
   B. Protein
   C. Carbohydrates
   D. Cholesterol
   E. Salts

2. Diabetic pregnancies often produce fetuses that are large for gestational age. This growth asymmetry is usually recognized at:
   A. 16–20 weeks
   B. 20–24 weeks
   C. 24–28 weeks
   D. 28–32 weeks
   E. 34–36 weeks

3. The placenta of a gestational diabetic is often edematous. The maximum placental thickness at term should not exceed:

   A. 2–3 cm

   B. 3–4 cm

   C. 4–5 cm

   D. 5–6 cm

   E. 7–8 cm

4. The insulin-dependent diabetic mother is at risk for having all of the following *except*:

   A. Monozygotic multiple gestations

   B. Intrauterine growth restriction

   C. Intrauterine fetal demise

   D. Congenital fetal anomalies

   E. Fetal hydrops

5. Of the following, which laboratory test will determine maternal glycemic control?

   A. Beta hCG

   B. SMA-12

   C. CEA

   D. HgBA1C

   E. MSAFP

6. A diabetic evaluation is recommended for all obstetric patients between:

   A. 16 and 20 weeks

   B. 20 and 24 weeks

   C. 24 and 28 weeks

   D. 28 and 32 weeks

   E. 34 and 36 weeks

7. The fetal anomaly most specifically associated with diabetes mellitus is:

   A. Femoral hypoplasia–unusual facies syndrome

   B. Caudal regression syndrome

   C. Prune belly syndrome

   D. Amniotic band syndrome

   E. Potter syndrome

8. Of the following, which diabetic patient would be at most risk for producing severe fetal anomalies?

   A. Gestational diabetic

   B. Type 1 diabetic

   C. Type 2 diabetic

   D. Class A diabetic

   E. Borderline diabetic

9. Of the following, which is *not* a common maternal complication of diabetes?

   A. Pregnancy-induced hypertension

   B. Postpartum hemorrhage

   C. Urinary tract infections

   D. Hyperemesis gravidarum

   E. Large for gestational age

10. Of the following statements, which is *not* true of color Doppler and waveform analysis in the diabetic patient?

    A. It is beginning to play a valuable role in evaluating high-risk pregnancies.

    B. It can provide conclusive evidence of the "at risk" pregnancy.

    C. It is extremely helpful in assisting with the diagnosis of heart defects.

    D. It aids in the physiologic evaluation of placental circulation.

    E. It can assist with evaluating fetal well-being.

11. Of the following, which is *not* a cause of nonimmune hydrops?

    A. Rubella

    B. Twin-to-twin transfusion

    C. Placental anomalies

    D. Fetal pulmonary disorders

    E. Rh isoimmunization

12. The hormone(s) responsible for gallstone formation during pregnancy is/are:

    A. Progesterone

    B. Estrogen

    C. Testosterone

    D. A and B

    E. B and C

13. Hyperemesis gravidarum is *not* associated with:

    A. Ectopic pregnancies

    B. Molar pregnancies

    C. Fertility assistance

    D. Multiple gestations

    E. Chorioadenoma destruens

14. If a patient presents with supine hypotensive syndrome, one should:

    A. Call the referring clinician immediately.

    B. Administer insulin and monitor blood pressure.

    C. Send the patient to the emergency room.

    D. Roll her into a left lateral decubitus position.

    E. Perform a targeted scan to rule out anomalies.

15. HELLP syndrome is a severe complication associated with:

    A. Pregnancy-induced hypertension

    B. Rh isoimmunization

    C. Maternal gallbladder disease

    D. Fetal anemia

    E. Supine hypotensive syndrome

16. Which hormone causes the maternal ureter to relax, contributing to hydronephrosis during pregnancy?

    A. Estrogen

    B. Progesterone

    C. Human choriogonadotropin

    D. Glycosylated hemoglobin

    E. Alpha-fetoprotein

17. Of the following, which would *not* be a cause of acute pain during pregnancy?

    A. Cholecystitis

    B. Degenerating fibroid

    C. Cystadenoma

    D. Ovarian torsion

    E. Urinary tract infections

18. Of the following, which is a cause of immune hydrops?

    A. Diabetes

    B. Rhesus (Rh) incompatibility

    C. Twin-to-twin transfusion

    D. Pregnancy-induced hypertension

    E. TORCH infections

19. Which of the following is a rare, lethal type of hydrops seen in patients of Asian descent?

    A. Alpha thalassemia

    B. Hemochromatosis

    C. Pernicious anemia

    D. Hyperalbuminemia

    E. Reticuloendotheliosis

20. Maternal blood pressure is considered elevated if it is:

    A. 110/60 mmHg

    B. 120/80 mmHg

    C. Over 120/80 mmHg

    D. Under 140/90 mmHg

    E. Over 140/90 mmHg

Answers

See Appendix F on page 615 for answers and explanations.

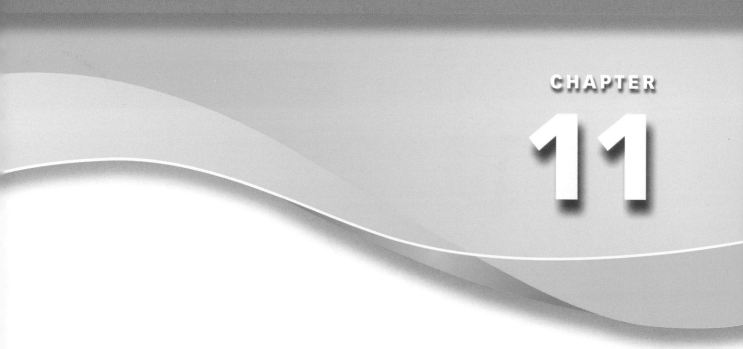

CHAPTER

11

Fetal Syndromes

Kathryn A. Gill, MS, RT, RDMS, FSDMS

OBJECTIVES

After completing this chapter you should be able to:

1. Define the term *syndrome* and list the more common syndromes identifiable by sonography.
2. Discuss maternal and paternal risk factors for producing a chromosomally abnormal fetus.
3. List the most common biochemical markers used to screen for genetic and chromosomal abnormalities.
4. Describe other tests utilized in genetic screening.
5. Explain how nuchal translucency is used as a screening parameter for chromosomal abnormalities.
6. Describe the sonographic findings associated with chromosomal abnormalities.

BETWEEN 3% AND 4% OF ALL NEWBORNS will have some type of defect, ranging from a simple birthmark to more serious anomalies that may require intervention. Of those born with a defect, 1% will have anomalies that cannot be corrected, and those usually involve the brain/central nervous system, face, and/or heart. Several fetal anomalies have been described in earlier chapters. These anomalies may occur as isolated defects or a fetus may present with multiple anomalies. This chapter focuses on pregnancies in which multiple fetal anomalies are present in a single fetus. When this occurs, there is a high likelihood that the fetus has a syndrome. The discussion is limited to those syndromes most commonly observed in radiology departments and private practices involved in obstetric care.

As defined in the *Encyclopedia and Dictionary of Medicine, Nursing, and Allied Health*, a **syndrome** is a "combination of symptoms resulting from a single cause or so commonly occurring together as to constitute a distinct clinical picture" (Figure 11-1). A **disorder** can be categorized as chromosomal, Mendelian (single-gene), teratogenic (environmental), or multifactorial (see Box 11-1). It is estimated that at least 10%–15% of all pregnancies are chromosomally abnormal, and chromosomal abnormalities are the most common cause of first trimester pregnancy loss. **Mendelian** or single-gene disorders are inherited as either **autosomal dominant** or **autosomal recessive** and include X-linked disorders, which are also recessive. Recessive disorders tend to be severer and are often fatal. Autosomal recessive disorders are transmitted if both parents carry the same recessive gene. The parents are not affected, but their offspring have an increased risk of 25%. With autosomal dominant disorders, one affected parent passes the disorder to 50% of his or her offspring. Symptoms may not present until well into adulthood, and the severity of the disease can vary significantly within the same family.

Figure 11-1. *Examples of syndromes:* **A** *Infant demonstrating multiple congenital anomalies, including an encephalocele, micro-cephaly, clinodactyly, clubfoot, and ambiguous sex.* **B** *Postmortem x-ray of a fetus demonstrating severe scoliosis, omphalocele, syn-dactyly, cleft defect of the face, and abnormal lower limb posture.*

A
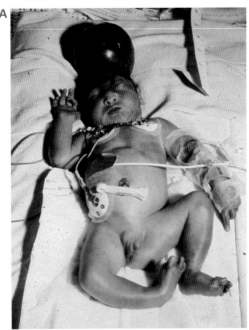

B
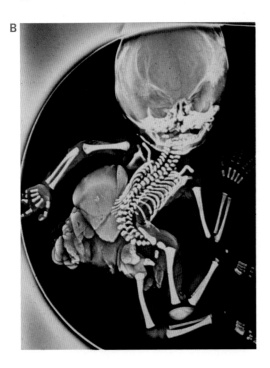

Box 11-1.	Types of disorders.
Chromosomal	
Mendelian	
Teratogenic	
Multifactorial	

Box 11-2.	Classifications for fetal defects.
Deformations	
Malformations	
Disruptions	

Table 11-1.   Chromosomally abnormal births by number of anomalies.

Number of Anomalies	% Chromosomally Abnormal
1	14
2	29
3	48
4	62
5–6	70
7	82
8	92

cause would be related to dysfunction of the kidneys, as seen with bilateral renal agenesis. A **malformation** occurs when the normal developmental process is altered, as happens with chromosomal abnormalities. **Disruptions** occur when something extrinsic affects the normal developmental process, such as synechiae or amniotic bands that cause amputations and deformities or hydranencephaly resulting from a vascular accident (Box 11-2).

The basic guidelines for obstetric scanning, if followed, allow us to identify many major fetal abnormalities. It is important to scan thoroughly and, if an abnormality is defined, to look for a second. Two or more anomalies associated with a single gestation increase the likelihood of a syndrome (Table 11-1).

Specific fetal defects themselves are further classified as deformations, malformations, and disruptions. **Deformations** are the result of mechanical forces that alter form, position, or shape. The deforming forces can be **intrinsic** or **extrinsic**. Oligohydramnios is infamous for causing deformations. An extrinsic cause would include premature rupture of membranes (PROM), while an intrinsic

Table 11-2.	Age risk in females for chromosomal abnormalities.

Age (Years)	Pregnancies Affected
35	1 in 250
40	1 in 55
45	1 in 14

Box 11-3.	Genetic diseases by population at risk.

African Americans: sickle cell anemia

Asian Americans: thalassemia

Ashkenazic Jews: Tay-Sachs and Canavan disease

Caucasians: cystic fibrosis

Males: hemophilia (rare in females)

Mediterranneans: thalassemia

RISK FACTORS

Advanced Maternal and Paternal Age

Mothers of **advanced maternal age** (**AMA**) are considered to be those 35 years of age or older at delivery. It is well documented that these patients are significantly more likely than younger mothers to give birth to infants with chromosomal abnormalities. These abnormalities are thought to be due to the incorrect separation of the chromosomes within the aged ova (Table 11-2). Although controversial, some studies have suggested an increase in chromosomal abnormalities with an increase in paternal age, but men do not seem to be affected until after age 55.

History of Chromosomal Abnormality

Some anomalies have a predisposition for recurrence, such as those associated with maternal metabolic disorders, while genetic disorders may be dictated by whether the parents are affected or are carriers. Family history is important in determining risk factors. Ethnicity may also play a role. African Americans have a higher incidence of sickle cell anemia, Caucasians of cystic fibrosis, Asians and those of Mediterranean descent of thalassemia, and Ashkenazic Jews of Tay-Sachs and **Canavan disease** (Box 11-3).

Teratogen Exposure

Organogenesis of the major organ systems occurs in the first eight weeks, with the most critical period being between the 15th and the 60th days of development. The **intraembryonic mesoderm**, the middle layer of the three fetal germ layers, which forms during this time, is the source of all connective tissues, including bone, cartilage,

Box 11-4.	Common teratogens.*

Alcohol

Androgenic agents

Antibiotics

Acutane

*For a complete list of teratogens, see Table 44 in Appendix A.

muscle, blood and blood vessels, lymphatics, lymphoid organs, pleura, pericardium, peritoneum, kidneys, and gonads. During this time, exposure to **teratogens**, or defect-causing agents, can cause serious malformations (Box 11-4). Six mechanisms of congenital malformations are associated with teratogens:

- Too little growth
- Too little resorption
- Too much resorption
- Resorption in the wrong place
- Normal growth in abnormal positions
- Local overgrowth of a tissue or structure

Teratogens include drugs (see Table 44 in Appendix A), chemicals, infections, by-products of maternal metabolic diseases, and ionizing radiation.

Multifactorial Risks

In some cases it is determined that anomalies are the result of multiple factors. In genetics, this is usually defined as arising from the interaction of several genes. When there are genetic factors and exposure to teratogens, the outcome can be quite severe.

BIOCHEMICAL MARKERS FOR GENETIC SCREENING

Alpha-Fetoprotein

Alpha-fetoprotein (**AFP**) is a plasma protein produced by the yolk sac and fetal liver and is best evaluated by measuring its presence in maternal serum between 16 and 18 weeks of gestation. It is expelled into the amniotic fluid and, through diffusion across the placenta, seeps into the maternal bloodstream. In 1972 Scottish scientists first reported that elevated AFP levels in amniotic fluid were associated with open neural tube defects, and shortly thereafter the same findings were confirmed for maternal serum AFP (MSAFP). An open structural fetal defect will allow abnormal amounts of AFP to spill into the amniotic fluid, causing an elevation. Other conditions associated with elevated AFP include fetal demise, placental abnormalities, bleeding, triploidy, renal disorders, sacrococcygeal teratomas, congenital cystic adenomatoid malformations (CCAMs), cystic hygromas, and congenital skin disorders. In patients with unexplained elevated MSAFP levels, the risk for fetal demise is increased from the time of testing to term, and the higher the level the greater the risk. In fetuses, the AFP concentration is very high, and because of the concentration gradient between fetus and mother even minimal placental compromise can result in an elevated MSAFP. **Congenital nephrosis**, an autosomal recessive disorder that necessitates a neonatal kidney transplant if the infant is to survive, is associated with extremely high levels of MSAFP. This condition is more common among Finnish populations. If the MSAFP and amniotic fluid AFP are elevated when the sonogram and acetylcholinesterase are normal, congenital nephrosis should be considered. In the 1980s, it was discovered that fetuses with Down syndrome exhibited abnormally low MSAFP levels.

Several variables affect AFP levels in maternal blood:

- Weight
- Race/ethnicity
- Gestational age
- Number of fetuses

Drawing a sample too early may result in false or unreliable readings. The most common cause of abnormal AFP levels is incorrect estimation of gestational age. If there is more than one fetus producing AFP, the maternal serum levels will naturally be higher than those for mothers of singletons. Obese patients have lower levels, while African American and Asian patients have slightly higher levels when compared to patients of other ethnicities. Diabetes can also be a cause of lower levels.

Another enzyme that can be extracted and analyzed in the amniotic fluid is **acetylcholinesterase** (**AChE**), an enzyme found in the central nervous system, muscle, and red blood cells. It catalyzes the hydrolysis of acetylcholine to choline and acetic acid. The acetic acid ester of choline is normally present in many parts of the body and has important physiologic functions. It is a neurotransmitter at cholinergic synapses in the central, sympathetic, and parasympathetic nervous systems. When elevated, AChE is associated with neural tube defects.

Human Chorionic Gonadotropin and Unconjugated Estriol

Human chorionic gonadotropin (hCG) is elevated (200%) in cases of Down syndrome, while **unconjugated estriol** (**uE3**) is significantly decreased (25%). Both are produced by the placenta. The **triple marker screening**, which tests for chromosomal anomalies by measuring hCG, estriol, and AFP levels, increases the chance for detecting Down syndrome by almost 90%. The triple screen is also helpful in identifying pregnancies affected by trisomy 18 because all three levels will be lower than normal. Low estriol levels can also be associated with anencephaly, presumably due to the absence, failure, or aplasia of the adrenal glands.

Other Testing Techniques for Genetic Screening

Amniocentesis

An **amniocentesis** is performed by inserting a long needle into the amniotic sac and withdrawing amniotic fluid, which contains cells shed by the fetus. These cells contain genetic information about the fetus and can identify those with disorders such as cystic fibrosis, sickle cell anemia, hemophilia A, **Duchenne muscular dystrophy**, Tay-Sachs disease, thalassemia, and polycystic kidney disease. The procedure can be performed as early as 13 weeks' gestation but is usually performed at around 16–18 weeks. Several studies have shown that performance of the procedure prior to 16 weeks increases the risk for pregnancy loss and limb defects. Amniocentesis can also indicate those fetuses with possible open neural tube and abdominal wall defects.

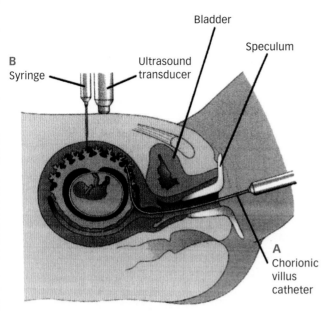

Figure 11-2. *Techniques for chorionic villus sampling.* **A** *Transcervical technique.* **B** *Transabdominal technique. Used with permission from Moore KL, Persaud TVN:* The Developing Human: Clinically Oriented Embryology, *8th Edition. Philadelphia, Saunders Elsevier, 2008, p 106.*

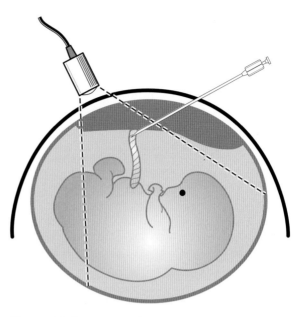

Figure 11-3. *Proper site for needle aspiration of umbilical vein.*

Chorionic Villus Sampling

Chorionic villus sampling (**CVS**) is a procedure that samples the placental tissue and is performed in the first trimester, usually between the 10th and 12th weeks of gestation. The most common technique is to insert a catheter through the maternal cervix (Figure 11-2). The trophoblastic cells are aspirated through a syringe. Although CVS can provide information about chromosomal and genetic disorders, it cannot detect defects such as neural tube disorders. Risks associated with the procedure include induced abortion and fetal limb abnormalities due to vascular compromise.

Percutaneous Umbilical Blood Sampling

Percutaneous umbilical blood sampling (**PUBS**), also known as **cordocentesis** or **fetal blood sampling**, allows for direct vascular access to the fetus. A fine-gauge needle is inserted into the fetal umbilical vein. This procedure can be performed for diagnostic as well as therapeutic purposes. Most clinicians use a 20- to 22-gauge spinal needle, inserting it near the cord insertion at the placenta (Figure 11-3). Other insertion sites can be used—into the fetal abdomen, for example, through a free loop of cord or even intracardiacally—but the cord will be stabler if one can localize a site approximately 1 cm from insertion into the placenta. Indications for performing PUBS include rapid karyotyping, confirming fetal infections,

confirming a cause for nonimmune hydrops, treating fetal arrhythmias, and performing fetal blood transfusions, to mention only a few. See Chapter 15 for additional information on amniocentesis, CVS, and PUBS.

FACIAL DEFORMITIES

The fetal face can offer a lot of information related to anomalies (Table 11-3). The eyes, nose, mouth, and ears are often affected, especially in chromosomally abnormal fetuses. Although several anomalies of the face can be identified with sonography, we see them only if the fetus presents them to us by settling into a cooperative position. The eyes begin development on the lateral aspects

Table 11-3.	Facial abnormalities.
Anophthalmia	Absence of one or both eyes
Microphthalmia	Abnormally small eyes
Hypertelorism	Eyes too far apart
Hypotelorism	Eyes too close together
Cyclopia	Single central eye/orbit
Clefts	Fusion abnormality creating a defect in lip/palate
Macroglossia	Abnormally large tongue that protrudes from open mouth
Micrognathia	Abnormally small mandible, recessed chin

of the face and migrate medially. The structures that form the nose migrate from a supralateral position to an inframedial position. The nose begins as two widely spaced structures above the level of the orbits that then migrate medially and inferiorly, fusing below the orbits in the normal midline position. Forebrain development and cleavage are related closely to development of the facial structures, so disruption in the process for one is often associated with a malformation of another.

Eyes

When evaluating the orbits, one should assess the individual orbital diameters, the interocular (inner orbital) distance (the distance between the orbits as measured from the inside edge of each orbit), and the binocular (outer orbital) distance (the distance from the lateral edge of one orbit to the lateral edge of the contralateral orbit). Charts have been published and can be used to estimate gestational age when fetal position precludes adequate imaging

Table 11-4.	Predicted biparietal diameter (BPD) and weeks' gestation from the inner (IOD) and outer (OOD) orbital distances.						
BPD (cm)	Gestation (wk)	IOD (cm)	OOD (cm)	BPD (cm)	Gestation (wk)	IOD (cm)	OOD (cm)
1.9	11.6	0.5	1.3	5.8	24.3	1.6	4.1
2.0	11.6	0.5	1.4	5.9	24.3	1.6	4.2
2.1	12.1	0.6	1.5	6.0	24.7	1.6	4.3
2.2	12.6	0.6	1.6	6.1	25.2	1.6	4.3
2.3	12.6	0.6	1.7	6.2	25.2	1.6	4.4
2.4	13.1	0.7	1.7	6.3	25.7	1.7	4.4
2.5	13.6	0.7	1.8	6.4	26.2	1.7	4.5
2.6	13.6	0.7	1.9	6.5	26.2	1.7	4.5
2.7	14.1	0.8	2.0	6.6	26.7	1.7	4.6
2.8	14.6	0.8	2.1	6.7	27.2	1.7	4.6
2.9	14.6	0.8	2.1	6.8	27.6	1.7	4.7
3.0	15.0	0.9	2.2	6.9	28.1	1.7	4.7
3.1	15.5	0.9	2.3	7.0	28.6	1.8	4.8
3.2	15.5	0.9	2.4	7.1	29.1	1.8	4.8
3.3	16.0	1.0	2.5	7.3	29.6	1.8	4.9
3.4	16.5	1.0	2.5	7.4	30.0	1.8	5.0
3.5	16.5	1.0	2.6	7.5	30.6	1.8	5.0
3.6	17.0	1.0	2.7	7.6	31.0	1.8	5.1
3.7	17.5	1.1	2.7	7.7	31.5	1.8	5.1
3.8	17.9	1.1	2.8	7.8	32.0	1.8	5.2
4.0	18.4	1.2	3.0	7.9	32.5	1.9	5.2
4.2	18.9	1.2	3.1	8.0	33.0	1.9	5.3
4.3	19.4	1.2	3.2	8.2	33.5	1.9	5.4
4.4	19.4	1.3	3.2	8.3	34.0	1.9	5.4
4.5	19.9	1.3	3.3	8.4	34.4	1.9	5.4
4.6	20.4	1.3	3.4	8.5	35.0	1.9	5.5
4.7	20.4	1.3	3.4	8.6	35.4	1.9	5.5
4.8	20.9	1.4	3.5	8.8	35.9	1.9	5.6
4.9	21.3	1.4	3.6	8.9	36.4	1.9	5.6
5.0	21.3	1.4	3.6	9.0	36.9	1.9	5.7
5.1	21.8	1.4	3.7	9.1	37.3	1.9	5.7
5.2	22.3	1.4	3.8	9.2	37.8	1.9	5.8
5.3	22.3	1.5	3.8	9.3	38.3	1.9	5.8
5.4	22.8	1.5	3.9	9.4	38.8	1.9	5.8
5.5	23.3	1.5	4.0	9.6	39.3	1.9	5.9
5.6	23.3	1.5	4.0	9.7	39.8	1.9	5.9
5.7	23.8	1.5	4.1				

Reprinted with permission from Mayden KL, Tortora M, Berkowitz RL, et al: Orbital diameters: a new parameter for prenatal diagnosis and dating. Am J Obstet Gynecol 144:289, 1982.

of the fetal head and brain anatomy (Table 11-4). By observing the spacing between the eyes, the practitioner can identify several facial anomalies or suspect features.

Hypotelorism

The condition of orbits spaced too close together is called **hypotelorism**. The space between the eyes should be the same distance as the ocular diameter, and both orbits should have the same measurement. Severe hypotelorism may be classified as **cyclopia**—a single central orbit. There is some variability in how these present. There can be two globes within a single large orbit, or the two orbits may simply be very close together, a condition called **ethmocephaly**. Hypotelorism/cyclopia may also be associated with a **proboscis**, a fleshy appendage that projects from the forehead. Holoprosencephaly is the most common condition associated with hypotelorism. **Cebocephaly** is a trunklike nasal structure with a single nostril (Figures 11-4 A and B).

Hypertelorism

The condition of orbits spaced too far apart is called **hypertelorism**. This can result from an abnormality in migration resulting in a midline or median cleft or, more commonly, from a mass. Although anterior encephaloceles are the least common type of fetal mass, they are considered the most common cause of hypertelorism (Figure 11-4C).

Microphthalmia/Anophthalmia

The condition leading to orbits that are too small is called **microphthalmia**. This condition can be unilateral or bilateral and is associated with a number of syndromes. Fetal alcohol syndrome is one of the more common. **Anophthalmia** is the congenital absence of the eyes and, without 3D/4D assistance, can be difficult to diagnose sonographically.

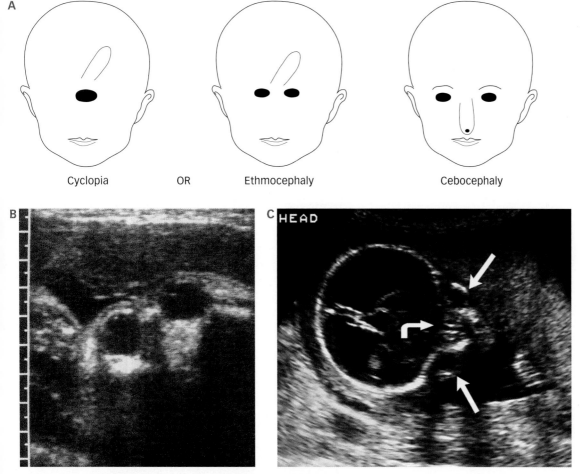

Figure 11-4. A Schematics of cyclopia, ethmocephaly, and cebocephaly. **B** Hypotelorism. Note that the orbits are too close together. Used with permission from De Lange M, Rouse GA: Ob/Gyn Sonography: An Illustrated Review. Pasadena, CA, Davies Publishing, 2004. **C** View of fetal orbits (straight arrows) showing hypertelorism. Note that the space between the orbits (curved arrow) is wider than the ocular diameters.

Facial Clefts

Cleft lip/cleft palate is considered an entity separate from the isolated cleft palate, median cleft lip syndrome, and the midline cleft associated with holoprosencephaly, all of which are different (Figures 11-5 A and B). When the maxillary processes and medial nasal process do not migrate and fuse normally, the cleft lip and palate occur. This is considered the most common congenital facial anomaly. Cleft defects can also be the result of an amniotic band. A lateral cleft lip can be unilateral or bilateral as well as isolated, with no hard palate defect. There seems to be some racial predisposition, with the highest incidence among Native Americans (3.6/1000 births), followed by Asians (1.5–2/1000), Caucasians (1/1000), and African Americans (0.3/1000). It is also more common in males. Recurrence rates increase if the mother had a cleft lip/palate and decrease if the father is affected. If parents are unaffected but siblings are, the risks increase with the number of affected siblings. Although a common anom-

aly, cleft lip and palate is often missed on sonographic examination, since evaluation of the fetal face is not part of the standard protocol.

If a fetus has an isolated cleft hard palate but a normal lip, it is unlikely that the defect will be readily identified because it is the lip defect that is most apparent sonographically. Nevertheless, 3D and 4D applications have improved our diagnostic capabilities, making it possible to reconstruct and view the anatomy from different angles (Figure 11-5C).

Micrognathia

A small mouth with recessed chin is called **micrognathia** and is the result of a small mandible. The associated polyhydramnios is thought to be secondary to a small oropharynx, which is obstructed by the tongue. This condition can be subtle and difficult to appreciate in some fetuses (Figure 11-6).

Macroglossia

An abnormally large, thick tongue is referred to as **macroglossia**. This defect can be associated with a number of syndromes, such as Beckwith-Wiedemann syndrome. The tongue persistently protrudes from the mouth (Figure 11-7). See the section on Beckwith-Wiedemann syndrome below.

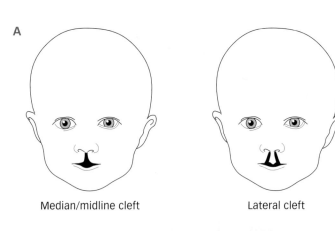

A

Median/midline cleft   Lateral cleft

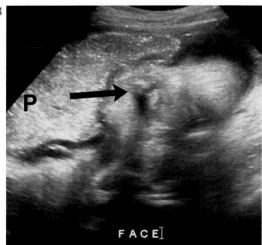

B

FACE

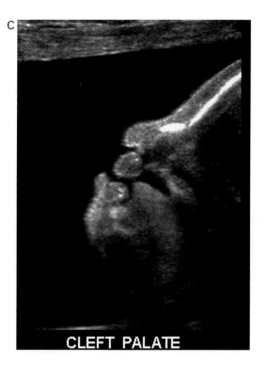

C

CLEFT PALATE

Figure 11-5. A *Schematics showing median (left) versus lateral cleft defects of the face.* **B** *Frontal view of fetal face showing cleft lip (arrow). P = placenta.* **C** *Profile of a fetus with a cleft lip/palate.*

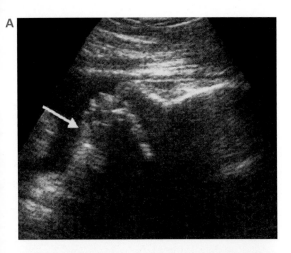

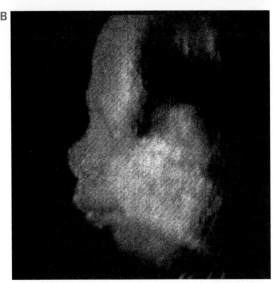

Figure 11-6. *Sonograms of fetuses with micrognathia:* **A** *2D. The arrow is pointing to the markedly recessed chin.* **B** *3D. Used with permission from De Lange M, Rouse GA: Ob/Gyn Sonography: An Illustrated Review. Pasadena, CA, Davies Publishing, 2004.*

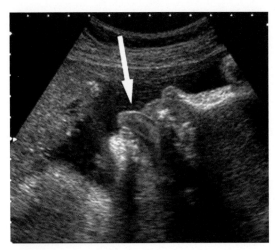

Figure 11-7. *Profile view of the fetal face showing macroglossia. The tongue (arrow) is seen protruding out of the mouth.*

Ears

Ears are not routinely imaged but can offer information regarding abnormalities. Low-set and/or deformed ears are often associated with chromosomal abnormalities, including trisomies 13, 18, and 21. Ears that look large and floppy or Yoda-like warrant further investigation (Figure 11-8).

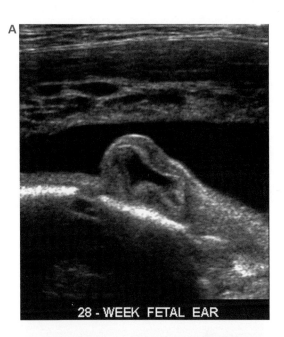

28 - WEEK FETAL EAR

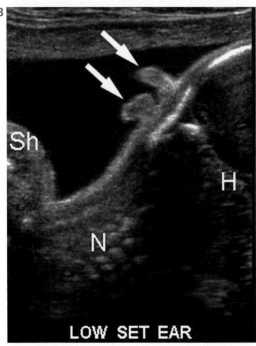

LOW SET EAR

Fig. 11-8. A *Sagittal view of a normal fetal ear.* **B** *Malformed fetal ears such as these (arrows) may be mistaken for encephaloceles or proboscises if the practitioner is not clear on orientation. Sh = shoulder, N = neck, H = head.*

ECHOGENIC BOWEL

Echogenic bowel usually refers to the central small-bowel patterns presenting as brightly white, having the same echogenicity as bone. This finding has been associated with a number of conditions, including cystic fibrosis, intrauterine infection, intra-amniotic bleeding, and chromosomal disorders. If echogenic bowel is seen in the absence of the fetal gallbladder, cystic fibrosis should be considered. Echogenic bowel in association with other anomalies is suggestive of chromosomal disorders such as trisomies 13, 18, and 21. If the patient has had a recent amniocentesis or episode of bleeding, the fetus will have swallowed bloody amniotic fluid, which can make the bowel more

echogenic. Finally, echogenic bowel has been seen in 18% of fetuses with growth restriction, and the finding has been associated with fetal demise (Figure 11-9).

HAND AND FOOT DEFORMITIES

Hand and foot deformities are frequently associated with chromosomal abnormalities, especially aneuploidy. For this reason, it is important to document any unusual observations related to them and then to look further for additional anomalies. If you see two or more anomalies in the same fetus, there is a high likelihood that you are dealing with a syndrome. See Table 11-5.

Clinodactyly and Camptodactyly

Clinodactyly is the overlapping of the digits. Up to 18% of normal fetuses will show mild clinodactyly, but 60% of fetuses with trisomy 21 (Down syndrome) and 50% with trisomy 18 (Edwards syndrome) will have it (Figure 11-10), and it will be most pronounced with Edwards syndrome. **Camptodactyly** is the permanent flexion of a finger.

Polydactyly

The presence of extra digits on the hands or feet is called **polydactyly**. Most cases are isolated findings, but polydactyly can be associated with a syndrome. The extra digit may consist of a fleshy appendage or a complete digit with bone. Preaxial polydactyly will be on the thumb or big toe side (radius/tibia) while postaxial polydactyly (the most common) is on the pinky side

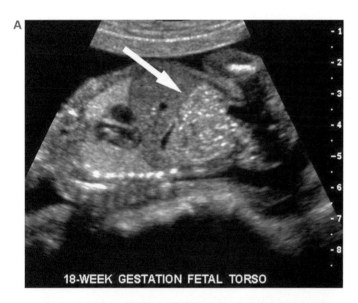

18-WEEK GESTATION FETAL TORSO

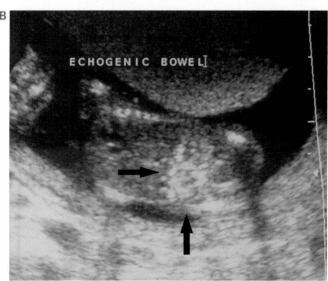

ECHOGENIC BOWEL

Figure 11-9. A *Normal bowel (arrow).* **B** *Echogenic bowel (arrows).*

Table 11-5.	Anomalies of the hand and foot.
Anomaly	**Definition**
Polydactyly	Extra digits
Clinodactyly	Overlapping digits
Syndactyly	Fused digits
Ectrodactyly	Lobster claw defect
Talipomanus	Clubhand
Talipes equinovarus	Clubfoot
Rocker bottom	Rounded sole of foot
Sandal toe	Wide-spaced big toe (between the big and second toes)

(ulna/fibula). Polydactyly can also be centrally located. This type carries a good prognosis and is usually familial (Figure 11-11).

Syndactyly

Syndactyly is fusion of the digits. It may simply be fusion by skin, such as webbing, or it may involve the fusion of bones. Second trimester growth restriction associated with fusion of the third and fourth fingers of the hand is suggestive of triploidy.

Abducted/Adducted Thumb

An **abducted thumb** is often referred to as the "hitchhiker" thumb and is associated with **diastrophic dwarfism**. This rare form of dwarfism involves short-limb skeletal dysplasia, clubfoot, ear swelling, and progressive spinal deformity and joint contractures, including the hitchhiker thumb. An **adducted thumb** is one that is turned inward toward the palm and has been associated with aqueductal stenosis.

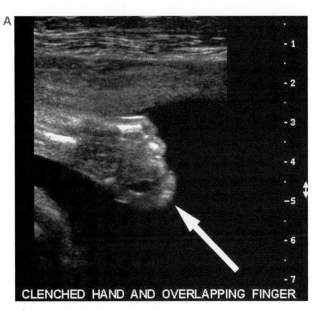
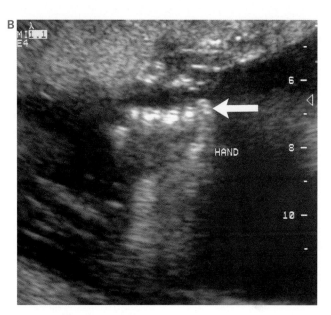

Figure 11-10. A This fetal hand is in a clenched position with a finger shown overlapping the others (arrow), showing clinodactyly. **B** Besides an extra digit, this fetal hand shows clinodactyly of the pinky finger (arrow).

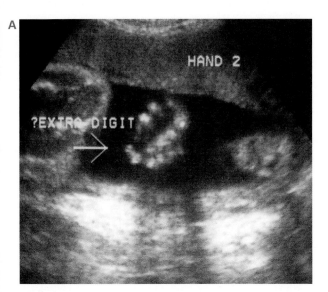
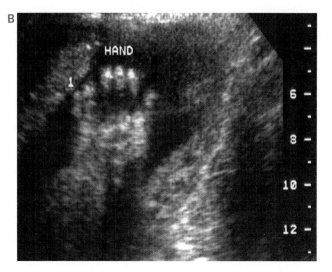

Figure 11-11. A and **B** Multiple digits are demonstrated on these fetal hands.

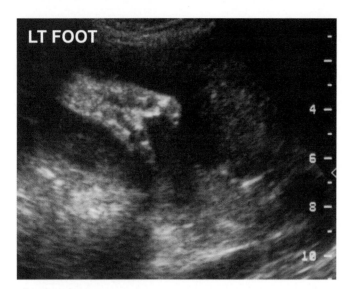

Figure 11-12. *Classic "lobster claw" foot.*

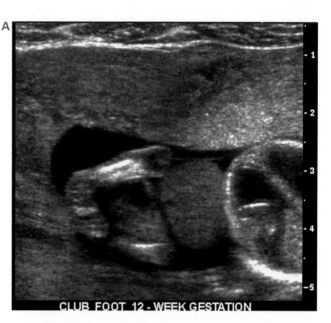

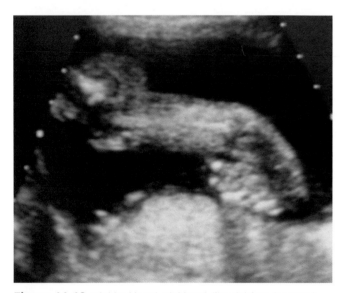

Figure 11-13. *Clubbed hand. Clubhand, like clubfoot, is turned inward. It may also be clenched, but its defining characteristic is that it is turned inward.*

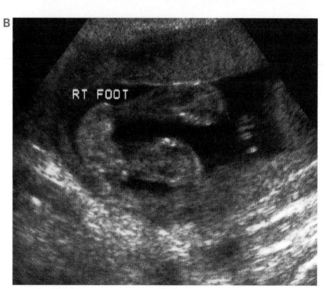

Figure 11-14. A *and* **B** *Two examples of clubfoot. Following page:* **C** *Schematic showing various types of talipes.*

Ectrodactyly

Also called the **lobster claw** deformity, **ectrodactyly** refers to a split hand or foot. As an isolated finding, it is in many cases found to be inherited from parents with only minimal manifestations (Figure 11-12).

Clubhand

Clubhand, also called **talipomanus**, can be radial or ulnar. The radial type (**radial aplasia**) is more common and usually associated with other abnormalities, while the ulnar type is associated with absence of the ulna but may also be an isolated finding (Figure 11-13).

Clubfoot

Often an isolated abnormality due to a cramped position in utero, the **clubfoot**, or **talipes**, is relatively common, occurring in 1 in 1000 births, with 15% having a familial association. A cramped fetal position in utero is usually the result of pathology (e.g., huge fibroids, uterine septum, multiple gestation) or variant anatomy (e.g., cubitus varas) and may be associated with oligohydramnios. The clubfoot may also be seen in association with more than 200 genetic, chromosomal, and sporadic syndromes. Although there are a variety of types, clubfoot mostly involves inversion and plantar flexion (Figure 11-14).

C

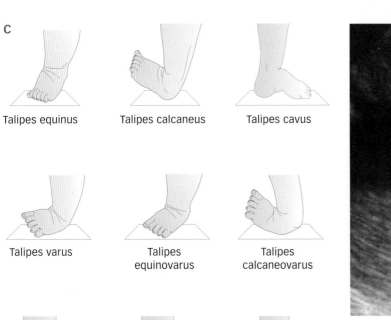

Talipes equinus   Talipes calcaneus   Talipes cavus

Talipes varus   Talipes equinovarus   Talipes calcaneovarus

Talipes valgus   Talipes cacaneovalgus   Talipes equinovalgus

Figure 11-14, continued.

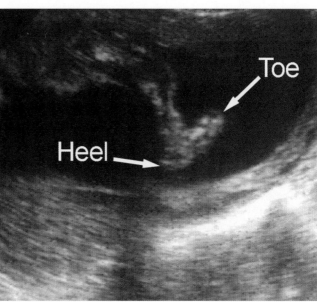

Figure 11-15. *Rocker bottom foot. Note how the heel extends past the calf and the rounded appearance of the sole of the foot.*

Rocker Bottom Foot

The **rocker bottom foot**, or **congenital vertical talus**, can result from an abnormally short Achilles tendon. The heel is prominent, extending beyond the calf, and the sole of the foot is convex in shape. The toes point upward like a pixie-toe shoe (Figure 11-15).

Sandal (Gap) Toe

When the large toe is widely spaced away from the others, it is called **sandal toe** or **sandal gap toe** (or **foot**) deformity. It may be familial but should raise concern to search for other anomalies that might associate it with a syndrome, such as Down syndrome (Figure 11-16).

ANEUPLOIDY

Aneuploidy is defined as the state of having chromosomes in a number that is not an exact multiple of the **haploid number** (23); 46 is the number normally present in humans. Most chromosomally abnormal pregnancies spontaneously abort, with estimations as high as 50%–60%. Only about 0.6% will progress and persist.

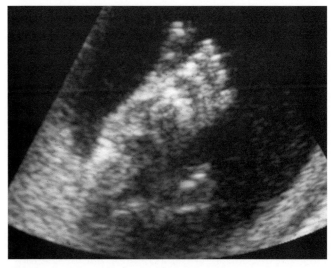

Figure 11-16. *Anterior view of a fetal foot with the sandal gap toe.*

Triploidy

Triploidy is rare, occurring in only 1%–2% of pregnancies. These fetuses have 69 chromosomes, a complete extra haploid set, instead of the normal 46. Most are thought to be the result of an egg fertilized by two sperm. The condition is fatal and pregnancies rarely progress to term, with most resulting in spontaneous abortion. Sonographic findings typically show a thickened placenta with multiple cystic areas similar to a molar pregnancy (Figure 11-17). If a fetus is present, it usually will have multiple anomalies, including those affecting the central nervous

Figure 11-17. *Example of a triploidy placenta demonstrating multiple cystic areas that create a "swiss cheese" appearance.*

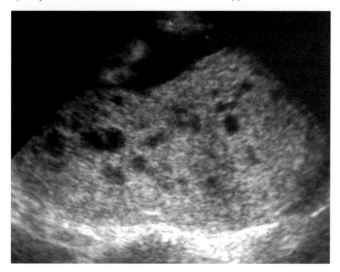

Box 11-5. Triploidy.

Intrauterine growth restriction (IUGR)

Ventriculomegaly, holoprosencephaly, Arnold-Chiari agenesis of the corpus calosum

Cleft lip/palate

Clubfoot, syndactyly

Neural tube defects

Congenital heart disease

Omphalocele, renal anomaly

Figure 11-18. A *Fetal head demonstrating alobar holoprosencephaly. The fused thalami are indicated by the arrow.* **B** *Frontal view of the fetal nose and mouth demonstrating a severe bilateral cleft defect of the lip.* **C** *The profile view shows flattening of the fetal face and abnormal nose and lips. Following page:* **D** *This fetal head demonstrates the "strawberry sign" with the broad, flat occiput and concave parietal bones. Reprinted with permission from TheFetus.net.* **E** *Specimen of an infant with trisomy 13.*

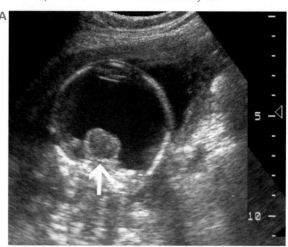

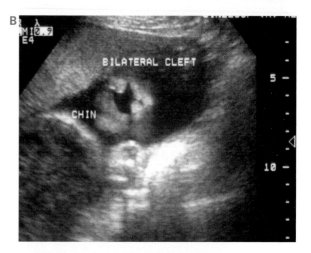

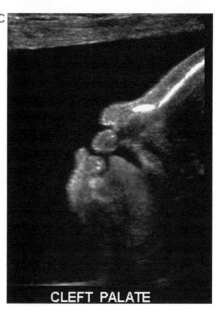

system, congenital heart disease, limb defects, and renal abnormalities (Box 11-5). Early onset of intrauterine growth restriction (IUGR) is a common finding, identifiable as early as the late first trimester (12–14 weeks).

Trisomy 13: Patau Syndrome

Considered the third most common trisomy, **trisomy 13**, or **Patau syndrome**, occurs in 1 in 5000 births and is generally not compatible with life. Most affected infants are stillborn, and the rest die between the first and sixth months of age. The syndrome is associated with alobar holoprosencephaly and severe cleft defects of the face (Figures 11-18 A and B). Profile views of the face show sloping of the forehead (Figure 11-18C) and micrognathia. Often described as having a "strawberry head," these fetuses present with facial, frontal lobe,

Figure 11-18, continued.

D

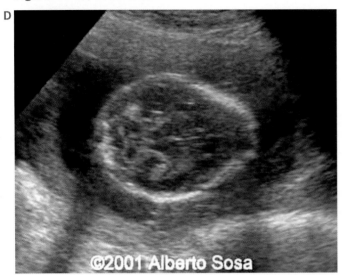

©2001 Alberto Sosa

Table 11-6.	Trisomy 13 (Patau syndrome).
Cranial:	Holoprosencephaly
	Encephalocele
	Facial clefts
Trunk:	Congenital heart defects
	Renal anomalies
	Abdominal wall defects
Extremities:	Polydactyly

E

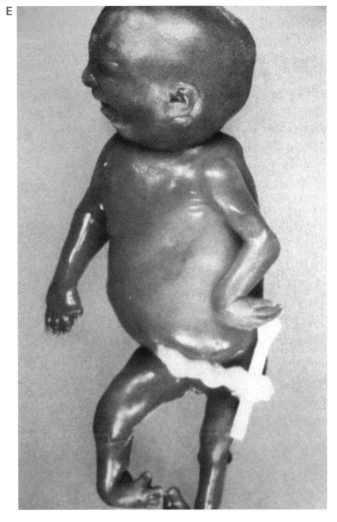

and occipital hypoplasia, resulting in a flat occiput and pointed frontal bones (Figure 11-18D). Microphthalmia and hypotelorism are also common. Recently, ear length has been studied; a short ear length can be associated with chromosomal abnormalities, particularly trisomies 13 and 18. Of fetuses with trisomy 13, 90% will have congenital heart disease, with ventricular septal defects among the most common; 80% have polydactyly. Other associated anomalies include infantile polycystic kidneys, horseshoe kidneys, and omphaloceles. Although amniotic fluid indices may vary in these cases, most will present with polyhydramnios in the third trimester and onset of growth restriction during the second trimester. (See Table 11-6.) As with many chromosomal abnormalities, hypotonia is usual. The triple screen is not helpful in detecting this syndrome (Figure 11-18E).

Trisomy 18: Edwards Syndrome

Trisomy 18, also known as **Edwards syndrome**, is the second most common trisomy, occurring in 1 in 3000–5000 births and with a male-to-female ratio of 1:3. It carries a dismal prognosis: About 50% of affected infants die within two months of delivery and only 10% live see their first birthdays. This syndrome is associated with early onset of severe growth restriction (80%) associated with polyhydramnios and congenital heart defects (90%), with deformities of the hands (clinodactyly, clenched fist, clubbed hand; Figure 11-19A) and feet (clubfoot and rocker bottom foot; Figures 11-19 B–E) being the most dramatic abnormal physical findings. Fetuses frequently show microcephaly with a prominent occiput, micrognathia, and short, malformed ears (Figure 11-19F). The so-called **strawberry head** has been associated with

Figure 11-19. A *View of the fetal arm extended, showing the clenched fist in a clubbed position.* **B** *and* **C** *Lower extremity of a fetus with a rocker bottom foot.* **D** *and* **E** *Lower extremity of a fetus showing a clubbed foot.* **F** *Abnormally shaped and low-set ear demonstrated on side of the fetal head.*

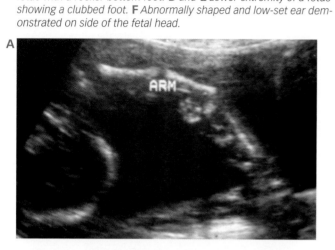

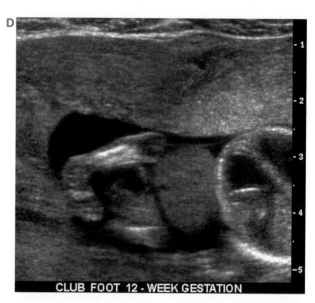

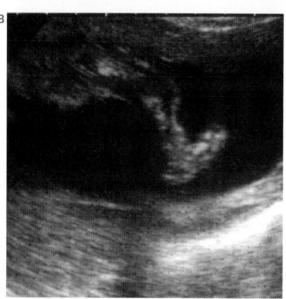

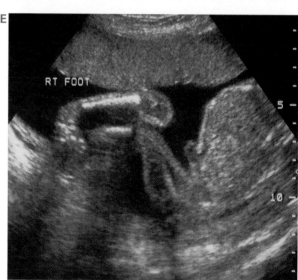

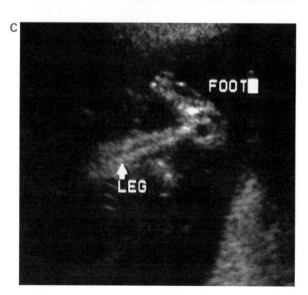

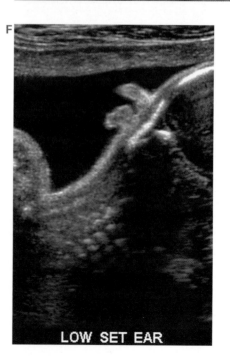

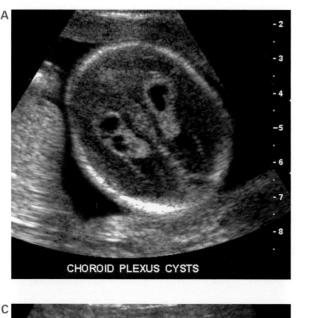

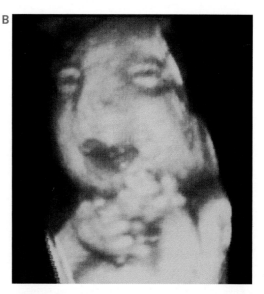

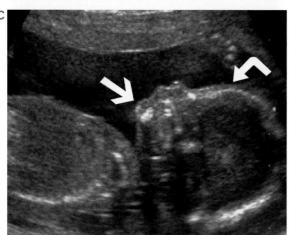

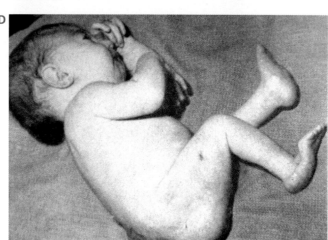

Figure 11-20. A *Bilateral choroid plexus cysts demonstrated in the brain of a fetus with trisomy 18.* **B** *3D imaging shows the facial features of a fetus with trisomy 18. Note the microcephaly, flat face, and abnormal mouth.* **C** *Profile view of a fetus with trisomy 18. The forehead is long and sloping (curved arrow) and the chin is recessed, indicating micrognathia. The back of the skull is also flat.* **D** *Infant with trisomy 18.*

Table 11-7.	Trisomy 18 (Edwards syndrome).
Cranial:	Choroid plexus cysts
	Micrognathia
Trunk:	Congenital heart defect
	Renal anomalies
	Omphalocele
	Diaphragmatic hernia
Extremities:	Clinodactyly
	Femoral shortening

trisomy 18, showing lateral flattening of the frontal bones of the skull (Figures 11-20 A–C). Choroid plexus cysts are relatively common and usually resolve in utero; however, those that measure more than 10 mm and persist after 24–26 weeks may be associated with a chromosomal abnormality when associated with other anomalies (Figure 11-20D). This is particularly true of trisomy 18. Other, less common abnormalities are listed in Table 11-7.

Trisomy 21: Down Syndrome

Considered to be the most common trisomy in humans, **Down syndrome**, **trisomy 21**, occurs in around 1 in 800 births. This incidence increases with maternal age: The risk factor for AMA mothers is about 1 in 75 pregnancies.

Still, using maternal age as a criterion will detect only 25%. The triple screen biochemical markers increase the detection rate by 60%. Much research has been devoted to identifying ultrasound markers that would help screen fetuses for Down syndrome, but many of these markers are very subtle and somewhat nonspecific, as they can resolve in utero. Most would agree that a fetus must have several of the markers before Down syndrome should be suggested relative to the obstetric sonogram. If sonographic criteria are added to the formula, detection accuracy for Down syndrome will increase an additional 20% (Box 11-6).

The prognosis for infants with Down syndrome varies depending on number and severity of associated anomalies. Cardiac anomalies are the most common cause of death during infancy, and only 40%–60% of Down syndrome children with cardiac disease live to age 10. Premature aging and early onset of **Alzheimer disease** (typically around age 30) are complications among patients who live into adulthood. Other concerns include an increased risk for developing leukemia and autoimmune phenomena such as thyroiditis and hypothyroidism. The average IQ range for children with Down syndrome is from 25 to 50, and IQ usually falls in adulthood. For additional information on Down syndrome in the second and third trimesters, see Chapter 4.

Sonographic Markers for Down Syndrome

Head and Brain Defects **Brachycephaly**, or **flat head syndrome**, is not usually considered a normal variant shape, as is **dolichocephaly** (when the head is longer relative to its width). Many fetuses with chromosomal abnormalities present with brachycephaly, indicated by a cephalic index greater than 86. Brachycephaly associated with Down syndrome is mild, however, and current cephalic indices do not apply and have not been established (Figures 11-21 A and B). Although choroid plexus cysts have been seen in fetuses with Down syndrome, this

Box 11-6.	Sonographic findings associated with Down syndrome.

Nuchal translucency, thickened nuchal fold

Brachycephaly, short/absent nasal bone

Heart defects, echogenic intracardiac foci

Duodenal atresia, mild pyelectasis

Echogenic bowel

Mild shortening of the femur/humerus

Iliac angle

Hypoplasia of middle phalanx of fifth digit

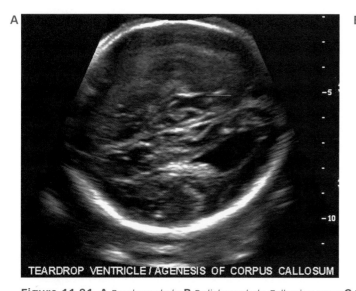

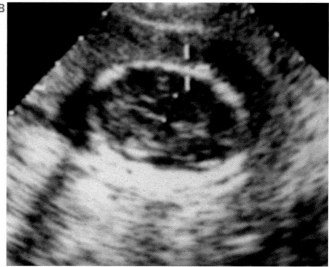

TEARDROP VENTRICLE / AGENESIS OF CORPUS CALLOSUM

Figure 11-21. A *Brachycephaly.* **B** *Dolichocephaly. Following page:* **C** *Transcerebellar measurements can be used to assist with screening for Down syndrome. The normal cerebellum is measured between the arrows.* **D** *This facial profile demonstrates macroglossia. Note how the tongue protrudes out of the mouth.* **E** *Fetal profile shows very short nasal bone (arrow) causing flattening of the face in a fetus with trisomy 21.* **F** *This facial profile shows no nasal bone (arrow). Although the nose is defined, the nasal bone is not. Note the broad sloping forehead.*

finding is more significant for trisomy 18 and does not raise the risk factor for trisomy 21. Transcerebellar measurements, however, are smaller with Down syndrome, and mild ventriculomegaly is not uncommon (Figure 11-21C).

Other markers associated with the head include macroglossia (Figure 11-21D) and an absent, short, or underossified nasal bone. When the profiles of these fetuses are imaged, the face will appear flattened. It has been suggested that by dividing the biparietal diameter (BPD) by the nasal bone length, one can establish a ratio, and a ratio of 11 or greater is associated with an increased risk for Down syndrome of 69% (Figures 11-21 E and F).

Thickened Nuchal Fold and Nuchal Translucency The **thickened nuchal fold** (thickening of tissue at the back of the fetus's neck) was one of the first sonographic markers identified for Down syndrome. It is identified at the cerebellar level of the fetal head and measured from the skull table of the occipital bone to the outer edge of the skin line

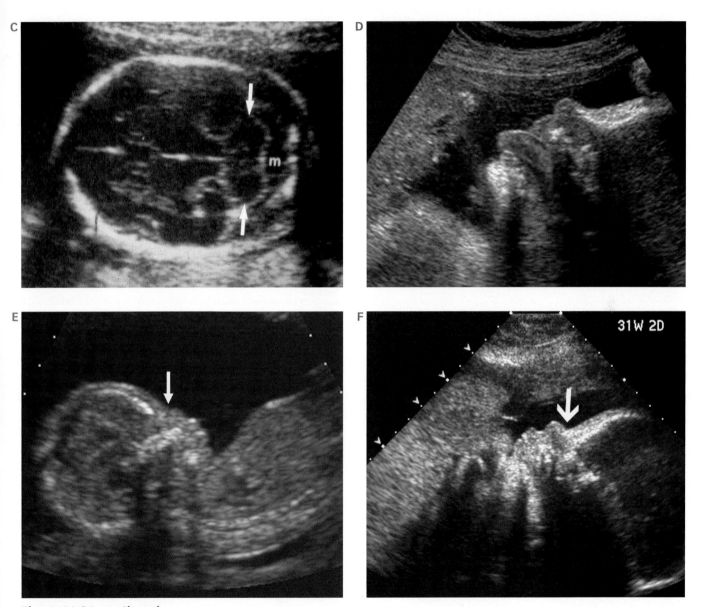

Figure 11-21, continued.

(Figure 11-22A). A measurement greater than 5 mm when maternal age is more than 35 years is a positive finding, with one of seven such fetuses having Down syndrome. Thickening is best seen between 15 and 20 weeks. It may resolve in the late second trimester and therefore lose accuracy for detection of the syndrome. Nuchal edema may progress into a cystic hygroma in about 10% of cases.

The **nuchal translucency** is a newer marker identified in the first trimester between 11 and 14 weeks. This translucency extends from the back of the head to the sacrum and should not measure more than 3 mm (Figure 11-22B).

A thick nuchal translucency has been associated with other chromosomal abnormalities as well as Down syndrome.

Heart Defects Structural cardiac defects are among the more common anomalies seen in Down syndrome patients with congenital heart disease, affecting approximately 50%. Defects of the atrioventricular canal and ventricular septum are most common (Figure 11-23). One of the screening markers suggesting chromosomal defects is the identification of an echogenic intracardiac focus. This finding can be normal, corresponding to the papillary muscles and echogenic chordae tendineae, and,

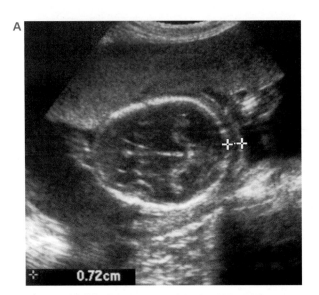

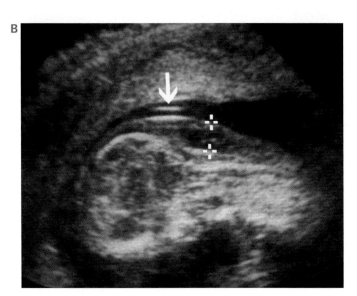

Figure 11-22. A *This image of the fetal head demonstrates a thickened nuchal fold between the calipers.* **B** *The first trimester nuchal translucency can be measured to rule out chromosomal abnormalities. One has to be careful not to mistake the normal amnion (arrow) for the nuchal structure.*

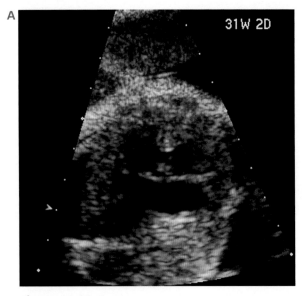

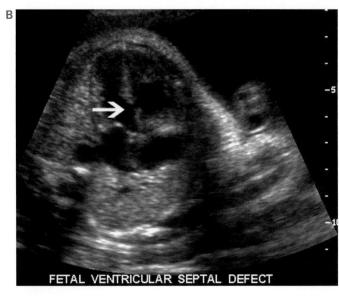

Figure 11-23. A *This four-chamber view shows what looks like a large single atrium, typical of an atrial septal defect.* **B** *This four-chamber view demonstrates a well-defined ventricular septal defect (arrow).*

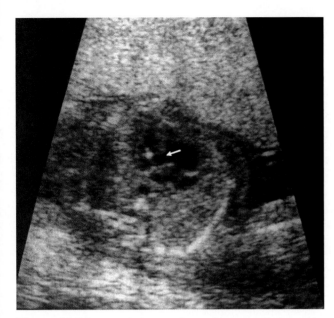

Figure 11-24. *Second trimester fetus with Down syndrome that has a complete atrioventricular canal with a large ventricular septal defect (arrow). Note that the left ventricle contains an echogenic intracardiac focus. Used with permission from Callen P: Ultrasonography in Obstetrics and Gynecology, 4th Edition. Philadelphia, Saunders, 2000, p 48.*

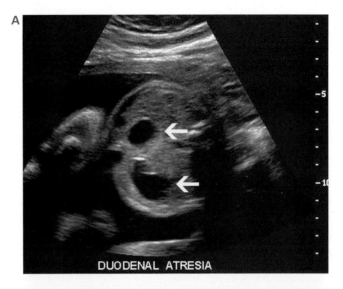

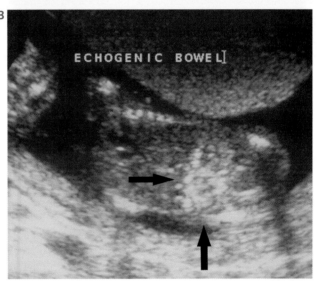

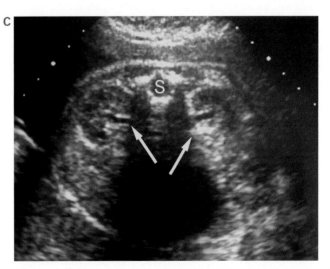

Figure 11-25. A *The typical "double bubble" sign is demonstrated (arrows), indicating duodenal atresia.* **B** *Longitudinal oblique view of fetal abdomen demonstrating bowel that is as echogenic as bone (arrows).* **C** *Transverse fetal abdomen through the level of the kidneys (arrows) demonstrates bilateral pyelectasis typically associated with Down syndrome. S = stomach.*

although it can be seen in either ventricle, it is seen mostly in the left ventricle. Echogenic foci that are right-sided or bilateral raise the suspicion for an associated chromosomal abnormality such as Down syndrome (Figure 11-24). Recently, there has been an association of first trimester tricuspid regurgitation with Down syndrome. When this finding is added to the first trimester findings of nuchal translucency and biochemical indicators, the detection rates have been estimated at 90%–95%.

Abdominal Defects Several abnormal abdominal findings have been associated with Down syndrome. The most common include duodenal atresia (Figure 11-25A), echogenic bowel (Figure 11-25B), and mild bilateral pyelectasis (Figure 11-25C). Sonographic identification of duodenal atresia carries a 30% risk for Down syndrome. This condition is associated with polyhydramnios as well as tracheoesophageal fistulas. It is important to remember, however, that this finding is not typically seen until after 22 weeks (usually at 22–26 weeks).

Although bowel patterns can be identified in fetuses and vary depending on gestational age, hyperechoic bowel is not common. When the small bowel is as echogenic as bone, the risk for Down syndrome is significantly increased. Echogenic bowel can also be associated with cystic fibrosis, cytomegalovirus (CMV), and severe early onset of IUGR.

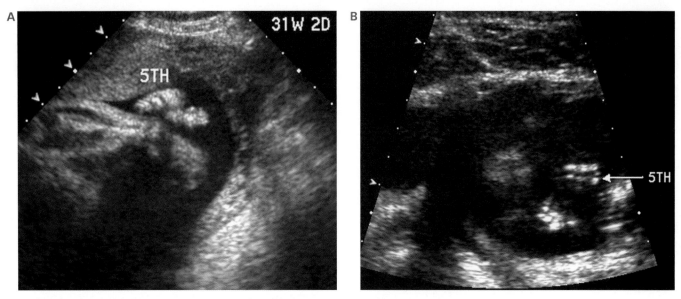

Figure 11-26. A and **B** *Images of the fetal fingers with the fifth digit labeled. Notice that the middle phalanx is quite short.*

Mild fetal renal pelvic dilatation has been associated with Down syndrome, but much controversy has arisen over the measurement threshold for normal. The dilatation is usually bilateral and measures around 4–5 mm in the greatest anteroposterior (AP) dimension. This may be considered normal physiologic dilatation in many sonography laboratories but should raise one's suspicion and warrant looking for additional markers. Down syndrome has also been associated with early-onset, late first or early second trimester development of posterior urethral valves (PUVs).

Skeletal Defects The effects of Down syndrome on the skeletal system have been well documented. The most common has to do with the hand. The middle phalanx of the fifth digit of the hand is shorter in patients with Down syndrome. This will cause overlapping of the little finger, which affects the posture of the hand (Figure 11-26).

Another observation that has been made in patients with trisomy 21 is that many have femurs that are slightly shorter when compared with those of normal patients. This holds true for the humerus as well. A biparietal diameter/femur length (BPD/FL) ratio greater than 1.5 would indicate a suspicious finding. Another, rather subtle finding is a mildly increased angle of the iliac bones. This measurement may be difficult to obtain accurately because of changes in scan planes; it is equally difficult to interpret and is therefore mostly subjective.

Table 11-8. Scoring system for Down syndrome.*	
Anomaly	2
Thickened nuchal fold	2
Short femur	1
Short humerus	1
Pyelectasis	1
Echogenic bowel	1
Echogenic intracardiac focus	1
Choroid plexus cyst	1

*A score > 2 provides a medical reason for an amniocentesis.

Scoring System for Down Syndrome
Most will agree that a diagnosis of trisomy 21 should never be based on a single isolated finding. Many researchers continue to search for a more definitive method of identifying this syndrome. As part of that work, Benacerraf and colleagues designed a scoring system that has worked well for diagnosing the Down syndrome fetus. Scores are tallied using the criteria in Table 11-8. A score of 2 or more provides a medical reason for performing an amniocentesis. Patients presenting with a score of 1 should be evaluated for amniocentesis based on their own risk factors combined with the associated risk for the specific marker. Absence of the nasal bone increases the risk

for Down syndrome, and several studies suggest that a short or hypoplastic nasal bone is also a risk factor. These authors have established that a BPD/nasal bone length ratio greater than 11 significantly increases the likelihood of Down syndrome, by about 50%.

TURNER SYNDROME

Turner syndrome, also known as **XO syndrome**, occurs sporadically in approximately 1 in 5000 births and is one of the most common causes of nonimmune hydrops. This chromosomal abnormality results in a fetus that lacks one of the sex chromosomes. Fetuses are usually either XX (female) or XY (male). With Turner syndrome, the fetus is XO, causing it to be phenotypically female. The most common anomalies associated with the syndrome include

lymphangiectasia (dilation of the lymphatic vessels) and cystic hygromas with or without fetal hydrops (Figures 11-27 A–C); 60% will show associated renal anomalies such as the horseshoe or pelvic kidney, while 20% will have a cardiac anomaly, the most common being coarctation of the aorta. Many conceptions affected by Turner syndrome spontaneously abort, and fetuses that develop hydrops frequently die in utero (Figures 11-27 D and E).

Turner syndrome, however, can be compatible with life. Individuals with Turner syndrome are shorter in stature and have the classic webbed neck from resolution in utero of a previous cystic hygroma. Other physical findings include streak ovaries resulting in sexual infantilism, low posterior hairline, and **cubitus valgus** (outward bending) of the arms. Since the ovaries degenerate after

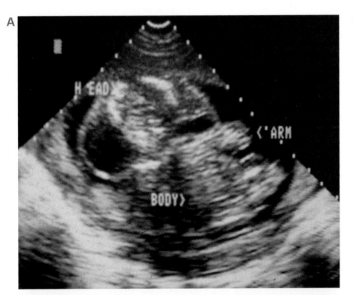

A

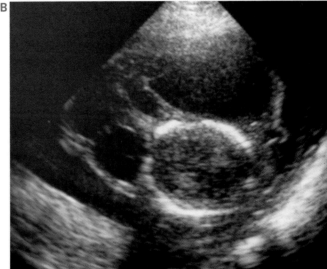

B

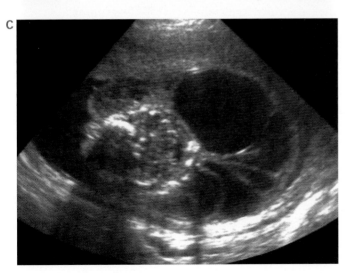

C

Figure 11-27. A Longitudinal view through a fetus demonstrating a cystic hygroma. **B** Transverse view of the fetal head showing the lobulated cystic hygroma. **C** Further down into the fetal abdomen, one can still see the extension of the cystic hygroma. (Figure continues . . .)

Figure 11-27, continued.
D and **E** *Anterior and posterior views of an aborted fetus with a cystic hygroma. This fetus proved to have Turner syndrome. Note the hydropic appearance.*

D

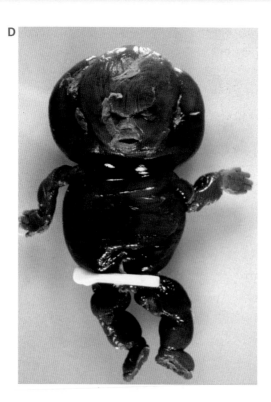

E

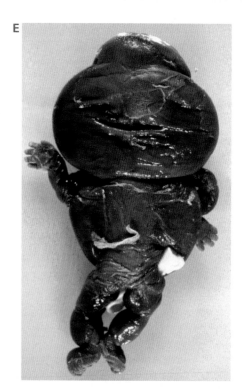

Table 11-9.	Turner syndrome.
Cranial:	Cystic hygromas
Trunk:	Pleural effusions
	Ascites
	Congenital heart defects
Extremities:	Lymph edema

delivery, these patients do not develop reproductively and therefore are infertile. Some 50% may present with mild mental retardation and hearing impairment. If a female newborn presents with edema of the hands and feet, Turner syndrome should be a consideration (Table 11-9).

Noonan syndrome will present as sonographically identical to Turner syndrome, with two exceptions. One is that Noonan syndrome fetuses can be male or female, whereas Turner syndrome is associated only with females. The second is that Noonan syndrome carries a greater hereditary risk as an autosomal dominant condition. When a Noonan syndrome fetus is male, he will often present with **cryptorchidism** (undescended testes) and micropenis. The most common cardiac defect is pulmonary stenosis. Look for a reduction in the size of the right ventricle.

MECKEL SYNDROME

Meckel syndrome, or **dysencephalia splanchnocystica**, is a rare genetic syndrome inherited in an autosomal recessive fashion. Occurring in less than 1 in 100,000 births, it has a slightly increased incidence among the Finnish population (1/9000). The disorder is lethal, and those fetuses born alive survive only a few days at most. This syndrome is often mistaken for Potter type I because of the associated infantile polycystic kidneys and severe oligohydramnios. These fetuses may also develop a **mesoblastic nephroma**, which is a hamartomatous tumor of the kidney that looks similar to a **Wilms tumor**.

The classic triad for diagnosing Meckel syndrome includes infantile polycystic kidneys (100%), a posterior encephalocele (80%), and polydactyly (75%). (See Figure 11-28.) The posterior encephalocele, if small, and polydactyly may be difficult to identify when associated with oligohydramnios. Clubbing of the feet, Potter facies (see Chapter 8), and pulmonary hypoplasia are usually secondary to oligohydramnios, and microcephaly is not uncommonly associated with the posterior encephalocele when large and brain-containing. A number of other central nervous system anomalies can also be seen with this condition, including Dandy-Walker abnormalities, ventriculomegaly, Arnold-Chiari malformations, and agenesis of the corpus callosum. Facial abnormalities may include microphthalmia, micrognathia, and cleft lip/palate (Table 11-10).

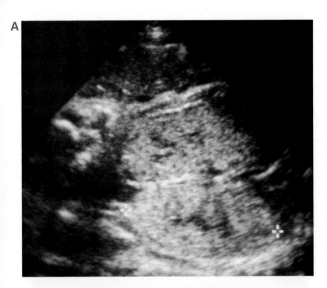

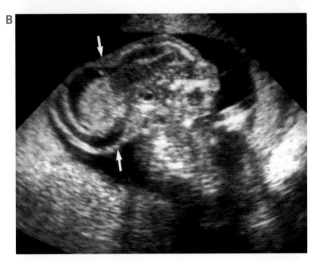

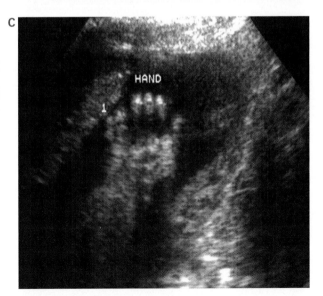

Figure 11-28. A *This image shows recessive polycystic kidney disease or infantile polycystic kidneys in long axis. They are large, filling the abdomen and brightly echogenic.* **B** *Profile view showing a fetus with a large, posterior encephalocele (arrows). Note the sloping forehead and recessed chin.* **C** *Fetal hand showing a sixth digit indicated by the numeral 1.*

Table 11-10.	Meckel syndrome.
Cranial:	Posterior encephalocele
	Facial clefts
	Microcephaly/hydrocephaly
Trunk:	Polycystic kidneys
	Congenital heart defects
	Pulmonary hypoplasia
Extremities:	Polydactyly/syndactyly/clinodactyly
	Clubfoot/rocker bottom foot

Box 11-7.	Prune belly (Eagle-Barrett) syndrome.
	Dysplastic/hydronephrotic kidneys
	Dilated bladder
	Megaureters
	Protuberant abdomen

PRUNE BELLY SYNDROME

Although the etiology of **prune belly syndrome**, also called **Eagle-Barrett syndrome**, is questionable, it is mostly thought to be associated with a bladder outlet obstruction including posterior urethral valves, with a male-to-female ratio of 20:1. It is characterized by abdominal wall distention due to gross dilatation of the fetal bladder, which causes obstruction of the entire urinary tract. Dilated ureters and bilateral hydronephrosis result, and over time cystic dysplasia of the kidneys may develop (Figure 11-29). See Box 11-7. The bladder distention is thought to inhibit the normal development of the abdominal musculature and prevents the testes from descending. The prognosis depends on lung development and the amount of renal destruction due to uropathy. If the process develops early in pregnancy the prognosis is poor. Clinical features can be classified as:

- *Category I:* Oligohydramnios, Potter facies, urinary tract dilatation, renal dysplasia, 33% stillborn.

- *Category II:* Typical external features, urinary tract dilatation, less severe renal dysplasia, survival beyond neonatal period.

- *Category III:* External features mild, mild dilatation of urinary tract, normal renal parenchyma.

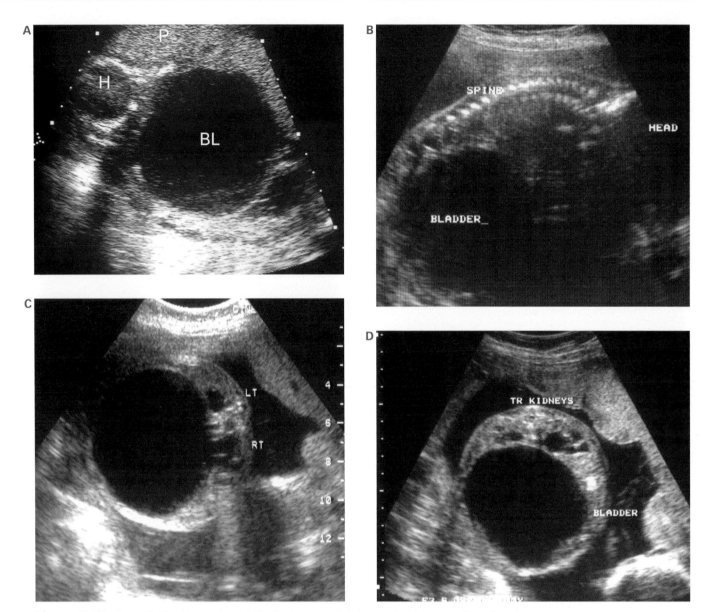

Figure 11-29. A *Longitudinal image through the fetal head and abdomen showing gross distention of the abdomen when compared to the fetal head. The large cystic area in the body is the overdistended fetal bladder. H = head, BL = bladder, P = placenta.* **B** *This fetus is lying face down with the spine up. Note how grossly distended the fetal bladder appears in this fetus with prune belly syndrome.* **C** *and* **D** *Transverse images through the fetal abdomen showing bilateral hydronephrosis and a huge, distended bladder typical of prune belly syndrome.*

The female counterpart of the prune belly syndrome is **megacystis microcolon malrotation intestinal hypoperistalsis syndrome**. This syndrome is rare, is usually fatal, and almost always affects females. The fetus presents with grossly distended abdomen; the bladder is enlarged and there is associated hydronephrosis with **hydroureters** (obstruction-caused distention of the ureters with urine or watery fluid). The microcolon is malrotated and there is little or no peristalsis of the bowel. In some cases, patients can be maintained with **total parenteral hyperalimentation**.

BECKWITH-WIEDEMANN SYNDROME

Considered mostly sporadic, **Beckwith-Wiedemann syndrome** occurs in 1 in 15,000 births and is associated with macrosomia, macroglossia, and organomegaly. Organ enlargement especially affects the kidneys, and the echogenicity of the renal cortex is often increased. Because severe polyhydramnios is usual, patients are at risk for preterm labor. Other anomalies that may be seen with the syndrome include omphalocele, ventral hernia, and cardiomegaly (Box 11-8). Patients with Beckwith-Wiedemann

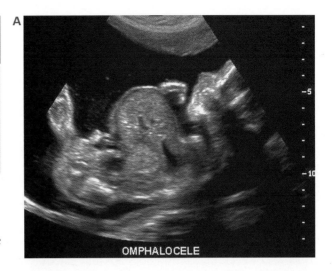

Box 11-8.   Beckwith-Wiedemann syndrome.

Macrosomia

Organomegaly

Macroglossia

Polyhydramnios

Omphalocele/ventral hernia

syndrome are at increased risk for developing hepatoblastomas, **neuroblastomas**, and Wilms tumors and therefore should be monitored closely.

PENTALOGY OF CANTRELL

Pentalogy of Cantrell, also known as **thoracoabdominal syndrome**, involves defects of the anterior chest and abdominal wall as well as congenital heart defects (Figure 11-30). It is a rare condition (affecting < 1/100,000) and carries a male-to-female predisposition of 2:1. In most cases the condition is lethal, although outcome depends on the severity of the cardiac abnormalities and the number of other associated anomalies. Fetuses almost always present with ectopia cordis, structural cardiac anomalies, and omphalocele. The cause may be associated with failure of the amnion and chorion to fuse (limb–body wall anomaly) or may be the result of a developmental defect. Five components are included, as indicated in Box 11-9.

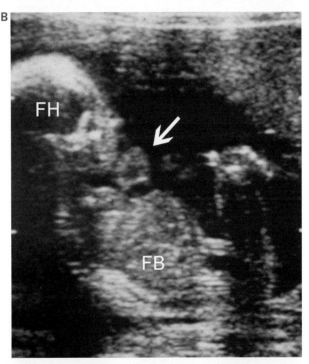

Box 11-9.   Pentalogy of Cantrell.

Defect of the lower sternum

Ectopia cordis

Congenital heart defects

Defect in the anterior diaphragm

Omphalocele

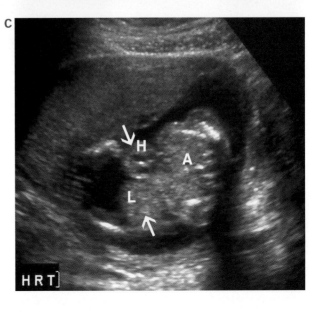

Figure 11-30. A *Longitudinal image of a fetus with an abdominal wall defect.* **B** *Longitudinal image demonstrating a fetus with ectopia cordis (arrow). FH = fetal head, FB = fetal body.* **C** *This fetus demonstrates most of its organs outside the abdomen (arrows), typical of limb–body wall complex. A = abdomen, L = liver, H = heart.*

CAUDAL REGRESSION SYNDROME

Caudal regression syndrome, also called **caudal aplasia/ dysplasia sequence**, refers to the partial or total absence of the lumbosacral spine and is associated with other anomalies of the lower extremities and gastrointestinal/ gastrourinary (GI/GU) tracts (Figure 11-31). While some of the urinary tract and bowel anomalies may not be compatible with life, prognosis depends on associated anomalies and the severity of those anomalies. This syndrome has been specifically associated with maternal diabetes, with about 16% of cases seen in infants of diabetic mothers. Although the literature has indicated detection as early as 9–11 weeks, the sacrum does not fully calcify until 22 weeks, which may make it difficult to confirm prior to this time (Box 11-10).

SIRENOMELIA

Sirenomelia, or **mermaid syndrome**, once thought to be related to caudal regression syndrome, is now suspected to evolve from a vascular incident resulting from a vitelline arterial steal causing a redirection of blood flow from the caudal structures. Both fetal legs may be fused or there may be a single lower extremity (Figure 11-32). This condition is often associated with bilateral renal agenesis and anogenital abnormalities. There is a male-to-female ratio

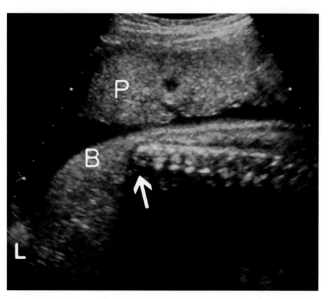

Figure 11-31. *Longitudinal image through the lumbosacral region of the spine of a fetus with caudal regression syndrome. Note how the spine abruptly ends (arrow) long before reaching the buttocks region. B = buttocks, L = leg, P = placenta.*

Box 11-10.	Caudal regression syndrome.

Total/partial absence of lumbosacral spine

Gastrointestinal/gastrourinary anomalies

Other anomalies of the lower extremities

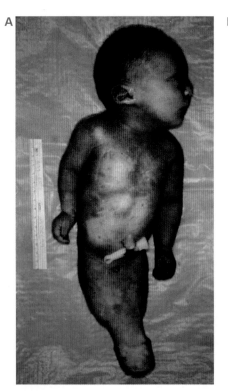
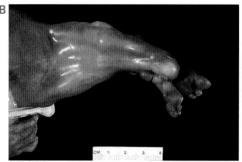
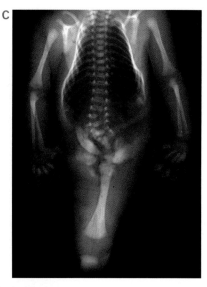

Figure 11-32. A *Postmortem specimen of an infant with sirenomelia (mermaid syndrome). Note the abnormal hands, facies, and low-set ears.* **B** *Lower limbs demonstrating the flipperlike feet associated with the mermaid syndrome.* **C** *Radiograph showing a single femur, abnormal lumbosacral spine, and deformed hands. The small chest is typical in fetuses with pulmonary hypoplasia due to severe oligohydramnios.*

of 3:1 and a significantly increased incidence (100–150 times) in monozygotic twins. Almost always fatal, sirenomelia is associated with severe oligohydramnios, which can make the diagnosis difficult. See Chapter 10 for additional information on sirenomelia.

FETAL ALCOHOL SYNDROME

Alcohol abuse is the most common drug abuse problem, affecting 1%–2% of women of childbearing age. Effects of **fetal alcohol syndrome** (**FAS**) on the fetus include pre- and postnatal growth deficiencies, flat face, small jaw, short upturned nose, hypertelorism, small orbits with squinty eyes, smooth **philtrum**, microcephaly, and hyperactivity (Figure 11-33, Box 11-11). Later, children may experience behavioral problems, learning disabilities, and mental retardation due to central nervous system damage. Other physical findings can include syndactyly, minor genital abnormalities, cardiac defects, hip dislocation, clubfoot, excessive hair during infancy, and abnormal pigmentations such as strawberry birthmarks.

AMNIOTIC BAND SYNDROME

The normal amnion and chorion usually fuse by the 12th week of gestation; certainly by 16 weeks the structures should be fused as one. Persistent separation of the amnion from the chorion should be documented and monitored, as the amnion can adhere to fetal parts, impeding movement, becoming entangled or wrapped around fetal structures, and causing deformities and/or disruption of normal development. This condition is called **amniotic band syndrome**. Severe anomalies—including anencephaly, encephalocele, limb–body wall anomaly, facial cleft defects, and amputations of limbs and digits—have been associated with amniotic band accidents. In the limb–body wall anomaly, the umbilical cord is quite short and the amnion adheres to the fetus, making it appear to be stuck to the placenta. It is not uncommon for many of the abdominal organs to develop outside the abdomen, totally disrupting normal anatomic development (Figure 11-34).

Discriminating Features

Short palpebral fissures
Flat midface
Short nose
Indistinct philtrum
Thin upper lip

Associated Features

Epicanthal folds
Low nasal bridge
Minor ear anomalies
Micrognathia

Figure 11-33. *Drawing demonstrating the classic facial features of fetal alcohol syndrome. National Institute on Alcohol Abuse and Alcoholism, adapted from Alcohol Health and Research World 18, 1994.*

Box 11-11.	Fetal alcohol syndrome (FAS).
	Microcephaly
	Micrognathia
	Microphthalmia
	Cleft lip/palate
	Smooth philtrum
	Malformed ears
	Atrial and ventricular septal defects
	Intrauterine growth restriction

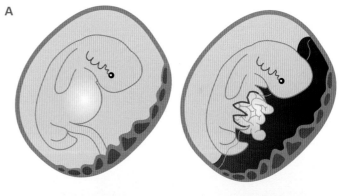

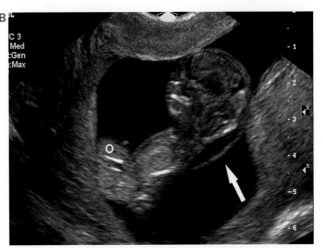

Figure 11-34. A *Drawing demonstrating the effect of a short umbilical cord contributing to the limb–body wall malformation.* **B** *Small fetus adhering to the placenta with abdominal contents developing outside the abdominal cavity. Note the thick nuchal translucency (arrow). O = omphalocele. (Figure continues . . .)*

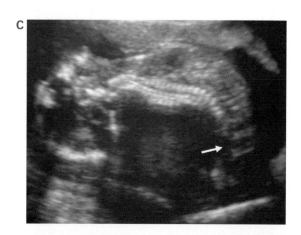

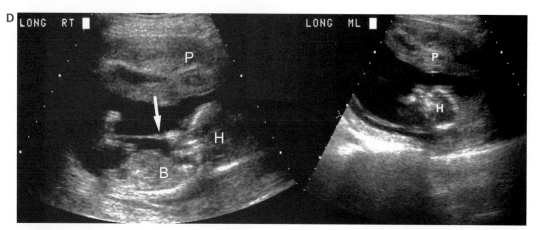

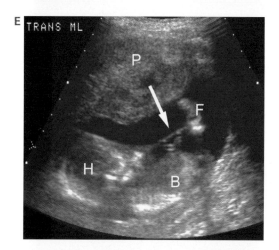

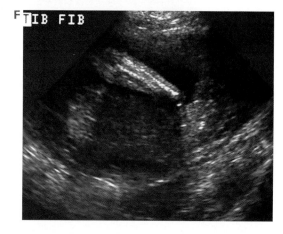

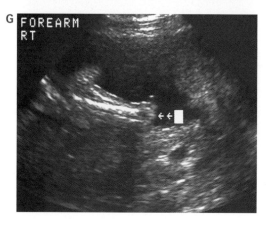

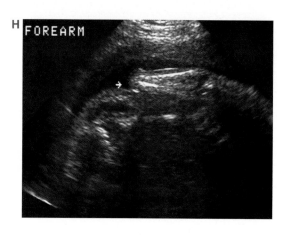

Figure 11-34, continued. C *Limb–body wall complex demonstrating a fetus adherent to the anterior placenta. It also has a single flipperlike appendage (arrow).* **D** *and* **E** *The strand of floating amniotic membrane (arrow) has adhered to fetal parts. H = head, B = body, F = foot, P = placenta.* **F, G,** *and* **H** *Fetal arms and legs missing hands and feet.*

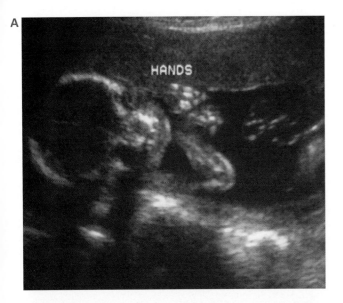

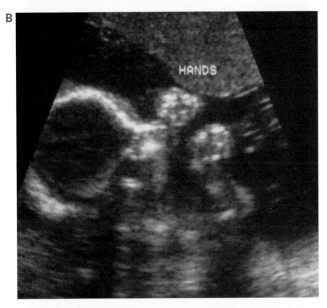

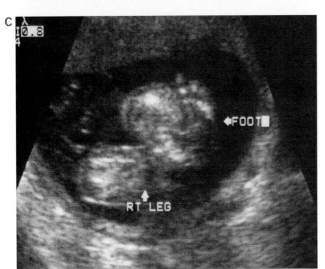

Figure 11-35. A *and* **B** *Fetal hands are fixed in a "praying mantis" position.* **C** *Fetal foot is turned back on the leg and in a fixed position.*

HOLT-ORAM SYNDROME

The major features of **Holt-Oram syndrome** include aplasia or hypoplasia of the radial structures and atrial septal defects in the heart. In many cases, the **radius**—the long bone in the forearm on the thumb side—is absent. The metacarpal and carpal bones in the hands and wrist can also be affected, causing positional and physical effects on the hand such as clubbing. Renal cystic dysplasia can also be observed in some cases. The images in Figure 11-35 show some of the limb deformities that can be seen with Holt-Oram.

SCANNING TIPS, GUIDELINES, AND PITFALLS

When multiple fetal anomalies are identified in a single fetus, the likelihood that chromosomal abnormalities exist is significantly increased. There are three areas that, when affected, add to that likelihood. They include the central nervous system, the fetal face, and fetal extremities, especially the hands and feet. Abnormalities of the hands and feet, as in sandal toe and polydactyly (Figures 11-36 and 11-10B), may be the most noticeable finding. Abnormal facies include a proboscis or an abnormal profile (Figure 11-37). Several syndromes are associated with micrognathia, cleft defects, microcephaly, and eye and ear abnormalities. Because of the similarities, they can be difficult to differentiate sonographically. Finally, be sure to evaluate the entire uterine cavity and adnexa. A placenta with molar changes may indicate a chromosomal abnormality, and the amniotic fluid level should

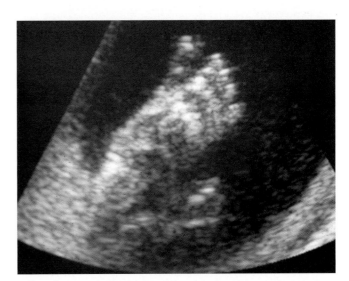

Figure 11-36. *Image of a fetal foot with a wide-spaced big toe, often referred to as the sandal toe. This finding can be associated with chromosomal disorders.*

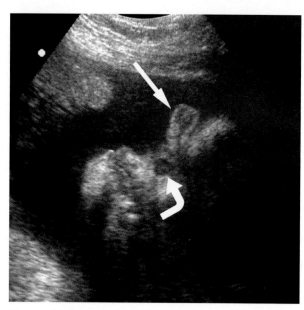

Figure 11-37. *This view shows the profile of a fetus with a proboscis (arrow). The overall profile is abnormally flat, showing no nasal features, and the orbit is quite small (curved arrow).*

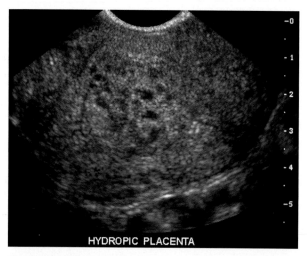

HYDROPIC PLACENTA

Figure 11-38. *Image of edematous placenta showing some molar changes.*

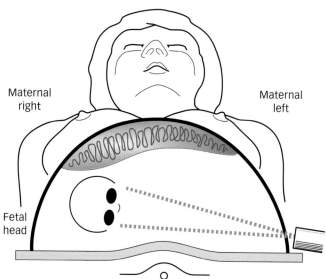

Figure 11-39. *Schematic showing how to obtain a profile view of the fetal face.*

always be assessed carefully; too much or too little can be associated with specific anomalies (Figure 11-38). When an abnormal finding is discovered, look for a second. If a second is discovered, look for a third. If a fetus demonstrates multiple anomalies, a perinatal consult and genetic counseling may be recommended.

1. When attempting to measure the nuchal translucency (NT) in the first trimester, be certain to magnify the image adequately so that the NT is well defined, thin, and clear. The fetal head, neck, and chest should be in a neutral position and fill the entire field of view. Reduce the depth so that the fetus is at the bottom of the image. Narrowing the sector width increases the number of scan lines, which increases resolution. Harmonics imaging does not improve the visualization of the nuchal translucency and should not be used. The calipers should be placed on the inner borders of the echolucent space and should be perpendicular to the long axis of the fetus.

2. Increasing contrast creates sharper, crisper lines. This can be accomplished by lowering the dynamic range and increasing edge enhancement. One might consider trying a cardiology setting designed for high-contrast imaging.

3. When imaging the nasal bone, you can use harmonics to better define and distinguish the bone from the overlying skin layer.

4. If the fetus is lying on its side or back, the fetal profile should be easy to access. To get the profile view of the fetal face, go to the side opposite from that on which the fetus is lying. If it lies on the maternal right facing the maternal left, go all the way over to the maternal left side laterally and angle the sound beam up underneath the fetus to image the profile of the face (Figure 11-39).

5. To obtain the frontal view of the fetal face, start with the profile and slide toward the tip of the nose and turn the transducer so that it sits right on the tip of the nose. Now the sound beam is shining (like a flashlight) right into the fetal face (Figure 11-40). The fetal face can offer much information relating to anomalies.

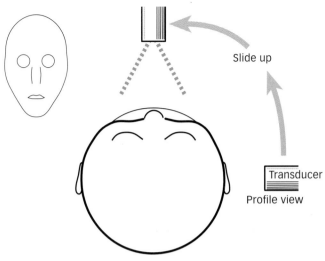

Figure 11-40. *Schematic showing how to obtain a frontal view of the fetal face.*

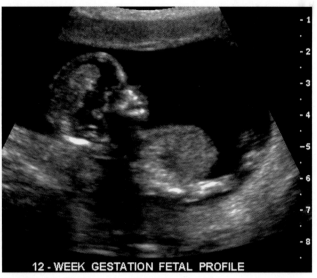

12 - WEEK GESTATION FETAL PROFILE

Figure 11-42. *Normal profile view of fetal face.*

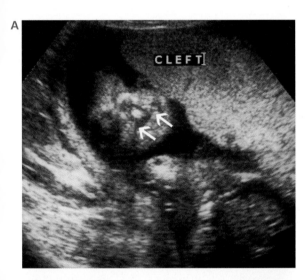

A

CLEFT

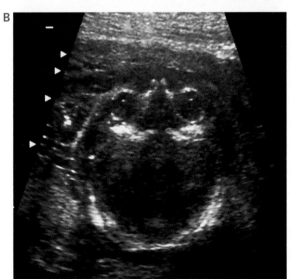

B

Figure 11-41. A *Frontal view of fetal face showing bilateral clefts.* **B** *Image demonstrates the proper view for measuring ocular diameters and distances.*

6. Coronal and transverse views of the face (Figure 11-41) allow the examiner to visualize the ears, eyes, nose, and lips.

7. The sagittal view of the face provides information about the shape of the forehead, occiput, nose, chin, and ear, while also allowing us to see movement of the mouth and tongue (Figure 11-42).

8. Before diagnosing a clubfoot, make sure the fetal foot is not pushed up against the uterine wall or other structures. Try to get the fetus to move to see if the foot relaxes into a normal position.

REFERENCES

Benacerraf BR: *Ultrasound of Fetal Syndromes*, 2nd Edition. New York, Churchill Livingstone, 2007.

Bromley B, Benacerraf B: Chromosomal abnormalities. In Rumack CM, Wilson SR, Charboneau JW, et al: *Diagnostic Ultrasound*, 4th Edition. St. Louis, Elsevier Mosby, 2011, pp 1119–1144.

Chervenak FA, Isaacson GC, Campbell S: *Ultrasound in Obstetrics and Gynecology*, Volume 2. Boston, Little Brown, 1993.

De Lange M, Rouse GA: *OB/GYN Sonography: An Illustrated Review*. Pasadena, CA, Davies Publishing, 2004.

Edwards A, Mulvey S, Wallace EM: The effect of image size on nuchal translucency measurement. Prenat Diagn 23:284–286, 2003.

Faiola A, Tsoi E, Huggon C, et al: Likelihood ratio for trisomy 21 in fetuses with tricuspid regurgitation at the 11 to 13 + 6-week scan. Ultrasound Obstet Gynecol 26:22–27, 2005. Published online in Wiley InterScience (www.interscience.wiley.com). DOI: 10.2002/uog.1922.

Falcon O, Auer M, Gerovassili A, et al: Screening for trisomy 21 by fetal tricuspid regurgitations, nuchal translucency and maternal serum free B-hCG and PAPP-A at 11 + 0 to 13 + 6 weeks. Ultrasound Obstet Gynecol 27:151–155, 2006. Published online in Wiley InterScience (www.interscience.wiley.com). DOI: 10.2002/uog.2699.

Finberg HJ: Aneuploidy detection in pregnancy: an evidence based approach. AIUM Ultrasound Bulletin 1:15–21, 2005.

Henningsen CG: Prenatal diagnosis of congenital anomalies. In Hagen-Ansert SL (ed): *Textbook of Diagnostic Sonography*, 7th Edition. St. Louis, Elsevier, 2011, pp 1190–1205.

Huggon IC, DeFigueiredo DB, Allan LD: Tricuspid regurgitation in the diagnosis of chromosomal abnormalities in the fetus at 11–14 weeks of gestation. Heart 89:1071–1073, 2003.

Kelly J: High maternal serum alpha fetoprotein: indicator of much more than neural tube defects. Pasadena, Genetics Institute, The Genetic Newsletter, Volume 2, Number 3, 1992.

Lee W, DeVore GR, Comstock CH, et al: Nasal bone evaluation in fetuses with Down syndrome during the second and third trimesters of pregnancy. J Ultrasound Med 22:55–60, 2003.

Leite JM, Granese R, Jeanty P, et al: Fetal syndromes. In Callen PW (ed): *Ultrasonography in Obstetrics and Gynecology*, 5th Edition. Philadelphia, Saunders Elsevier, 2008, pp 112–180.

Miller, BF, O'Toole MT: *Encyclopedia & Dictionary of Medicine, Nursing & Allied Health*, 7th Edition. Philadelphia, Saunders, 2005.

Nicolaides KH, Sebire NJ, Snijders RJM: *The 11–14 Week Scan: The Diagnosis of Fetal Abnormalities.* New York, Parthenon, 1999.

Sanders RC, Blackmon LR, Hogge WA, et al: *Structural Fetal Abnormalities: The Total Picture*, 2nd Edition. St. Louis, Mosby, 2002.

Yeo L, Guzman ER, Ananth CV, et al: Prenatal detection of fetal aneuploidy by sonographic ear length. J Ultrasound Med 22:565–576, 2003.

SELF-ASSESSMENT EXERCISES

Questions

1. Alpha-fetoprotein (AFP) is produced by:
   A. Fetal kidneys
   B. Fetal liver
   C. Fetal adrenal glands
   D. Placental tissue
   E. Maternal ovaries

2. A low AFP level would *not* suggest:
   A. Down syndrome
   B. Pseudocyesis
   C. Fetal demise
   D. Molar pregnancy
   E. Congenital nephrosis

3. Chorionic villus sampling (CVS) is best performed at:
   A. 4–6 weeks
   B. 10–12 weeks
   C. 14–16 weeks
   D. 16–18 weeks
   E. After 20 weeks

4. Trisomy 21 is also known as:
   A. Patau syndrome
   B. Edwards syndrome
   C. Potter syndrome
   D. Down syndrome
   E. Meckel syndrome

5. Caudal regression syndrome has been specifically associated with:
   A. Diabetes mellitus
   B. Rh isoimmunization

C. Pregnancy-induced hypertension (PIH)

D. Hyperemesis gravidarum

E. Sickle cell anemia

6. The triad of infantile polycystic kidneys, a posterior encephalocele, and polydactyly suggests:

   A. Eagle-Barrett syndrome

   B. Classic Potter syndrome

   C. Potter type I

   D. Potter type II

   E. Meckel syndrome

7. What is the probability that disorders inherited in an autosomal recessive fashion will be passed on?

   A. 0%

   B. 25%

   C. 50%

   D. 75%

   E. 100%

8. Turner syndrome is often associated with:

   A. Cystic hygromas

   B. Sacrococcygeal teratomas

   C. Macroglossia

   D. Spina bifida

   E. Omphaloceles

9. Chorionic villus sampling (CVS) will *not* diagnose:

   A. Chromosomal disorders

   B. Genetic disorders

   C. Neural tube defects

   D. Fetal gender

   E. Blood disorders

10. Of the following, which is *not* considered compatible with life?

    A. Turner syndrome

    B. Beckwith-Wiedemann syndrome

    C. Down syndrome

    D. Prune belly syndrome

    E. Patau syndrome

11. This image of the fetal head demonstrates:

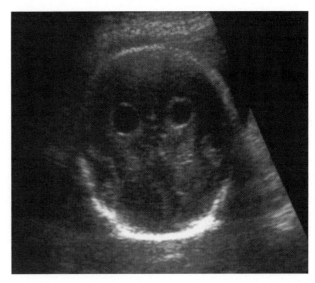

    A. Choroid plexus cysts

    B. Small orbital diameters

    C. Bilateral hydrocephalus

    D. Vein of Galen aneurysms

    E. Normal ventricular atria

12. This image of the fetal upper extremity was taken from the same fetus imaged in Question 11. What would most likely be suspected with these two findings?

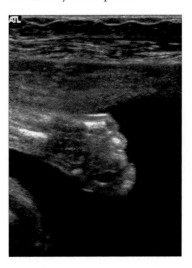

    A. Triploidy

    B. Trisomy 13

    C. Trisomy 18

    D. Trisomy 21

    E. Aneuploidy

13. Holoprosencephaly is often associated with:

A. Trisomy 13

B. Trisomy 18

C. Trisomy 21

D. Triploidy

E. Aneuploidy

14. When the fetal eyes are too close together it is called:

A. Anophthalmia

B. Cyclopia

C. Hypertelorism

D. Hypotelorism

E. Microphthalmia

15. The common term for talipes equinovarus is:

A. Sandal toe

B. Rocker bottom foot

C. Acheiropodia

D. Ectrodactyly

E. Clubfoot

Answers

See Appendix F on page 615 for answers and explanations.

Doppler Applications in Obstetric and Gynecologic Sonography

Jim Baun, BS, RDMS, RVT, FSDMS

OBJECTIVES

After completing this chapter you should be able to:

1. Describe normal female pelvic vascular anatomy and hemodynamics.

2. Explain the hemodynamic changes that occur in the presence of ovarian pathology.

3. Describe normal hemodynamic states in the uterine arteries in gravid patients.

4. Identify normal and abnormal Doppler spectral waveforms obtained from the umbilical and cerebral arteries in the fetus.

5. Explain how Doppler waveforms reflect the hemodynamic changes occurring in the presence of failed first trimester gestations.

6. Understand the significance of resistivity and pulsatility changes observed in both maternal and fetal arteries throughout normal and abnormal pregnancies.

7. Develop sonographic examination protocols for a complete Doppler evaluation of the gravid patient.

DOPPLER ULTRASOUND APPLICATIONS enhance obstetric and gynecologic sonographic examinations by adding a physiologic element to the traditional two-dimensional anatomic display. More specifically, Doppler display modalities provide information about **hemodynamics**, the movement of blood in and around human soft tissues and organs. By applying basic physical principles of the Doppler effect to echo information received by a sonographic imaging system, practitioners can extract information about movement of blood and use it to formulate a more complete analysis of the living tissues being examined. Doppler ultrasound applications have proven very useful in studying nongravid pelvic anatomy, i.e., the uterus and ovaries, as well the gravid uterus and its contents. It has become a standard component in the diagnostic armamentarium used for evaluating high-risk pregnancies, particularly those that may result in compromise of normal fetal growth and development.

PHYSICAL FOUNDATION OF DOPPLER ULTRASOUND

The Doppler Effect

The **Doppler effect** describes the change in frequency that occurs when energy interacts with motion. Austrian mathematician and physicist Christian Doppler first described the predictable relationship between movement and energy in 1842 when he observed a shift in the frequency of light emitted from moving stars compared with those that remained stationary. Under telescopic observation, some stars appeared to emit light from the blue end of the electromagnetic spectrum, while others emitted light from the red end of the spectrum. Professor Doppler posited that the frequency of light, which determines its perceived color, is affected by the star's motion; the frequency of emitted light increases as the star (energy source) moves toward the observer's eye (receiver) and decreases as it moves away. In other words, the wavelength of an energy source moving toward the observer is shorter compared to a stationary object, while that of an energy source moving away from the observer is longer. Doppler concluded that movement away from the receiver is perceived as lower frequency/longer wavelength (red in the realm of visible light) and movement toward the receiver is perceived as higher frequency/shorter wavelength (blue). The particulars of Doppler's astronomical observations can be extrapolated to other types of energy as they, too, interact with movement. While acoustic energy is mechanical and not electromagnetic in nature, it nonetheless demonstrates the Doppler effect when either the source or the receiver of the sound moves in relation to the other. The classic example of the audible acoustic Doppler effect is the perceived change in pitch of a train whistle or ambulance siren as the vehicle moves first toward and then away from a listener; the pitch (frequency) is higher as the sound source approaches the receiver (listener's ear) and lower as it continues on past.

Mathematically, the Doppler shifted frequency (F_d) is simply the difference between the frequency of the outgoing ultrasound beam (F_i) and the returning echoes (F_r):

$$F_d = F_i - F_r$$

where:

F_d = Doppler frequency shift
F_i = incident frequency
F_r = reflected frequency

Example: If the central incident frequency is 5 MHz and the receiver detects a 4.5 MHz returning frequency, the Doppler shift is 0.5 MHz. If the receiver detects a 5.5 MHz returning frequency, the Doppler shift is −0.5 MHz. Conveniently, in medical applications, Doppler frequencies fall within the range of human hearing (20–20,000 Hz). This makes fetal monitoring devices and Doppler stethoscopes easy to design. They also rely on continuous-wave Doppler technology, not the pulse-echo principles used in Doppler imaging applications.

The Doppler effect, as applied in diagnostic medical sonography, takes this phenomenon down to the cellular level. In the human body, it is the change in frequency that occurs as a high-frequency ultrasound beam encounters the microscopic red blood cells that scatter it like headlights in a fog. The redirected acoustic energy experiences a phase and frequency shift during the scattering phenomenon. That portion of Rayleigh-scattered energy coming back toward the transducer is compared to the phase and frequency of that which went out. The difference is the **Doppler frequency**, or **Doppler shift** (F_d). It can be a positive or a negative value depending on whether the flow is toward or away from the emitted ultrasound beam. Just like Professor Doppler's observations in astronomy, movement toward a receiver creates a positive frequency shift, movement away a negative shift.

Two critical bits of information are present in the returning Doppler signal: **polarity**, which is the positive/negative value that correlates with direction of flow, and Doppler **frequency**. The Doppler frequency is converted through a restatement of the Doppler formula into the velocity values that permit quantitative spectral analysis, which provides the diagnostic criteria we use in most obstetric and gynecologic vascular studies. The Doppler signal contains the raw data that the imaging system uses to create all of the Doppler display modalities—audio, spectral, color, and power. Processing circuits process the signal differently, but it is all the same information displayed simultaneously in real time.

The Doppler Formula

While the basic concept of Doppler frequency change is expressed in the foregoing formula, there are several other factors that affect the actual characteristics of the Doppler signal. It is worthwhile to take a look at the Doppler formula in its more complete expression, as it demonstrates the significance of several physical factors that are pertinent to clinical practice. The variables in the Doppler formula consist of those that are sonographer-controllable and those that are not. The uncontrollable variables are the speed of sound (C), which is a universal constant, and the velocity of the moving red blood cells (V), the product of hemodynamics. Both incident frequency (F_i), emitted by the sonographer's selected probe, and Doppler angle, determined by probe position and electronic beam steering, are controllable.

Doppler Formula

$$F_d = \frac{2F_i V \times \cos \theta}{C}$$

where:

F_d = Doppler frequency shift
F_i = incident frequency
V = velocity of reflectors
C = velocity of sound
$\cos \theta$ = angle of incidence

The two sonographer-controllable variables are incident frequency and Doppler angle ($\cos \theta$). Incident frequency (F_i) from the Doppler formula translates into the transducer frequency used by the sonographer. There is a wide range of transducer frequencies used in obstetric and gynecologic applications. They vary from 2.5 MHz deep-penetrating transabdominal obstetric probes to 15 MHz transvaginal devices. In addition to its importance to the contrast resolution of the gray-scale image, transducer frequency equally affects the color Doppler image resolution and limits the maximum frequency that can be displayed. This limitation—the **Nyquist limit**—can become a factor in deciding which transducer to use, particularly in the higher frequency range. When incoming Doppler frequencies exceed the Nyquist limit, aliasing artifact occurs, improperly placing information on the wrong side of the baseline.

To correct for aliasing:

Reduce imaging depth.

Increase transducer frequency.

Doppler Angle

The issue of "Doppler angle" that comes up so often in peripheral vascular imaging studies centers on the other sonographer-controllable variable in the Doppler for-mula, i.e., **cos θ**. A cosine is a number associated with an angle. Values between 0 and 1 are assigned to angles between 90º and 0º. As the angle approaches 90º, the cosine approaches zero. Looking at the Doppler formula demonstrates that the entire calculated Doppler frequency is modified by cos θ. At 90º, cos θ is zero, which produces a final Doppler frequency (F_d) of zero. Not very useful information. At 0º, cos θ is unity, or one, the complete and unadulterated Doppler shift. In theory a zero degree angle is desirable, which, however, is obtainable only by inserting the transducer into the blood vessel and measuring the bolus of blood coming down the bore. Not a very noninvasive method.

Generally, as the angle between the steered ultrasound beam and the streamline of blood approaches zero, the reliability of the Doppler signal increases. Conversely, as the Doppler angle approaches 90º, the reliability of the velocity measurements becomes unusable in clinical studies. As a rule, maintaining a Doppler angle of less than 60º and measuring along the central stream in the vessel as demonstrated by color Doppler imaging will yield the best range of usable Doppler signals. Most diagnostic criteria used in obstetric and gynecologic Doppler ultrasound studies are ratios measured from a single waveform and, as such, are angle-independent. The magnitude of difference between peak systolic velocity (PSV) and end-diastolic velocity (EDV) in a particular waveform remains constant as the velocity scale upon which it is displayed changes with operator control adjustments. Ratios and indices, which measure resistive and pulsatile characteristics of flow instead of Bernoulli velocity values, can be accurately measured from **spectral waveforms** obtained from virtually any angle other than 90º.

Continuous-Wave vs. Pulsed Doppler

Ultrasound can be used in two ways to produce Doppler signals. The simplest method is **continuous-wave (CW) Doppler**, which is used in fetal monitoring devices and handheld Doppler stethoscopes (Figure 12-1). CW Doppler devices usually have two transducer crystals, one emitting a continuous stream of ultrasound while the other continuously listens for returning echoes. The region common to the transmitted beam and the focused depth of the receiving transducer is called the **sensitivity zone**. Reflectors and scatterers positioned within the sensitivity zone create the Doppler shift that is converted into an audio signal or sent to a waveform recorder.

A

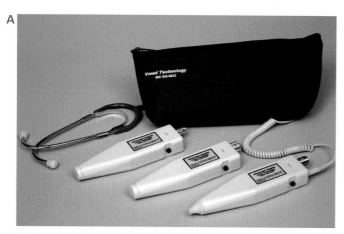

B

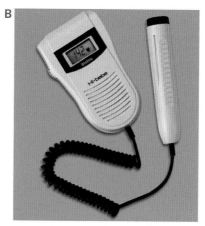

Figure 12-1. *Continuous-wave (CW) Doppler instruments.* **A** *Doppler stethoscopes for many and varied clinical applications.* **B** *Handheld obstetric CW Doppler.*

Pulsed Doppler is more complicated. It is based on the pulse-echo principles of ultrasound imaging systems that can locate the depth of specific acoustic phenomena by measuring the time it takes echoes to return after the initial pulse is generated. This is sonar on a cellular level. With the pulse-echo technique, an acoustic pulse is emitted from the transducer array. An onboard clock controls the time elapsed before listening for returning information and, using the range formula, codes this returned information with a depth dimension. Each returning echo itself is encoded with frequency, amplitude, phase, and polarity information. The combined depth and Doppler signal information can be sent to either a spectral waveform generator or a color Doppler image display.

CLINICAL UTILITY OF DOPPLER ULTRASOUND

In clinical applications, Doppler information is hemodynamic information. It is the sound, the sight, and the measurements of blood flow in the arterial and venous conduits that constitute the human circulatory system. Returning echo information is captured by the transducer array and directed across different circuits to produce one of the three main Doppler display modalities: audio, spectral Doppler (SD), and color Doppler imaging (CDI). Each modality displays the same hemodynamic information and, in a true **triplex system**, all three formats are displayed simultaneously and in real time. The characteristics of each Doppler ultrasound display modality are discussed below.

Advances in acoustic engineering have created contemporary ultrasound imaging systems that can accurately sample and analyze blood flow down to submillimeter magnitude. Such an exacting instrument requires operator understanding of the system controls that permit accurate hemodynamic reporting.

What kinds of clinical questions can Doppler ultrasound answer? Doppler ultrasound finds its utility in evaluating blood flow. A little gel, a little pushing, and a lot of useful hemodynamic information can be obtained quickly and noninvasively. Hemodynamic parameters that can be assessed with Doppler ultrasound include presence of flow, arterial vs. venous flow, and direction of flow:

- **Presence of Flow**. Presence of flow is a fundamental hemodynamic characteristic. If the structure being examined is truly a vascular structure, then flow, whether arterial or venous, should be detected with Doppler interrogation. Color Doppler imaging is superb at performing this function even down to very slow flow states (1–5 cm/s) in very small vessels (<1 mm). Here again, Doppler threshold, baseline, and gain settings must be optimized to confidently exclude the presence of blood flow in a diseased or obstructed vessel.

- **Arterial vs. Venous Flow**. Occupying the two hemodynamically distinct sides of the human circulatory system, arteries and veins yield entirely different types of Doppler hemodynamic patterns. The blast of kinetic energy delivered by the left ventricle during systole pulsates through the arterial network, creating Doppler spectral waveforms with dramatic highs and lows. When mapped over time, these velocity changes correspond to the contractile states of the heart with landmarks occurring at peak systole, early diastole, and end diastole.

Direction of Flow

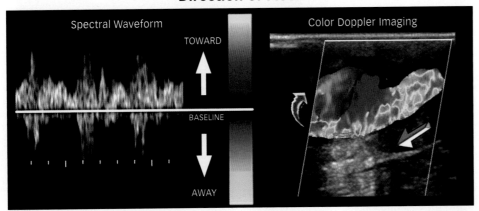

Figure 12-2. *Direction of flow. Spectral waveform (left).*

On the venous side of the circulation, the blood is pumped by the skeletal muscles and sucked upward by the right atrium, producing a Doppler signal that is spontaneous, slow, and phasic. The pressure changes in the chest and abdominal cavities that accompany breathing rhythmically augment and depress flow as deoxygenated blood makes its way back toward the heart. Venous Doppler signals display spontaneous, phasic flow that looks and sounds relaxed and un-rushed compared to the pulsatile, high-velocity jetting of the arteries.

- **Direction of Flow.** The formula (above) demonstrates that the Doppler signal has a positive or negative polarity created by the directional flow of the blood being sampled. Flow coming toward the transducer produces a positive Doppler shift; flow going away produces a negative Doppler shift. This polarity $(+/-)$ information is translated back into directional information and output to the three Doppler display formats: Stereo speakers split the audio signal into right and left channels, a red/blue hue is assigned by the color Doppler circuitry, and spectral waveform pixels are plotted either above or below the horizontal baseline. Understanding flow direction is fundamental to interpreting Doppler ultrasound studies. The accompanying illustration demonstrates how flow direction is mapped on a triplex ultrasound image (Figure 12-2).

Arterial Doppler Characteristics

Pulsatility

The defining characteristic of an arterial Doppler signal is its pulsatility. Driven by the kinetic energy of the left ventricle, the velocity of blood in an artery fluctuates over

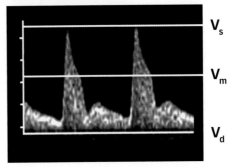

Figure 12-3. *Velocity measurements from a uterine artery Doppler waveform. V_s = peak systolic velocity, V_m = mean systolic velocity, V_d = end-diastolic velocity.*

the cardiac cycle. Peak systole is the point of maximum contraction of the left ventricle that produces the highest velocity in an artery conducting a laminar column of flow. **Peak systolic velocity** (**PSV**) is a value that is used in virtually all Doppler spectral waveform diagnostic criteria. As an absolute value, or when measured above and below a stenosis, PSV can be useful in estimating the degree of narrowing in an artery. As used in the resistivity and pulsatility indices discussed below, PSV represents the maximum flow state used in calculating the degree of resistance and pulsatility (Figure 12-3).

Diastolic flow occurs between the two systolic peaks on a Doppler spectral waveform. The velocity of flow just before the beginning of the systolic upsweep is measured as **end-diastolic velocity** (**EDV**). By relating PSV and EDV in various ways, one can obtain numeric values that reflect hemodynamic states in the downstream vascular beds such as the placenta, the fetus, the uterus, and the ovaries. These measurements provide an idea of how much and how easily blood can flow into the tissue bed being examined.

If blood continues its forward flow throughout the cardiac cycle, the tissue bed is receiving a constant, uninterrupted supply of oxygen and nutrients to support its metabolically active state. Waveforms representing a continuous forward flow of blood are called **monophasic**, meaning they go in one direction. Monophasic waveforms are the type encountered in obstetric Doppler applications and, with cyclical variation, in the uterine and ovarian arteries.

In the larger, main pelvic arteries—i.e., the common, internal, and external iliac arteries—Doppler spectral waveforms tell a different story. The predominant vascular bed supplied by the infra-aortic arterial tree is skeletal muscle. The large gluteal, thigh, and calf muscle groups at rest require only viability-sustaining levels of blood, which is reflected in the highly resistive Doppler waveforms of these arteries. Categorized as triphasic, these waveforms represent the rapid stream of forward flow during systole followed by a rebounding flow reversal before the forward flow finale in late diastole. Loss of triphasicity in the iliac arteries is a Doppler hallmark of patients with lower extremity peripheral arterial disease (Figure 12-4).

The Diastolic Notch

Another Doppler waveform characteristic encountered in obstetric applications is the diastolic notch. A **diastolic notch** represents an early diastolic flow restriction to the bolus of blood directed at the uterus during systole. While mild notching may be associated with a normal pregnancy, more dramatic types of notching suggest an initial restriction to flow by a vascularly compromised placental circulation (Figure 12-5).

Resistivity Index

The **resistivity index** (**RI**) is a spectral waveform–derived indicator of the relative resistance to flow into a tissue bed (Figure 12-6). Waveform velocities obtained at peak systole (V_s) and end diastole (V_d) are used to calculate the index of resistance. The accompanying formula shows that resistivity, as measured by the RI, is almost solely a function of the end-diastolic velocity (V_d).

$$RI = \frac{V_s - V_d}{V_s}$$

Peak systolic velocity (V_s) is included in both the numerator and the denominator, effectively canceling it out. What remains is the effect of V_d. This is consistent with what one would expect considering the characteristics of high- and low-resistance hemodynamic patterns

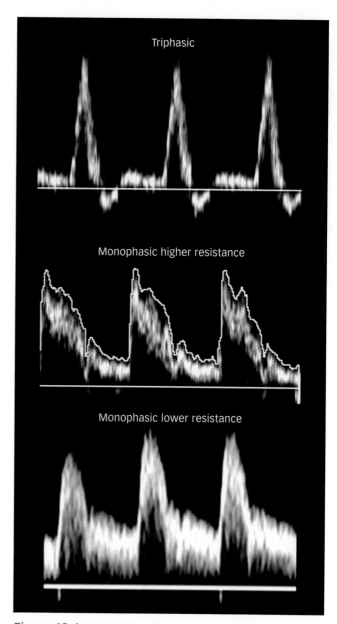

Figure 12-4. *Arterial phasicity waveform examples.*

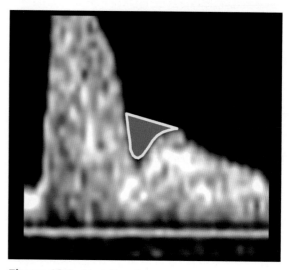

Figure 12-5. *Diastolic notch.*

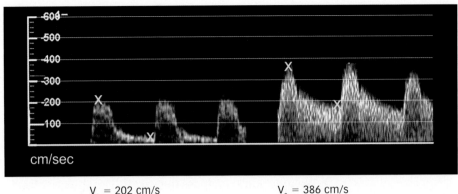

Figure 12-6. *Resistivity index examples.*

$V_s = 202$ cm/s
$V_d = 38$ cm/s
$RI = \dfrac{202 - 38}{202}$
$RI = 0.81$

$V_s = 386$ cm/s
$V_d = 168$ cm/s
$RI = \dfrac{386 - 168}{386}$
$RI = 0.56$

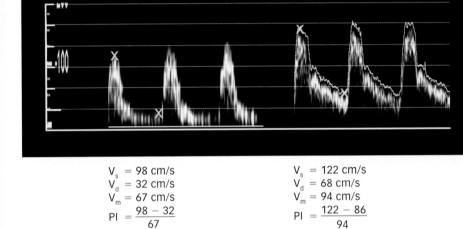

Figure 12-7. *Pulsatility index examples.*

$V_s = 98$ cm/s
$V_d = 32$ cm/s
$V_m = 67$ cm/s
$PI = \dfrac{98 - 32}{67}$
$PI = 0.98$

$V_s = 122$ cm/s
$V_d = 68$ cm/s
$V_m = 94$ cm/s
$PI = \dfrac{122 - 86}{94}$
$PI = 0.38$

as discussed above. Low-resistance vascular beds need and get fresh blood throughout the cardiac cycle. This is expressed in the RI formula as persistent, higher-velocity flow measured at end diastole (V_d). High-resistance vascular beds resist perfusion as expressed in near-zero, or even retrograde, flow at end diastole.

Pulsatility Index

The **pulsatility index** (**PI**) is a Doppler value that provides a sensitive index of diastolic runoff into a tissue bed (Figure 12-7). Pulsatility is the difference between peak systolic velocity (V_s) and late diastolic peak velocities (V_d) divided by mean diastolic flow (V_m). High peak systolic and low end-diastolic flow velocities produce good pulsatility; low peak systolic and high end-diastolic flow velocities produce poor pulsatility.

$$PI = \frac{V_s - V_d}{V_m}$$

Venous Doppler Characteristics

Doppler ultrasound demonstrates the following characteristics of normal venous hemodynamics (Figure 12-8):

- **Spontaneous flow** is the regular, rhythmic movement of blood through a vein powered by the normal pressure changes occurring throughout the cardiac and respiratory cycles.

- **Competence** refers to the Doppler demonstration of unidirectional, forward flow of blood through the veins.

- **Phasic with respiration**. Normal venous flow varies in volume and velocity over the stages of respiration. During inspiration, as intra-abdominal pressure increases, venous signals in the lower extremity decrease or stop; during expiration, as intra-abdominal pressure decreases, venous signals return in a slightly augmented state. These flow patterns are reversed in the upper extremity, where venous flow normally increases with inspiration and decreases with expiration.

- **Provocative Maneuver Response**:

Proximal Compression. The purpose of applying external pressure to a vein above the area of Doppler interrogation is to induce flow reversal in vessels with incompetent valves. The response to proximal compression in a vein with competent valvular structure and function is no response. In normal long veins of the leg there may be a short (<1 second) flow reversal at maximum compression. Flow reversal lasting longer

is consistent with some level of venous insufficiency. The accompanying illustration demonstrates an abnormal response with quick, sharp reflux induced by proximal compression in an incompetent femoral vein.

Augmentation with Distal Compression. External compression of the leg veins by the examiner's hand or by a rapid inflation pressure cuff causes a dramatic increase in (augmentation of) flow volume through the vein above the site of applied pressure. Upon release, flow volume quickly returns to normal. The absence of augmentation with distal compression suggests venous obstruction.

Valsalva Maneuver. Following the performance of a **Valsalva maneuver**, venous flow in the lower extremity normally increases. Augmentation *during* the maneuver represents retrograde flow (venous reflux) and suggests valvular incompetence.

- **Nonpulsatility.** Normal systemic venous hemodynamics is nonpulsatile. The presence of pulsatility in a venous Doppler display indicates pathology, usually on the right-sided circulation. Some pathologic entities that can induce pulsatility include venous or pulmonary hypertension, congestive heart failure, excessive intrathoracic fluid, and the presence of an arteriovenous fistula. Pulsatile energy from the heart can also be transmitted to veins in close proximity to the right atrium and is frequently seen in the inferior vena cava and the hepatic veins. This should not be considered an abnormal finding.

GYNECOLOGIC APPLICATIONS

Vascular Anatomy of the Pelvis and Female Reproductive Organs

Pelvic Veins

The deep and superficial regions of the pelvis are drained, respectively, by veins originating in the external and supporting soft tissue structures and by those originating in the deep parenchymal organs. While there are many anatomic variations on the exact architecture of the two venous systems, it is a fair generalization to say that the superficial regions in the pelvis drain via the external iliac vein while the deep regions drain via the internal iliac vein.

After passing beneath the inguinal ligament, the common femoral vein (CFV) enters the pelvic cavity and empties into the external iliac vein (Figure 12-9). Several

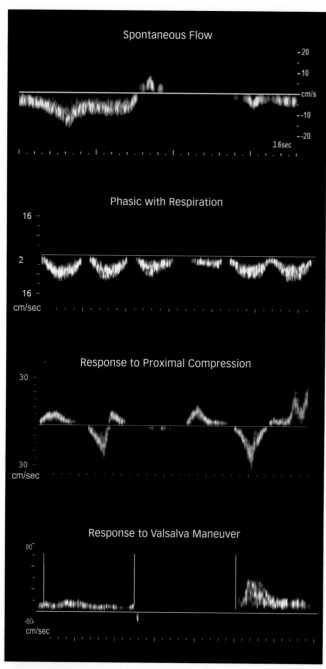

Figure 12-8. *Venous Doppler characteristics from top: spontaneous flow, phasic with respiration, proximal compression, and Valsalva maneuver.*

Figure 12-9. A *Female pelvic venous anatomy.* **B** *Doppler ultrasound images demonstrating hemodynamic patterns in the parauterine venous vasculature.*

A

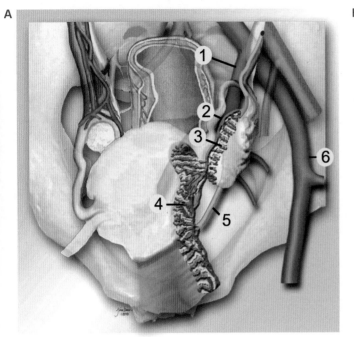

1 = internal iliac vein 4 = uterine plexus
2 = ovarian vein 5 = uterine vein
3 = ovarian plexus 6 = external iliac vein

B

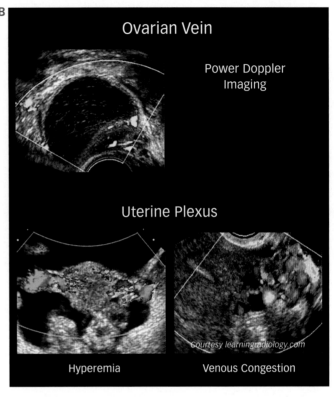

centimeters along its course, after fusing with the internal iliac (hypogastric) vein, it becomes the common iliac vein, which empties into the inferior vena cava. There is slight variation between the two sides. On the right the common femoral vein initially lies medial to the artery, but as it proceeds cephalad the vein moves increasingly posterior to the artery. On the left side, the common femoral vein lies medial to the artery throughout its entire course. The common iliac vein contains one or two bicuspid valves.

Veins of the Female Reproductive Organs

The internal iliac vein provides outflow for tributaries draining both deep and superficial regions of the pelvis. The deep tributaries drain the bladder, rectum, gluteal, sacral and pudendal regions, and internal reproductive organs. In the female reproductive tract, uterine and vaginal venous outflow is accommodated by the interconnected uterine and vaginal plexuses that lie along adjacent surfaces of each organ. Outflow from the uterus empties into the **ipsilateral** uterine vein and ultimately into the internal iliac vein; venous outflow from the ovary empties into the ovarian vein, which empties into the IVC or renal vein by way of the gonadal vein. Valves are occasionally found in these veins. The right ovarian vein travels through the suspensory ligament of the ovary and

Box 12-1.	Tributaries of the internal iliac vein.

Gluteal veins	Pudendal veins
Sacral veins	Hemorrhoidal vein
Vesicular vein	Spermatic vein (m)
Uterine vein (f)	Vaginal vein (f)

f = female, m = male

generally joins the IVC directly. The left ovarian vein typically empties into the left renal vein instead of the inferior vena cava. In the male reproductive tract, the spermatic veins (male gonadal veins, testicular veins) drain the corresponding testicle and epididymis. Tributaries of the internal iliac vein include those in Box 12-1.

Pelvic Arteries

Blood supply to the pelvic organs is provided by major branches of the distal abdominal aorta. The aorta bifurcates at the level of the third lumbar vertebra (L3) into right and left **common iliac arteries** (**CIA**). See Figure 12-10. These vessels course along the pelvic sidewall and exit the pelvis via the iliac fossae. The CIA bifurcates into

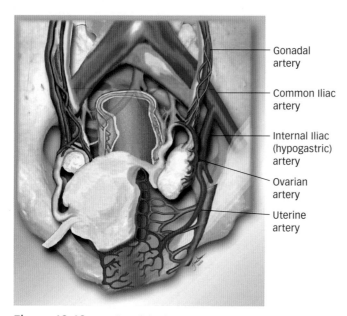

Figure 12-10. *Arteries of the female pelvis.*

Gonadal artery

Common Iliac artery

Internal Iliac (hypogastric) artery

Ovarian artery

Uterine artery

Box 12-2.	Ovarian artery resistance.	
Nondominant ovary		0.96
Follicular phase		0.86
Luteal phase		0.83

the **external** and **internal iliac (hypogastric) arteries**. The hypogastric dives deep into the pelvis and gives rise to branches which supply the uterus, cervix, and vagina. The **uterine artery** attaches to the upper third of the cervix and continues its course upward along the lateral aspect of the uterus. The **vaginal arteries** arise separately from the hypogastric artery.

The Ovarian Artery and Its Hemodynamics

Since the embryonic ovaries originate in the abdominal cavity and descend into the pelvis during gestation, they bring their original blood supply with them. The **ovarian arteries**, frequently called **gonadal arteries**, originate directly from the abdominal aorta or, alternatively, from the renal artery. The primary source of blood to the ovary is the ovarian artery. It courses through folds of the suspensory ligaments and pierces the ovary at its hilus. Branches radiate circumferentially from the hilus into the ovarian parenchyma. When blood supply through the ovarian artery is reduced by >50%, blood flow to the ovary is maintained by collateral flow from the uterine artery.

Hemodynamic alterations occur in both the ovary and—as a result of physiologic changes in the distal vascular bed that are reflected upstream—the ovarian artery. The dominant ovary is the one that, under the direction of pituitary hormones, begins the process of follicular maturation in preparation for ovulation. Neovascularization occurs in the ovarian parenchyma surrounding the developing follicles, which reduces the resistance of the entire ovary. Doppler resistance values in the ovarian artery de-

crease steadily across the follicular and ovulatory phases of the menstrual cycle (Box 12-2). Following ovulation, Doppler resistance patterns quickly return to a quiescent, less hemodynamically active state that is characterized by more highly resistant spectral waveforms. Resistance values in a nondominant ovary remain high throughout a typical 28-day cycle (Figure 12-11).

Ovarian Pathology

Ovarian artery Doppler studies provide general information about the perfusional state of an ovary based on the resistivity values obtained from the ovarian artery. Low-resistance flow in the ovarian artery is an indicator of robust metabolic activity in the ovary itself. Enhanced metabolic activity is present in both normal hormonally induced physiologic changes and most significant pathologic states, such as neoplasia, ectopic pregnancy, and pelvic inflammatory masses. The use of ovarian artery Doppler data, as an isolated diagnostic criterion, is not reliable in differentiating normal from abnormal; however, used in conjunction with related sonographic imaging findings and clinical lab values, it can be a useful adjunct.

One useful and revelatory role that color Doppler imaging does play in gynecologic applications is in detecting the presence of blood flow within the internal architecture of an adnexal mass. Color flow, particularly organized arterial flow patterns in septations or within the echogenic areas of a complex mass, argue toward it being a living neoplasm, differentiating it from the dead, lysed blood in a hemorrhagic cyst or the complex-appearing pus in a pelvic abscess (Figure 12-12).

Ovarian Torsion

Ovarian torsion is an acute gynecologic condition characterized by the twisting of the ovary and its vasculature along the ovarian ligamentous axis. When the fallopian tube twists with the ovary, the condition is referred to as **adnexal torsion**. The mechanical compression of both arterial inflow and venous outflow of the ovary disrupts the hemodynamic status of the ovary, acutely threatening

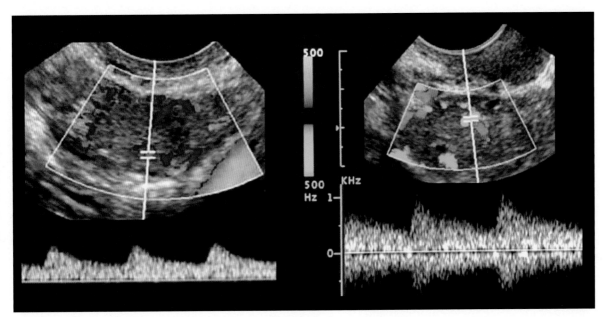

Figure 12-11. *Ovarian artery. Early follicular phase (left). Ovulatory phase (right).*

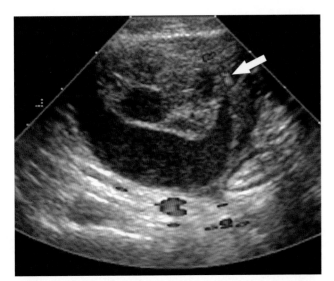

Figure 12-12. *Color Doppler imaging demonstrates blood flow in the ovarian parenchyma (arrow) but not in the complex, partially lysed thrombus in a benign ovarian cyst.*

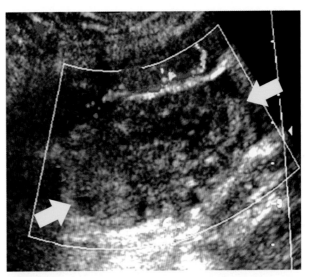

Figure 12-13. *Ovarian torsion. Ovaries (yellow arrows).*

its viability. Torsion is more common in ovaries containing a mass, which can serve as a fulcrum for levering the usually little organ out of its normal, burrowed-in position in the ovarian fossa.

As it does in many aspects of clinical medicine, sonography provides an essential piece of the diagnostic puzzle but, in itself, lacks the specificity to diagnose ovarian torsion on its own merit. Ovarian enlargement is the most common sonographic finding in patients with ovarian torsion (Figure 12-13). It is secondary to the edema caused by venous and lymphatic drainage obstruction and to the increased likelihood that an ovarian mass was the culprit for the torsion in the first place. The addition of color flow Doppler imaging may be useful but it does not yield pathognomonic information. Blood flow may be identifiable in cases of ovarian torsion arising from collateral flow into the ovary via branches of the uterine artery, and in scenarios where the ultrasound study is performed during a transient period of detorsing of the ovary. Of course, absence of flow in the ovarian hilar vessels and within the ovarian parenchyma itself is strong evidence of an ischemic ovary and supports the diagnosis of adnexal torsion.

To be certain that color Doppler imaging parameters are set appropriately for demonstrating ovarian intraparenchymal flow, scan the contralateral ovary, optimize baseline, scale, and gain settings, and *then* proceed to scan the ovary in question.

Ovarian Vein Thrombosis

Ovarian vein thrombosis is characterized by the *in situ* clotting of blood in the main venous outflow conduit of the ovary. It most commonly occurs in postpartum women but also has a propensity to arise in women with other types of pelvic pathology. Comorbidities in the pelvic region and the classic Virchow's triad (hypercoagulability, endothelial injury, and venous stasis) cause the blood in the ovarian vein to clot where it stands. The subsequent bulking up of the intraluminal thrombus and the associated inflammation of the vein itself give rise to the tubular, hypoechoic structure extending cephalad out of the adnexa that can sometimes be seen during sonographic examination (Figure 12-14). Differential diagnoses of this appearance, however, are many and include appendicitis, hydroureter, lymphadenopathy, and fallopian tube pathology. Compounded by its imaging pitfalls—particularly interposing and adjacent loops of bowel—and its lack of specificity in diagnosing ovarian vein thrombosis, Doppler ultrasonography is not a useful imaging modality in delineating the differential diagnoses of ovarian vein thrombosis. Magnetic resonance imaging (MRI) remains the superior imaging method in directing the clinician toward a proper diagnosis.

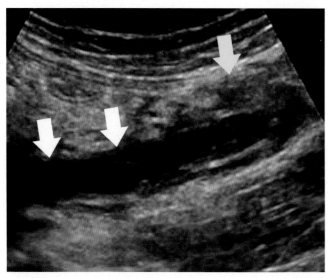

Figure 12-14. *Thrombosed ovarian vein (white arrows). Ovary (yellow arrow).*

OBSTETRIC APPLICATIONS

Hemodynamics

Doppler ultrasound applications in obstetrics attempt to predict which pregnancies will be complicated by common obstetric morbidities such as intrauterine growth restriction (IUGR) and pre-eclampsia. Both of these conditions result from placental insufficiency, a condition in which there is inadequate exchange of oxygen and nutrients between the fetus and the mother. Lacking the metabolites necessary for normal growth and development, the fetus becomes compromised, creating the hallmark sonographic picture of a small-for-gestational-age (SGA) fetus in an oligohydramniotic sac. Placental insufficiency may be caused by both fetal and maternal factors; each, however, results in similar histopathologic changes. Anomalous development of the vascular architecture or infiltration of microscopic branches of the spiral arteries by invading trophoblastic tissue thickens the walls and narrows the lumens of the small arteries in the placental bed. The resulting loss of vessel compliance increases the impedance to flow into the placenta on both maternal and fetal sides of the circulation.

The increased resistance reduces the volume of blood available for metabolic exchange. Chronic impairment of oxygen and nutrient delivery to the gestation compromises the normal growth of the fetus.

These altered hemodynamic states can be found in the uterine arteries, which are the main sources of blood to the gravid uterus. They are also found in components of the fetal circulation, such as the umbilical and middle cerebral arteries. In both instances, the normally low-resistance arterial flow characteristic of the robust perfusion that takes place throughout a normal gestation is restricted by physiologic or pathologic changes. The associated hemodynamic changes are similar on both sides of the maternofetal circulation; the low-resistance waveforms become increasingly resistive as the pregnancy progresses. This is reflected by an increase in both the pulsatility index and the resistivity index values obtained from uterine and umbilical arteries and becomes particularly evident with the appearance of hallmark spectral waveform anomalies—diastolic notching and flow reversal. Doppler ultrasound is one of several tools that allow the clinician to manage patients with known or suspected complications of pregnancy.

Box 12-3.	Indications for fetal Doppler examination.	
Hypertensive disorders	Suspected IUGR	
Diabetic disorders	Known IUGR (serial surveillance)	
Other maternal comorbidities	Rh isoimmunization	
Placental abnormalities	Fetal comorbidity	
	Multiple gestation complications	

Indications for fetal Doppler examination are listed in Box 12-3.

Bioeffects

Little has been reported in the medical literature on the **bioeffects** of high-frequency ultrasound exposure in human embryos and fetuses. Obvious ethical implications precluded the design of *in vivo* human studies. However, several experiments in other mammalian embryos suggest there are no significant or appreciable adverse effects from ultrasound energies used during routine imaging.

On the other hand, since there are documented variations in both tissue temperature (as measured by the **thermal index** [**TI**]) and nonthermal mechanisms observed in studies of the central nervous system (as measured by the **mechanical index** [**MI**]), prudent use of ultrasound in all trimesters of pregnancy is imperative. Exposure should be kept as low as reasonably achievable (ALARA) because of the potential for tissue heating. Higher energy deposition in tissue is of particular concern for pulsed Doppler and color flow imaging used in first trimester ultrasound with a long transvesical path (> 5 cm), and in second or third trimester exams when bone is in the focal zone, as well as when scanning tissue with minimal perfusion (embryonic) or patients who are febrile.

Doppler Ultrasound in Failed Pregnancy

Trophoblastic tissue is some of the most metabolically active tissue found in the human body. As a conceptus evolves from a small sphere of cells into a fully formed fetus by the end of the first trimester, there is rapid and abundant growth of new micro- and macrovascular networks necessary to support a normal and successful gestation. Trophoblastic hemodynamic patterns reflect the continuous need for oxygen and metabolites that

the rapidly proliferating tissue requires. There is robust, unimpeded forward flow of blood into trophoblastic tissue beds. Spectral Doppler waveforms are characterized by high-velocity, high-amplitude values throughout the cardiac cycle. Color Doppler imaging typically presents bright and aliased filling of the vascular rete associated with trophoblastic tissue.

Trophoblastic tissue is normally found within the uterine cavity in association with an intrauterine gestation. However, pathologic trophoblastic tissue, both within and outside of the uterus, presents as hemodynamically similar. Identification of a sonographically complex mass, without evidence of an intact gestational sac in a patient with discriminatory levels of serum beta-hCG, is strong evidence that the mass is the gestation. Located outside of the uterus, the mass is an ectopic pregnancy; within the uterus, it is a failed gestation. The presence and identification of trophoblastic hemodynamic patterns in soft tissue areas of the pelvis are clinically useful in:

- Localizing a gestational event in a woman suspected of having an ectopic pregnancy.

- Early diagnosis of primary gestational trophoblastic disease.

- Detecting retained products of conception in the uterus following a normal or failed intrauterine pregnancy.

Ectopic Pregnancy

Ectopic pregnancy, the implantation of a conceptus anywhere outside of the central uterine cavity, is a condition that requires quick and accurate diagnosis to reduce the very real risk of maternal mortality and to help minimize the serious clinical and reproductive sequelae associated with its complications. While Doppler ultrasound interrogation of the uterus and parauterine structures can help illuminate solid, perfused structures from the myriad loops of interposing bowel, it adds little to improving or enhancing the diagnosis of ectopic pregnancy. The role of sonography in the diagnosis of extrauterine gestations is to provide a diagnosis of exclusion. In patients with discriminatory levels of serum beta-hCG, the presence of an empty uterus is sufficient evidence for most clinicians to initiate treatment. The identification of an adnexal or cul-de-sac mass and free fluid, particularly one associated with trophoblastic hemodynamic patterns, cements the diagnosis and may help localize the anatomic site of implantation.

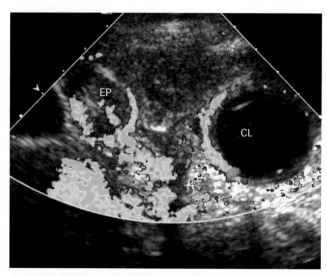

Figure 12-15. *Ectopic pregnancy (EP) in right adnexa. Corpus luteum cyst (CL) in left adnexa. Note orientation.*

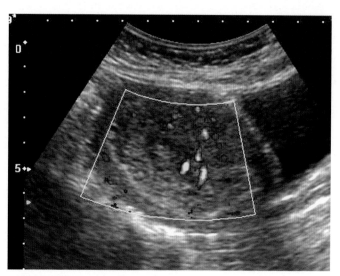

Figure 12-16. *Gestational trophoblastic disease. Power Doppler imaging demonstrates robust flow around the periphery of a hydatidiform mole.*

Intact ectopic pregnancies have been seen with regularity in clinical ultrasound practice since the introduction of high-resolution endovaginal probes. In addition to cardiovascular tube activity demonstrable in the embryo, an organized semicircle of preplacental trophoblastic vasculature surrounding the gestation reflects a dramatic color Doppler "ring of fire." The accompanying image (Figure 12-15) also demonstrates the similarity of the color Doppler appearance of the vasculature perfusing the ectopic pregnancy to that of the corpus luteum cyst of pregnancy. Both are metabolically active structures requiring a continuous supply of arterial blood.

Gestational Trophoblastic Neoplasia

Not all types of abnormal trophoblastic tissue are related to a concomitant pregnancy. Gestational trophoblastic neoplasia (GTN) is a spectrum of pathologic entities resulting from the excessive proliferation of trophoblastic tissue. Traditional classification of GTN divided it into hydatidiform mole, invasive mole, and choriocarcinoma. More specific histologic schemata have been developed and are used in the clinical management of GTN. From a hemodynamic perspective, however, these three entities demonstrate the spectrum of possibilities when trophoblastic cells from the placenta turn malignant. The most common type of GTN is **complete hydatidiform mole**, in which the uterine cavity is filled with grape-like clusters of hydropic villi. There is no identifiable placental or embryonic tissue present. While the preponderance of a hydatidiform mole is cystic in nature, high-amplitude flow associated with trophoblastic tissue permits demonstration

of the vascular component of the mass, particularly when using low-threshold color and **power Doppler** imaging methods (Figure 12-16). An **invasive mole** (chorioadenoma destruens) burrows into the myometrium at the site of implantation and is histologically identical to a complete mole. Similarly, there may be foci of high-amplitude, low-resistance arterial flow seen within the uterus and/or myometrium using color or power Doppler. **Choriocarcinoma** is a solid tumor consisting of sheets of trophoblastic cells alternating with layers of hemorrhage. It appears sonographically as an irregularly marginated solid mass within the uterus. There are no remarkable hemodynamic characteristics observable with Doppler imaging.

Retained Products of Conception

Retained products of conception (RPOCs) are residual fragments of fetal, placental, and/or vascular tissue remaining after an early pregnancy loss or, in some cases, even after a normal, full parturition. RPOCs are more frequently associated with the early termination of pregnancy, either spontaneous or elective. The sonographic and Doppler ultrasound appearance of RPOCs is dependent upon how much and what types of products remain *in situ*. Thrombosis, fresh and lysed blood, and ischemic tissue will yield a complex sonographic appearance but lack active hemodynamics. Remnants of trophoblastic and placental tissue that retain their vascular connections to the uterus will also present as a sonographically complex mass, but robust blood flow will be easily demonstrated within and around these masses (Figure 12-17).

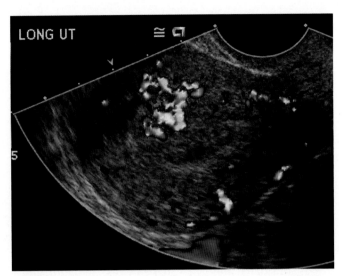

Figure 12-17. *Retained products of conception. Color Doppler imaging demonstrates enhanced flow patterns typical of trophoblastic tissue remaining in the uterus after a spontaneous abortion.*

1st trimester

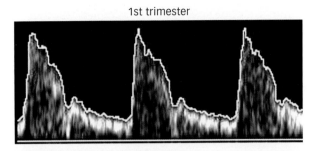

Mid-trimester

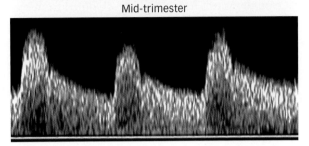

Figure 12-18. *Uterine artery spectral waveforms.*

Uterine Artery Doppler

Uterine artery Doppler studies provide a snapshot of the hemodynamic status of a uterus and its contents. There are profoundly different perfusional requirements and associated hemodynamic changes between a gravid and nongravid uterus. Few clinical applications for Doppler ultrasound are found in the regular practice of gynecology; its utility lies mainly in obstetrics.

Nongravid Uterine Hemodynamics

Rhythmic changes in uterine blood flow during the menstrual cycle are mediated by fluctuating levels of progesterone and estrogens in the blood. The periarterial sympathetic vasoconstrictor nerves respond to these ovarian steroids, regulating arterial inflow to the uterus; estrogens decrease the vasoconstrictor effects while progesterone increases them. In clinical terms, estrogen allows more blood flow into the uterus, progesterone less. This phenomenon can be demonstrated by the variations found in uterine artery resistance in hormonally disparate women. Uterine artery flow in women on **hormone replacement therapy** (**HRT**)—which always includes an estrogen component and sometimes contains a progesterone component—demonstrates a lowly resistive hemodynamic pattern in the uterine artery. Postmenopausal women not on HRT enter into a physiologic state characterized by chronic estrogen depletion. Uterine artery Doppler demonstrates a highly resistive flow pattern with no cyclical variations.

Gravid Uterine Hemodynamics

In pregnant patients, the hemodynamic status of the uterine artery undergoes significant and dramatic changes. During the first trimester, the rapidly growing trophoblastic tissue implanted in the highly vascularized endometrium requires a substantial increase in blood flow to provide for the metabolic needs of the conceptus. This is reflected in a reduction in both the pulsatility and resistivity values. By the mid-trimester, resistance in the uterine artery has decreased and will remain so for the remainder of the gestation (Figure 12-18). Some groups have studied these hemodynamic changes and have found a positive association between an adequate supply of blood, as measured with various Doppler parameters, and the ultimate success of the pregnancy. Specific, predictive values, however, have not been standardized or widely accepted in clinical practice.

Placental Hemodynamics

By the mid-second and third trimesters, the placenta has become the hemodynamic workhorse of the gestation. The fetus depends entirely upon the properly formed and functional apposition of the microscopic endpoints of both maternal and fetal tissue. Fetal chorionic villi project into tiny pools of maternal blood that bathe the cells with the requisite mix of oxygen and nutrients. The maternal blood filling the villi arrives from main uterine arteries that arborize into the **spiral arteries** that squirt blood into the many intervillous spaces. A normal placenta is a large vascular mass offering little resistance to the bolus of blood pumping into the pelvis at a rate of approximately

600 cc/min. A uterine artery PI of 1.7 is typical throughout the second and third trimesters. Blood depleted of its vital components and laden with metabolic waste products drains from placental cotyledons though the placental veins to be carried back to the maternal heart via the retroperitoneal venous vasculature.

Doppler Methods—Uterine Artery

Spectral Doppler waveforms should be obtained from one or both uterine arteries as they course toward the uterus and attach at the level of the cervix (Figure 12-19). There are three criteria that can be gleaned from a Doppler spectral waveform that add valuable information about the hemodynamic status of the uterus and, by extension, to the pregnancy itself: the pulsatility index, the resistivity index, and spectral "notching."

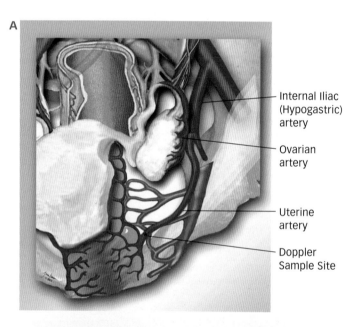

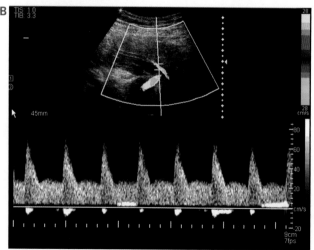

Figure 12-19. A *Uterine artery Doppler sample site.* **B** *Sample volume and waveform.*

Pulsatility Index The pulsatility index (PI) from the uterine artery has been used in several attempts to predict adverse outcomes in patients at risk for a compromised pregnancy. There is broad agreement that an increased PI after 34 weeks has a statistical association with obstetric complications such as maternal or fetal disease, delivery of small-for-gestational-age (SGA) infants, premature labor, and the necessity of labor induction. Abnormal uterine artery pulsatility values are a better predictor of pre-eclampsia than they are of IUGR.

Resistivity Index Measured using the standard RI formula (see page 376), the RI is a general and nonspecific detector of increased placental resistance. A value greater than 0.58 is considered abnormal after 24 weeks' gestation and is evidence that fetal outcome may be compromised as the pregnancy progresses. Nevertheless, when RI is used alone its prognostic value is less than that of diastolic notching.

Diastolic Notching The appearance of a rapid vertical deflection of the spectral waveform at the beginning of diastole is referred to as diastolic notching. The "notch" results from a momentary, reactive vasospasm that is triggered as receding blood volume and pressure decline at the end of systole. This criterion is more reliable in predicting adverse fetal outcomes as it occurs in the middle of the cardiac cycle, not at end-diastole, where a waveform may appear normal and produce a normal RI value. The appearance of a diastolic notch is of prognostic value only after 24 weeks' gestation. Prior to that, it may be seen as a normal spectral variant (Figure 12-20).

Of the three criteria standing alone, diastolic notching has a better record of predicting adverse fetal outcomes than does RI. When two of three Doppler spectral abnormalities are observed in the same pregnancy, fetal compromise is nearly assured.

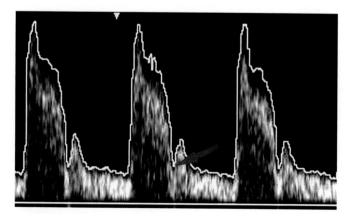

Figure 12-20. *Diastolic notch.*

Umbilical Arterial Doppler

While uterine artery Doppler provides information about the resistance that the uterus and its contents maintain against the hemodynamic pressure exerted on them by the maternal circulation, spectral Doppler interrogation of the umbilical arteries provides information about the resistance the placenta presents to the fetal side of the circulation. The resistance on both sides of the circulation is determined by the structural integrity and vascular capacitance of the placenta. Increased resistance caused by a compromise in either of these elements can be identified with Doppler ultrasound. Umbilical artery Doppler is a noninvasive method of assessing fetal physiologic status by studying hemodynamic patterns and alterations that can be predictive of untoward pregnancy outcomes. Because Doppler interrogation sites in a fetus are more accessible and varied than the uterine artery, umbilical artery Doppler is the method of choice in obstetric Doppler ultrasound applications.

Umbilical Artery Hemodynamics

Deoxygenated blood is pumped by the fetal heart through the **umbilical arteries** to the placenta. Beyond the cord insertion, the paired umbilical arteries spread across the placental surface, penetrating the parenchyma and ultimately giving rise to the myriad arborized branches that terminate in each chorionic villus. Following the physiologic exchange that takes places within the villus, oxygenated, nutrient-rich blood returns to the fetus via the single **umbilical vein**. Factors that influence hemodynamic patterns found in umbilical arteries include the morphologic and functional status of the distal vascular bed, i.e., the placenta itself, and the cardiovascular status of the fetus.

As previously described, a normal placenta is a large mass of physiologically active tissue arranged within a complex interwoven vascular network that must handle an ever-increasing volume of blood as a gestation advances. As one would expect, normal umbilical artery spectral Doppler waveforms demonstrate low resistance throughout gestation. In the umbilical arteries, powered by the 160–200 beats per minute of a normal fetal heart, there is constant forward flow of blood toward the placenta throughout the cardiac cycle. Because of the rapidity of the heart rate, diastolic flow never reaches zero, describing a condition in which there is always a forward flow component above which systolic accelerations take place (Figure 12-21).

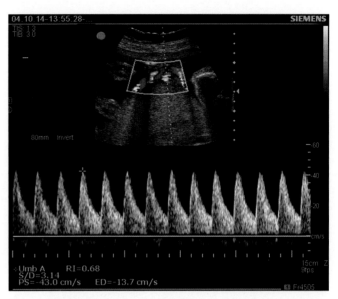

Figure 12-21. *Normal umbilical artery Doppler waveform.*

Doppler Methods—Umbilical Artery

Doppler signals are obtained from either umbilical artery in the mid-portion of the cord or near its insertion on the placental surface. Because the diagnostic criteria used in Doppler studies of the umbilical artery are ratios of values obtained from the same spectral waveform, Doppler angle is irrelevant—obviating the need for time-consuming and error-inducing angle correction. Whichever numeric ratio is used, the hallmark hemodynamic change observed in umbilical artery Doppler studies is an increase in resistance (Figure 12-22). Recall the hemodynamic rule of thumb: As pregnancy progresses, resistance decreases. On serial sonographic examination, Doppler measures of resistance decrease or they may stabilize and remain constant from exam to exam. Both findings are normal. What is never normal is evidence of increasing resistance, as reflected by stunted diastolic flow and the consequent increase in either PI or RI.

A significant increase in placental resistance can severely compromise a pregnancy. Underlying maternal comorbidities and risk factors, particularly gestational hypertensive states and diabetes, damage the delicately intertwined apposition of trophoblastic and vascular tissue that forms the functional villi of the placenta. As vascular channels constrict and become clogged with metabolic detritus, blood pressure in the distal vascular bed increases. This increased pressure is transmitted upstream to the umbilical artery and its chorionic surface branches and is reflected in the associated spectral Doppler waveforms.

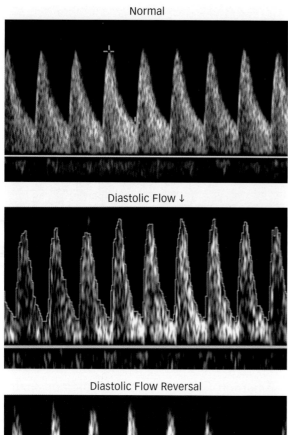

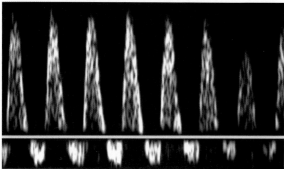

Figure 12-22. *Increasing resistance demonstrated with serial Doppler studies.*

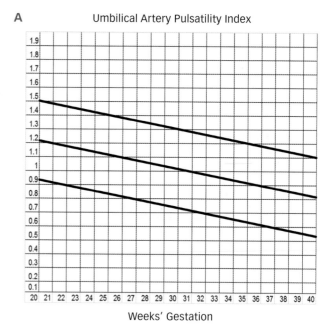

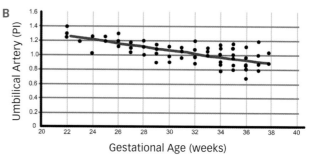

Figure 12-23. A *and* **B** *Nomograms: Obstetric Doppler parameters.*

Umbilical artery hemodynamics, as reflected by Doppler ultrasound findings, can be summarized as follows:

- Relatively high resistance to flow is normally observed in the early second trimester of pregnancy.
- Resistance decreases with advancing gestational age.
- Highly resistive waveforms are always abnormal.
- A persistence of reduced diastolic flow on serial sonograms is associated with a poor pregnancy outcome.
- Diastolic flow reversal = severely compromised fetus.

In clinical obstetric practice, nomograms that are adapted to gestational age are available for the **systolic-to-diastolic (S/D) ratio**, resistivity index (RI), and pulsatility index (PI) upon which serial resistivity values can be plotted (Figure 12-23).

Ductus Venosus and Umbilical Vein Doppler

The **ductus venosus** (**DV**) is a regulator of oxygen to the fetus. It can open and close as necessary and is mediated by the fetal autonomic nervous system. Half the oxygenated blood returning from the placenta can be directed through the ductus venosus. Thus, as fetal compromise increases, the ductus venosus can dilate to shunt blood directly to the fetal heart. During hypoxia, pressure in the umbilical vein increases and more blood is shunted through the ductus venosus. In fetal compromise, as much as 70% of blood returning from the placenta is directed into the inferior vena cava through the ductus venosus. Increased pulsatility in the venous circulation is the result of cardiac compromise from increased cardiac afterload.

Umbilical vein pulsations are a common finding in the early, normal pregnancy and are associated with fetal breathing. However, when the fetus is acutely compromised, increased pressure in the fetal heart creates a notching in the umbilical venous waveform. This is a severe finding of tremendous clinical significance (described on page 386).

Middle Cerebral Artery Doppler

Doppler evaluation of the fetal **middle cerebral arteries** (MCAs) plays a crucial role in both the assessment of growth-restricted fetuses and the management of fetuses with anemia. Intracerebral hemodynamic changes signal the onset of "brain sparing"— the physiologic response that preferentially shunts blood to the brain when there is not an adequate supply to support the entire fetus, a hallmark of IUGR. The reduced viscosity of blood in anemic fetuses creates the elevated peak systolic velocities found in their cerebral arteries. Contemporary high-resolution color Doppler imaging systems make the identification of intracranial vascular anatomy a reliable and reproducible way of studying fetal physiologic changes in high-risk pregnancies.

Cerebral-Umbilical Ratio and Velocimetry

In addition to the more familiar hemodynamic measures of distal vascular bed resistance (RI, PI, S/D ratio), Doppler studies of the MCA rely on two values that contribute to the identification of a compromised pregnancy: velocimetry (PSV) and the cerebral-umbilical ratio (CU). **Velocimetry** is the measurement of blood flow velocities in the MCA and is useful in identifying anemic fetuses. Viscosity of blood is a prime determinant of its flow capabilities and maintains an inversely proportional relationship with velocity: As viscosity increases, velocity decreases; as viscosity decreases, velocity increases. The reduced viscosity of red cell–deficient blood in anemic fetuses yields the elevated peak systolic velocities that are characteristic Doppler findings in the fetal MCA.

The **cerebral-umbilical ratio** is an indicator of relative resistance between the fetus and the placenta.

$$CU = \frac{CRI}{URI}$$

Shifts in blood from the placenta toward the fetal brain, reflected as an increase in the CU ratio, are strong evidence that brain-sparing is under way. The main pitfall of the CU ratio is that it is equally dependent on the RI of the placenta. Structural or functional abnormalities of the placenta can increase the umbilical artery RI (URI), which, by virtue of its inversely proportional nature, will decrease the CU ratio. Still, when used as a piece in the overall clinical management of a patient with a high-risk pregnancy, the CU ratio can help identify fetal cerebral hemodynamic changes that are associated with an increased risk of fetal compromise.

Doppler Methods of Cerebral Resistivity (CRI, URI, and CU)

The **cerebral resistivity index** (**CRI**) is calculated on a Doppler spectral waveform obtained from one of the two fetal middle cerebral arteries. Doppler ultrasound interrogation of intracranial fetal circulation begins in the same axial plane that is used to measure the biparietal diameter (BPD). With color Doppler engaged, the ultrasound beam is directed toward the base of the skull, where the circle of Willis and its component arteries will be readily found. The MCA is easily demonstrated as a major branch arising from the circle at the level of the lesser wing of the sphenoid bone. Spectral Doppler signals are obtained from the MCA approximately 1 cm above its takeoff from the circle (Figure 12-24). Slight adjustments in transducer position and reducing the baseline and threshold levels

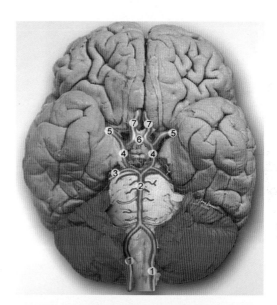

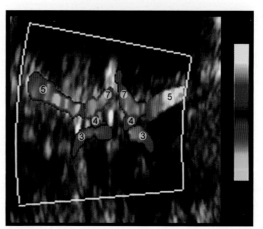

Figure 12-24. *Circle of Willis. Vertebral artery (1), basilar artery (2), posterior cerebral artery (3), posterior communicating artery (4), internal carotid artery (5), anterior communicating artery (6), and anterior cerebral artery (7).*

help to optimize the color Doppler image, which is used to localize the spectral interrogation site. The RI is calculated using standard methods.

Similarly, the **umbilical artery resistivity index (URI)** is calculated from a spectral waveform obtained from the umbilical artery in the manner described above. The two RI values set against each other yield the cerebral-umbilical

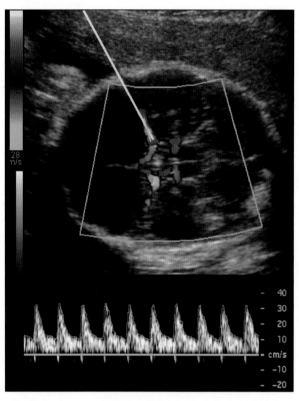

Figure 12-25. *Cerebral artery velocimetry.*

(CU) ratio, which describes the relative impedance to blood flow between the placenta and the fetus. In a normal pregnancy, there is a general parity between cerebral and placental flow with a CU of about 1.0. Fetuses with CU values of less than 1.0 or falling below the 5th percentile are more likely to be compromised.

Doppler Methods—Velocimetry
Measurement of peak systolic velocity is obtained from the same location in the MCA as that used in calculating the cerebral resistivity index. The angle of insonation between the central portion of the ultrasound beam and the proximal segment of the MCA should be kept as close to zero (<10°) as possible, which provides the highest-amplitude Doppler signal and the most correct PSV values. Doppler interrogation of the MCA closest to the transducer usually yields better results and, since cerebral flow velocities have been noted to change significantly during physiologically active states, the study is best done when the fetus is asleep and quiet (Figure 12-25).

The primary diagnostic criterion in MCA Doppler studies is the relationship between the PSV and the velocity averaged over the entire concurrent cardiac cycle, i.e., the average, or mean, velocity (V_{MEAN}). An increase of MCA PSV over V_{MEAN} by ≥ 1.5 SD carries a high statistical association between severe anemia and isoimmunized pregnancy. Elevated cerebral PSVs have also been reported in various medical conditions such as fetal compromise (both growth restriction and hypoxia), twin-twin transfusion syndrome, and fetal intracranial lesions such as tumors and intracranial hemorrhage (Figure 12-26).

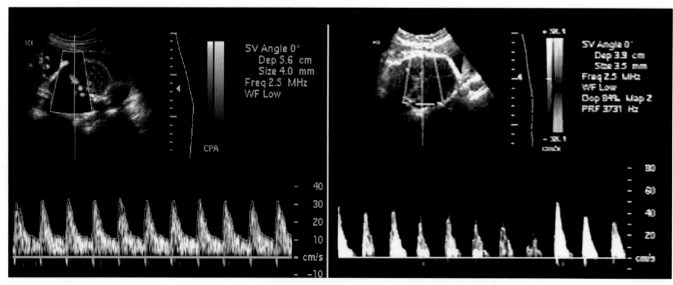

Figure 12-26. *Cerebral (MCA) Doppler spectral waveforms. Normal (left) and compromised fetus (right).*

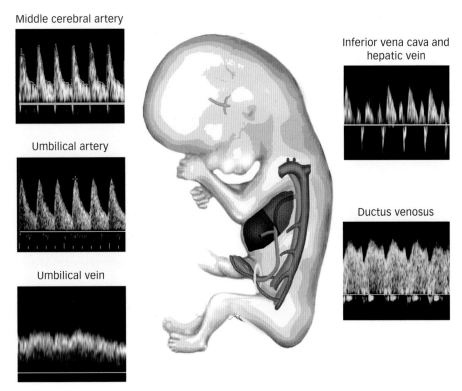

Figure 12-27. *Normal Doppler spectral waveforms in the fetus.*

SCANNING TIPS, GUIDELINES, AND PITFALLS

1. Adjacent vascular structures can be confused with the vessel of interest. The close physical proximity and small size of the myriad arterial and venous vascular structures in the pelvis create a challenge to the examiner in accurately localizing and identifying vessels of interest. A thorough knowledge of anatomy and a sensitive color Doppler instrument are requisite. In obstetric patients exhibiting a centrally located placenta, sampling should be done on each side.

2. The uterine artery is localized by identifying the common iliac artery and following it to its bifurcation into internal and external iliac arteries. The uterine artery arises from the internal iliac artery, lies just beyond the bifurcation, and courses medially toward the lower uterine segment. The ideal uterine artery Doppler signal is obtained about 1 cm into the vessel.

3. Do Doppler exams in a quiescent pregnancy. Umbilical artery waveform measurements should not be made during periods of fetal activity, breathing, or uterine contractions. Middle cerebral artery Doppler waveforms should be obtained when the fetus is quiescent and/or sleeping. Fetal activity momentarily increases both systolic and diastolic pressures and can skew Doppler ratios.

4. At least three measurements should be obtained and the mean result calculated for each of the indices (S/D, PI, and RI).

5. A low-pass filter should be used (50–100 Hz) to eliminate low frequencies produced by arterial wall pulsations.

6. Umbilical artery Doppler spectral waveforms should be obtained near the placental end of the cord.

7. Middle cerebral artery: When viewing the brain stem in the axial view, one can observe an oblique cross-section of the internal carotid artery at the bifurcation into the anterior and middle cerebral arteries anterior to the cerebral peduncles. The MCA is located caudal to the cerebral peduncles at the same level as the pons, medulla oblongata, and greater paired wings of the sphenoid. Measurements should not be taken during fetal breathing or movement, and the mother should be comfortably positioned to avoid supine hypotensive syndrome. Color Doppler can be used to help identify the circle of Willis. The angle of insonation should be 0 degree, and the Doppler gate should be close to the origin of the internal carotid artery. For the most accurate peak systolic velocity, angle correct to ≤ 10 degrees.

8. A summary of normal Doppler waveforms in the fetus can be found in Figure 12-27.

REFERENCES

1. Brown AS, Reid AD, Leamen L, et al: Biological effects of high-frequency ultrasound exposure during mouse organogenesis. Ultrasound Med Biol 9:1223–1232, 2004.

2. Bly S, Van den Hof MC: Obstetric ultrasound biological effects and safety. J Obstet Gynaecol Can 6:572–580, 2005.

SELF-ASSESSMENT EXERCISES

Questions

1. The primary vessels supplying blood to the pelvic organs are the:
   A. Gonadal arteries
   B. Internal iliac arteries
   C. Spermatic arteries
   D. External iliac arteries

2. All of the following Doppler ultrasound findings can be associated with ovarian torsion *except*:
   A. Ovarian hyperemia
   B. Ovarian enlargement
   C. Ovarian mass
   D. Absent ovarian parenchymal blood flow

3. All of the following Doppler ultrasound studies can be useful in helping to predict fetal growth restriction *except*:
   A. Umbilical artery Doppler
   B. Fetal cerebral artery Doppler
   C. Uterine artery Doppler
   D. Internal iliac artery Doppler

4. The various Doppler ultrasound modalities used in assessing pelvic organs can demonstrate all of the hemodynamic parameters listed below *except*:
   A. Pressure of flow
   B. Presence of flow
   C. Flow direction
   D. Pulsatility of flow

5. The Doppler criterion that provides the best indicator of diastolic runoff into a distal vascular bed is the:
   A. S/D ratio
   B. End-diastolic velocity
   C. Resistivity index
   D. Pulsatility index

6. The diastolic notch is best described as:
   A. Flow reversal in early diastole
   B. Flow reversal in late diastole
   C. Early diastolic flow reduction
   D. Late diastolic flow reduction

7. Spectral Doppler waveforms obtained from arteries supplying trophoblastic tissue will demonstrate:
   A. High-amplitude, low-resistance flow
   B. High-amplitude, high-resistance flow
   C. High-amplitude, triphasic flow
   D. Low-amplitude, monophasic flow

8. Hemodynamic changes occur in the uterine arteries in response to cyclical variations in hormone levels. As the uterus cycles toward menstruation, how do blood flow patterns change?
   A. The resistance decreases.
   B. The resistance increases.
   C. The pulsatility increases.
   D. There is no discernible change.

9. Which of the following is not a Doppler ultrasound finding associated with a compromised pregnancy?
   A. Flow reversal in diastole
   B. Increasing resistance on serial surveillance
   C. Decreasing resistance on serial surveillance
   D. Diastolic notching

10. In performing a uterine artery Doppler study, the spectral range gate (sample volume) should be placed:
    A. Near its origin at the internal iliac artery
    B. Mid-vessel, with strongest color signal
    C. Near the cervix
    D. Anywhere along its course

Answers

See Appendix F on page 616 for answers and explanations.

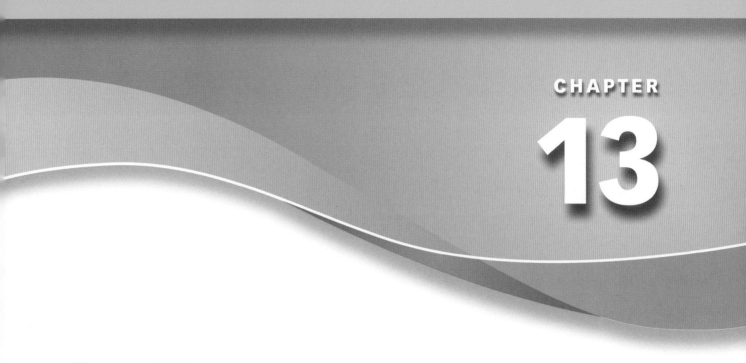

Infertility

George Koulianos, MD, FACOG, and Kathryn A. Gill, MS, RT, RDMS, FSDMS

OBJECTIVES

After completing this chapter you should be able to:

1. Define infertility and list male and female factors that affect fertility.

2. Discuss the various tests performed to identify a fertility problem.

3. List and describe the various techniques of fertility assistance.

4. Explain why age is a significant factor affecting female fertility.

5. Describe how sonography is used to monitor follicular development.

INFERTILITY IS DEFINED AS THE INABILITY to achieve pregnancy after one year of unprotected intercourse for women under 35 and six months for those over 35 years old. Once thought to be solely a female condition, infertility can be the result of male as well as female contributing factors and affects about 80 million couples worldwide. Approximately 10% of the reproductive-age population have problems conceiving. Factors that may play a role in increasing the number of couples seeking evaluation and treatment include delay in starting a family for any num-

ber of reasons and improved success rates with assisted reproductive technologies. In about 20% of couples, both the man and the woman have conditions that contribute to infertility, whereas for 40% of couples infertility is related only to male or female factors.

Several male factors can affect fertility, including varicoceles (40%), cryptorchidism, obstruction, testicular failure, semen disorders, endocrine disorders, infection, and genetic and idiopathic factors (Box 13-1). Both maternal and paternal age can affect fertility. The age factor is not

Box 13-1.	Male factors contributing to infertility.
	Varicoceles (40%)
	Cryptorchidism
	Obstruction
	Testicular failure
	Semen disorders
	Endocrine disorders
	Infections
	Genetic factors
	Idiopathic factors

as sensitive in males, however, although reports have indicated that fathers over the age of 50 have a greater risk of contributing to birth defects such as Down syndrome and achondroplasia as well as a higher incidence of intrauterine fetal death.

GYNECOLOGIC FACTORS IN INFERTILITY

Because the focus of this volume is on gynecologic sonography, this chapter considers female factors that contribute to infertility. These include ovarian/ovulatory dysfunction (40%), tubal disorders, and peritoneal and uterine factors (Box 13-2). In addition, age is a particularly important factor for females. Pregnancy rates begin to decline in the mid-30s, and the slope becomes steeper with advancing age. It is well documented that women over the age of 40 have much lower pregnancy rates and higher incidences of miscarriage and offspring with Down syndrome compared to women younger than 40. It seems that a woman's best chance for fertility is between the ages of 18 and 30 years. If we review what we know about the ovary and follicular development, we understand better why this happens.

In the female fetus, the ovaries contain approximately 7 million eggs, but at term the number has decreased to between 1 million and 2 million. By puberty, the normal female will be down to about 400,000 eggs, and those will steadily decline with age at a rate of about 1000 per month. Fertility rates are halved in the decade following age 25. Not only does the number of eggs rapidly diminish after age 35, but the quality of the eggs also deteriorates, contributing to an increased risk for birth defects. By age 40, fertility is 15% of what it was at age 25, and there is only a 1% chance of success after age 44.

ULTRASOUND IMAGING AND LABORATORY TESTS

For these reasons, women pursuing in vitro fertilization undergo a battery of tests to help determine the number and quality of their eggs. These tests include ultrasound imaging and various blood analyses (Box 13-3).

Ovarian Reserve

Assessment of **ovarian reserve**—the number of remaining eggs and therefore the fertility potential—involves determining the number of **antral follicles** (fluid-filled

Box 13-2.	Female factors contributing to infertility.
Ovarian/ovulatory dysfunction (40%)	
Tubal disorders	
Peritoneal factors	
Uterine factors	

Box 13-3.	Tests to determine number/quality of eggs.
Follicle-stimulating hormone (FSH)	
Estradiol	
Clomiphene citrate challenge test (CCCT)	
Sonography for ovarian volume/antral follicles	

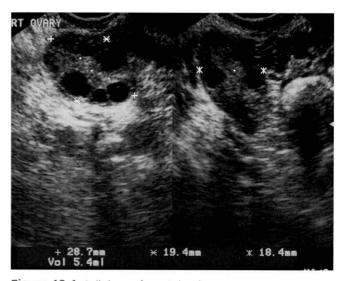

Figure 13-1. *Split-image format showing proper measurements taken to calculate ovarian volume.*

areas on the ovary where eggs grow) and calculating ovarian volume. Ovarian volumes are easily calculated by taking an average of the longitudinal, transverse, and anterior/posterior (AP) measurements of the ovary (Figure 13-1). The formula for calculating ovarian volume is V = (longitudinal × AP × transverse measurements) × 0.523 cc. Some ultrasound systems have ovarian volume calculation packages programmed into the system, or one can simply refer to a chart (Table 13-1; see also Appendix A, Table 6).

Table 13-1.   Adult ovarian volumes.

Parameter		
Age (decade)	No. of Ovaries	Mean Volume (cm³ ± SD)
1	19	1.7 ± 1.4
2	83	7.8 ± 4.4
3	308	10.2 ± 6.2
4	358	9.5 ± 5.4
5	206	9.0 ± 5.8
6	57	6.2 ± 5.7
7	44	6.0 ± 3.8
Menstrual Status		
	No. of Ovaries	Mean Volume (cm³ ± SD)
Menstruating	866	9.8 ± 5.8
Postmenopausal	100	5.8 ± 3.6

Reprinted with permission from Cohen HL, Tice HM, Mandel FS: Ovarian volumes measured by ultrasound: bigger than we think. Radiology 177:189–192, 1990.

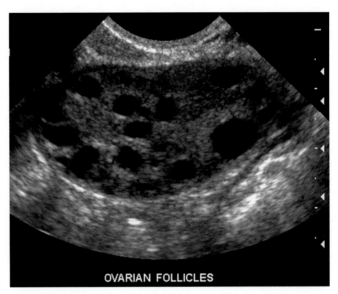

Figure 13-2. *Long-axis transvaginal view of a normal ovary demonstrating multiple antral follicles.*

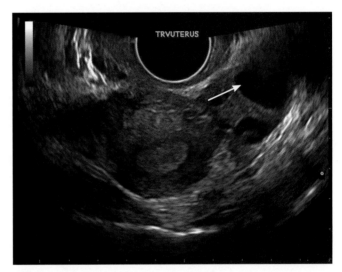

Figure 13-3. *Transvaginal image showing a dominant follicle (arrow).*

A normal ovary has, on average, 11.6 ± 6.2 antral follicles. Patients with diminished ovarian reserve usually have 4.2 ± 3.3 follicles on days 2–3 of a baseline cycle. Antral follicle counts are the best predictors of the ovary's response to ovulatory stimulation. Normal cycles begin with the follicle measuring 5–6 mm in diameter (Figure 13-2). These follicles grow about 2 mm per day until one clearly becomes dominant on days 6–7 (menstrual dates) of the cycle (Figure 13-3). The egg is nurtured to maturity by the brain (follicle-stimulating hormone is secreted by the pituitary gland) and the follicle (which secretes estradiol, the most potent naturally occurring estrogen). The oocyte itself is microscopic and cannot be imaged sonographically. Nevertheless, the **cumulus oophorus**—the mass of epithelial granulosa cells that surrounds the oocyte in the vesicular ovarian follicle—may be detected as a cyst-like structure on the wall of the dominant follicle. It will be about 1 mm in diameter (Figure 13-4). Visualization of the cumulus oophorus indicates follicle maturity and suggests that ovulation will occur within 36 hours. Sonographic indications of ovulation include identifica-

tion of fluid in the cul-de-sac and development of the follicle into the corpus luteum (Figure 13-5A). A corpus luteum may be two to three times larger than the original follicle and contain debris (Figures 13-5 B and C).

Evaluation of ovaries for infertility baseline and monitoring should be performed with transvaginal technique. The technology offers much better resolution and more accurate measurements that are more easily reproduced.

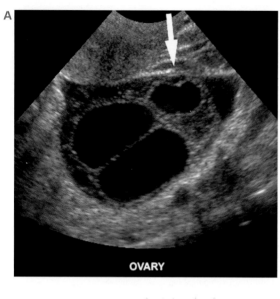

A

OVARY

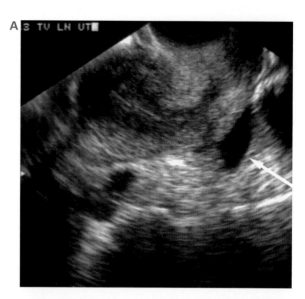

A

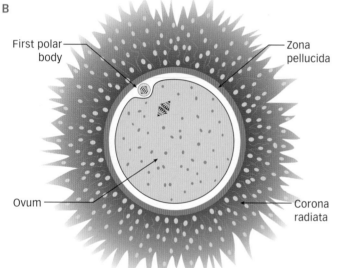

B

First polar body

Zona pellucida

Ovum

Corona radiata

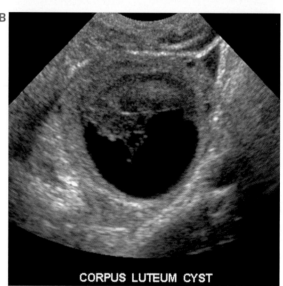

B

CORPUS LUTEUM CYST

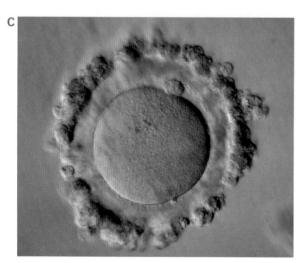

C

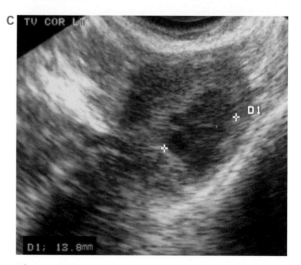

C

D1

D1; 13.8mm

Figure 13-4. A *This ovary contains a follicle demonstrating the cumulus oophorus (arrow).* **B** *Drawing of an oocyte.* **C** *Mature oocyte with visible polar body and with coronal cells still attached to the zona pellucida.*

Figure 13-5. A *A small amount of fluid is seen behind the cervix (arrow) after ovulation.* **B** *Transvaginal image of a corpus luteum cyst containing some hemorrhagic debris.* **C** *Transvaginal image of a hemorrhagic corpus luteum cyst (calipers) showing very irregular edges and almost solid in appearance.*

Blood Analysis

Follicle-Stimulating Hormone Level

The "cycle day 3 FSH" is a blood test that measures the level of **follicle-stimulating hormone** (**FSH**) on the third day of the menstrual cycle (third day of bleeding). If the FSH is high, the brain has to work harder to stimulate the ovaries; therefore an abnormally high FSH can cause infertility. The cutoff value for diminished reserve will vary from laboratory to laboratory, depending on the hormone analyzer that is used and the respective programs' success rates. However, an FSH level greater than 12–15 is usually considered abnormal.

Estradiol Level

An **estradiol** level is also drawn on day 3 of the cycle. FSH and estradiol should be at their lowest levels on this day. It is important to perform both evaluations because a high estradiol level can suppress the FSH. If only the FSH is drawn, one might think the level is normal when it is not. Timing of this test is important: Readings will be worthless after day 5 of the cycle because the growing follicles are producing hormones that signal the pituitary gland to decrease FSH and the levels will be lower as time elapses. An estradiol level greater than 80 is considered abnormal.

Clomiphene Citrate Challenge Test

The **clomiphene citrate challenge test** (**CCCT**) involves drawing day 5 FSH and estradiol levels and prescribing 100 mg of clomiphene citrate for five days starting on day 5 of the cycle. This is followed by determining the FSH level on day 10. If a patient has a normal ovarian reserve, the day 10 FSH level is usually lower than or equal to that of day 3. If it is higher than day 3 FSH, it is abnormal.

Clomiphene or **clomifene** (marketed under the brand name Clomid) and clomiphene citrate (marketed as Clomid and Serophene) are oral agents that will stimulate the ovary to develop follicles (**agonist**) and can also decrease the amount of cervical mucus and endometrial proliferation (**antagonist**). The antagonistic effects do not always occur. However, when they do they usually are the result of higher doses. For this reason one should also monitor endometrial thickness when performing studies to monitor follicular development. Studies show that pregnancy rates are lower in patients demonstrating endometria measuring less than 6 mm on the day of human chorionic gonadotropin (hCG) administration.

If a patient does not respond to clomiphene, injectable gonadotropins (marketed under trade names such as Repronex, Follistim, Gonal-F, Bravelle, and Menopur) can be attempted. These drugs are all either FSH or a combination of FSH and luteinizing hormone (LH) derived from the urine of menopausal women or generated via recombinant technology. Because these drugs are associated with ovarian hyperstimulation and high-order multiple gestations, careful monitoring is mandatory. Side effects include abdominal distention and pain, bloating, fatigue, restlessness, and mood swings.

Because patients with polycystic ovary syndrome (PCOS) typically have abnormally low levels of insulin in the blood, Metformin (Glucophage) may also be used to induce ovulation because of the relationship between elevated insulin levels and insulin resistance.

OVULATORY FACTORS

Anovulation

One of the first steps in ruling out a female factor for infertility is to confirm ovulation—that is, rule out **anovulation** (failure of the ovary to release an oocyte). This can be assessed by charting **basal body temperature** (**BBT**, or core body temperature), by testing with over-the-counter urinary ovulation predictor kits, and by observing follicular collapse with sonography. Another sonographic sign ruling out anovulation is the identification of a small amount of free fluid in the posterior cul-de-sac. Of the three assessments, BBT charting is most commonly and sonography least commonly relied upon. The BBT is elevated when a woman ovulates. To monitor her BBT, a patient should take her temperature early in the morning, prior to getting out of bed, when the BBT is at its lowest for the day. When ovulation occurs, the ovary begins producing progesterone, which also elevates the BBT by about 0.5 degree Fahrenheit. An infertility patient must monitor her cycles and chart her BBT over several months to determine her individual ovulation patterns (Table 13-2). For this method to be effective menstrual cycles must be regular, within a few days of each other.

PCOS, also known as Stein-Leventhal syndrome, is the most common cause of anovulation. Patients with PCOS typically present with fluctuating FSH/LH, irregular or absent menstrual cycles, and elevated androgen levels, which produce hirsutism. Excessive production of androgens by the ovary inhibits normal follicular development and maturation. PCOS patients typically are hypoinsulinemic, which also causes a tendency toward obesity. The

Table 13-2. Basal body temperature and cervical mucus chart.

Name: _____

Dates covered: ___ / ___ / ___ to ___ / ___ / ___

Cycle Day	1	2	3	4	5	6	7	8	9	10	11	12	13	14	15	16	17	18	19	20	21	22	23	24	25	26	27	28	29	30	31	32	33	34	35	36	37	38	39	40	41	42	43	44	45
Day of week																																													
Date																																													
Time																																													
99.1																																													
99.0																																													
98.9																																													
98.8																																													
98.7																																													
98.6																																													
98.5																																													
98.4																																													
98.3																																													
98.2																																													
98.1																																													
98.0																																													
97.9																																													
97.8																																													
97.7																																													
97.6																																													
97.5																																													
97.4																																													
97.3																																													
97.2																																													
97.1																																													
97.0																																													
96.9																																													
CM*																																													
Intercourse																																													
Cervical Mucus textures																																													

*CM = cervical mucus: P=period, D=dry, M=mucus, E=eggwhite

Notes: (List any changes to your routine)

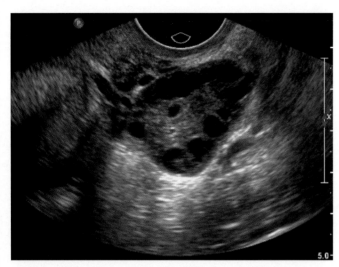

Figure 13-6. *Image of a polycystic ovary with tiny immature peripheral follicles and ovarian parenchyma seen centrally. Courtesy of Jill D. Trotter, BS, RT(R), RDMS, RVT.*

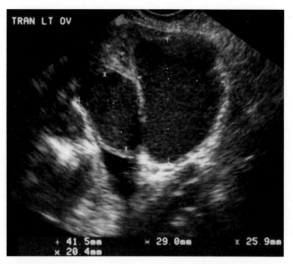

Figure 13-7. *Image of the left adnexa demonstrating endometriomas (calipers).*

hyperinsulinemia of PCOS stimulates the ovary to make additional androgens, perpetuating the anovulation and hirsutism frequently seen in these patients. The condition affects both ovaries, resulting in bilaterally enlarged ovaries that exhibit multiple small (2–5 mm) follicles situated peripherally (Figure 13-6). Because estrogen levels are often high, the patient has a thickened endometrium.

Treatment involves administration of ovulatory stimulants. If fertility is not achieved, surgical procedures such as the wedge resection or ovarian drilling can be performed. With **ovarian drilling**, a laser or electrosurgical needle is used to puncture the ovary several times. Within a few days, there is usually a dramatic decrease in androgen levels. The procedure is successful in restoring ovulatory function in 80% of patients, but it is temporary, lasting only about 6 months. Those patients who did not respond to ovarian stimulants prior to the procedure often will be responsive to the drugs afterward. The **wedge resection** removes a portion of ovary and is associated with the highest pregnancy rates in patients who have lower insulin levels and are less obese. Currently, these procedures are of only historical importance and are infrequently used. For the most part they have been replaced by insulin-sensitizing drugs, such as Metformin.

Peritoneal Factors

Anything that inhibits the egg from being transported through the fallopian tube will result in infertility. Tubal blockage is most frequently the result of scarring and adhesions but can also be due to conditions that do not allow the tube to function normally, such as exposure to diethylstilbestrol (DES). Conditions that cause scarring include pelvic inflammatory disease, endometriosis, and invasive tubal procedures such as tubal reanastomosis or surgical removal of an unruptured tubal ectopic pregnancy.

In the general population 7%–10% of women have endometriosis and, of those women who are infertile, 20%–50% are infertile because of endometriosis. Diffuse endometriosis can be difficult to appreciate on sonographic evaluation; the diagnosis requires visual diagnosis. Endometriomas, however, are well defined with sonography (Figure 13-7) and when identified suggest the patient has at least moderate disease, according to the staging system established by the American Society for Reproductive Medicine (see ASRM clinical data sheet in Appendix C). A diagnosis of endometriosis almost always assures one that pregnancy will be difficult to achieve without assistance. When it is determined that tubal disease is the cause of infertility, IVF is often the therapy of choice because success rates are high.

Cervical/Uterine Factors

Some cervical factors that affect female fertility, such as the quality and toxicity of the cervical mucus, cannot be evaluated with sonography. However, secondary effects of infection, congenital anomalies, and trauma allow us to monitor the cervix for preterm dilation causing spontaneous habitual abortions (Figure 13-8A).

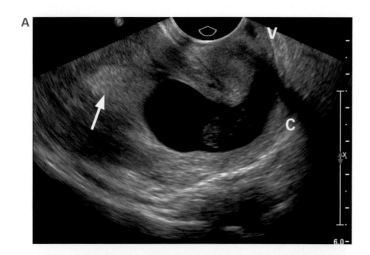

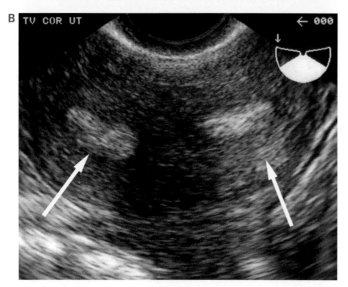

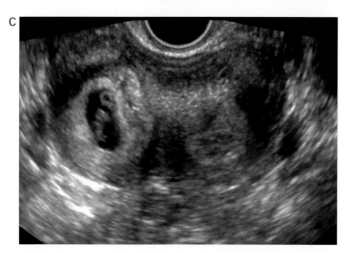

Figure 13-8. A *Longitudinal image demonstrating an impending abortion with the products of conception within the endocervical canal. The endometrial canal is indicated by the arrow. V = vagina, C = cervix.* **B** *Transverse transvaginal image shows a bicornuate uterus demonstrating two decidualized endometrial echoes (arrows).* **C** *Bicornuate uterus demonstrating a gestational sac in the right horn. Parts A and C courtesy of Jill D. Trotter, BS, RT(R), RDMS, RVT.*

Many uterine factors affect a woman's ability to maintain pregnancy. One of the most common has to do with insufficient decidualization of the endometrium secondary to the inability of the corpus luteum to produce adequate amounts of progesterone. This is referred to as a **luteal phase deficiency**. Monitoring the endometrial thickness with hormone levels can help identify this common cause of pregnancy loss.

Structural anomalies and pathologies of the uterus can also affect implantation and normal growth and development of an embryo. These include congenital malformations as the result of DES exposure or failure of normal müllerian duct fusion as well as acquired conditions such as uterine synechiae (adhesions) and fibroids (Figure 13-8B).

It is not uncommon for the endometrium along the septum of a bicornuate or septated uterus to be insufficient to maintain a cleaving embryo. This is also true for patients with an infantile uterus. However, with regard to the various types of duplications, the septated uterus is more significant than the bicornuate (Figure 13-8C) for causing fertility difficulties. Wide-spaced endometrial canals would not be considered clinically significant for infertility or pregnancy failure. Endometrial canals that appear to be very close together would be more bothersome and typical for a septated uterus.

Traditionally, the uterus was evaluated by hysterography. A radiopaque dye would be introduced into the uterus and allowed to flow into the fallopian tubes. X-ray imaging allows for evaluation of both uterine and tubal abnormalities with this technique (Figure 13-9). Sonohysterography (see Chapter 2) has begun to replace the radiographic procedure, at least when imaging of the internal uterine cavity is most important. This procedure does not require the assistance of the radiography department and can easily be done in the physician's office. Endometrial polyps, uterine synechiae, and submucosal fibroids can be readily identified with this technique. Although polyps and fibroids are relatively benign conditions in the nonpregnant patient, they can act as intrauterine contraceptive devices for women trying to become pregnant. If a patient does achieve pregnancy, fibroids can compete with the pregnancy for blood supply and result in demise and abortion (Figure 13-10). Another thing to consider when analyzing causes of pregnancy loss and infertility is always infection. With regard to the uterus, anything that causes slight widening or opening of the cavity can allow bacteria to enter and colonize, creating a hostile environment for a cleaving embryo.

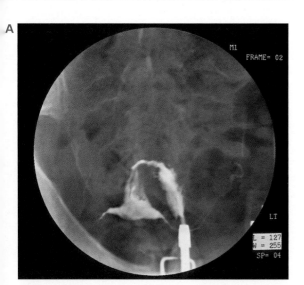

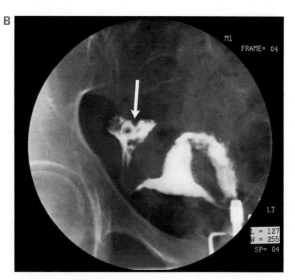

Figure 13-9. A *Hysterogram showing contrast media filling the uterine cavity and spilling into the fallopian tubes to indicate they are not obstructed. Note the severe retroflexion of the uterus.* **B** *The fallopian tube is seen all the way to the fimbriated end (arrow).*

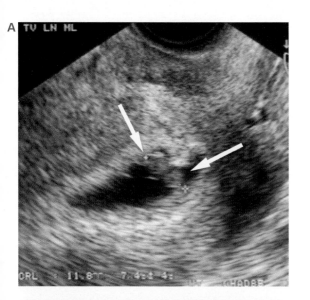

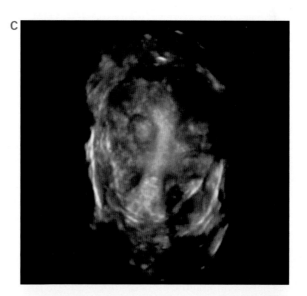

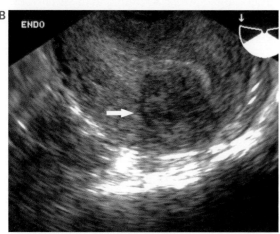

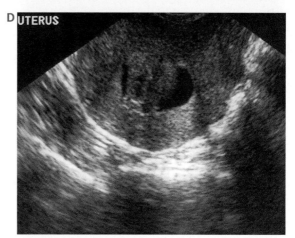

Figure 13-10. A *Sonohysterogram showing two endometrial polyps (arrows).* **B** *Transvaginal image showing a fibroid (arrow) impinging on the endometrial cavity.* **C** *3-D reconstruction of the endometrial cavity during sonohysterogram identifying a submucosal fibroid laterally. Courtesy of Jill D. Trotter, BS, RT(R), RDMS, RVT.* **D** *Sonohysterogram showing an intracavitary fibroid.*

ASSISTED REPRODUCTIVE TECHNOLOGY

Any procedure or treatment that involves surgically removing eggs from the patient's ovaries and combining those eggs with sperm in order to help achieve pregnancy is referred to as **assisted reproductive technology** (**ART**). The most common procedures include donor embryo transfer, gamete intrafallopian transfer, zygote intrafallopian transfer, and in vitro fertilization. **Donor embryo transfer** (**DET**) is the use of a donor egg, which is usually fertilized with the sperm of the patient's partner, although both sperm and egg can be donated. **Gamete intrafallopian transfer** (**GIFT**), developed in 1984, involves removing the patient's eggs and combining them with sperm. This mixture is immediately injected into the fallopian tube so that fertilization takes place in the patient's fallopian tube. GIFT has for the most part been replaced by IVF, since IVF success rates now are much higher than those seen with GIFT. **Zygote intrafallopian transfer** (**ZIFT**) involves the same procedure as GIFT; however, the eggs are allowed to be fertilized in a Petri dish before they are reintroduced into the fallopian tubes, usually the day after they are retrieved. There are few indications for ZIFT, and fewer than 1% of all ART cycles use GIFT or ZIFT. Women with scarred or damaged tubes are not good candidates for the GIFT or ZIFT procedures, as they are more susceptible to ectopic pregnancy.

The procedure involves using a special embryo transfer catheter with a metal band at the end, which serves as an echogenic sonographic marker on the image. The physician swabs the cervical mucus away so it will not impede movement of the embryos. Sometimes the mucus will act like a rubber band, slinging the embryos out of the uterus. The embryos are introduced into the uterus within a culture medium (approximately 10–20 microliters). A small amount of air is introduced before and after the embryos so that they do not slip out on the way in. These air bubbles also allow for visualization of where the embryos go once they are transferred. The embryos should be placed approximately 1–1.5 cm from the uterine fundus (Figure 13-11A).

In vitro fertilization (**IVF**) is probably the most widely recognized procedure for infertility. Patients are carefully stimulated and monitored with injectable gonadotrophins. Eggs are retrieved and fertilized in the laboratory. The fertilized eggs undergo multiple cell divisions and the

Figure 13-11. A *Ultrasound-guided embryo transfer. Note the echogenic catheter within the endometrial cavity that shadows near the fundus. In the bottom image, the catheter has been slightly withdrawn. (Figure continues . . .)*

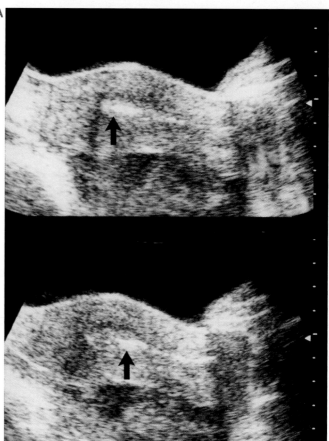

resulting embryos are then transferred into the uterine cavity for implantation. In 1978, the first "test-tube baby" was born in England. Today the overall success rate of IVF is about 50%, and as of 2012 the average cost of one IVF cycle in the United States, according to the American Society for Reproductive Medicine, was $12,400 (not including additional services such as use of donor eggs).

An IVF procedure requires that the ovaries be chemically shut down with a gonadotropin-releasing hormone (GnRH) agonist. Once this is accomplished, the ovaries will be stimulated with drugs that cause the release of FSH and LH. These trigger follicular development. Egg harvesting is performed under ultrasound guidance prior to ovulation. A 16- or 17-gauge needle is typically used to aspirate the eggs from the follicles (Figure 13-11B). On average, 5–15 eggs are retrieved and fertilized. Because it is assumed that not all zygotes or blastocysts

Figure 13-11, continued. B *Image showing the tip of a 16-gauge needle within a follicle for egg retrieval.* **C–E** *Day 1:* **C** *Endometrium. Courtesy of Jill D. Trotter, BS, RT(R), RDMS, RVT.* **D** *Follicles of right ovary.* **E** *Follicle of left ovary.* **F–J** *Day 5:* **F** *Endometrium. (Figure continues . . .)*

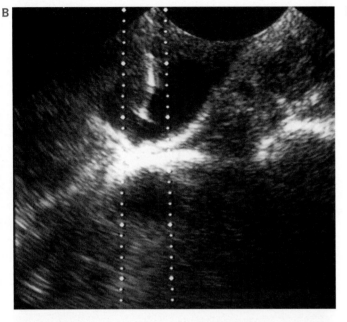

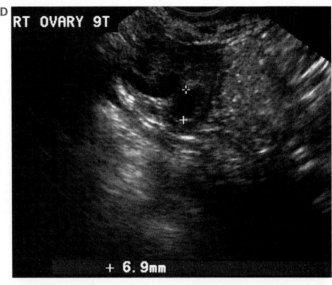

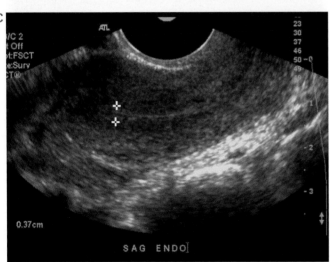

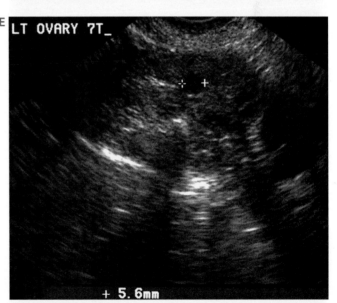

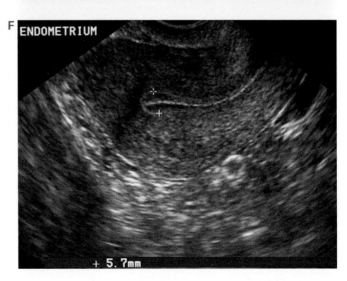

will survive, multiple fertilized eggs, usually no more than four, are introduced into the uterine cavity. The number of embryos that are transferred depends on the patient's age, number of previous tries, and embryo quality. Couples have the option of cryopreservation of the remaining embryos for use at a future date. The images in Figures 13-11 C–O show how the normal progression of follicular development and endometrial proliferation should appear during a single cycle, beginning with the baseline study.

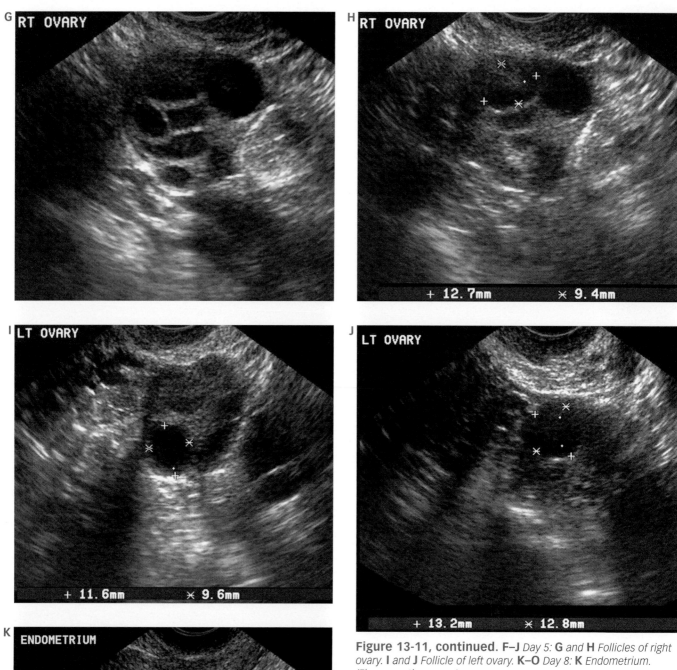

Figure 13-11, continued. F–J Day 5: **G** and **H** Follicles of right ovary. **I** and **J** Follicle of left ovary. **K–O** Day 8: **K** Endometrium. (Figure continues . . .)

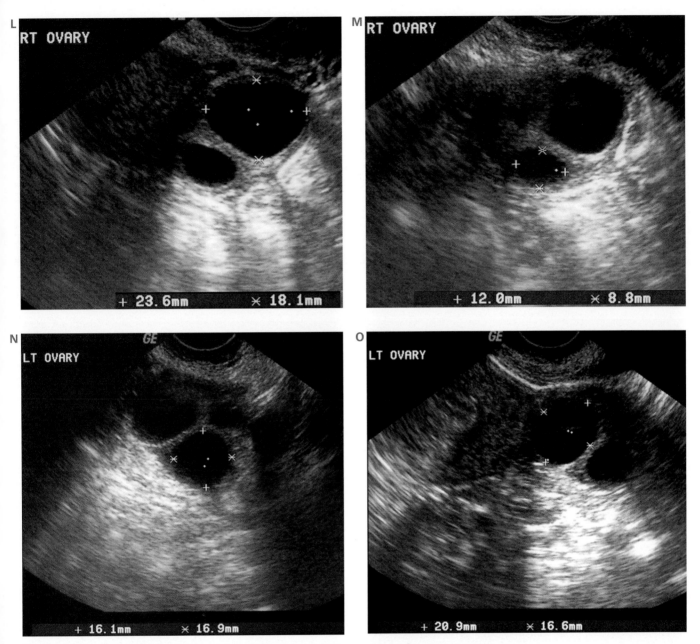

Figure 13-11, continued. K–O *Day 8:* **L** *and* **M** *Follicle of right ovary.* **N** *and* **O** *Follicle of left ovary.*

IVF is not without risks. Although rare, fatalities have resulted, and anesthetics can lead to serious adverse reactions. Deep vein thrombosis of the arms and legs has been associated with the high levels of estrogen used for ovarian stimulation. This condition is serious, as a clot can break away and travel to the lungs, causing a pulmonary embolism, which can be life-threatening. Thrombosis and embolism can also be associated with **ovarian hyperstimulation**, a common concern especially when injectable fertility drugs are used to induce follicular development (Figure 13-12A). Patients utilizing ART are at increased risk for ectopic pregnancy as well. Since multiple zygotes/embryos must be introduced to ensure that at least one survives, some zygotes/embryos may implant in sites outside the endometrial cavity. Heterotopic pregnancies, considered rare naturally, are most often seen in association with ART (Figures 13-12 B and C). Finally multiple gestations are not uncommon, since multiple fertilized eggs are reintroduced into the uterus. For this reason clinicians typically limit the number of embryos transferred (Figures 13-12 D and E).

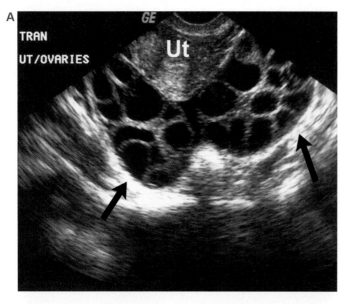

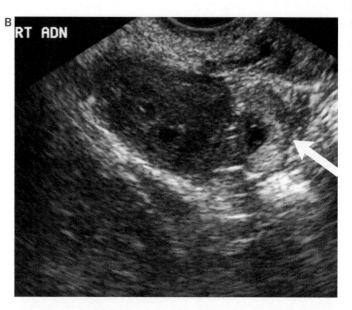

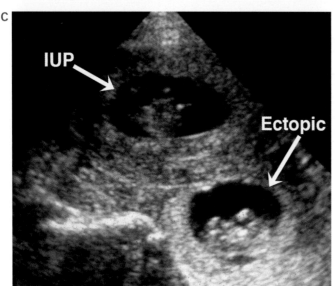

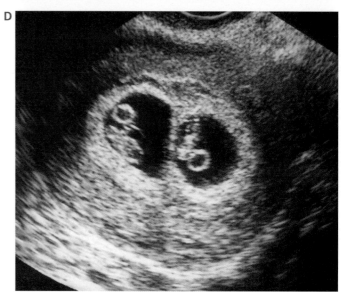

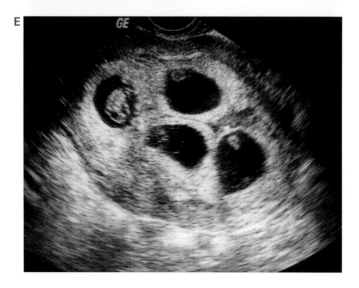

Figure 13-12. A *This transverse image shows bilateral ovarian hyperstimulation (arrows). Ut = uterus.* **B** *Ectopic pregnancy is seen adjacent to the right ovary (arrow). Note the yolk sac within the tubal ring.* **C** *Heterotopic pregnancy. IUP = intrauterine pregnancy.* **D** *Twin intrauterine gestational sacs both containing a yolk sac and embryo.* **E** *Transverse image demonstrating a quadruplet pregnancy.*

Selective Reduction

The risks of multifetal gestations for both mothers and fetuses have been well documented, and risks are particularly pronounced for pregnancies involving three or more fetuses. ART success rates have increased significantly. Today there are three times more triplets born than seen 30 years ago, and most are the result of fertility assistance. The process required to accomplish a successful term pregnancy is time-consuming (sometimes taking years) and expensive (costing thousands of dollars per cycle), involving costs that insurance does not cover. Patients with multifetal pregnancies must consider the likelihood of a successful outcome based on the number of fetuses they are carrying.

Selective reduction is the termination of one or more fetuses of a multifetal pregnancy of three or more fetuses. The philosophy of selective reduction is to give the remaining fetus(es) the best chance possible to develop normally and progress to term. The procedure is controversial and for most parents a difficult option to consider. Usually performed between 9 and 12 weeks under ultrasound guidance, it involves injection of potassium chloride or air into the heart of the selected fetus(es) and results in their demise and subsequent resorption. The procedure can be performed transabdominally or endovaginally and, although it will improve the chances of survival for the remaining fetuses, is not without risks. Risks include infection, spontaneous abortion, and permanent damage to the remaining fetus(es). There may also be subsequent psychological trauma for the parents.

SCANNING TIPS, GUIDELINES, AND PITFALLS

1. First and foremost, it is important that the sonography practitioner take his or her time to be thorough and not rush through procedures. Accurate measurements are critical to the overall outcome of the process.

2. Documentation for procedures should be thorough and consistent. Each follicle should be measured and documented on a form with all pertinent clinical information (Figure 13-13).

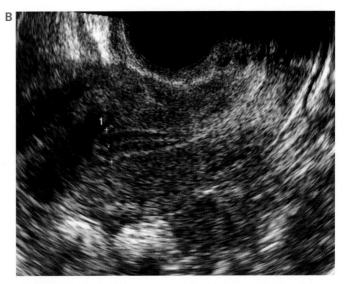

Figure 13-13. A *Example of a form used to track endometrium and follicular development.* **B** *Example of endometrial thickness. (Figure continues . . .)*

Figure 13-13, continued. C *Left ovary with multiple follicles.* **D** *Right ovary with cumulous oophorus (arrow). Each follicle measured should be documented on the form (13-13A).*

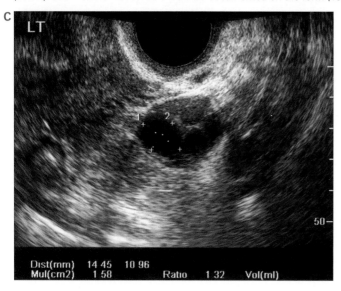

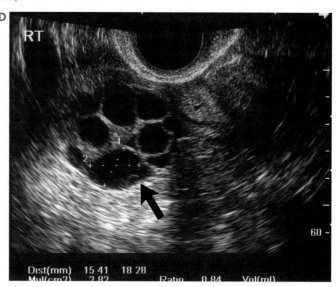

3. Ultrasound-guided embryo transfer has become fairly routine in the fertility clinic environment, and ultrasound guidance is performed transabdominally. The patient should partially fill her bladder in order to straighten the plane of the uterus and allow for better visualization. A special catheter with a metal band at the tip is used so the sonography practitioner can identify the echogenic tip and can visually follow it into and along the uterine cavity.

4. Practitioners should read the American Institute of Ultrasound in Medicine's "Practice Guideline for Ultrasonography in Reproductive Medicine" (Appendix B) for additional guidelines.

REFERENCES

Barnhart K, Christos C: The use of ultrasound in the evaluation and treatment of the infertile woman. In Benson CB, Arger PH, Bluth EI: *Ultrasonography in Obstetrics and Gynecology: A Practical Approach.* New York, Thieme, 2000, pp 69–80.

Evans MI, Dommergues M, Timor-Tritsch I, et al: Transabdominal vs. transcervical and transvaginal multifetal pregnancy reduction: international collaborative experience of more than one thousand cases. Am J Obstet Gynecol 170:902–909 [IS] [Medline], 1994.

Feigin K, Rosenblatt R, Kutcher R, et al: Sonohysterography in the evaluation of infertility. Applied Radiology Jan:14–20, 2000.

Fleischer AC, Herzog J, Vasquez JM, et al: Transvaginal sonography scanning in gynecologic infertility. In Fleischer AC, Toy EC, Lee W, et al: *Sonography in Obstetrics and Gynecology, Principles and Practice,* 7th Edition. New York, McGraw-Hill Medical, 2011.

Fleischer AC, Vasquez J: Transvaginal sonography scanning in gynecologic infertility. In Fleischer AC, Manning FA, Jeanty P, et al: *Sonography in Obstetrics and Gynecology: Principles and Practice,* 5th Edition. Stamford, CT, Appleton & Lange, 1996, pp 914–928.

Frates MC: Infertility. In Benson CB, Arger PH, Bluth EI: *Ultrasonography in Obstetrics and Gynecology: A Practical Approach.* New York, Thieme, 2007, pp 39–49.

Lynch L, Berkowitz RL, Chitkara U, et al: First trimester transabdominal multifetal pregnancy reduction: a report of 65 cases. Obstet Gynecol 75:735–738, 1990.

Mitchell A, Trampe B, Lebovic D: The role of ultrasound in evaluating female infertility. In Hagen-Ansert SL (ed): *Textbook of Diagnostic Sonography,* 7th Edition. St. Louis, Elsevier, 2012, pp 1039–1046.

Pierson RA: Ultrasonographic imaging in infertility. In Callen PW (ed): *Ultrasonography in Obstetrics and Gynecology*, 5th Edition. Philadelphia, Saunders Elsevier, 2008, pp 986–1019.

Timor-Tritsch IE, Peisner DB, Monteagudo A, et al: Multifetal pregnancy reduction by transvaginal puncture: evaluation of the technique used in 134 cases. Am J Obstet Gynecol 168:799–804, [ISI] [Medline], 1993.

Valentin L, Callen PW: Ultrasound evaluation of the adnexa (ovary and fallopian tubes). In Callen PW (ed): *Ultrasonography in Obstetrics and Gynecology*, 5th Edition. Philadelphia, Saunders Elsevier, 2008, pp 968–985.

SELF-ASSESSMENT EXERCISES

Questions

1. The most common cause of male infertility is:

    A. Cryptorchidism

    B. Testicular failure

    C. Varicoceles

    D. Spermatic cord obstruction

    E. Endocrine disorders

2. If the follicle-stimulating hormone (FSH) is too high, it can result in:

    A. Ovarian hyperstimulation

    B. Hyperemesis gravidarum

    C. Multiple gestations

    D. Abnormal bleeding

    E. Infertility

3. Estradiol and FSH levels will be at their lowest on which day of the cycle?

    A. Day 1

    B. Day 2

    C. Day 3

    D. Day 4

    E. Day 5

4. All of the following are considered uterine factors for infertility *except*:

    A. Bicornuate malformation

    B. Synechiae

    C. Luteal phase deficiency

    D. Leiomyomas

    E. Endometriosis

5. When a radiopaque dye is introduced into the uterus and fallopian tubes for visualization on x-rays, the procedure is called a:

    A. Sonohysterogram

    B. Hysteroscope

    C. Hysterogram

    D. Laparoscopy

    E. Endoscope

6. Patients undergoing ART procedures are at increased risk for:

    A. Ectopic pregnancy

    B. Pelvic infection

    C. Endometriosis

    D. Cancer

    E. Uterine rupture

7. The abbreviation that refers to placing an egg into the fallopian tube after it has been fertilized in a Petri dish is:

    A. ART

    B. GIFT

    C. IVF

    D. ZIFT

    E. BBT

8. Adhesions within the endometrial cavity are referred to as:

    A. Polyps

    B. Synechiae

    C. Mucosa

    D. Adenomyosis

    E. Antagonists

9. An increase in the basal body temperature indicates that:

A. Ovulation has occurred.

B. Fertilization is certain.

C. The patient has an infection.

D. Fertilization has occurred.

E. Ovulation will occur in 48 hours.

10. The most potent naturally occurring estrogen in humans is:

A. Clomiphene

B. H

C. LH

D. Progesterone

E. Estradiol

Answers

See Appendix F on page 617 for answers and explanations.

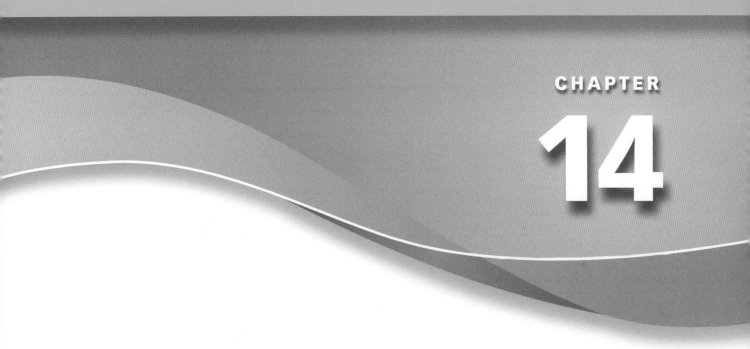

Volume Sonography

George Bega, MD, and Daniel A. Merton, BS, RDMS, FSDMS, FAIUM

OBJECTIVES

After completing this chapter you should be able to:

1. List the various methods used to acquire volume sonography data.

2. Describe the benefits that volume sonography has as compared to conventional two-dimensional sonography.

3. Describe the image display options provided by volume sonography.

4. List the most common obstetric and gynecologic applications of volume sonography.

5. List the primary technical limitations of volume sonography.

INTRODUCTION

DIAGNOSTIC MEDICAL ULTRASOUND (sonography) is widely recognized as the gold-standard imaging modality for assessment of the pregnant uterus, including the fetus, as demonstrated elsewhere in this textbook. High-resolution two-dimensional ultrasound imaging (2D ultrasound) is routinely used for a wide variety of clinical indications in obstetrics and gynecology. When clinicians employ conventional 2D sonography to evaluate anatomy, they routinely use 2D tomographic ultrasound information to mentally develop a three-dimensional (3D) concept of the region or structures of interest. Nevertheless, clinicians and even imaging experts can at times have difficulty comprehending the true spatial relationships of the anatomy from the information provided in 2D tomographic or planar images. This is particularly true when dealing with complex or unusual anatomic malformations such as fetal congenital cardiac anomalies.

Volume sonography or **volumetric sonography** (**VS**)—the acquisition and use of a volume of ultrasound data as opposed to individual 2D images—is a relatively new advancement in ultrasound technology that has been found to have distinct advantages over conventional 2D sonography. The advantages of volume sonography over 2D sonography include visualization of image planes not possible in conventional 2D imaging, improved visualization of depth in normal and abnormal anatomy, enhanced evaluation of complex anatomic structures, reduced scanning time, and more effective workflow. Volume sonography data are also suited to off-site analysis via teleradiology, as the volume data are digitally saved and stored. Thus, volume sonography has the ability to enhance not only the depiction of sonographic data but also image acquisition methods as well as how the data can be reviewed on- or off-site to enhance the overall diagnostic imaging processes.

Research in volume sonography technology began in the early 1970s, but not until the 1990s did VS-capable systems become commercially available, allowing more investigations to be conducted on its use for clinical applications. Technological developments in transducers and advances in computer signal processing and image display techniques have made possible the acquisition of volumes of ultrasound data with even more advanced display capabilities. Furthermore, the **real-time** 3D sonographic imaging systems (also known as **four-dimensional**, or **4D, sonography**), which were first available only for echocardiography, are now being utilized for noncardiac applications, including obstetric and gynecologic examinations. Additional advances in technology coupled with user experience will no doubt lead to even greater utilization of volume sonography in the future.

Volume sonography can depict the anatomy of interest as images that are either static or in motion (i.e., digitally captured cine loops) in fully interactive uniplanar, biplanar, and multiplanar displays as well as 3D renderings. Imaging practitioners in radiology environments are already familiar with the use of volume imaging and rendering techniques in computed tomography (CT) and magnetic resonance imaging (MRI). Ultrasound volume acquisition and display technologies provide clinicians and researchers with volume imaging tools that can be applied to sonographic applications.

Currently, volume sonography is most commonly utilized clinically for cardiological and obstetric applications. In addition, many reports have described its potential benefits for other applications, including neonatal brain, gynecologic, musculoskeletal, and interventional procedures. New applications are emerging at an astonishing rate. Systems are now available that can acquire both anatomic **gray-scale** (B-mode) sonography and color flow imaging (CFI) volume data.

TECHNOLOGY AND DATA ACQUISITION

Volume sonography presents new challenges to both the engineers developing the technology and the practitioners using it clinically. One major technological obstacle of volume sonography is the need to acquire a large amount of imaging data in a relatively short amount of time. Fortunately, advances in computer technology have made significant progress in overcoming this potential problem.

Volume scanners obtain multiple consecutive 2D image slices that are compiled to create a volume of data having three dimensions (or four dimensions when the data are viewed in real time). This is done by sweeping the ultrasound beam through a **region of interest** (**ROI**) either manually (when the operator physically moves or pivots the transducer) or automatically in one of several ways, as described below. Four main techniques are used to acquire volume data: the free-hand technique, the use of conventional 2D probes with position sensors attached, the use of dedicated volume (mechanized) probes, and the use of electronic matrix array volume probes (Table 14-1).

Free-Hand Technique

The free-hand technique acquires volume data using conventional 2D probes. This technique has been used with both on-board systems (whereby the volume data acquisition, storage, and manipulation are done on the ultrasound system) and off-line systems that use conventional 2D probes (whereby the ultrasound data are sent from the scanner to an off-line volume-rendering computer system). Although these free-hand methods are economical and can be implemented either in or attached to existing systems, their main drawback is that volume sonographic data acquired using these methods typically cannot be used for accurate measurement of structures and are likely to suffer from acquisition-related artifacts, especially of moving targets.

Off-Line Volume Sonography

Free-hand acquisition techniques are traditionally used to image parts of the anatomy that do not move (e.g., the nonpregnant uterus and adnexa) and generally are of limited value in the imaging of moving targets. With the off-line systems (Figure 14-1), the volume data obtained are downloaded to an off-line computer workstation equipped with specialized software for subsequent volume sonographic image reconstruction and analysis. A variety of technological approaches have been developed in order to optimize the accuracy of the acquired VS data. One off-line volume sonography system utilizes an electromagnetic position sensor that is attached to a conventional 2D probe, while a separate transmitter is placed

Table 14-1. Different types of volume sonography data acquisition systems.

Acquisition Method	Advantages	Disadvantages
Free-hand	Economical. Can be implemented into existing systems.	Volume data cannot be used for measurements. Data are more susceptible to acquisition artifacts.
Probe position sensor	Can be externally attached to the existing 2D systems or integrated into the mechanized probes. Improved image registration. Measurements and calculations can be performed on VS data.	Articulated arms or probe holders are cumbersome to use. Requires connection of the scanner to an off-line computer workstation.
Dedicated mechanized probe	Reliable volume data. Accurate VS data are provided without manual movement of probe. Fast acquisition speeds to capture moving targets.	Dedicated VS probes are slightly larger and heavier and more expensive than 2D probes. Generally does not provide the resolution of high-end 2D probes.
Matrix array probe	Fast frame rates, reasonable image spatial resolution, focus on the elevational plane, small footprint probes. Simultaneous visualization of two orthogonal planes without resolution loss.	Very expensive. Limited probe configurations (only lower frequencies) and availability. Narrow apertures.

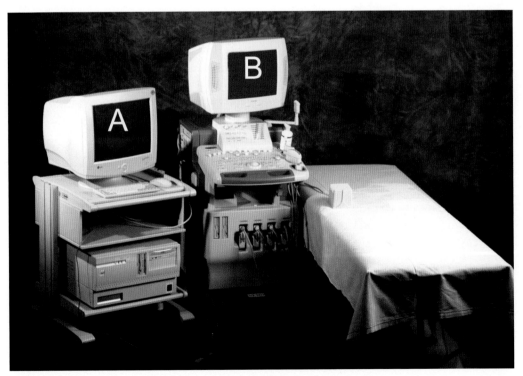

Figure 14-1. *Traditional off-line system setup. A computer workstation (A) commonly equipped with a video frame grabber card connects to the main 2D ultrasound machine (B) via its video-out port. Ultrasound volumes are acquired with the 2D ultrasound machine (B), and postprocessed and displayed at the off-line workstation (A). In the examination table there is a position-sensing device used to improve the registration process.*

near the patient. The sensor then provides the computer with information on position (in space and time) to register the acquired volume data accurately.

Dedicated Volume Probes

Dedicated mechanized volume probes (probes with a mechanical drive contained within the probe case itself) are commonly referred to as **volume probes**. When the volume sonography acquisition control is activated by the operator, a motor drive automatically sweeps the transducer elements through the region of interest (volume box) at an operator-selected speed and angle while the probe is held stationary. The main advantage of this method is that it provides a volume of data that are more accurate spatially and temporally, thereby allowing more accurate linear and volume measurements as well as more precise spatial relationships of structure, which in turn provide more accurate 3D renderings (Figures 14-2 and 14-3).

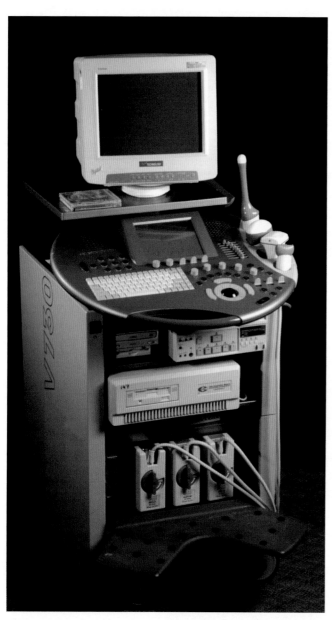

Figure 14-2. *Although the GE Voluson (GE Healthcare, Waukesha, Wisconsin) shown here is considered a dedicated volume ultrasound system, it can also perform conventional 2D ultrasound imaging.*

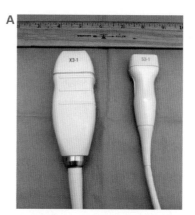

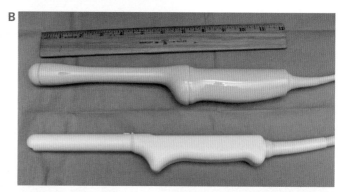

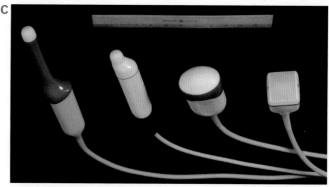

Figure 14-3. *Several ultrasound volume probes.* **A** *2D matrix array probe on the left and a conventional 2D probe on the right.* **B** *A transvaginal volume probe on top and a conventional 2D probe below.* **C** *From left to right, volume probes for transvaginal, transfontanelar, transabdominal, and breast imaging.*

Matrix array transducers (which are also dedicated volume probes) are composed of a very high number of transducer elements (typically 1000–6000). Because these transducers permit volume acquisitions, they provide the ability to focus the beams not only in the axial and lateral planes but also in the elevational plane, significantly increasing the overall quality of the acquired volume images. In addition, these transducers provide very fast frame rates without significant deterioration in image quality. Beam steering is employed to allow operators to select the size of the region to be evaluated and from which to obtain volume data. The information is typically displayed in biplanar or orthogonal multiplanar displays as well as in rendered 3D or 4D displays. A significant advantage of 2D matrix arrays is the simultaneous visualization of two orthogonal planes without resolution loss, as these probes have the unique ability to focus in the elevational plane. Matrix array volume sonography technology is still in its infancy and continued improvements can be expected to advance its imaging capabilities and resultant clinical potential (Figure 14-3).

These dedicated volume acquisition methods—mechanized probes and matrix arrays—are considered more reliable than free-hand methods, especially for imaging moving targets. As the operator's hand remains stationary and the transducer elements are swept through the region of interest, the volume data are acquired. Advances in technology have enabled the acquisition to take place quickly, allowing real-time depiction of fetal motion, cardiac activity, and blood flow for assessment of the associated structures.

Display Methods

Regardless of the acquisition technique used, ultimately the VS data must be displayed and made available for user manipulation in order to be diagnostically useful. Generally speaking, computer processing is used to interpolate the individual 2D slices to create what could be considered a seamless volume data set containing individual volume elements called **voxels**. The manner of acquisition has a significant impact on the degree to which the data set can be viewed, manipulated, and utilized.

The display methods used for volume sonography have become increasingly similar to those used in CT and MRI. Volume sonography data can be displayed and manipulated in a variety of ways. **Multiplanar displays** simultaneously show three orthogonal 2D planes (i.e., longitudinal, transverse, and coronal) through the volume. Using the multiplanar display, the operator can interactively navigate and explore the volume of data as desired by scrolling through the various planes in any of the three views or by rotating the volume in order to obtain an optimal view of the structures of interest, even when they are in planes other than conventional views.

The operator may choose to analyze and manipulate the volume data after the patient is discharged and spend as much time as needed to view any desired 2D plane of section in order to examine anatomy, obtain measurements, or otherwise analyze the data obtained. The digitally stored volume data can also be displayed as true 3D images using a variety of rendering algorithms. Rendering algorithms include **maximum-intensity projections** (which preferentially display tissues or structures that are high in echo intensity, useful in showing bony structures such as the fetal spine) and **minimum-intensity projections** (which preferentially display tissues or structures that are low in echo intensity, or **anechoic**, useful for demonstrating fluid-filled structures such as the fetal bladder or a cyst). **Surface rendering** is commonly used to display soft tissues such as the surface tissues of the fetal face. Rendering algorithms work best when a high degree of ultrasound interface difference is present, such as amniotic fluid around the fetal face or soft tissue against bone. Volume renderings provide lifelike images of anatomic structures, which are often more easily comprehended by patients and practitioners than are individual conventional 2D images.

The volume data set provides a new means to review sonographic scans for formal interpretation and reporting, to create individual 2D still images, and to analyze data for other purposes. Using the volume data set, the reviewer can perform a "virtual scan" by scrolling through the data in any plane desired. The multiplanar display can also be studied simultaneously with a rendered image, which allows important correlation of the planar images with the volume rendering.

A useful feature of a 3D display is the ability to create a short movie clip in which the rendered 3D volumes are viewed as they rotate. Movie clips can be recorded on videotape or digitally archived (e.g., in an audio video interleaved or AVI file) for later review or for presentations. This capability significantly enhances depth perception and gives a true 3D perspective of both normal and abnormal structures.

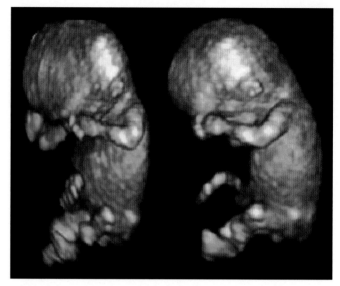

Figure 14-4. *Surface rendered views of a fetus at 11 weeks' gestation.*

OBSTETRIC APPLICATIONS

The First Trimester

Transvaginal (endovaginal) sonography is widely considered the standard approach for imaging the first trimester pregnancy. (See Box 14-1.) Nevertheless, anatomic factors may limit the manipulation of the vaginal probe and therefore the scan planes that can be obtained. Volume sonography overcomes this limitation because any plane, even a plane that is normally unobtainable with 2D sonography (e.g., a plane perpendicular to the ultrasound beam direction, such as a true coronal cross section of an ovary or the uterus), can be derived from the volume data set. In addition, rendered 3D images of the developing embryo provide depth visualization. Accurate volume measurements of the gestational sac and other structures are possible.

Fetal nuchal translucency measurement between 10 and 14 weeks' gestation has been shown to be an effective screening method for chromosomal anomalies. The exact mid-sagittal plane for assessing the nuchal region may be difficult to obtain with 2D sonography, however, because of a less than optimal fetal position. Volume sonography assists in achieving the required imaging plane and may also assist in detailed morphologic characterization of the increased nuchal translucency. Volume sonography in the first trimester, especially using the transvaginal approach, can demonstrate normal and abnormal embryonic and early fetal anatomy in exquisite detail (Figure 14-4). Published reports indicate that detailed imaging of the yolk

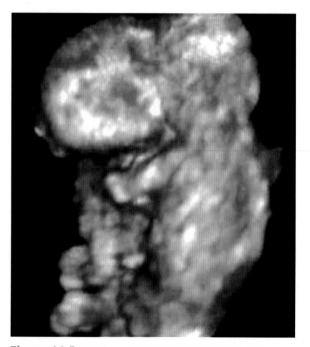

Figure 14-5. *Rendered view of conjoined twins at 11 weeks' gestation.*

sac, vitelline (omphalomesenteric) duct, umbilical cord, fetal trunk, head, face, spine, extremities, and even genitalia are possible (Figures 14-5 and 14-6). This advanced imaging technique provides opportunities for earlier and potentially more accurate diagnoses in the first trimester and may reduce the need for more invasive studies such as chorionic villus sampling (see Chapter 15). Nevertheless, additional research on the use of volume sonography for first trimester pregnancies is required.

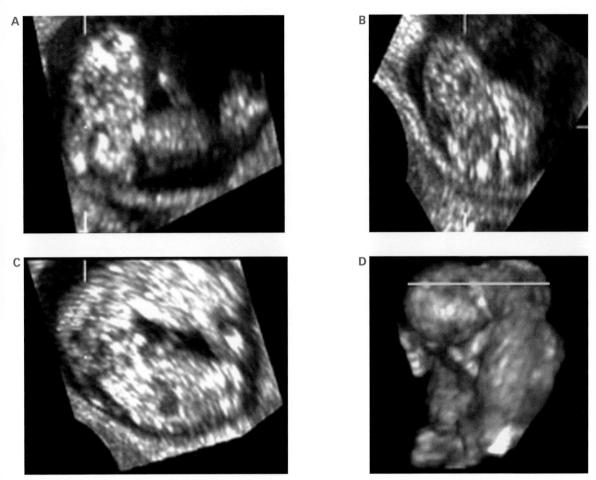

Figure 14-6. *Multiplanar (**A, B, C**) and rendered (**D**) views of conjoined twins (same as in Figure 14-5) at 11 weeks' gestation.* **B** *The multiplanar view shows an axial plane through the fetal heads that demonstrates brain sharing. This view can assist in evaluating the fetal orbits, the fetal midface, the upper and lower lips, and ear location and morphology.*

The Second and Third Trimesters

Compared to the first trimester evaluations, more detailed fetal anatomic assessments can be performed with volume sonography during the second trimester, including assessment of the major organs, facial features, genitalia, and skeletal components (see Box 14-2 and Chapter 4).

By displaying soft tissue information in a surface-rendering mode, volume sonography provides unique and clinically useful images of facial features (Figures 14-7, 14-8, 14-9, and 14-10). The anatomy of cranial sutures and fontanels in the developing fetus can be difficult to display with 2D sonography, as are other curved bony structures such as the ribs. Many authors have demonstrated that volume sonography offers clearer visualization of cranial structures and bony plates, allowing improved understanding of cranial anatomy and detection of craniosynostosis or abnormal cranial contours such as cloverleaf skull. Several

Box 14-2. **Second trimester applications and benefits of volume sonography.**

Assessment of major organs.

Improved visualization and evaluation of facial features, including cranial sutures, fontanels, bony plates, and other curved bony structures.

Clearer visualization and improved assessment of fetal spine and thorax.

Evaluation of limbs, hands, and feet.

Increased accuracy of gender determination and ambiguous genitalia.

Thorough evaluation of abdominal wall defects and their contents.

Unique visualization and improved assessment of the thoracic and abdominal cavities.

Thorough visualization and improved evaluation of the fetal brain.

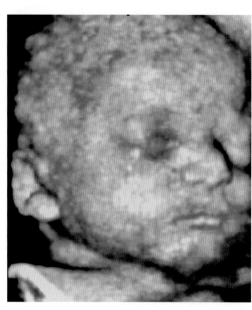

Figure 14-7. *Rendered view of a normal fetal face at 27 weeks. Note the amount of detail that the surface rendered views provide.*

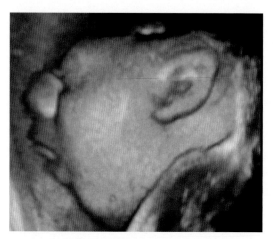

Figure 14-9. *Three-dimensional surface rendered view of a fetus at 31 weeks with anencephaly demonstrating absence of the calvarium.*

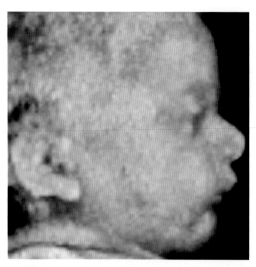

Figure 14-8. *Profile view of the same fetus as in Figure 14-7. Note the unique visualization of the fetal profile as well as the fetal ear in the same view, thanks to the depth that VS displays. This view can reliably assess the level and the posterior rotation of the fetal ears in relation to the fetal profile plane. Additionally, this view can assist in evaluating fetal frontal bones for frontal bossing, nasal bridge shape, tip of the nose, height of the filtrum, upper and lower lips, and chin to rule out micrognathia.*

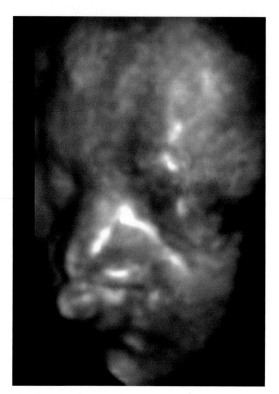

Figure 14-10. *Rendered image of premaxillary protrusion in a bilateral cleft lip and palate.*

authors have reported improved visualization of the fetal face in pregnancies at high risk for dysmorphology syndromes caused by exposure to teratogens such as phenytoin (Dilantin), fetal alcohol syndrome, and chromosomal abnormalities (Figures 14-7, 14-8, and 14-9). Cleft lips and palate, micrognathia, malformed ears, and frontal bossing have all been reported to be better displayed and analyzed by the use of volume sonography (Figure 14-10).

Obtaining detailed structural information regarding the fetal spine and thorax is important in evaluating fetuses at risk for skeletal dysplasia, abnormalities leading to a small thorax and subsequent pulmonary hypoplasia, and neural tube defects. These and other types of skeletal abnormalities affecting the thorax and spine—such as scoliosis, spinal disruption, hemivertebrae, butterfly vertebrae, and rib abnormalities—can be assessed much better with the use of volume sonography.

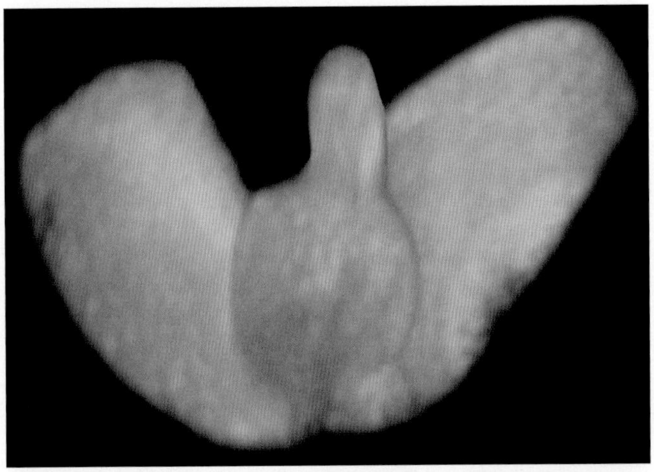

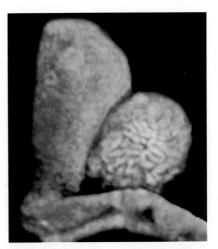

Figure 14-11. *Male genitals in a 24-week fetus. Note the amount of detail in depicting the normal anatomy of the perineum, penis, and testes.*

Figure 14-12. *Surface rendered view of a fetus with gastroschisis. Note that the abdominal mass has bowel loops in it.*

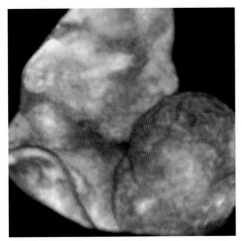

Figure 14-13. *Surface rendered view of a fetus with a giant omphalocele (more than 80% of the liver's volume is outside the abdomen).*

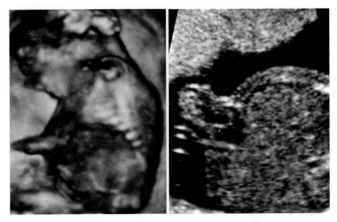

Figure 14-14. *Surface rendering of ectopia cordis and anencephaly on the left and 2D axial cross section of the fetal chest on the right.*

Sonographic evaluations of the limbs, hands, and feet are also facilitated with volume sonography, which allows the examiner to standardize the orientation of the limb, thereby enabling a detailed examination of the relationships of the distal forearm bones, metacarpals, fingers, and thumbs, as well as evaluation of the axis. Several reports have shown the utility of volume sonography in detecting isolated cases of abnormal extremities such as clubfoot, polydactyly, claw-hand, and phocomelia.

Fetal gender can be readily identified with volume sonography in the late first and early second trimesters, because the diagnostic mid-sagittal plane can usually be obtained from the volume data set (Figure 14-11). Prenatal diagnosis of ambiguous genitalia with volume sonography has been reported using surface rendered images.

Abdominal wall defects can be thoroughly evaluated with both multiplanar and rendered views. The real impact of volume sonography is in detailing the location, type, and extent of these anomalies. The contents of a herniated mass in the anterior abdominal wall could reveal liver, bowel, or both (Figures 14-12 and 14-13). Volume sonography assists in depicting the presence of these structures in rendered views, identifies the presence or absence of a covering membrane, identifies the abdominal wall defect itself and/or rules out a herniation via the umbilical insertion, and even assists in identification of the umbilical cord insertion (to the herniated mass or normal insertion) via color or power Doppler rendering to differentiate gastroschisis from omphalocele. The same principles apply to bladder exstrophy and ectopia cordis (Figure 14-14).

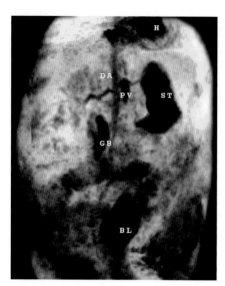

Figure 14-15. *Minimum-intensity projection rendered view of a normal fetal chest and abdomen. H = heart, DA = descending aorta, PV = portal vein, ST = stomach, GB = gallbladder, BL = bladder.*

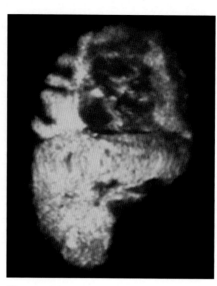

Figure 14-16. *Normal surface rendered view of the fetal liver at 27 weeks' gestation.*

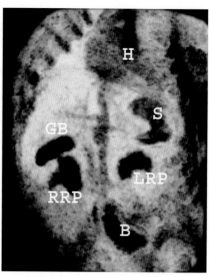

Figure 14-17. *Minimum-intensity projection rendered view of a normal fetal chest and abdomen with presence of bilateral hydronephrosis. H = heart, S = stomach, GB = gallbladder, RRP = right renal pelvis, LRP = left renal pelvis, B = bladder.*

Volume sonography provides unique information on the abdominal and chest cavity by displaying several key anatomic landmarks, both fluid-filled hypoechoic structures (such as stomach, heart, gallbladder, and vessels) and liver, bowel, and kidneys (Figures 14-15, 14-16, and 14-17). These views enable the operator to clearly establish the anatomic relationships between different structures and precisely pinpoint the location and extent of anomalies.

The most common rendering algorithms used are not just surface rendering but also minimum-intensity projection and inverse rendering.

The fetal brain can be thoroughly visualized with volume sonography, as planes that are nonconventional for 2D ultrasound, such as sagittal and coronal views, can be visualized and evaluated (Figure 14-18). In coronal views, useful scan planes of the brain—such as the cerebellum,

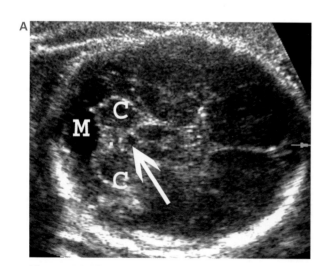

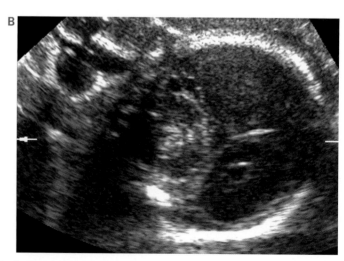

Figure 14-18. *Multiplanar display of the posterior fossa of the fetal brain.* **A** *Axial view of the cerebellum, cisterna magna, and fourth ventricle (long arrow). C = cerebellum, M = cisterna magna.* **B** *Coronal view of the posterior fossa. Following page:* **C** *Sagittal view through the cerebellar vermis. Short arrows show the antero-posterior and craniocaudal dimensions of the vermis. Volume sonography allows visualization of the vermis in a sagittal view that is not commonly obtained with 2D ultrasound. M = cisterna magna, SP = septum pellucidum, V = vermis.*

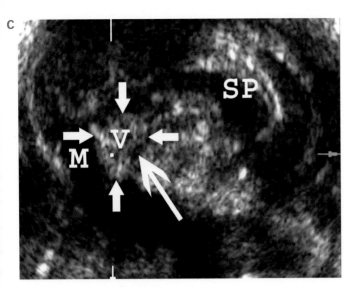

Figure 14-18, continued.

thalami, third and fourth ventricles, corpus callosum, and anterior and posterior horns of the ventricular system—are visualized. In the sagittal views, volume sonography allows visualization of the vermis, third and fourth ventricles, corpus callosum, and septa pellucida, views that may not be easily obtained using 2D ultrasound (Figure 14-19).

The Pregnant Cervix

The coronal view of the cervix is a unique view that is obtained only with volume sonography and provides new information on the shape and dimensions of the endocervical canal (Figure 14-20). The visualization of the funnel is also improved by using 3D ultrasound, as

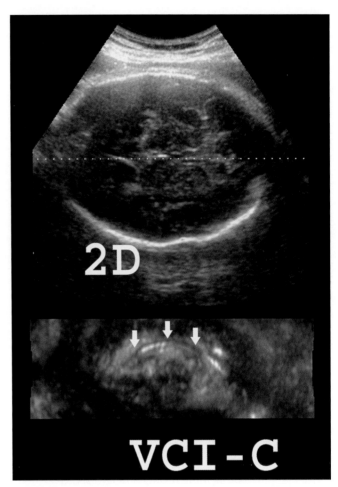

Figure 14-19. *Virtual contrast imaging in the C plane (VCI-C) of the corpus callosum. A 2D ultrasound axial view of the fetal brain at the BPD level (top) has a dotted line that represents the location of the perpendicular scanning plane. The mid-sagittal plane obtained via VCI-C (bottom) demonstrates the corpus callosum (arrows).*

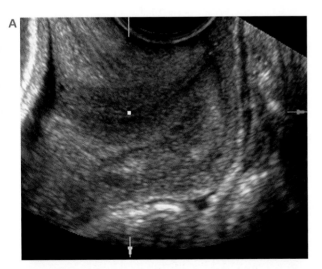

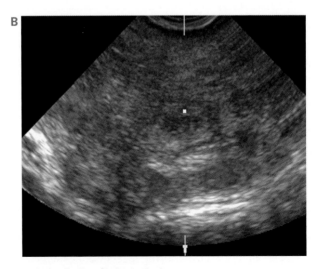

Figure 14-20. *Ultrasound image of a normal cervix displayed in the multiplanar display. A The sagittal plane of the cervix that corresponds to the acquisition plane of this volume. B The computer-generated axial plane of the cervix cut precisely at the level of the cross-planar point (the square dot) 90 degrees from the sagittal plane. (Figure continues . . .)*

C

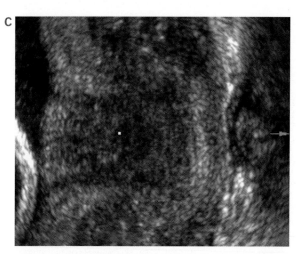

Figure 14-20, continued. C *The coronal plane of the cervix, again precisely 90 degrees from the sagittal plane coronally. Note that these three planes simultaneously shown (sagittal, axial, and coronal) are interactively linked to one another in a 90 degree (orthogonal) relationship. The evaluation of the cervix is not limited to the sagittal plane only but extends with the axial and coronal planes. Note that cervical length and width are shown in both sagittal and coronal planes.*

the funnel can be evaluated in all three planes: sagittal, axial, and coronal. The coronal funnel width is the true width of the funnel, as the commonly known funnel width as seen with 2D ultrasound represents the true funnel height. The coronal funnel and endocervical canal widths are not necessarily the same value as their respective sagittal values and as such may provide additional, new, and potentially useful information. Three-dimensional ultrasound makes it possible to obtain an axial plane through the cervix at the level of the cerclage, demonstrating the entire stitch. This view is not obtainable with conventional 2D ultrasound. New display and acquisition methods enable the operator to view the cervix in multiple slices in operator-selectable distances such as CT- or MRI-like displays or to image the sagittal and coronal views of the cervix in real time, such as with virtual contrast imaging (VCI). Imaging the cervix using volume sonography not only provides additional views of the cervix but also assists in standardizing the evaluation of the cervix by obtaining important views (e.g., the mid-sagittal view of the cervix) in a controlled fashion.

Potential New Fetal Biometric Assessments

Organ volume measurements obtained by 2D sonography have not been widely utilized during assessment of fetal growth and organ abnormalities, primarily because of the limitations of 2D sonography in estimating volumes of irregular structures. However, with volume sonography it

is possible to measure the volume of fetal organs, and the accuracy of VS volume measurements has been demonstrated.

The feasibility of calculating volumes of the following structures has been reported: gestational sac, fetal lungs and fetal heart from second trimester to term, placental volume, liver volume, and fetal arm and thigh volume for estimation of the fetal weight. These fetal biometric data could offer new possibilities in assessing fetal growth and development. In addition, fetal limb volumetry is being studied as a means to improve prediction of estimated fetal weight. Furthermore, several authors have reported the feasibility of accurately measuring fetal lung volume and growth over time. Lung volume nomograms have been published showing that lung volume increases with gestational age and fetal weight.

Fetal Echocardiography

An advantage of volume sonography over 2D sonography is the ability to obtain different views from one stored volume data set. For example, one technically adequate volume scan acquired in the four-chamber view of the heart yields a volume from which the operator can obtain not only the standard four-chamber view but also views of the outflow tracts, valves, and ductal and aortic arches. Because the cardiac volumes are stored digitally, a thorough examination of the fetal cardiac anatomy, including its connections to the pulmonary and great vessels, can be accomplished after the patient is discharged. Views that may not be readily obtainable with 2D imaging as a result of fetal position may be extracted from the stored cardiac volume data (Figures 14-21, 14-22, 14-23, and 14-24). Volumes sent digitally over networks allow for consultation with experts in fetal echocardiography. Thus, volume sonography holds the potential to improve the detection of cardiac defects in routine fetal screening.

The time required to obtain volume data has improved significantly over the last several years. In the past, it was generally believed that increases in acquisition speeds (frame acquisition rates) would have a great impact in volume sonography used for fetal echocardiography. While most commercially available volume ultrasound machines today can achieve speeds of acquisition over 30 frames per second (what is commonly considered as real-time imaging), in acquiring fetal heart volumes, these higher frame rates do not necessarily translate into higher-quality or more diagnostic volumes, with

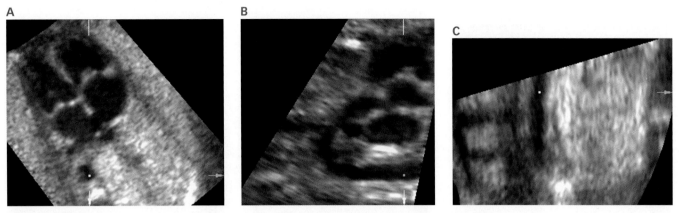

Figure 14-21. *Multiplanar view of the fetal heart acquired at the level of the four-chamber view (4CHV).* **A** *The 4CHV in an axial plane. Note that the cross-planar point rests over the descending aorta.* **B** *Aortic arch.* **C** *Long axis of the descending aorta.*

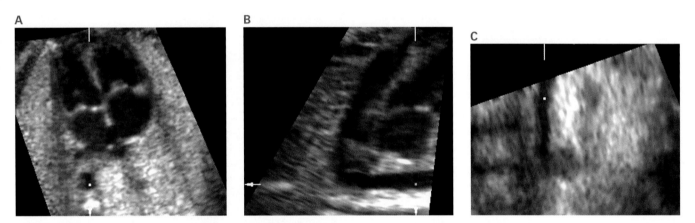

Figure 14-22. *Multiplanar view of the fetal heart acquired at the level of the four-chamber view (4CHV).* **A** *The 4CHV in an axial plane rotated around the cross-planar point at the descending aorta for about 30 degrees as compared to the view in Figure 14-21.* **B** *This maneuver is performed to visualize the ductal arch.* **C** *Coronal view of the long axis of the descending aorta, corresponding to the cross-planar point in windows A and B.*

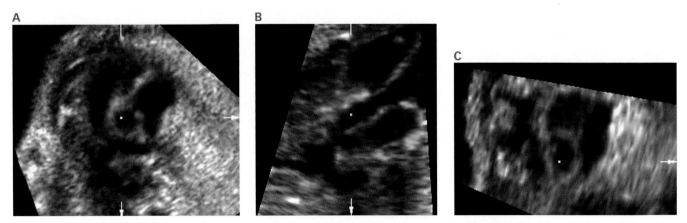

Figure 14-23. *Multiplanar view of the fetal heart after reformatting showing the orthogonal relationships between the short and long axes of the aorta.* **A** *Branching of the pulmonary arteries, ductal continuation, and a short axis of the aorta in an axial view.* **B** *Left ventricular outflow tract (LVOT) is visualized as the cross-planar point in A is at the short axis of the aorta.* **C** *Coronal image in relation to the short axis of the aorta in A as depicted by the cross-planar point.*

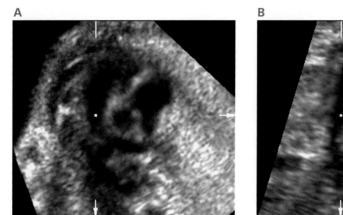
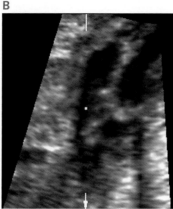
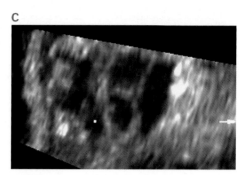

Figure 14-24. *Multiplanar view of the fetal heart after reformatting showing the orthogonal relationships between the axial and sagittal views of the pulmonary artery.* **A** *Branching of the pulmonary arteries, ductal continuation, and a short axis of the aorta in an axial view.* **B** *Right ventricular outflow tract (RVOT) is visualized as the cross-planar point in A is at the level of the pulmonary artery.* **C** *Coronal cut through the pulmonary artery and aorta.*

the current mechanically steered probes. Indeed, the opposite is true. Slower acquisition speeds yield higher-quality information, as they allow the probe to acquire a greater number of 2D frames to be incorporated into the volume. To overcome this obstacle, a special, very slow volume acquisition technology was introduced. This technology is called spatio-temporal image correlation (STIC), nowadays available in almost all volume ultrasound machines. With STIC an extra slow (by volume sonography standards) acquisition of 7.5–15 seconds is performed over a predefined area of the fetal heart, typically at the level of the four-chamber view. The acquisition angle ranges from 15 to 40 degrees, and it too is user-selectable. After the acquisition, postprocessing of spatial and temporal data is performed so the individual 2D images that constitute the volume data set are correlated in time and space. This information is displayed in a classic multiplanar view and/or in a cine sequence depicting heart motion with total control on interactive reslicing and/or rendering, the same as in a static volume. Typically in gray scale, this type of acquisition can achieve very high frame rates (even 150 frames/second or more) due to the relatively small region of interest.

The STIC technique was initially introduced only in gray scale, but advances in this technology permit acquisition of fetal heart volumes with STIC in gray scale and color Doppler imaging or power Doppler imaging modes (Figures 14-25, 14-26, and 14-27). This development has created a whole new area in evaluating the fetal heart with volume sonography (Figures 14-28, 14-29, and 14-30).

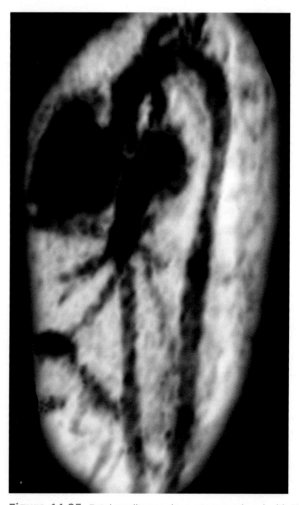

Figure 14-25. *Fetal cardiovascular system rendered with 3D minimum-intensity projection rendering in STIC. This is a unique technique for visualizing the vascular system without color or power Doppler that has none of the drawbacks of these techniques, such as dependence on the direction of flow or bleeding artifacts.*

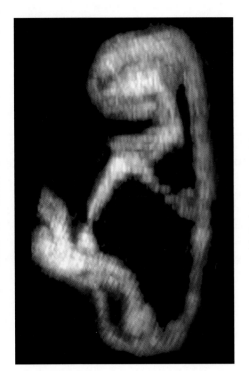

Figure 14-26. *3D STIC B flow rendered view at 25 weeks' gestation. This view not only shows unique spatial relationships of the heart and arterial and venous system but also gives real-time blood flow information. This is a true volume display and can be rotated up to 360 degrees to better appreciate the anatomy.*

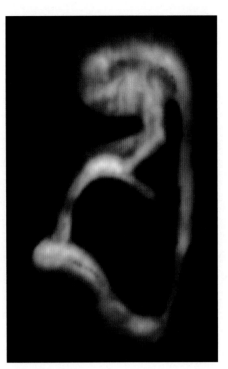

Figure 14-27. *3D STIC power Doppler rendered view at 25 weeks' gestation. This view shows the spatial relationships of the heart and arterial and venous system and gives real-time blood flow information. This view is a true volume display and can be rotated up to 360 degrees to better appreciate the anatomy.*

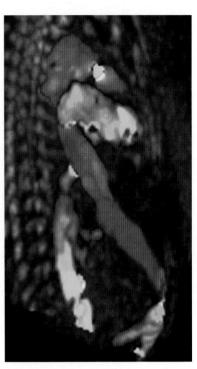

Figure 14-28. *Absent ductus venosus in a Noonan syndrome fetus at 24 weeks' gestation. This view is a 3D glass mode rendering acquired with STIC and color Doppler. The umbilical vein enters straight and directly to the right atrium, bypassing the fetal liver.*

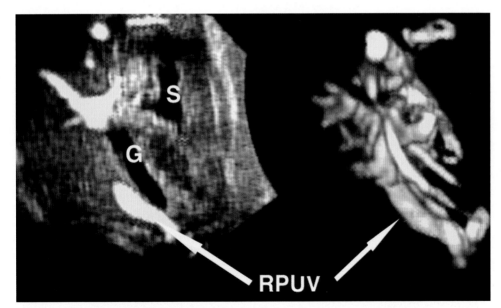

Figure 14-29. *Right persistent umbilical vein (RPUV) in a 2D power Doppler axial view on the left and 3D power Doppler rendered view on the right (dual view). The normal left umbilical vein is missing and instead a persistent right umbilical vein is seen around the gallbladder. G = gallbladder, S = stomach.*

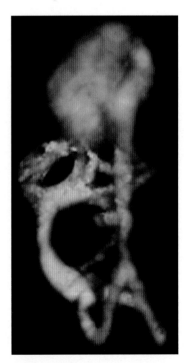

Figure 14-30. *Right persistent umbilical vein (RPUV) in a STIC 3D power Doppler rendered view. Note that ductus venosus is present and comes from the RPUV.*

When used for fetal heart scanning STIC represents a significant development in volume sonography that has the potential to perform a full fetal echocardiography examination utilizing a single fetal heart volume acquired at the level of the four-chamber view.

Studies done before and after the introduction of STIC have demonstrated that a volume scan of the fetal heart can provide all the diagnostic data usually necessary for fetal echocardiographic examinations. Several reports have demonstrated the value of STIC for the evaluation of the fetal heart. Chaoui and colleagues (2004) published a comprehensive prospective study that examined the potential of color Doppler STIC in the evaluation of 35 normal fetuses and 27 fetuses with congenital heart defects (CHDs) examined between 18 and 35 weeks' gestation. Volume acquisition was achieved by initiating the image-capture sequence from the transverse four-chamber view. Volumes were stored for later off-line evaluation using a personal computer–based workstation in a multiplanar mode and as spatial volume rendering. Successful acquisition was possible in all 62 cases. Spatial volume rendering was attempted in 18 fetuses with congenital heart defects. In four normal fetuses there was inadequate visualization using color Doppler STIC because the region of interest was perpendicular to the ultrasound beam. In two fetuses with congenital heart defects, inadequate visualization was related to an enlarged heart in late gestation, for which the entire cardiac volume could not be acquired. The third case was an 18-week fetus with complex CHDs, including transposed great vessels in which artifacts were related to confluent color signals as a result of low resolution in the reconstructed plane. The study concluded that STIC in combination with color Doppler imaging is a promising new tool for multiplanar rendering of the fetal heart.

While the promise of the STIC technique is clear, a number of potential pitfalls are worth mentioning. The acquisition is still relatively slow, 7.5–15 seconds, so fetal breathing and gross body movement commonly occur during the process. After the acquisition is obtained, a careful evaluation of all planes demonstrated in the multiplanar display is crucial to ensure that no artifacts are present. Adjusting the volume box tightly around the region of interest helps, generally increasing the frame rate. The best frame rates recommended are the ones above 15 Hz, typically with higher rates for smaller hearts and slower rates for larger hearts. The acquisition angle is also important, with optimal angles ranging from 15 to 30 degrees, and these too are related to the gestational age. The earlier the gestational age, the narrower the angle of acquisition should be.

Psychological Aspects of Volume Sonography in Obstetrics

In a study involving 20 high-risk women at 24 to 32 weeks of pregnancy, volume sonography had a positive influence on the patients' perception of the fetus. The mothers reported more motivation to endure pregnancy-related difficulties, reduced anxiety, and improved capacity to cope. Improved bonding between the mother and the fetus has the potential to help mothers refrain from smoking and other risky behaviors during pregnancy. The ability to show patients and their families comprehensible images of the fetus can also provide greater reassurance of the health of the fetus and facilitate counseling in cases of fetal anomalies.

GYNECOLOGIC APPLICATIONS

The use of conventional 2D sonography has proven to be a valuable means of evaluating the female pelvis (see Chapter 2). Although the transabdominal scanning approach (through a full urinary bladder) has been used for many years, transvaginal sonography has made more detailed evaluations possible while avoiding the need to have a patient fill her urinary bladder (see Chapter 1).

After insertion into the vagina, the transvaginal probe is in closer proximity to the major pelvic structures, including the uterus and ovaries. Therefore a higher transducer frequency can be utilized for transvaginal examinations, providing a higher level of spatial resolution and detail than that provided by the transabdominal approach. An additional benefit of transvaginal sonography is that the transducer can be used to manually probe specific areas and structures within the female pelvis (similar to the examiner's fingers during a digital pelvic examination), which can be useful to determine which structures may be causing the patient discomfort or pain, as well as to evaluate for pelvic adhesions or other processes that could result in a lack of normal mobility of the pelvic organs. Numerous reports have described the benefits of the transvaginal approach over that of the transabdominal technique, and in many sonography laboratories a transvaginal examination alone is performed for the vast majority of cases. Nevertheless, in some instances a transabdominal sonographic examination may still be necessary (e.g., for evaluation of structures located higher in the pelvis and beyond the view of the transvaginal probe or for examinations of virginal or particularly modest females).

The use of volume sonography, including multiplanar, 3D, and 4D imaging, has been shown to have unique advantages over conventional 2D sonography, including the ability to improve the depiction of spatial relationships of structures as well as to acquire images in planes of section that would otherwise be difficult or impossible to obtain using 2D imaging (Box 14-3). This is particularly true for the transvaginal examination because of the limited ability to manipulate the transvaginal probe within the confines of the vagina. Additionally, volume sonography has the potential to provide more accurate volume estimations and allows retrospective review of the imaging data in arbitrary planes.

Currently, volume sonography scanning is used primarily as an adjunct to a conventional 2D sonography gynecologic examination. Nevertheless, additional clinical experience and advances in ultrasound as well as picture archiving and communications systems (PACS) may lead to the use of volume sonography as the primary means of performing clinical sonographic examinations. In the future the volume sonography scan may replace the 2D examination, similarly to the way transvaginal examinations have nearly obviated the use of full-bladder scanning for gynecologic applications. Investigations into the use of volume sonography for gynecologic applications focus primarily on the assessment of uterine masses (e.g., myomas) and congenital malformations, infertility, and the detection and characterization of adnexal masses.

The Uterus

Both transabdominal and transvaginal 2D sonography of the uterus have significant limitations in the amount of planar sections that can be obtained. Transabdominally, the bony pelvis prevents scanning from the pelvic sidewall; therefore, the coronal plane through the long axis of the uterus typically cannot be obtained. Likewise, the restricted range of mobility of the vaginal probe limits the views obtainable transvaginally. As a result, the information obtained with 2D sonography of the uterus may be limited. For example, the inability to image the coronal plane through the fundus limits the ability to assess the fundal contour and thus to diagnose or exclude uterine anomalies. As has been mentioned, the main advantage of volume sonography acquisitions in gynecology is the fact that volume acquisition allows the operator to obtain image planes that simply cannot be acquired with conventional 2D techniques. The reason is very simple: These planes are commonly perpendicular or near perpendicular to the ultrasound beam and cannot be obtained regardless of how much the operator angles the probe. However, these planes (e.g., the coronal plane) yield a significant amount of information, especially in the evaluation of uterine abnormalities.

Volume sonography permits detailed interactive assessment of the uterus in conventional longitudinal and transverse image planes as well as in unlimited oblique and coronal planes that can be useful to demonstrate both horns of the endometrial cavity and endometrial lining simultaneously (Figure 14-31).

Congenital uterine abnormalities, including septate, arcuate, and bicornuate configurations, typically are better appreciated using the multiplanar display provided by volume sonography (Figures 14-32, 14-33A–D). Differentiation of the specific congenital configuration when present is important for management of patients, particularly those being evaluated for infertility. The improved depiction of the endometrial lining and canal provided by volume sonography can also be useful for evaluation of

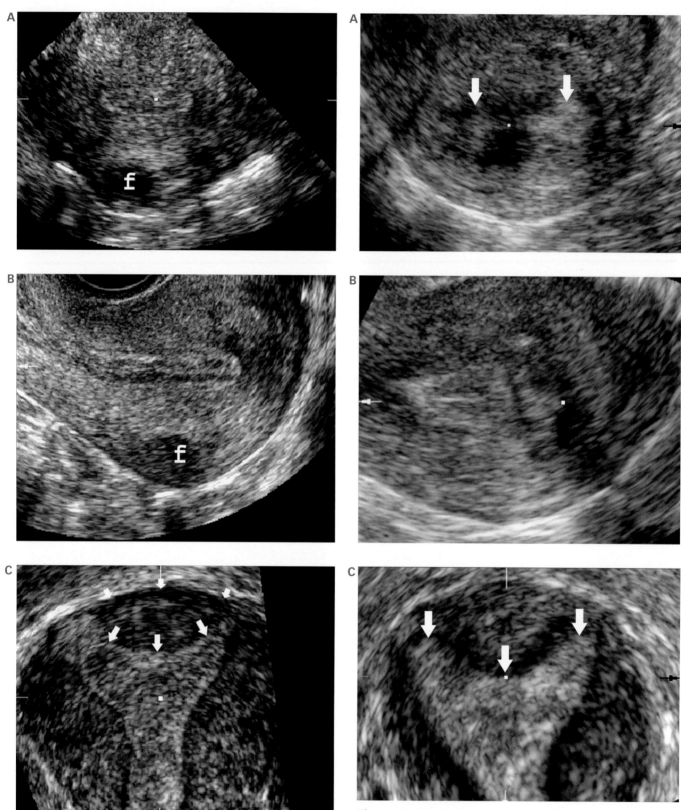

Figure 14-31. *Multiplanar views of the uterus.* **A** *Transverse view through the uterus.* **B** *Sagittal view through the uterus. f = subserosal fibroid.* **C** *Coronal view of the uterus. The shorter arrows display the external contour of the uterus. The longer arrows display the upper level of the triangular-shaped endometrial canal.*

Figure 14-32. *Multiplanar views of an arcuate uterus.* **A** *Transverse view through the uterus showing the classic "double echo complex' (arrows).* **B** *Sagittal view through the uterus.* **C** *Coronal view of the uterus. The arrows point to the arcuate shape of the endometrial canal. Note the normal shape of the external uterine wall.*

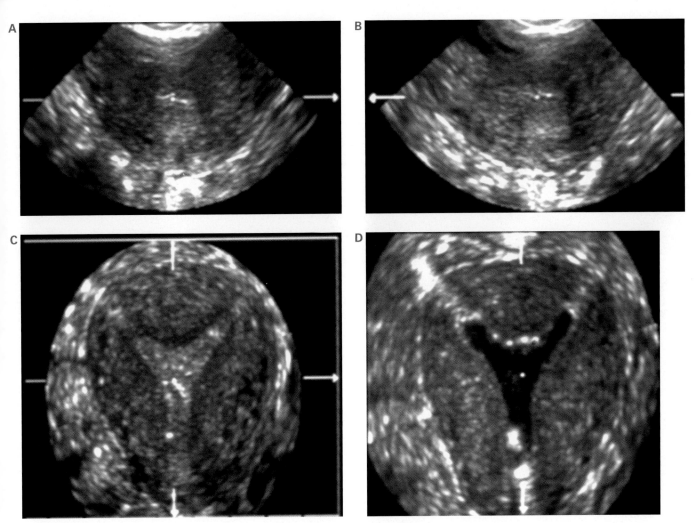

Figure 14-33. *Multiplanar and rendered views of an arcuate uterus.* **A** *Transverse view through the uterus.* **B** *Sagittal view through the uterus.* **C** *Coronal view of the uterus. Note the arcuate shape of the endometrial canal and the normal shape of the external uterine wall.* **D** *Rendered coronal view of this same patient after saline infusion (SHG). Note the bright echogenic spots at the upper end of the endometrial cavity, consistent with small polyps.*

patients presenting with dysfunctional uterine bleeding (DUB), patients who have experienced repeated miscarriages, and other indications. In these cases, neoplasms (e.g., polyps) can be detected and assessed from the stored volume data set. The use of volume sonography has been found to be advantageous for identification of the precise location of endometrial polyps and to determine the effect of fibroids on the endometrial lining, including their depth beneath the mucosa (Figures 14-33D and 14-34). This information can be of great value during the planning stages for surgical management of patients with these and other uterine abnormalities.

The definitive diagnosis of endometrial cancer typically requires endometrial biopsy or dilation and curettage.

Two-dimensional ultrasound has been used as a screening method for patients at high risk. However, volume sonography can improve the ability to detect endometrial abnormalities.

The normal uterus, as seen in the coronal plane, has a flat or slight upwardly convex fundal contour. The endometrium is normally triangular in shape at the fundus. The echogenicity of the endometrium varies during the menstrual cycle, but generally the endometrium is more echogenic than the myometrium. The normal endometrium should be of homogeneous echotexture and the endometrial-myometrial junction should be distinct. A coronal view of the uterine body and fundus that is not in the true mid-coronal plane may give the false impression

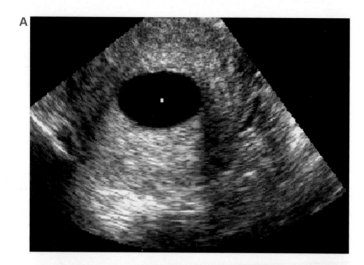

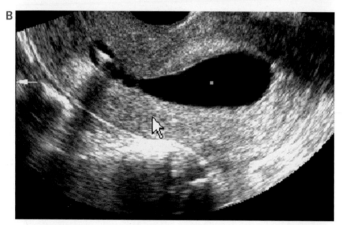

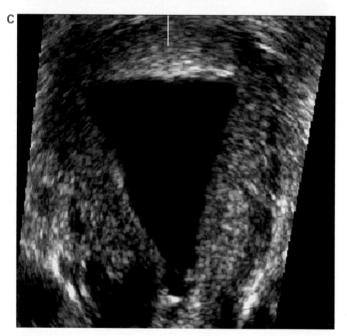

Figure 14-34. *Multiplanar views of the uterus with saline infusion (SHG). **A** Transverse view through the uterus. **B** Sagittal view through the uterus. **C** Coronal view. Note the visualization of the endometrial cavity in all three planes.*

of an arcuate uterus or may obscure the presence of this or other uterine deformities. Because of ante- or retro-flexion of the uterus with respect to the cervix, it is clear that the coronal plane through the center of the uterine cavity is often not the same as the coronal plane through the center of the cervical canal. Therefore, a mid-coronal view of the uterus is not likely to give a true mid-coronal view of the cervical canal. The normal nulliparous uterus is usually encompassed in a single volume acquisition. However, even the normal-sized uterus may be positioned such that more than one volume is required to allow assessment of the entire cervix and uterine body.

The double endometrial echo-complex seen in a transverse view of the fundus with 2D imaging is generally indicative of a uterine anomaly, most commonly a septate or bicornuate uterus. However, an arcuate uterus (a very mild form of uterine anomaly) may also display two endometrial echoes in an axial slice through the fundus. Therefore, while some information can be deduced from the appearance of the upper uterus and the upper endometrial echoes, it is usually not possible to confidently evaluate the shape of the uterine fundus or of the endometrium with a 2D scanning approach. Traditionally, patients have been initially screened by means of **hysterosalpingography**, which images only the uterine cavity (lumen). When indicated, patients would receive a hysteroscopic examination, which has been considered the gold standard for the assessment of the uterine cavity. **Hysteroscopy** is limited to the evaluation of the endometrial surface of the uterus and does not provide detailed information on the myometrium or serosal surface, which is important to make a clear distinction between a bicornuate and septate uterus. For this purpose, laparoscopic assessment of the external contour of the uterus would be required. Volume sonography, especially when combined with sonohysterography (described below), provides detailed information about the myometrium, the endometrial and serosal surfaces, and the contours of the uterus. Thus, transvaginal volume sonography may obviate the need for other diagnostic modalities, such as MRI, hysteroscopy, and hysterosalpingography, as well as invasive procedures that may otherwise be necessary to derive a diagnosis. Furthermore, the coronal view of the uterus allows precise measurement of the distance between the mid-fundus and a line connecting the two internal tubal ostia. Fedele and colleagues (1991) emphasized the importance of these measurements to distinguish between bicornuate and septate uteri and hence to determine which patients should be treated by hysteroscopic metroplasty.

Uterine myomas can also be assessed using volume sonography, particularly with an transvaginal approach. The multiplanar display, by demonstrating the anatomy in three orthogonal views, allows precise localization of a myoma with respect to the endometrial cavity, which assists in determining the optimal surgical approach (hysteroscopic resection or abdominal myomectomy). The multiplanar display is also useful in some cases for differentiating adnexal lesions close to the uterus from lesions within or originating from the uterus. In our experience this may obviate MRI in selected cases.

The Endometrium

Transvaginal sonography has an important role to play in assessing the endometrium. The multiplanar display provided by volume sonography permits clear visualization of the triangular-shaped endometrium and depicts the cornual angles, the myometrial-endometrial border, and the entire cervical canal. The coronal plane, in particular, is helpful in demonstrating focal changes (such as polyps or cysts) in or adjacent to the endometrium.

Depiction of the coronal plane through the uterus provided by volume sonography can allow a more comprehensive assessment of the location of intrauterine devices (IUDs). Lee, Eppel, and colleagues (1997) reported the visualization of TCu380A IUDs in 96 women. Complete visualization of all parts of the IUD was possible in 95% of cases; volume sonography enabled visualization of the entire IUD (i.e., the shaft and the arms within the cavity) on a single image.

Wu and colleagues (1997) demonstrated the value of volume sonography for identification of retained intrauterine fetal bones after a therapeutic abortion in the second trimester. The multiplanar capability of volume sonography, along with the rendering features that highlight bony structures (i.e., maximum-intensity projections), demonstrated the retained fragments with clarity, and hysteroscopic removal was then performed.

Sonohysterography

Transvaginal sonography is sensitive in detecting small uterine masses and endometrial abnormalities, but the exact location (with respect to the uterine cavity or lining) and nature of lesions are often difficult to ascertain. Furthermore, in the presence of fibroids, the endometrial echo complex may be difficult to visualize. Uterine anomalies may be suspected on transvaginal sonography, but specific diagnosis often requires additional imaging or surgical exploration (hysteroscopy or laparoscopy).

Sonographic evaluation of the endometrial canal can be markedly improved by the installation of sterile saline to dilate the canal via sonohysterography (SHG). Sonohysterography permits detailed simultaneous evaluation of the uterine cavity, the endometrial lining, and the myometrium. Although a detailed explanation of sonohysterographic technique is beyond the scope of this chapter, the potential benefits of volume sonography over conventional 2D sonography are many and will be discussed here.

The technique of performing **volume sonohysterography** with a dedicated volume ultrasound system is similar to conventional sonohysterography (see Chapter 2). A sterile, specially designed dual-channel catheter is used to distend the uterine cavity with sterile saline while imaging the uterus with real-time transvaginal 2D sonography. When optimal distention of the cavity is achieved an appropriately sized volume box is chosen and the volume mode is activated. During volume acquisition the transvaginal probe is held stationary and the patient is instructed not to move as the transducer sweeps through the region of interest. Typically, one to three volumes are obtained in rapid succession so that the duration of uterine distention is less than two minutes to minimize patient discomfort (see Figure 14-34). With the advent of 4D imaging, multiplanar views or 3D renderings are displayed and updated rapidly (at or near real-time frame rates). Several volume data sets can be acquired and then saved for later analysis. Using 4D sonography, it is possible to image and record dynamic events such as catheter insertion and withdrawal during distention of the lower uterine segment and cervical canal, locations that may be difficult to examine. In addition, 4D sonography may be useful during evaluation of fallopian tube patency and for guiding interventions; however, additional studies are required to evaluate these possible roles of volume sonography.

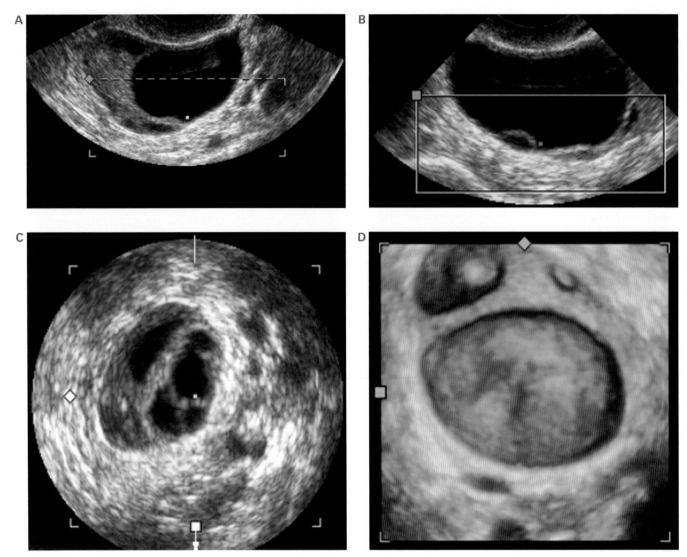

Figure 14-35. *Multiplanar and rendered views of a complex multicystic ovarian mass. The mass is shown* **A** *in long axis,* **B** *in the transverse plane, and* **C** *in the coronal plane. The operator-selected rendering boxes shown in* **A** *and* **B** *define the volume rendering shown in window* **D***.*

The Adnexa and Ovaries: Applications in Infertility

Volume sonography has been found to be of value in the assessment of female patients undergoing therapy for infertility (Figure 14-35). Assessment of ovarian volume prior to stimulation has been shown to be a useful predictor of the ultimate response to hormonal therapy, including the risk of hyperstimulation. Published reports also indicate that volume sonography can be useful to monitor follicular development during hormonal treatments. The volume of a developing follicle as determined by volume sonography has been shown to reflect its actual size more accurately than linear (i.e., multiple diameter) measure-

ments obtained with 2D imaging (Figure 14-36). This is because the volume of the follicle will remain constant even in cases where its overall shape and contour are asymmetrical. In addition, determination of the maturity of follicles may be improved with the use of volume sonography for detecting the cumulus oophorus, as well as increased blood flow (detected with color flow imaging) around the developing follicle.

A relatively common finding in patients who suffer from infertility is polycystic ovary syndrome (PCOS), which typically results in enlarged ovaries containing many immature follicles. In these cases volume sonography can provide accurate measurements of total ovarian volume

A
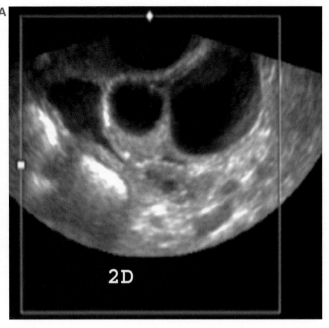

B
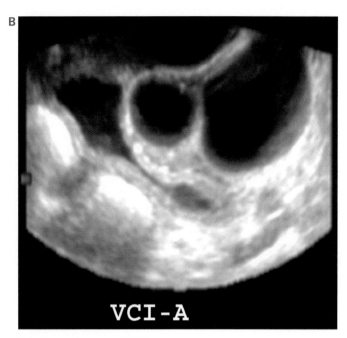

Figure 14-36. *Virtual contrast imaging (VCI).* **A** *2D visualization of a multicystic ovarian mass.* **B** *VCI improves the delineation of tissue interfaces and improves contrast resolution.*

as well as identify the hypertrophic stroma, which is one characteristic of an ovary in a patient with polycystic ovary syndrome.

Real-time volume sonography shows promise for guiding invasive procedures such as egg retrievals and cyst aspirations. More accurate needle placement and more complete cyst aspirations can be performed because the needle can be simultaneously viewed in a multiplanar projection, which provides improved assessment of the anatomy and the effectiveness of the procedure at the time of treatment.

VOLUME COLOR FLOW SONOGRAPHY

Just as **gray-scale volume sonography** can improve the depiction of anatomic structures and the spatial relationship of structures, **volume color flow imaging** (**CFI**) can also improve the depiction of blood flow in both normal and abnormal vessels.

Technique

One of the most common problems sonography professionals encounter in their learning curve for acquiring volume CFI data is optimization of the various system parameters (both Doppler and volume parameters).

While there is no fixed recipe for every occasion, the basic principles pertaining to 2D color flow imaging should be understood and employed, as these will also help to optimize volume CFI data acquisitions. Typically, because the acquisition of volume data requires movement of the probe or the beam through a region of interest, it is often necessary to reduce the level of color flow sensitivity to avoid artifacts related to tissue or probe motion.

Some of the basic principles and techniques of performing color flow imaging (both color Doppler imaging and power Doppler imaging) evaluations are:

- Using low Doppler beam-to-vessel angles (i.e., directing the transmitted Doppler beam as parallel to the vessel as possible).

- Optimizing the CFI gain setting to improve functional lumen fill-in while avoiding color "blooming" artifacts.

- Adjusting the CFI wall filter (the wall filter should be set as low as possible to improve flow sensitivity but high enough to avoid motion artifacts).

- Setting the dynamic motion differentiation to avoid background noise signals.

- Adjusting the scale setting (pulse repetition frequency, or PRF) and baseline position to maximize flow sensitivity but avoid aliasing artifacts.

The practitioner should begin the examination with 2D gray-scale sonography, employing the highest possible frame rate. That translates into a volume with the highest quality, as there will be more frames in a volume. Also, the examiner should keep the overall field of view as shallow and narrow as possible (based on the width and depth of the region of interest). Factors that affect the frame rates of volume sonography include the size of the volume region of interest in both the axial and lateral dimensions (one should use the smallest region of interest that includes the necessary anatomy) and the number of focal zones employed (fewer focal zones will improve frame rates). Tissue harmonic imaging (THI) can help to reduce speckle or noise on the gray-scale image (i.e., to display blood vessels as anechoic structures), but it is important to know that on some platforms tissue harmonic imaging reduces frame rates.

Flow Volume and Perfusion Studies

Volume color flow imaging has the potential to provide accurate volume flow measurements. Multiple studies have shown that volume flow measurements are feasible, and nomograms of several different organ systems in the fetus have been generated. An interesting aspect of obtaining color flow imaging volumes is that this information can estimate the overall blood supply of a given organ or anatomic region. Equipment manufacturers continuously improve the capabilities of their products, including the ability to quantify blood flow. One of the most useful programs is the 3D shell imaging method. In this method a power Doppler imaging volume data set is acquired and then a volume of interest (VOI) inside the initial acquired volume is manually defined by the operator. Inside the volume of interest, gray-scale and/or color histograms can be evaluated together or separately and expressed as a mean relative value. From these measure-

ments a variety of ratios and indices can be derived to quantify blood flow. The potential clinical value of these flow volume quantification methods is better estimation of blood flow within the area of interest (e.g., the placenta or a tumor).

It is important that, while these measurements provide a useful means of quantifying relative blood flow and vascularity in the acquired volumes, their information is based on digitized color voxel information. The accuracy of this information is likely to improve with advances in the technology. Published nomograms for vascularity based on the acquisition of data using one platform typically cannot be used for imaging with other systems or with different generations of the same system because of the potential variability in color sensitivity. Nevertheless, the information obtained can provide important qualitative assessment of vascularization and blood flow changes in both normal and abnormal physiologic states.

Volume color flow imaging has been shown to be of value for evaluation of a variety to structures. Studies have indicated its usefulness in imaging the vascularity of tumors (chorioangiomas, teratomas, hygromas, lung sequestration), the fetal brain (vein of Galen aneurysms, agenesis of the corpus cavernosum, vascular malformations), kidneys (agenesis of the kidneys, renal arteries), fetal abdominal vessels, umbilical cord anomalies, and placental disorders (Figures 14-37 and 14-38).

Lee and colleagues (2004) demonstrated that volume color flow imaging could visualize placental angiogenesis (as early as 7.1 weeks' gestation), cerebral and neck vessels (as early as 12.9 weeks' gestation), intracranial vessels, cord insertion, placenta, and vasa previa. In another interesting study, Kalache and colleagues (2003) described the use of 3D power Doppler sonography for the identification of vascular congenital anomalies of the fetal portosystemic

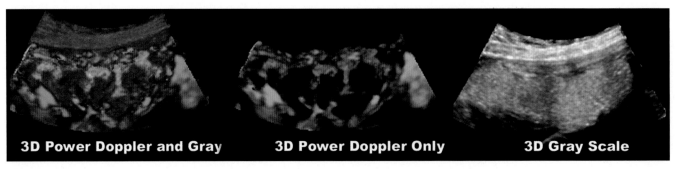

3D Power Doppler and Gray   **3D Power Doppler Only**   **3D Gray Scale**

Figure 14-37. *3D gray-scale and power Doppler views of the placenta showing placental vascular tree.*

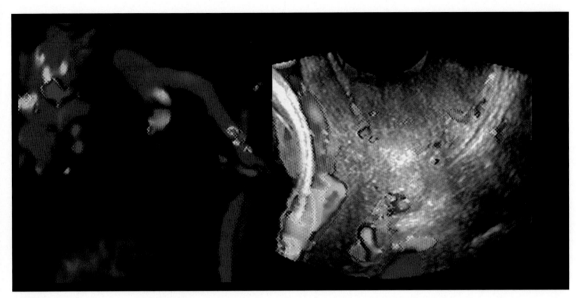

Figure 14-38. *3D color Doppler of vasa previa at 22 weeks' gestation showing the relationship between the vasa previa and the internal os of the cervix on the right.*

and umbilical venous systems. They correctly identified eight out of 310 fetuses with portosystemic venous malformations.

Shih and colleagues reported their experiences evaluating placental blood flow with volume color flow imaging. They found that volume power Doppler imaging (PDI) allowed a more accurate diagnosis of placenta accreta and its variants (increta and percreta). The authors found that 3D PDI detection of numerous coherent vessels was the single best criterion for the diagnosis of placenta accreta, with a sensitivity of 97% and a specificity of 92%.

NETWORKING WITH VOLUME SONOGRAPHY

Volume sonography lends itself to teleradiology. Because the volume data set is stored digitally, it can be transmitted to workstations within a given institution via an intranet as well as to other institutions that may be located around the world for expert consultation. The digitally stored volumes can be accessed and analyzed by physicians and sonographers for diagnostic purposes as well as to enhance sonography training. The ability to perform "virtual scans" via review and analysis of the volume data shows strong potential. There is little doubt that volume sonography used for off-site interpretation is not yet firmly established, but it will have a substantial impact on the way clinical sonography is performed. Using this technology, one would expect that in the future primary

clinical sites in remote areas would have access to expert interpretation and consultation, enabling high-quality, cost-effective medical care.

VOLUME SONOGRAPHY ARTIFACTS, LIMITATIONS, AND PITFALLS

It must be emphasized that volume sonography information is based on the compilation and manipulation of multiple consecutive 2D images. Therefore, volume sonography remains susceptible to many of the same artifacts and limitations that affect 2D sonography, such as unfavorable patient body habitus, fetal movement, and decreased amniotic fluid. In fact, these problems can be compounded when performing volume sonography.

When utilizing volume sonography, practitioners may encounter two types of artifacts: (1) acoustic artifacts that also occur with conventional imaging (e.g., acoustic shadowing, enhancement, refraction, reverberation, attenuation, and motion artifacts) and (2) artifacts that are unique to volume sonography. It is important to recognize and understand artifacts in order to avoid misinterpretations (see Chapter 1).

Artifacts that are unique to volume sonography can be divided into acquisition artifacts, rendering artifacts, and editing artifacts, as described in detail in a review article by Nelson and colleagues (2000). The most common **acquisition artifacts** encountered in obstetrics and gynecology are motion artifacts. They typically originate from sudden fetal motion during a relatively slow data acquisition. In gynecology, pulsating pelvic vessels or even the patient's breathing can affect the quality of the volume data. In imaging the uterus, one of the most commonly seen artifacts is the **enhancement artifact**, in which the echogenic endometrium appears to spread beyond the endometrial/myometrial interface, causing the adjacent myometrium to appear artifactually hyperechoic. Another problem commonly encountered in obstetric and gynecologic volume sonography is related to the limited size of the volume region of interest. There is a finite size of the volume region of interest, which varies depending on the specific system and probe employed. In some cases, it may be necessary to acquire two volumes in order to obtain all the anatomic structures or regions needed for diagnosis. For this reason, the multiplanar display should be quickly reviewed immediately after the acquisition to ensure that portions of a structure have not been excluded from the volume data set. Likewise, a very large fetus or adnexal mass may not be imaged completely in a single volume data set obtained transvaginally. Because the size of the volume region of interest on an abdominal volume probe is typically larger, a transabdominal acquisition of the fetus or adnexal mass may allow acquisition of the entire structure in one data set. Another potential pitfall in volume sonography of the pelvis involves spatial orientation within the volume data. During the preliminary real-time survey the operator must determine the orientation of the fetus or the uterus (e.g., anteverted or retroverted), as this may not be apparent on the saved volumes. Also, if the acquired volume is manipulated prior to digital storage, the correct orientation of the structures within the volume may not be apparent on later review of the volume. Likewise, the saved volumes of the extremities and/or adnexa must be annotated with respect to left and right because one cannot reliably determine this from review of the volume at a later time.

There are also technical issues and artifacts that are specific to volume sonography. For example, within the volume data set, resolution is typically lower in the planes that are orthogonal to the acquisition plane. Although recent improvements have resulted in faster volume data acquisition, less bulky and lighter probes, and better segmentation software, there remains a need for even higher resolution, improved software, and automated volume measurements to overcome problems related to these and other **rendering artifacts**.

Editing artifacts result when imaging data (e.g., a portion of a structure such as the fetal lip) is removed from a rendered image. Editing artifacts can make normal structures appear abnormal, leading to a misdiagnosis.

While volume sonography might improve the examiner's overall comprehension of anatomy, it does not make up for poor scanning technique. Problems affecting 2D sonography on a given patient will often also adversely affect volume sonography image quality and diagnostic utility. As is often the case, experience with this new technology is needed in order to identify situations that will prevent even the most competent professional from obtaining high-quality volume scans. Further research is needed to develop standardized techniques and methods for optimal acquisition, display, and rendering of 3D ultrasound data.

SCANNING TIPS, GUIDELINES, AND PITFALLS

The diagnostic quality of color flow imaging volume acquisitions can be improved by using the following techniques and parameter adjustments:

1. Start with the slowest acquisition speed practical in order to leave time for the transducer to acquire the maximum amount of information. Typically a slower speed of acquisition will improve the quality of the obtained volume.

2. Ask the patient not to move during the acquisition and acquire volumes of fetuses when they are in quiet states; patient or fetal movement may result in color flow imaging artifacts.

3. Analyze the volume data immediately after the acquisition for artifacts that can result from fetal breathing, respiration, or movement. Pay particular attention to the multiplanar views that are orthogonal to the acquired plane, since those are the computer-generated views and may be more susceptible to artifacts.

4. When possible, obtain volume data using different acquisition angles to determine which approach provides the best display. For example, color flow imaging volumes of the uterine vasculature can be obtained in a plane along the uterine axis (longitudinal) or a plane perpendicular to its axis (cross-sectional). Acquire a volume data set using both approaches and see how they compare to each other. In some cases vessels seen on one acquisition may not be seen on

the other acquisition. Thus, the two acquisitions will complement each other.

5. To access the fetal face, there must be adequate fluid in front of the fetal face, and one should be able to obtain a good fetal profile using 2D imaging. Once you have obtained the fetal profile in the mid-sagittal plane, place your ROI over the profile and begin the render start line above the profile. The ROI box should be sized appropriately and positioned as close to the fetal structures as possible. Now your 3D sweep can be performed.

6. It is helpful whenever possible to perform the 3D and 4D sweeps with the ultrasound beam positioned at a 90-degree angle to the structure of interest.

REFERENCES

Alcazar JL, Galan MJ, Garcia-Manero M, et al: Three-dimensional sonographic morphologic assessment in complex adnexal masses. J Ultrasound Med 22:249–254, 2003.

Alcazar JL, Iturra A, Sedda F, et al: Three-dimensional volume off-line analysis as compared to real-time ultrasound for assessing adnexal masses. Eur J Obstet Gynecol 161:92-95, 2012.

Athanasiou S, Khullar V, Boos K, et al: Imaging the urethral sphincter with three-dimensional ultrasound. Obstet Gynecol 94:295–301, 1999.

Bega G, Kuhlman K, Lev-Toaff A, et al: Application of three-dimensional ultrasonography in the evaluation of the fetal heart. J Ultrasound Med 20:307–313, 2001.

Bega G, Lev-Toaff A, Kuhlman K, et al: Three-dimensional multiplanar transvaginal ultrasound of the cervix in pregnancy. Ultrasound Obstet Gynecol 16:351–358, 2000.

Bega G, Lev-Toaff A, Kuhlman K, et al: Three-dimensional ultrasonographic imaging in obstetrics: present and future applications. J Ultrasound Med 20:391–408, 2001.

Bega G, Lev-Toaff AS, O'Kane P, et al: Three-dimensional ultrasonography in gynecology: technical aspects and clinical applications. J Ultrasound Med 22:1249–1269, 2003.

Bega G, Wapner R, Lev-Toaff A, et al: Diagnosis of conjoined twins at 10 weeks using three-dimensional ultrasound: a case report. Ultrasound Obstet Gynecol 16:388–390, 2000.

Benacerraf BR: The future of ultrasound: viewing the dark side of the moon? Ultrasound Obstet Gynecol 23:211–215, 2004.

Benacerraf BR: The role of three-dimensional ultrasound in the evaluation of the fetus. In Callen P (ed): *Ultrasonography in Obstetrics and Gyncecology*, 5th Edition. St. Louis, Saunders Elsevier, 2008, pp 830–862.

Benacerraf BR: Tomographic sonography of the fetus: is it accurate enough to be a frontline screen for fetal malformation? J Ultrasound Med 25:687–689, 2006.

Benacerraf BR, Benson CB, Abuhamad AZ, et al: Three- and 4-dimensional ultrasound in obstetrics and gynecology: proceedings of the American Institute of Ultrasound in Medicine consensus conference. J Ultrasound Med 24:1587–1597, 2005.

Benacerraf BR, Sadow PM, Barnewolt CE, et al: Cleft of the secondary palate without cleft lip diagnosed with three-dimensional ultrasound and magnetic resonance imaging in a fetus with Fryns' syndrome. Ultrasound Obstet Gynecol 27:566–570, 2006.

Benacerraf BR, Shipp TD, Bromley B: How sonographic tomography will change the face of obstetric sonography: a pilot study. J Ultrasound Med 24:371–378, 2005.

Benacerraf BR, Shipp TD, Bromley B: Improving the efficiency of gynecologic sonography with 3-dimensional volumes: a pilot study. J Ultrasound Med 25:165–171, 2006.

Benacerraf BR, Shipp TD, Bromley B: Three-dimensional ultrasound of the fetus: volume imaging. Radiology 238:988–996, 2006.

Benoit B, Chaoui R: Three-dimensional ultrasound with maximal mode rendering: a novel technique for the diagnosis of bilateral or unilateral absence or hypoplasia of nasal bones in second-trimester screening for Down syndrome. Ultrasound Obstet Gynecol 25:19–24, 2005.

Bernard JP, Lecuru F, Darles C, et al: Saline contrast sonohysterography as first line investigation for women with uterine bleeding. Ultrasound Obstet Gynecol 10:121–125, 1997.

Bhaduri M, Fong K, Toi A, et al: Fetal anatomic survey using three-dimensional ultrasound in conjunction with first-trimester nuchal translucency screening. Prenat Diagn 30:267–273, 2010.

Bonilla-Musoles, Raga R, Osborne NG, et al: Three-dimensional hysterosonography for the study of endometrial tumors: comparison with conventional transvaginal sonography, hysterosalpingography, and hysteroscopy. Gynecol Oncol 65:245–252, 1997.

Bromley B, Shipp TD, Benacerraf BR: Structural anomalies in early embryonic death: a 3-dimensional pictorial essay. J Ultrasound Med 29:445–453, 2010.

Bronz L, Suter T, Rusca T: The value of transvaginal sonography with and without saline instillation in the diagnosis of uterine pathology in pre- and postmenopausal women with abnormal bleeding or suspect sonographic findings. Ultrasound Obstet Gynecol 9:53–58, 1997.

Chang FM, Hsu KF, Ko HC, et al: Fetal heart volume assessment by three-dimensional ultrasound. Ultrasound Obstet Gynecol 9:42–48, 1997.

Chaoui R, Heling KS: New developments in fetal heart scanning: three- and four-dimensional fetal echocardiography. Semin Fetal Neonatal Med 10:567–577, 2005.

Chaoui R, Heling KS: Three-dimensional ultrasound in prenatal diagnosis. Curr Opin Obstet Gynecol 18:192–202, 2006.

Chaoui R, Hoffmann J, Heling KS: Three-dimensional (3D) and 4D color Doppler fetal echocardiography using spatio-temporal image correlation (STIC). Ultrasound Obstet Gynecol 23:535–545, 2004.

Chaoui R, Levaillant JM, Benoit B, et al: Three-dimensional sonographic description of abnormal metopic suture in second- and third-trimester fetuses. Ultrasound Obstet Gynecol 26:761–764, 2005.

Chase DM, Crade M, Basu T, et al: Preoperative diagnosis of ovarian malignancy: preliminary results of the use of 3-dimensional vascular ultrasound. Int J Gynecol Cancer 19:354–360, 2009.

Cho HY, Kwon JY, Kim YH, et al: Comparison of nuchal translucency measurements obtained using Volume NT(TM) and two- and three-dimensional ultrasound. Ultrasound Obstet Gynecol 39:175-180, 2012.

Coyne L, Jayaprakasan K, Raine-Fenning N: 3D ultrasound in gynecology and reproductive medicine. Women's Health 4:501–516, 2008.

Dolz M, Osborne NG, Blanes J, et al: Polycystic ovarian syndrome: assessment with color Doppler angiography and three-dimensional ultrasonography. J Ultrasound Med 18:303–313, 1999.

Faro C, Benoit B, Wegrzyn P, et al: Three-dimensional sonographic description of the fetal frontal bones and metopic suture. Ultrasound Obstet Gynecol 26:618–621, 2005.

Faro C, Chaoui R, Wegrzyn P, et al: Metopic suture in fetuses with Apert syndrome at 22–27 weeks of gestation. Ultrasound Obstet Gynecol 27:28–33, 2006.

Faro C, Wegrzyn P, Benoit B, et al: Metopic suture in fetuses with holoprosencephaly at 11 + 0 to 13 + 6 weeks of gestation. Ultrasound Obstet Gynecol 27:162–166, 2006.

Faro C, Wegrzyn P, Benoit B, et al: Metopic suture in fetuses with trisomy 21 at 11 + 0 to 13 + 6 weeks of gestation. Ultrasound Obstet Gynecol 27:286–289, 2006.

Fedele L, Dorta M, Brioschi D, et al: Re-examination of the anatomic indications for hysteroscopic metroplasty. Eur J Obstet Gynecol Reprod Biol 39:127–131, 1991.

Feichtinger W: Follicle aspiration with interactive three-dimensional digital imaging (Voluson): a step toward real-time puncturing under three-dimensional ultrasound control. Fertil Steril 70:374–377, 1998.

Goncalves LF, Espinoza J, Kusanovic JP, et al: Applications of 2-dimensional matrix array for 3- and 4-dimensional examination of the fetus: a pictorial essay. J Ultrasound Med 25:745–755, 2006.

Goncalves LF, Espinoza J, Lee W, et al: Should the frontal bone be visualized in midline sagittal views of the facial profile to assess the fetal nasal bones during the first trimester? Ultrasound Obstet Gynecol 25:90–92, 2005.

Goncalves LF, Espinoza J, Lee W, et al: Three- and four-dimensional reconstruction of the aortic and ductal arches using inversion mode: a new rendering algorithm for visualization of fluid-filled anatomic structures. Ultrasound Obstet Gynecol 24:696–698, 2004.

Goncalves LF, Espinoza J, Mazor M, et al: Newer imaging modalities in the prenatal diagnosis of skeletal dysplasias. Ultrasound Obstet Gynecol 24:115–120, 2004.

Goncalves LF, Espinoza J, Romero R, et al: Four-dimensional fetal echocardiography with spatiotemporal image correlation (STIC): a systematic study of standard cardiac views assessed by different observers. J Matern Fetal Neonatal Med 17:323–331, 2005.

Goncalves LF, Espinoza J, Romero R, et al: Four-dimensional ultrasonography of the fetal heart using a novel tomographic ultrasound imaging display. J Perinat Med 34:39–55, 2006.

Goncalves LF, Espinoza J, Romero R, et al: A systematic approach to prenatal diagnosis of transposition of the great arteries using 4-dimensional ultrasonography with spatiotemporal image correlation. J Ultrasound Med 23:1225–1231, 2004.

Goncalves LF, Lee W, Espinoza J, et al: Examination of the fetal heart by four-dimensional (4D) ultrasound with spatio-temporal image correlation (STIC). Ultrasound Obstet Gynecol 27:336–348, 2006.

Goncalves LF, Lee W, Espinoza J, et al: Three- and 4-dimensional ultrasound in obstetric practice: does it help? J Ultrasound Med 24:1599–1624, 2005.

Goncalves LF, Nien JK, Espinoza J, et al: What does 2-dimensional imaging add to 3- and 4-dimensional obstetric ultrasonography? J Ultrasound Med 25:691–699, 2006.

Grigore M, Mare A: Applications of 3-D ultrasound in female infertility. Rev Med Chir Soc Med Nat Iasi 113:1113–1119, 2009.

Jarvela IY, Sladkevicius P, Kelly S, et al: Three-dimensional sonographic and power Doppler characterization of ovaries in late follicular phase. Ultrasound Obstet Gynecol 20:281–285, 2002.

Joshi M, Ganesan K, Munshi HN, Ganesan S, Lawande A: Ultrasound of adnexal masses. Semin Ultrasound CT MR 29:72–97, 2008.

Kalache K, Romero R, Goncalves LF, et al: Three-dimensional color power imaging of the fetal hepatic circulation. Am J Obstet Gynecol 189:1401–1406, 2003.

Kupesic S: The present and future role of three-dimensional ultrasound in assisted conception. Ultrasound Obstet Gynecol 18:191–194, 2001.

Kurjak A, Jackson D: An Atlas of Three- and Four-Dimensional Sonography in Obstetrics and Gynecology. London, Taylor & Francis, 2004.

Kyei-Mensah A, Machonochie N, Zaidi J, et al: Transvaginal three-dimensional ultrasound: reproducibility of ovarian and endometrial volume measurements. Fertil Steril 66:718–722, 1996.

Kyei-Mensah A, Zaidi J, Pittrof R, et al: Transvaginal three-dimensional ultrasound: accuracy of follicular volume measurements. Fertil Steril 65:371–376, 1996.

Laudy J, Janssen M, Struyk P, et al: Three-dimensional ultrasonography of normal fetal lung volume: a preliminary study. Ultrasound Obstet Gynecol 11:13–16, 1998.

Lee A, Eppel C, Sam A, Kratochwil A, et al: Intrauterine device localization by three-dimensional transvaginal sonography. Ultrasound Obstet Gynecol 10:289–292, 1997.

Lee W, Comstock CH, Kirk J, et al: Birth weight prediction by three-dimensional ultrasonographic volumes of the fetal thigh and abdomen. J Ultrasound Med 16:799–805, 1997.

Lee W, Deter RL, McNie B, et al: Individualized growth assessment of fetal soft tissue using fractional thigh volume. Ultrasound Obstet Gynecol 24:766–774, 2004.

Leventhal M, Pretorius D, Budorick N, et al: Three-dimensional ultrasonography of the normal fetal heart: comparison with two-dimensional imaging. J Ultrasound Med 17:341–348, 1998.

Lev-Toaff AS, Ozhan S, Pretorius D, et al: Three-dimensional multiplanar ultrasound for fetal gender assignment: value of the mid-sagittal plane. Ultrasound Obstet Gynecol 16:345–350, 2000.

Lev-Toaff A, Pinheiro L, Bega G, et al: Three-dimensional multiplanar sonohysterography: comparison with conventional two-dimensional sonohysterography and x-ray hysterosalpingography. J Ultrasound Med 20:295–306, 2001.

Liang RI, Chang FM, Yao BL, et al: Predicting birth weight by upper-arm volume with use of three-dimensional ultrasonography. Obstet Gynecol 177:632–638, 1997.

Maier B, Steiner H, Wieneroither H, et al: The psychological impact of three-dimensional fetal imaging on the fetomaternal relationship. In Baba K, Jurkovic D (eds): *Three-Dimensional Ultrasound in Obstetrics and Gynecology.* New York, Parthenon, 1997, pp 67–74.

Merz E, Bahlmann F, Weber G: Volume scanning in the evaluation of fetal malformations: a new dimension in prenatal diagnosis. Ultrasound Obstet Gynecol 5:222–227, 1995.

Merz E, Weber G, Bahlmann F, et al: Application of transvaginal and abdominal three-dimensional ultrasound for the detection or exclusion of malformations of the fetal face. Ultrasound Obstet Gynecol 9:237–243, 1997.

Meyer-Wittkopf M, Cook A, McLennan A, et al: Evaluation of three-dimensional ultrasonography and magnetic resonance imaging in assessment of congenital heart anomalies in fetal cardiac specimens. Ultrasound Obstet Gynecol 8:303–308, 1996.

Monteagudo A, Timor-Tritsch IE: Normal sonographic development of the central nervous system from the second trimester onwards using 2D, 3D and transvaginal sonography. Prenat Diagn 29:326–339, 2009.

Muscat M, Chavez M, Demishev M, et al: Intra- and inter-observer variability in the evaluation of first trimester placental volume by 3D ultrasound. Am J Obstet Gynecol 206:S165–S166, 2012.

Nelson TR, Downey D, Pretorius DH, et al: *Three-Dimensional Ultrasound.* Philadelphia, Lippincott Williams and Wilkins, 1999.

Nelson TR, Pretorius DH: Three-dimensional ultrasound of fetal surface features. Ultrasound Obstet Gynecol 2:166–174, 1992.

Nelson TR, Pretorius DH: Visualization of the fetal thoracic skeleton with three-dimensional sonography. AJR 164:1485–1488, 1995.

Nelson TR, Pretorius DH, Hull A, et al: Sources and impact of artifacts on clinical three-dimensional ultrasound imaging. Ultrasound Obstet Gynecol 16:374–383, 2000.

Nelson TR, Pretorius DH, Lev-Toaff A, et al: Feasibility of performing a virtual patient examination using three-dimensional ultrasonographic data acquired at remote locations. J Ultrasound Med 20:941–952, 2001.

Nelson TR, Pretorius DH, Sklansky M, et al: Three-dimensional echocardiographic evaluation of fetal heart anatomy and function: acquisition, analysis, and display. J Ultrasound Med 15:1–9, 1996.

Ness A, Bega G, Wood DC, et al: Massive fetal ileal duplication requiring antenatal intervention. J Ultrasound Med 25:785–790, 2006.

Poehl M, Hohlagschwandtner M, Doerner V, et al: Cumulus assessment by three-dimensional ultrasound for in vitro fertilization. Ultrasound Obstet Gynecol 16:251–253, 2000.

Pohls UG, Rempen A: Fetal lung volumetry by three-dimensional ultrasound. Ultrasound Obstet Gynecol 11:6–12, 1998.

Pretorius DH: Maternal smoking habit modification via fetal visualization. University of California Tobacco Related Disease Research Program. Annual report to the California State Legislature, 1996, p 76.

Pretorius DH, Nelson TR: Prenatal visualization of cranial sutures and fontanelles with three-dimensional ultrasonography. J Ultrasound Med 13:871–876, 1994.

Riccabona M, Pretorius DH, Nelson TR, et al: Three-dimensional ultrasound: display modalities in obstetrics. J Clin Ultrasound 25:157–167, 1997.

Sabogal JC, Becker E, Bega G, et al: Reproducibility of fetal lung volume measurements with 3-dimensional ultrasonography. J Ultrasound Med 23:347–352, 2004.

Shih JC, Palacios Jaraquemada JM, Su YN, et al: Role of three-dimensional power Doppler in the antenatal diagnosis of placenta accreta: comparison with gray-scale and color Doppler techniques. Ultrasound Obstet Gynecol 33:193–203, 2009.

Shipp TD, Bromley B, Benacerraf B: Is 3-dimensional volume sonography an effective alternative method to the standard 2-dimensional technique of measuring the nuchal translucency? J Clin Ultrasound 34:118–122, 2006.

Sklansky MS, Nelson TR, Pretorius DH: Three-dimensional fetal echocardiography: gated versus non-gated techniques. J Ultrasound Med 17:451–457, 1995.

Sladkevicius P, Ojha K, Campbell S, et al: Three-dimensional power Doppler imaging in the assessment of Fallopian tube patency. Ultrasound Obstet Gynecol 16: 644–647, 2000.

Sleurs E, Goncalves LF, Johnson A, et al: First-trimester three-dimensional ultrasonographic findings in a fetus with frontonasal malformation. J Matern Fetal Neonatal Med 16:187–197, 2004.

Soto E, Richani K, Goncalves LF, et al: Three-dimensional ultrasound in the prenatal diagnosis of cleidocranial dysplasia associated with B-cell immunodeficiency. Ultrasound Obstet Gynecol 27:574–579, 2006.

Steiner H, Staudach A, Spitzer D, et al: Three-dimensional ultrasound in obstetrics and gynaecology: technique, possibilities and limitations. Hum Reprod 9:1773–1778, 1994.

Stephenson SR: 3D and 4D sonography history and theory. J Diag Med Sonography 21:392–399, 2005.

Sur S, Clewes J, Jayaprakasan K, et al: Linear and volumetric ultrasound measures of embryo growth and their predictive value for first trimester miscarriage. Ultrasound Obstet Gynecol 38:61-61, 2011.

Turan S, Turan O, Baschat AA: Three- and four-dimensional fetal echocardiography. Fetal Diagn Ther 25:361–372, 2009.

Umek WH, Obermair A, Stutterecker D, et al: Three-dimensional ultrasound of the female urethra: comparing transvaginal and transrectal scanning. Ultrasound Obstet Gynecol 17:425–430, 2001.

Van Mieghem T, DeKoninck P, Steenhaut P, et al: Methods for prenatal assessment of fetal cardiac function. Prenat Diagn 29:1193–1203, 2009.

Wisher D: 3D and 4d evaluation of fetal anomalies. In Hagen-Ansert SL (ed): *Textbook of Diagnostic Sonography*, 7th Edition. St. Louis, Elsevier, 2012, pp 1206–1219.

Wisser J, Schar G, Kurmanavicius J, et al: Use of 3D ultrasound as a new approach to assessment of obstetric trauma to the pelvic floor. J Ultrasound Med 20:15–18, 1999.

Wu MH, Hsu CC, Lin YS: Three-dimensional ultrasound and hysteroscopy in the evaluation of intrauterine retained fetal bones. J Clin Ultrasound 25:93–95, 1997.

Yagel S, Cohen SM, Messing B, Valsky DV: Three-dimensional and four-dimensional ultrasound applications in fetal medicine. Curr Opin Obstet Gynecol 21:167–174, 2009.

Yuh EL, Jeffrey RB, Birdwell RL, et al: Virtual endoscopy using perspective volume-rendered three-dimensional sonographic data: technique and clinical applications. AJR 172:1193–1197, 1999.

Zosmer N, Jurkovic D, Jauniaux E, et al: Selection and identification of standard cardiac views from three-dimensional volume scans of the fetal thorax. J Ultrasound Med 15:25–32, 1996.

SELF-ASSESSMENT EXERCISES

Questions

1. The volume data acquisition technology that provides the best spatial relationships of structure and more accurate 3D renderings is:

   A. Off-line system analysis

   B. Free-hand technique using conventional 2D probes

   C. 2D probes with position sensors

   D. Dedicated mechanized volume probes

2. Of the following, which is best for demonstrating bony structures?

   A. Surface rendering

   B. Maximum-intensity projections

   C. Minimum-intensity projections

   D. Multiplanar viewing

3. Of the following statements, which is true for 3D imaging?

   A. Anomalies that cannot be seen with 2D images are well demonstrated with 3D.

   B. 3D imaging has no real value in the first trimester, as fetal skin and subcutaneous tissues are not developed enough to visualize.

   C. The fetal heart cannot be evaluated with 3D/4D due to motion artifacts.

   D. Volume sonography is mostly used in the cardiology and obstetric specialties.

4. The individual volume elements that create the volume data set obtained from 2D slices are called:

    A. Voxels

    B. Pixels

    C. RAM

    D. Frames

5. Soft tissues of the fetal face are well displayed when using the following mode:

    A. Maximum-intensity

    B. Brightness

    C. Surface rendering

    D. Multiplanar

6. A volume scan of the fetal heart acquired in the four-chamber plane will allow one also to demonstrate:

    A. Aortic and ductal arches

    B. Outflow tracts

    C. A and B

    D. None of the above

7. The pitfalls of spatio-temporal image correlation (STIC) include all of the following *except*:

    A. Decreased image quality

    B. Slower acquisition time

    C. Common motion artifacts

    D. The narrow angle required for acquisition

8. Which of the following statements would be incorrect for 3D/4D imaging?

    A. The overall field of view should be as shallow as possible.

    B. Use the lowest frame rate possible.

    C. Use the slowest possible acquisition speed.

    D. The field of view should be as narrow as possible.

9. All of the following can limit the quality of 3D obstetric imaging *except*:

    A. Polyhydramnios

    B. Patient body habitus

    C. Fetal position

    D. Fetal movement

10. Which of the following is the most common artifact encountered in obstetrics and gynecology?

    A. Acquisition

    B. Rendering

    C. Editing

    D. Motion

Answers

See Appendix F on page 617 for answers and explanations.

Invasive Procedures

Bryan T. Oshiro, MD, and Kathryn A. Gill, MS, RT, RDMS, FSDMS

OBJECTIVES

After completing this chapter you should be able to:

1. List the indications and timing for performing an amniocentesis based on the procedure's different purposes.

2. Describe how to localize fluid for an amniocentesis, including techniques used for twin pregnancies.

3. Explain the therapeutic and diagnostic capabilities of cordocentesis.

4. Describe the procedures and purposes for performing amnioreduction as opposed to amnioinfusion.

5. Identify the two techniques used for guiding the needle in fetal blood sampling.

6. List the steps in preparing patients for intrauterine fetal transfusion and discuss how they differ from those for cordocentesis.

7. Discuss the obstetric uses of minimally invasive ultrasound-guided procedures.

THE MODERN HISTORY OF INVASIVE OBSTETRIC PROCEDURES begins with amniocentesis, which was first performed during the 1880s for decompression of polyhydramnios. The technique has been used for a variety of reasons over the years (Table 15-1). Placenta localization was first achieved in 1930 by injecting a radiographic contrast medium into the amniotic fluid. The English obstetrician Douglas Bevis pioneered the use of amniocentesis for prenatal diagnosis when he published a paper in *The Lancet* in 1952 describing the use of amniocentesis to predict hemolytic disease in neonates born to Rh-sensitized women. However, not until 1961, when Albert William Liley published a paper describing his use of the spectrophotometric measurement of bilirubin in the amniotic fluid, did the use of amniocentesis in the management Rh-sensitized pregnancies become widespread. By the mid-1960s it was demonstrated that amniocytes could be cultured to determine fetal karyotype. Subsequently, the use of amniocentesis was expanded for a variety of prenatal problems, including testing for aneuploidy, intrauterine infections, and lung maturity.

AMNIOCENTESIS

Amniocentesis is a procedure in which a needle is inserted into the uterus through the abdomen and a sample of amniotic fluid is withdrawn under sonographic guidance. It is the most common invasive prenatal diagnostic test used during pregnancy. Performing the

Table 15-1.   History of amniocentesis.

Years	Purpose
1880s	Amniocentesis is first performed to relieve polyhydramnios.
1950s	Amniocentesis is first used to measure bilirubin in amniotic fluid for monitoring Rh disease.
1961	Liley describes spectrophotometric measurement of bilirubin in the amniotic fluid.
1966	Steele and Breg demonstrate the feasibility of culturing/karyotyping fetal cells.
1967	The first reported abnormal karyotype is diagnosed prenatally.
1968	Valenti et al. first detect prenatal trisomy 21.
1968	Nadler first detects a prenatal metabolic disorder (galactosemia).
1972	Brock and Sutcliff use AFP for detection of neural tube defects.
Late 1970s–1980s	DNA technology emerges; CVS and PUBS are introduced.

Box 15-1.   Indications for amniocentesis.

Advanced maternal age (≥35 years)
Previous fetus with an aneuploidy
Parental balanced translocation
X-linked recessive disorders
Other genetic disorders
Fetal anomaly
Confirmation of lung maturity
Evaluation for intrauterine infection
Rh isoimmunization
Polyhydramnios
Fetal sex/paternity

amniocentesis under sonographic guidance is associated with a higher rate of successful taps and a lower rate of bloody taps (from 2.4% to 0.8%). Sonography also assists in avoiding the **dry tap** (a failure in obtaining amniotic fluid), since we can actually see the location of fluid, fetus, and placenta. An amniocentesis can be performed for a variety of reasons. Indications for a genetic amniocentesis include patients who have had a previous infant with a chromosomal abnormality or neural tube defect, an abnormal maternal serum alpha-fetoprotein (MSAFP) or quad marker screen, and/or a family history of genetic or central nervous system anomalies and Down syndrome. Amniocentesis can also be performed to check for fetal lung maturity, intrauterine infections, and the Rh status of the fetus (Box 15-1). For patients at risk for aneuploidy, due to either advanced maternal age (≥35 years) or an abnormal maternal serum screening test, a genetic amniocentesis is generally offered and performed between 15 and 20 weeks' gestation.

Several considerations apply to timing the amniocentesis for genetic counseling as opposed to fetal lung maturity. If the genetic amniocentesis is attempted prior to 15 weeks' gestation, fetal cells may not be adequate in number or mature enough to grow for a reliable reading. Also, the

amnion and chorion may not be fused enough until after 15 weeks to withdraw fluid safely. Studies have shown that performing the amniocentesis prior to 14 weeks increases the miscarriage rate to 2.7%. An amniocentesis performed for fetal lung maturity is usually performed after 36 weeks' gestation. Therefore a sonogram to check gestational age is often performed prior to the procedure.

Complications

Risk factors associated with the amniocentesis include miscarriage, cramping, bleeding, leakage of amniotic fluid (1%–2%), needle injuries, and Rh sensitization, the last two of which are rare. Traditionally, the pregnancy loss rate after a mid-trimester amniocentesis has been quoted as approximately 0.5%, based on three nonrandomized retrospective studies from the United States, Canada, and Great Britain from the 1970s. However, data from Eddleman et al. (2006), a large prospective multicenter clinical study evaluating the risk for aneuploidy using first and second trimester screening, found the amniocentesis-related fetal loss rate to be much lower, 0.06%. A recent review article reported the total risk for procedure-related complications of amniocentesis and chorionic villus sampling to be approximately 1.9%. Other potential complications are rare and include premature rupture of membranes, chorioamnionitis (0.1%), and placental abruption and sepsis. When amniocentesis is performed after 20 weeks' gestation, there is an additional risk of preterm labor.

Traversing the placenta when performing the amniocentesis does not appear to increase the risk of pregnancy

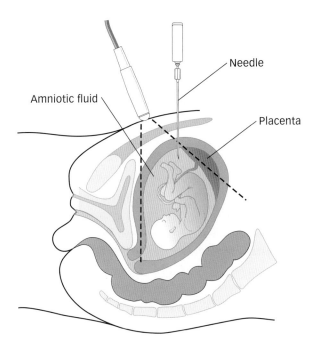

Figure 15-1. *Amniocentesis.*

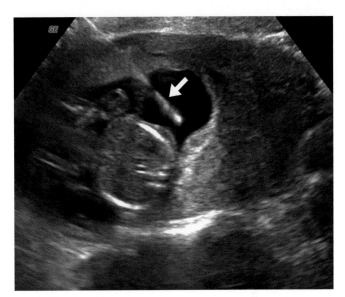

Figure 15-2. *Sonogram demonstrating needle placement (arrow) into the amniotic fluid.*

loss but sometimes can be problematic in the Rh-negative (Rh–) patient. Rh sensitization is rare today because of the routine administration of Rh immune globulin during pregnancy. Rh immune globulin is administered to unsensitized Rh– patients after amniocentesis in order to prevent Rh sensitization. An exception is made for patients whose partners are known to be Rh–, as their fetuses will also be Rh–. If the placenta must be traversed, it is recommended that one choose a site where the placenta is the thinnest and always try to avoid the umbilical cord insertion site. Puncturing the placenta increases the risk of bleeding, and a bloody tap can impair the results. Needle injuries can occur when the fetus moves into the tip of the needle, which is another reason sonographic guidance is important.

Technique

Prior to the procedure, a sonogram is performed to assess fetal viability, the gestational age, fetal number, location of placenta, fetal anatomy, amount of amniotic fluid, and any uterine abnormality. Sonography is used to localize the largest pocket of amniotic fluid (Figure 15-1). Next, the skin of the abdomen is cleansed, usually with an antiseptic, betadine, or iodine preparation (Box 15-2). A topical anesthetic may be applied to lessen the pain of puncturing the skin, but the uterine wall cannot be anesthetized. A 20-gauge spinal needle is then introduced into the amniotic cavity under direct ultrasound guidance

(Figure 15-2). The patient may feel an aching or cramping pain as the needle passes through the uterine wall. The first 1–2 ml of the aspirated fluid are discarded to avoid contamination of the fluid with maternal blood or other tissues. The amount of fluid removed varies depending on the diagnostic test. For example, 5–10 ml of fluid are adequate to perform a lung maturity test, but approximately 1 ml of fluid per week of gestation is obtained for chromosome analysis. With normal fetal renal function, the amniotic fluid aspirated will be replaced in less than a day. Results of the karyotype may take 2–4 weeks, but fluorescence in situ hybridization (FISH) techniques applied to uncultured amniocytes can be used to diagnose certain aneuploidies within 1–2 days. Results for lung maturity can be obtained within a few hours. Sonography is used to confirm fetal cardiac activity before and after the procedure has been completed.

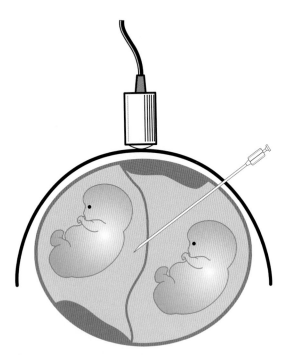

Figure 15-3. *Single-puncture technique for performing amniocentesis on diamniotic twin gestation.*

Amniocentesis in Multiples

Multiple gestation pregnancies pose an additional challenge in that one must be careful to obtain distinct amniotic fluid samples from each sac. The technique is the same as that for a singleton except that indigo carmine dye is injected after fluid is removed from the first sac. Another site is usually required to enter the sac of the other fetus. If the aspirated fluid is clear, then you know you have not inadvertently entered the first sac. If the fluid is blue, the needle should be removed and another site should be chosen after careful evaluation to establish the correct target sac. If there are triplets, the practitioner should again inject indigo carmine dye into the sac after the amniocentesis in the sac of the second fetus before attempting the amniocentesis in the sac of the next fetus.

Another technique for performing an amniocentesis on twins is the **single-puncture method**. The needle insertion site is determined by the position of the separating membrane (Figure 15-3). Once the first specimen has been obtained, the needle is simply advanced through the membrane into the second sac. Fluid is then aspirated from the second sac. The first milliliter of fluid drawn from the second sac will be discarded so the sample is not contaminated by the fluid from the first aspiration. The advantage of this technique is that only one puncture site is required, reducing the risk for potential complications due to mul-

tiple needle insertions. A disadvantage of this technique is that it may increase the risk of rupturing the membranes between the twins and causing a monoamniotic cavity.

CHORIONIC VILLUS SAMPLING

Chorionic villus sampling (**CVS**) is a prenatal test that can detect genetic or hereditary disorders such as Tay-Sachs disease, cystic fibrosis, and chromosomal anomalies. Advantages include the ability to perform the test earlier than the amniocentesis and the ability to receive results within 48 hours in most cases and no longer than 7 days for more complex analyses. CVS is usually performed between weeks 10 and 14 of pregnancy. If the results are abnormal patients can opt for a simple, safe method of termination. CVS results are quite accurate, with false-positive results occurring in fewer than 1% of cases. The disadvantage of CVS is that it will not identify open neural tube or abdominal wall defects. The risks associated with the procedure are similar to those for amniocentesis and include miscarriage, bleeding, cramping, and Rh sensitization.

There are two techniques for performing CVS, transcervical and transabdominal (Figure 15-4). If the placenta is in a favorable position, a catheter can be inserted through the cervical os after the vagina and cervix have been cleaned with an antiseptic solution. The catheter is directed toward the maternal side of the placenta, where chorionic villi are gently suctioned. This method is contraindicated in patients with some cervical or uterine abnormalities, an active genital infection, or chronic cervicitis. The transabdominal technique is similar to amniocentesis, except the needle is inserted into the placenta.

AMNIOREDUCTION

Amnioreduction is indicated in cases of severe polyhydramnios, which causes maternal respiratory difficulty, severe maternal discomfort, or preterm-labor insomnia. It is also indicated in cases of twin-to-twin transfusion. The technique is similar to that of an amniocentesis. However, as the amount of fluid removed may be a liter or more, the needle is usually attached to a vacuum suction bottle. The needle used should be one with a flexible rubber sheath such as a Yueh catheter. The risks include premature rupture of membranes, preterm labor, infection, and placental abruption. (See Figure 15-5.)

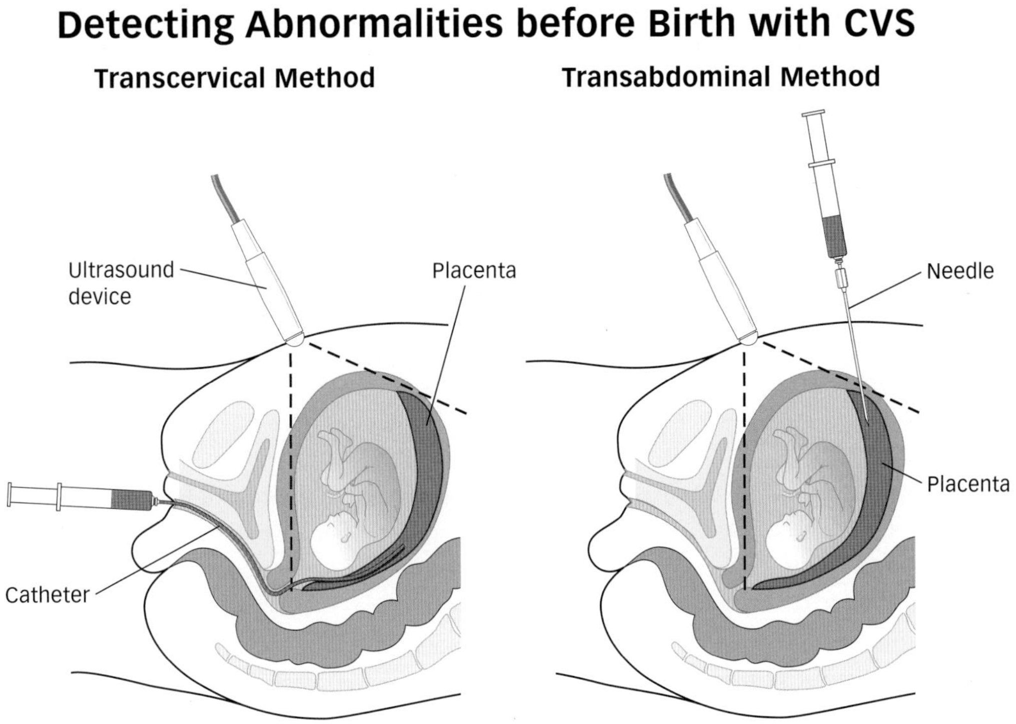

Detecting Abnormalities before Birth with CVS

Transcervical Method

Transabdominal Method

Ultrasound device

Placenta

Needle

Placenta

Catheter

Figure 15-4. *Drawings demonstrating the transabdominal and transcervical techniques for performing chorionic villus sampling.*

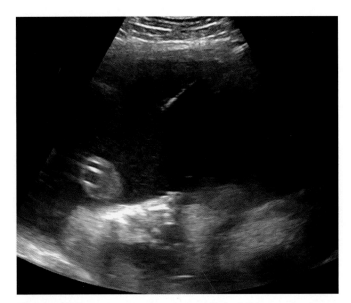

Figure 15-5. *Amnioreduction. The needle is visible entering from the top right of the image.*

AMNIOINFUSION

Amnioinfusion is a technique whereby fluid, typically normal saline, is infused into the uterine cavity to allow better visualization of the fetus in cases of severe oligohydramnios or in cases of **anhydramnios**, when no amniotic fluid is present. Indigo carmine may also be injected into the amniotic cavity if premature rupture of membranes is suspected and cannot be confirmed by usual methods. In such a situation, a vial of indigo carmine is infused along with approximately 100 cc of normal saline. A tampon is then placed in the vagina and removed after an hour. If there is rupture of membranes, the tampon will be stained blue. The primary risks of infusing fluid into the amniotic cavity are infection, premature rupture of membranes, and preterm labor. Infusing fluid will facilitate fetal lung maturation. If there is no fluid, the lungs will not develop properly. Lung fluid triggers lung development.

FETAL BLOOD SAMPLING

Fetal blood sampling—also known as **cordocentesis** or **percutaneous umbilical blood sampling** (**PUBS**)—is a technique in which a needle is inserted into the umbilical vein to obtain fetal blood for testing purposes. Valenti reported the first fetal blood sampling for the diagnosis of fetal hemoglobinopathy in 1973, but not until the following year was sonography used to direct the insertion of the fetoscope for fetal blood sampling. In 1983 Daffos pioneered the use of sonographic guidance to needle the cord, and since that time this technique has become the standard method for gaining access to fetal blood.

Box 15-3.	Indications for fetal blood sampling.

Rapid karyotyping
Red blood cell alloimmunization
Intrauterine infection
Neonatal alloimmune thrombocytopenia
Fetal anemia
Rh disease
Other blood problems
Administration of medications

Box 15-4.	Potential complications of fetal blood sampling.

Bleeding
Bradycardia
Cord hematoma
Fetal loss
Infection
Preterm labor
Rupture of membranes

Fetal blood sampling should be restricted to those cases in which fetal diagnosis cannot be obtained by another method or if rapid karyotype analysis is desired. (Nevertheless, even rapid diagnosis for the common aneuploidies is available by amniocentesis through the use of FISH techniques.) The most common indications today are to diagnose or treat severe fetal anemia, thrombocytopenia, Rh disease, and other blood problems, and administer some fetal medications (Box 15-3).

Complications and Risks

Serious complications occur in approximately 2% of procedures. Pregnancy loss is the most serious complication, occurring in approximately 1%–2% of procedures. However, the loss rate varies according to factors such as the reason for the procedure. For example, a report of 343 mid-trimester cordocentesis cases showed that fetal loses occurred only in cases in which there were either hydrops (6/36) or multiple anomalies (2/98). There were no losses in the 209 cases in which no fetal abnormalities were identified. Other factors may include the technical competence of the practitioner, the difficulty of the procedure, and the gestational age of the fetus. A list of potential complications of fetal blood sampling appears in Box 15-4.

Procedure

A fetal blood sampling procedure is technically more challenging than amniocentesis and requires an experienced team. The procedure can be done in an outpatient suite if the fetus is previable, but it should be performed in proximity to an operating room once the fetus is viable. The patient and fetus will need to be monitored before and after the procedure to evaluate fetal well-being, preterm labor, and pain. An anesthesiologist may need to administer conscious sedation, and in the case of fetal hemorrhage or sustained fetal bradycardia, the patient may need to be delivered by immediate cesarean section. Box 15-5 lists some of the preparatory steps and procedures required to carry out a fetal blood sampling procedure.

Once the patient has consented, an intravenous line is placed and blood samples obtained. Some practitioners choose to administer antibiotics or tocolytic agents prior to the procedure. Many practitioners do not do this routinely, however, finding it unnecessary under most circumstances.

An ultrasound examination is performed to evaluate the best site for the fetal blood sampling procedure. The cord insertion into the placenta is the preferred site because it provides a fixed segment of cord. It is easiest if the placenta is anterior so the fetus does not hinder the approach to the cord. The umbilical vein is the vessel of choice. Compared to the umbilical artery, the umbilical vein is larger, does not spasm upon entry, and bleeds less.

Once the site is located, the abdomen is prepped with an antiseptic solution and draped. Local anesthesia of the skin is optional but may help during prolonged procedures. Maternal sedation is also helpful in cases of prolonged procedures. A 20- or 22-gauge spinal needle is generally used for the procedure. Needles with hyperechoic tips help in placement, as they are easier to see sonographically.

The procedure can be performed using a two-person method in which an assistant holds the ultrasound transducer and guides the operator during the procedure. When a single-person technique is used, the operator guides the needle him- or herself.

There are also two techniques to guide the needle to the target vessel: a parallel approach whereby the needle is inserted at the end of the probe and the needle can be

Box 15-5. Materials and personnel needed for fetal blood sampling.

1. **Informed consent:** The patient should be fully apprised as to the risks and benefits of the procedure. After viability, discuss the possible need for an emergent cesarean section and obtain consent for this procedure as well.

2. **Intravenous access:** Intravenous access is recommended as there may be a need to provide the patient with analgesics, fluids, or antibiotics.

3. **Ultrasound equipment:** A high-resolution ultrasound with color flow and pulsed Doppler is essential.

4. **Needle:** A 20- or 22-gauge spinal needle is generally used for fetal blood sampling. An echogenic spinal needle may be helpful in localizing the needle during the procedure.

5. **Other equipment and supplies:**

   - Heparinized tuberculin syringes
   - Normal saline
   - 1% lidocaine
   - Pancuronium or vecuronium
   - Syringes
   - Sterile transducer cover with sterile ultrasound gel
   - Antiseptic solution
   - Sterile drapes
   - Point-of-care hemoglobin analyzer (optional)

6. **Physical environment/personnel:**

   - Fetal procedure room and/or operating room
   - Neonatal intensive care unit
   - Pre- and postprocedure fetal monitoring capability
   - Laboratory
   - Sonographer
   - Sonography assistant (optional)
   - Anesthesiologist
   - OB nurse
   - OB surgeon (stand-by)

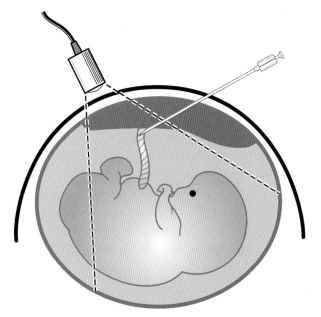

Figure 15-6. *Technique for performing an umbilical blood sampling (parallel approach).*

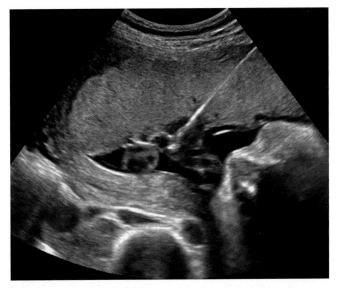

Figure 15-7. *Sonogram of percutaneous blood sampling using parallel approach.*

tracked all the way to the target vessel, and a perpendicular approach whereby the needle is inserted along the lateral edge of the transducer, with the transducer nearly vertical to the target vessel. In addition, some practitioners use a needle guide that is fixed to the end of the transducer. The freehand parallel approach is shown in Figures 15-6 and 15-7.

Once the patient is appropriately prepped and draped, a sterile transducer cover is placed over the transducer. The target vessel is identified and the needle is advanced within a few millimeters of the vessel. After confirmation of the appropriate angle to the target vessel, the needle is advanced until it touches the vessel. Then the needle is advanced into the vessel. Entry into the vessel is accompanied by a popping sensation as the vessel wall is penetrated. Once the needle tip is seen within the vessel, the stylet is removed and backflow of blood to the needle hub is observed. A heparin-coated tuberculin syringe is then placed onto the hub of the needle with gentle aspiration to collect a sample for analysis. Occasionally the addition of a small amount of negative pressure by aspiration using a tuberculin syringe is necessary for the blood to start flowing. Typically if blood is not obtained the needle should be withdrawn slowly with a slight amount of suction. Turning the needle may help direct the bevel away from the vessel wall and allow for aspiration of blood.

Once the sample is withdrawn a small amount of normal saline can be infused. This creates turbulence that can be seen by sonography, confirming proper placement of the needle within the vessel. The fetal sample should have laboratory confirmation as to its origins. The mean corpuscular volume (MCH) of fetal red blood cells varies slightly by gestational age but generally is greater than 110 fL, whereas adult values are around 85 fL.

Once the procedure is completed, the needle is withdrawn with firm pressure under direct sonographic guidance. The puncture site is evaluated for cessation of bleeding. The fetal heart rate is also evaluated and should be in the normal range before the patient is moved. The patient is also monitored for tetanic contractions or preterm labor. Typically the patient is ready for discharge after one hour of monitoring.

Alternate Sampling Sites

In cases in which the fetal cord is not accessible, vessels within the fetus may be directly accessible. The most common are the portal vein and intrahepatic portion of the umbilical vein. The risk of fetal loss from this procedure seems to be equivalent to that of cordocentesis. Less commonly, the fetal heart is sampled. Cardiocentesis appears to have a higher fetal loss rate and is not commonly performed.

INTRAUTERINE FETAL TRANSFUSION

The risk of hemolytic disease of the newborn has decreased significantly with the universal screening of the Rh factor in pregnancy and the administration of Rh immune globulin to nonsensitized Rh– women. Nevertheless, there continues to be a need for **intrauterine fetal transfusion** for fetal anemias from a variety of causes. Most commonly fetal anemia is the result of red blood cell alloimmunization or parvovirus infection. Intravascular transfusion is rarely successful prior to 18 weeks' gestation. Prior to this age, medical management may be helpful in temporizing the condition until an intravascular transfusion can be performed.

Preparation

The requirements and set-up for intrauterine fetal transfusion are similar to those for fetal blood sampling, but in addition blood must be available for immediate transfusion. Type O negative blood is usually used. Maternal blood can be used and has the advantage of decreasing the risk of additional sensitization to new red cell antigens. The patient also must have a type and crossmatch performed. In addition to the usual crossmatch procedures, the blood must be cytomegalovirus-negative, washed, and spun down to a hematocrit of around 80%–85%.

The amount of volume to be transfused can be calculated by the following formula: Volume transfused (ml) = fetal blood volume (ml) × (final hematocrit – initial hematocrit) ÷ hematocrit of the donor blood. The fetal blood volume is calculated from the estimated fetal weight in grams multiplied by 0.14. There are useful websites (such as Perinatology.com) with online calculators that simplify the calculation process.

Procedure

After being taken to the procedure room, the patient is prepped and draped in sterile fashion. Continuous sonographic guidance is critical for the success of the procedure and gaining access to the fetal circulation. The laboratory is alerted in advance that a fetal procedure is being performed and is able to provide results within 5 minutes. Once the fetal vessel is accessed, a sample of fetal blood is withdrawn and sent to the laboratory for a complete blood count. A portable hemoglobinometer is useful in approximating the degree of fetal anemia, allowing the team to start the transfusion while awaiting laboratory confirmation.

Once a sample is removed, the fetus can be paralyzed using a short-acting paralytic agent such as pancuronium or vecuronium to minimize fetal movement during the procedure. After the degree of fetal anemia is determined, blood is transfused.

The fetal heart rate is evaluated periodically during the procedure and the cord visualized to confirm proper needle placement within the vessel during the entire procedure. The streaming of transfused blood within the cord should be seen; if not, the procedure should be stopped and proper placement confirmed by gentle aspiration through the needle and injection of small amounts of normal saline. In addition, the transfusion should be stopped if fetal bradycardia is noted. If bradycardia persists, the procedure should be abandoned and consideration made to deliver the patient immediately by cesarean section if the fetus is viable.

After the transfusion is completed, a sample of fetal blood is obtained to confirm the fetal hematocrit. The patient is monitored until fetal well-being is documented.

The fetal hematocrit decreases by approximately 1% per day. Therefore, fetuses are transfused approximately 14 days after the first transfusion. Most centers transfuse the patient up to 35 weeks' gestation and deliver the patient within 3 weeks of the last transfusion. Observation of fetal tachycardia during transfusion is not uncommon. Bradycardia, however, is worrisome and carries a poorer prognosis. If fetal demise occurs within 24 hours postprocedure, the cause of death is usually associated with the procedure. Fetal demise occurring 24 or more hours postprocedure is thought to be the result of the fetus's overall condition.

MINIMALLY INVASIVE FETAL SURGERY

Advancements in fetal ultrasound technology have made it possible to perform lifesaving procedures in fetuses while minimizing the risk to the mother by avoiding an open procedure. It is now possible to intervene in cases of bladder outlet obstruction, pleural effusions, and cystic chest masses by placing specially designed catheters to shunt fluid outside the fetus into the amniotic cavity.

Bladder Aspiration

Bladder outlet obstruction is most commonly caused by the presence of posterior urethral valves that occlude the egress of urine from the bladder in male fetuses. This occurs in approximately 1 in 5000 pregnancies. This condition results in severe enlargement of the bladder, hydronephrosis, and anhydramnios. If untreated the condition is fatal, as adequate amniotic fluid is necessary for proper fetal lung development. The treatment is the placement of a vesicoamniotic shunt. Candidates for the procedure are fetuses with normal karyotypes and evidence of adequate renal function.

The technique is the same as described above under amniocentesis and is fairly simple. An injection site should be identified directly over the fetal bladder and away from maternal vessels. The placenta should be avoided and the needle trajectory should be as short as possible. Intrave-

nous (IV) sedation should be administered for maternal and fetal sedation. The maternal abdomen is prepped as for other invasive procedures. A 20-gauge spinal needle is introduced into the fetal bladder under continuous sonographic guidance and the fetal urine is aspirated. Complications are rare but include infection and fetal trauma.

Bladder Shunt

The placement of a vesicoamniotic shunt involves a unique challenge, as there is very little if any amniotic fluid surrounding the fetus. In such cases an amnioinfusion is first performed to allow enough space around the fetus to deploy the shunt successfully.

The patient should be prepped in a fashion similar to that used for an amnioinfusion procedure. The fetus is then imaged and the skin at the site of catheter insertion is anesthetized with local anesthetic. Then the introducer is inserted into the fetal bladder under direct ultrasound guidance. It is important to confirm the presence of an adequate amount of urine in the bladder before starting the procedure. Once the catheter is deployed appropriately, the curved "pigtails" should be seen entirely within the bladder and outside the fetal abdominal wall (Figure 15-8). It is not uncommon to have persistent hydronephrosis and hydroureter even weeks after the shunt is

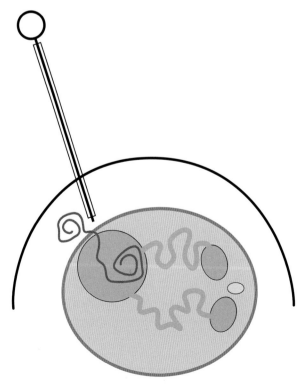

Figure 15-8. *Technique of bladder shunting.*

placed. Complications of the procedure include infection, premature rupture of the membranes, preterm labor, and occlusion or migration of the shunt. In one instance, the author has seen the fetus grab and pull the shunt completely out of the bladder soon after the shunt was inserted!

Hydrocephalus Shunt

Treatment for obstructive hydrocephalus in utero has had mixed results and is currently not performed in the United States.

Thoracoamniotic Shunt

Shunting to drain cysts or eliminate plural effusions into the amniotic cavity is a fairly simple procedure for the perinatal specialist and can be done in an outpatient setting. The procedure is similar to the placement of a vesicoamniotic shunt. However, as there is a normal amount of amniotic fluid, amnioinfusion prior to the placement of the shunt is unnecessary. Insertion of the cannula is made through the fetal chest wall in the mid-thoracic region on the side where the effusion or cyst is seen.

SCANNING TIPS, GUIDELINES, AND PITFALLS

The sonographer is responsible for making sure everything is set up for a procedure and should be knowledgeable about preparing a sterile environment and maintaining sterile technique. It is always wise to ensure that the informed consent form has been signed prior to starting any procedure.

Amniocentesis

1. In amniocentesis it is critical that an adequate amniotic fluid pocket is first identified. The needle and target must be aligned during entry into the amniotic fluid pocket and under constant view during the procedure. In the case of a transplacental needle insertion, the needle insertion site should be evaluated for possible blood streaming and monitored to make sure the bleeding stops.

2. When selecting a site for needle puncture during amniocentesis, the sonographer should attempt to stay

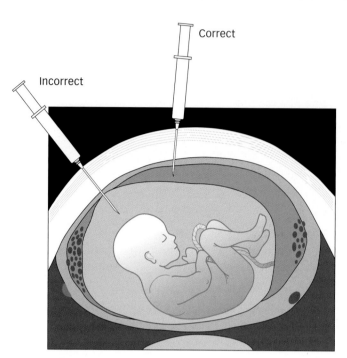

Figure 15-9. *Correct and incorrect placement of needle for amniocentesis.*

as close to the midline as possible. Lateral punctures should be avoided as well so that uterine vessels and maternal bowel are not punctured (Figure 15-9). If a suprapubic tap is attempted, one should be cautious not to puncture a full maternal bladder. Urine and amniotic fluid can look similar when aspirated.

3. Needle diameter for amniocentesis should not be larger than 20 gauge. Larger needle diameters increase the risk of bleeding as well as fluid flow from the puncture site.

4. Tenting (the elevation of the amnion by a needle when the membranes have not fused) and nonadhesion of the amniotic membrane can increase the risk of amniotic rupture. Therefore, amniocentesis should be delayed until the membranes are completely fused to the uterine wall. This generally occurs by 15 weeks, but in some instances fusion may not occur until 16–17 weeks. In addition, to avoid tenting, especially in the second trimester, a quick needle insertion is recommended.

5. The site of needle insertion for amniocentesis should always be documented on film with calipers in order to show the proper depth.

Cordocentesis

6. During cordocentesis, it is important for the sonographer to keep the transducer aimed at the target vessel. An experienced practitioner can usually bring the needle into the plane of the ultrasound beam.

7. The sonographer must periodically assess the fetal heart rate during cordocentesis and be able to come back and locate the needle within the cord and assess appropriate needle placement.

8. It is essential that the sonographer and the operator communicate constantly during cordocentesis. The sonographer must keep the ultrasound transducer steady during the procedure so the operator does not lose site of either the needle or the target vessel.

9. Some recommend fetal monitoring, including a quick check for fetal viability and heart rate one hour after the cordocentesis procedure.

Shunts

10. Prior to any type of shunt procedure, the patient should have a targeted examination to rule out associated anomalies and to determine the exact cause of the abnormality to be treated. If the decided course of action will not have much effect on the outcome for the fetus, it would not be prudent to submit the patient to an invasive procedure.

REFERENCES

An assessment of the hazards of amniocentesis. Report to the Medical Research Council by their Working Party on Amniocentesis. Br J Obstet Gynaecol 85(supp 2):1–41, 1978.

Ayadi S, Carbillon L, Varlet C, et al: Fetal sepsis due to *Escherichia coli* after second-trimester amniocentesis. Fetal Diagn Ther 13:98–99, 1998.

Bevus DCA: The antenatal prediction of hemolytic disease of the newborn. Lancet 1:395–398, 1952.

Chinnaiya A, Venkat A, Dawn C, et al: Intrahepatic vein fetal blood sampling: current role in prenatal diagnoses. J Obstet Gynaecol Res 24:239–246, 1998.

Clewell WH: Hydrocephalus shunt. In Chervenak FA, Isaacson GC, Campbell S: *Ultrasound in Obstetrics and Gynecology*, Volume 2. Boston, Little Brown, 1993, pp 1283–1287.

Daffos F, Capella-Pavlosvsky M, Forestier F: A new procedure for fetal blood sampling in utero: preliminary results of fifty-three cases. Am J Obstet Gynecol 146:985–987, 1983.

Davies NP, Nicolaides KH: Amniocentesis. In Chervenak FA, Isaacson GC, Campbell S: *Ultrasound in Obstetrics and Gynecology*, Volume 2. Boston, Little Brown, 1993, pp 1245–1250.

Eddleman KA, Malone FD, Sullivan L, et al: Pregnancy loss rates after midtrimester amniocentesis. Obstet Gynecol 108:1067–1072, 2006.

Forestier F, Daffos F, Catherine N, et al: Developmental hematopoiesis in normal human fetal blood. Blood 77:2360–2363, 1991.

Goldman JA, Peleg D: Massive extraperitoneal bleeding: a rare complication of amniocentesis. Acta Obstet Gynecol Scand 59:283–284, 1980.

Hamar B: Ultrasound-guided invasive fetal procedures. In Rumack CM, Wilson SR, Charboneau JW, et al: *Diagnostic Ultrasound*, 4th Edition. St. Louis, Elsevier Mosby, 2011, pp 1543–1552.

Henningsen CG: Prenatal diagnosis of congenital anomalies. In Hagen-Ansert SL (ed): *Textbook of Diagnostic Sonography*, 7th Edition. St. Louis, Elsevier, 2012, pp 1190–1194.

Hobbins JC, Mahoney MJ, Goldstein LA: New method of intrauterine evaluation by the combined use of fetoscopy and ultrasound. Am J Obstet Gynecol 118:1069–1072, 1974.

Hodor JG, Poggi SH, Spong CY, et al: Risk of third-trimester amniocentesis: a case-controlled study. Am J Perinatol 23:177–180, 2006.

Hogge WA, Buffone GJ, Hogge JS: Prenatal diagnosis of cytomegalovirus (CMV) infection: a preliminary report. Prenat Diagn 13:131–136, 1993.

Liley AW: Liquor amnio analysis in management of pregnancy complicated by Rhesus immunization. Am J Obstet Gynecol 82:1359–1370, 1961.

Martin JA, Hamilton BE, Sutton PD, et al: Births: final data for 2003. Natl Vital Stat Rep 545:1–116, 2005.

Midtrimester amniocentesis for prenatal diagnosis: safety and accuracy. JAMA 236:1471–1476, 1976.

Nadler HL: Antenatal detection of hereditary disorders. Pediatrics 42:912–918, 1968.

Nicolini U, Nicolaidis P, Fisk NM, et al: Fetal blood sampling from the intrahepatic vein: analysis of safety and clinical experience with 214 procedures. Obstet Gynecol 76:47–53, 1990.

Nicolini U, Rodeck CH: Fetal urinary diversion. In Chervenak FA, Isaacson GC, Campbell S: *Ultrasound in Obstetrics and Gynecology*, Volume 2. Boston, Little Brown, 1993, pp 1277–1282.

Nicolini U, Santolaya J, Ojo OE, et al: The fetal intrahepatic umbilical vein as an alternative to cord needling for prenatal diagnosis and therapy. Prenat Diagn 8:665–671, 1988.

Norton ME: Genetics and prenatal diagnosis. In Callen P (ed): *Ultrasonography in Obstetrics and Gynecology*, 5th Edition. St. Louis, Saunders Elsevier, 2008, pp 48–52.

Patrick JE, Perry TB, Kinch RA: Fetoscopy and fetal blood sampling: a percutaneous approach. Am J Obstet Gynecol 119:539–542, 1974.

Ruma MS, Moise KJ, Kim E, et al: Combined plasmapheresis and intravenous immune globulin for treatment of severe maternal red cell alloimmunization. Am J Obstet Gynecol 196:138.e1–e6, 2007.

Schonewille H, Klumper F, van de Watering LM, et al: High additional maternal red cell alloimmunization after Rhesus- and K-matched intrauterine intravascular transfusions for hemolytic disease of the fetus. Am J Obstet Gynecol 196:143.e1–143.e6, 2007.

Simon NV, Williams GH, Fairbrother PF, et al: Prediction of fetal lung maturity by amniotic fluid fluorescence polarization, L:S ratio, and phosphatidyl glycerol. Obstet Gynecol 57:295–300, 1981.

Simpson NE, Dallaire L, Miller JR, et al: Prenatal diagnosis of genetic disease in Canada: report of a collaborative study. Can Med Assoc J 115:739–748, 1976.

Steele MW, Breg W Jr: Chromosome analysis of human amniotic-fluid cells. Lancet 1:383–385, 1966.

Thor JA, Helfgott AW, King EA, et al: Maternal death after second-trimester genetic amniocentesis. Obstet Gynecol 105:1213–1215, 2005.

Valenti C: Antenatal detection of hemoglobinopathies: a preliminary report. Am J Obstet Gynecol 114:851–853, 1973.

Valenti C, Kehaty T: Culture of cells obtained by amniocentesis. J Lab Clin Med 73:355–358, 1969.

Weiner CP, Wenstrom KD, Sipes SL, et al: Risk factors for cordocentesis and fetal intravascular transfusion. Am J Obstet Gynecol 165:1020–1025, 1991.

Wilson RD, Farquharson DF, Wittmann BK, et al: Overall pregnancy loss rate as important as procedure loss rate. Fetal Diagn Ther 9:142–148, 1994.

SELF-ASSESSMENT EXERCISES

Questions

1. Of the following, which would *not* be an indication for chorionic villus sampling?

   A. To perform a karyotype

   B. To identify an inherited disorder

   C. To rule out Down syndrome

   D. To rule out spina bifida

   E. To look at chromosomes

2. Which of the following complications is *not* associated with an amniocentesis?

   A. Pre-eclampsia

   B. Rupture of membranes

   C. Preterm labor

   D. Fetal death

   E. Bleeding and cramping

3. What is *not* an indication for amnioreduction?
   A. Twin-to-twin transfusion syndrome due to mono-chorionicity
   B. Fetal hydrops due to Rh sensitization
   C. Maternal difficulty breathing due to polyhydramnios
   D. Maternal insomnia due to polyhydramnios
   E. Maternal discomfort due to polyhydramnios

4. Of the following, which is an indication for percutaneous umbilical blood sampling?
   A. Rapid karyotyping
   B. Evaluation for fetal anemia
   C. Evaluation for fetal infection
   D. Evaluation for fetal thrombocytopenia
   E. All of the above

5. The following are complications of fetal blood sampling except:
   A. Bradycardia
   B. Infection
   C. Twin-to-twin transfusion syndrome
   D. Fetal loss
   E. Cord hematoma

6. Fetal blood transfusion is rarely successful before how many weeks' gestation?
   A. 18 weeks
   B. 20 weeks
   C. 22 weeks
   D. 24 weeks
   E. 26 weeks

7. In cases of fetal transfusion for fetal anemia, the amount of daily decrease in the hematocrit is approximately what percentage?
   A. 1%
   B. 2%
   C. 3%
   D. 4%
   E. 5%

8. When should a fetal transfusion be stopped?
   A. When blood streaming is seen in the umbilical vein
   B. When fetal tachycardia is noted
   C. When fetal bradycardia is noted
   D. When the baby moves around
   E. When fetal respiration stops

9. Of the following, which would *not* be a reason for performing an amnioinfusion?
   A. To test for premature rupture of membranes
   B. To better visualize the fetal anatomy in cases of oligohydramnios
   C. To facilitate an amniocentesis
   D. To facilitate shunt placement for bladder outlet obstruction
   E. To facilitate fetal lung maturity

10. In which situation would a fetal shunt procedure be indicated?
    A. Hydranencephaly
    B. Pleural effusion
    C. Polycystic kidneys
    D. Duodenal atresia
    E. All of the above

11. Of the following, which cannot be identified with chorionic villus sampling?
    A. Hemophilia
    B. Down syndrome
    C. Tay-Sachs disease
    D. Trisomy 13
    E. Spina bifida

12. Tenting refers to:

   A. Proliferation of placental tissue between the amnions in a twin pregnancy

   B. The elevation of the amnion by a needle when the membranes have not fused

   C. Discoloration of amniotic fluid when blue dye is introduced

   D. Use of a stent with a triangular tip

   E. A fishing and camping expedition

13. Which needle choice would be best for performing an amniocentesis?

   A. 16 gauge

   B. 8 gauge

   C. 20 gauge

   D. 22 gauge

   E. Size is irrelevant.

Answers

See Appendix F on page 618 for answers and explanations.

The Sonographer's Role in the Grieving Process

Kathryn A. Gill, MS, RT, RDMS, FSDMS

OBJECTIVES

After completing this chapter you should be able to:

1. Describe the difference between bereavement and mourning.

2. List and explain the four phases of bereavement.

3. Discuss the types of losses experienced by the terminally ill.

4. Give examples of situations in which grief counseling techniques might be helpful in dealing with sonography patients.

5. Discuss what should and should not be said to a patient who has experienced a failed pregnancy.

SONOGRAPHY PRACTITIONERS COME FROM A VARIETY of educational and professional backgrounds. We are a diverse group with very different experiences and levels of knowledge. Many of us never received training in how to deal with loss, death, and dying, yet we are faced with these issues all too frequently in our daily work. The sonography practitioner needs to be acutely aware of the process of grieving and realize that a loss can be defined in many ways. Understanding the phases of bereavement allows

us to appreciate why patients react as they do, provides us with the knowledge to help them through their difficult time, and helps us recognize their need for both immediate and ongoing support. A patient who has suffered a spontaneous abortion or an ectopic pregnancy and returns to the sonography department with a subsequent pregnancy only a few months later, for example, may still require help dealing with the first loss.

When a patient is terminally ill—as when a cancer has recurred, diminishing the likelihood of survival—she experiences multiple losses. Five major losses are experienced by the dying patient:

- Loss of control
- Loss of identity
- Loss of achievement
- Loss of social worth
- Loss of relationships

Healthcare providers become controlling influences in the life of the dying patient and must be sensitive to the potential for reducing the patient's identity to a chart number, test, or procedure. The patient has often already lost the ability to work and provide for a family, significantly affecting his or her sense of identity and social value. The dying patient is also vulnerable to radical changes in even close relationships with family and friends, as many of us find it difficult to be around those who are dying or have experienced significant loss. Therefore the healthcare provider must be aware of patients' mental and emotional status as well as their physical condition.

Another way of looking at loss is to think of it as a type of death. **Social death** occurs when an illness or handicap causes one's world to shrink in terms of relationships with friends, coworkers, and family. **Psychological death** involves personality changes when the patient is forced to face the implications of his or her condition. **Biologic death** occurs when life support equipment must be employed. **Physiologic death** is the actual failure of vital organs. All of these forms of loss/death evoke emotions and initiate the phases of bereavement.

While the forms of loss and death listed above are universally recognized, other losses often go unacknowledged. The loss of a child in utero, for example, is often dismissed. Society does not expect a woman who has lost a fetus to experience much grief, especially if she has other children on whom to concentrate. This attitude can make women who have experienced miscarriage, abortion, or other serious complications from their pregnancies vulnerable to pathologic grief. For example, a woman carrying twins, one of whom dies in utero, may be so debilitated by grief that she has difficulty attaching with the surviving twin. A woman who loses her breast or uterus to cancer, although her prognosis for survival may be good, will often feel the loss of her identity, especially if she equates her femininity and self-worth with her physical appearance or ability to produce a child. Such losses, although they may be less obvious than the more widely recognized losses identified earlier, are still felt as intensely and may prompt equally intense grief.

As sonography practitioners most of us find it uncomfortable to talk about a loss with our patients. We tend to avoid the subject or the individual altogether. However, it is important to understand and manage the emotional impact of our patients' conditions without ignoring them and in a way that will support the best outcomes for them. This chapter provides some guidelines for how the sonography practitioner who is faced with a patient experiencing a loss can help that individual to deal with grief issues in a professional and supportive manner.

THE TERMINOLOGY OF GRIEF

In order to understand the grief process, we must know the proper definitions of terms that are often used interchangeably, such as *loss, grief, mourning,* and *bereavement.*

LOSS

A **loss** is the result of any event that changes the status quo, such as the absence of something that was there before, often, but not limited to, someone or something one loves. We usually think of a loss in negative terms, such as a death, divorce, or unemployment, but losses can also result from apparently positive events. Moving into a new house may mean losing old friends or good neighbors. A new baby in the family may mean the loss of privacy through having to share one's room with a sibling.

In the context of obstetrics and gynecology, a woman still in her reproductive years may suffer the **physical loss** of her fertility if a gynecologic cancer necessitates a hysterectomy. A young nulliparous woman who has suffered from chronic pelvic inflammatory disease may discover she is incapable of becoming pregnant because her fallopian tubes have been damaged beyond repair. A patient who has undergone multiple elective abortions may find that uterine synechiae have made it impossible for her to retain a pregnancy after she has decided that a family is her goal. The dreams of these women are suddenly dashed.

Symbolic losses—including loss of independence, control, identity, self-esteem, or intimacy as the result of a disability or hospitalization—often follow and compound physical losses. Losing a body part to cancer or trauma carries with it a number of symbolic losses. For example, a woman who has had a mastectomy suffers a loss of family and home environment during her hospital stay. She also loses control and independence during her recuperative period. The physical loss of the body part may affect her identity as a woman and her feeling of self-esteem. She may become more inhibited during intimacy, losing the ability to express her sexuality.

Loss has been described in terms of time as well. The loss of a parent equates with losing part of one's past, the loss of a spouse with losing part of one's present, and the loss of a pregnancy with losing part of one's future.

Grief

A loss is what happens. **Grief** is how it makes one feel—the emotional response to the loss. Grief happens whether we know it, like it, want it, or need it. It happens whether we feel it or appreciate it; it happens whether we are ready for it or not. We do not choose to grieve, but we can choose how we deal with grief.

In her groundbreaking book *On Death and Dying* (1969), Elisabeth Kübler-Ross identified five stages of grief:

1. *Denial:* a phase during which the individual cannot consciously accept that the traumatic event is actually real—a coping mechanism that allows people to process the impact of the event but a stage in which some individuals can become stuck.

2. *Anger:* a stage during which the individual recognizes the reality of the situation but reacts by seeking and blaming a cause, often others (even loved ones) but also him- or herself.

3. *Bargaining:* a stage when the individual seeks a solution or alternative that will provide hope when a solution may be unavailable, such as undergoing alternative treatments that may not be indicated or are ineffective.

4. *Depression:* a phase in which the patient recognizes that there is no solution to the problem (e.g., acknowledges the certainty of death) and loses interest in continuing, often typified by sadness, silence, fear, isolating behaviors, and detachment from others.

5. *Acceptance:* the last stage, in which the individual is able to come to terms with the reality of his or her situation, recognize and follow through on available options, and/or accept the inevitability of death and participate in remaining life, even helping others to prepare for their losses.

Successfully negotiating all the stages of grieving is essential for mental and physical health, and it is a social process that is best shared. A Swedish proverb says, "Shared joy is double joy; shared sorrow is half-sorrow." A social support system is critical, and lack of support can be a significant handicap when attempting to overcome grief. David Spiegel, a Stanford University psychiatrist, conducted an interesting study to determine if emotional support truly aids in healing. He selected 50 women who were being treated for metastatic breast cancer to participate in weekly support group meetings. His data revealed that at the end of one year these women had experienced 50% less pain, were less depressed, and felt more positive than the control group, which had received only conventional treatment. Better yet, the support group members survived twice as long. Truly our lives depend on the nurturance, empathy, and understanding we get from others.

People have many misconceptions about grief. Several years ago, a newspaper article reported the results of a survey asking individuals how long they thought it would take to "get over" the death of a spouse, a pet, and a failed pregnancy. The results were quite interesting, if unscientific. Most indicated that it takes only six months to mourn a spouse but one year for a pet. When asked how long it takes to grieve a miscarriage, most said about one month. The fact that respondents rated the time to grieve a failed pregnancy as significantly less than that for a lost pet is revealing, suggesting a general miscomprehension regarding the impact a failed pregnancy can have on a woman.

During a grief counseling training session, couples who had experienced pregnancy losses were asked what their emotional response to a miscarriage or ectopic pregnancy was after one year. In response, 75% said they felt they had lost a baby, while only 25% took the attitude that the loss was just "one of those things," a part of life. *The fact is that grief is experienced in relation to the significance of the attachment to those who experience the loss, not those who have not.*

The failure to understand this key aspect of grief has led to several myths about it, which can be held by even the most empathetic healthcare providers. Some of these myths are listed in Box 16-1.

Myths 1 and 2 state that all losses are the same and all people grieve the same way. In fact perceptions of loss and how people deal with those losses are as different as individual fingerprints. There are no defined criteria that describe a normal method of grieving, nor is there a set time line. Even partners who have experienced a pregnancy loss may not react in the same way, at the same time, or with the same intensity.

Myths 3, 4, 8, and 11 are related to the amount of time required for grieving. Myths 3 and 4 state that grief declines steadily over time, eventually is resolved, and never comes back. Myths 8 and 11 indicate that the length and intensity of grief are equivalent to the intensity of love for

Box 16-1. Myths about grief.

1. All losses are the same.
2. All people grieve the same.
3. Grief declines steadily over time.
4. Grief is eventually resolved and never comes back.
5. A pregnancy loss is not as difficult as the loss of a child or other loved one.
6. Children need to be protected from grief.
7. Grief is personal and it is not important to have social support.
8. It takes a couple of months to "get over it."
9. Children grieve like adults.
10. Parents feel crazy only if they are going crazy.
11. The length and intensity of grief are equivalent to the intensity of the love for the deceased.
12. Parents do not have a relationship with a fetus.

the deceased and that it usually takes about two months to "get over" a loss. As we will see in reviewing the various phases of bereavement, grief is experienced in waves, waxing and waning over different time frames. The phases of bereavement may occur one by one or all at once. There are no set patterns.

Myths 5 and 12 tell us that parents do not establish a relationship with a fetus and a pregnancy loss is therefore not as difficult to deal with as other losses because the parents have never known the fetus as an infant. The truth is that miscarriages can be among the worst losses, as they do not receive the same social support from friends and family. There is no ritual for a miscarriage, as there is for the death of an infant, child, or adult. Funerals are not performed, and few hold a memorial service after such an event.

Myths 6 and 9 say that children grieve like adults and that they should be protected from grief. However, death is part of life, and more harm can be done when grieving is suppressed. Children, like adults, respond in many different ways. A child's understanding of death varies according to age. Some will need reassurance, some absolution. One thing is certain, however: All need nurturance. It is important to be open and honest with children. They should be supported and encouraged in their own grief process, and we need to answer their questions in simple terms that are appropriate to their level of understanding.

Finally, Myths 7 and 10 say that grief is personal and not to be shared, suggesting that those in grief should keep their feelings to themselves. Myth 10 suggests that those who are feeling confused or disoriented are mentally unstable. Because we are all different and react differently to similar circumstances, we must understand that almost any feeling associated with grief can be normal. Family members, friends, and others who provide social support (including healthcare providers) need to let us know that our feelings are "normal"—no matter how crazy they may make us feel (or could be perceived) at the time.

Mourning and Bereavement

Mourning and bereavement go hand in hand. **Mourning** is the process that resolves the conflicts associated with loss. There are two sides to mourning, one painful and one soothing. The pain comes from the separation from the deceased or absence of the thing we loved—the actual loss. However, mourning can also soothe us when it helps us to renew closeness with the deceased through memories, often with the aid of pictures, videos, letters, emails, and other mementos that remind us of the joy we experienced with our loved one in the past.

Bereavement is the process of experiencing and mourning a loss, including its signs and symptoms. Bereavement can be devastating to one's health, causing anxiety and depression, excessive weight loss or gain, difficulty swallowing, blurred vision, skin rashes, and menstrual disturbances. Patients may also note alterations in libido, vomiting, fatigue, headaches, dizziness, and fainting. Other symptoms include excessive sweating, chest pain, heart palpitations, and even an increased incidence of infection.

Several authorities have defined the patterns of mourning and bereavement by dividing them into four phases:

1. Shock and numbness
2. Searching and yearning
3. Disorientation and disorganization
4. Reorganization and resolution

These phases can occur one at a time, all at once, or in any variation in between. Although the pace at which one moves through or experiences the phases varies from person to person, generally the entire process spans two years. The intensity of symptoms can fluctuate over time, and feelings do not necessarily fade steadily over time.

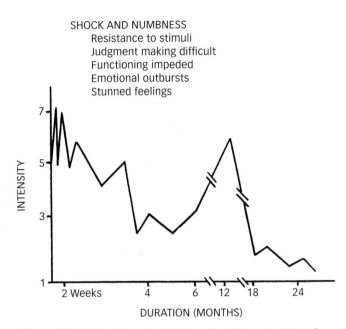

Figure 16-1. *Graph showing the intensity of characteristics of shock and numbness during the two years following the death of a loved one. Reprinted with permission from Davidson GW:* Understanding Mourning. *Minneapolis, Augsburg Fortress, 1984.*

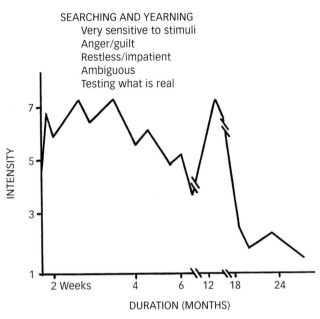

Figure 16-2. *Graph showing the intensity of characteristics of searching and yearning during the two years following the death of a loved one. Reprinted with permission from Davidson GW:* Understanding Mourning. *Minneapolis, Augsburg Fortress, 1984.*

Phase 1: Shock and Numbness

Shock and numbness are present initially and may continue for many months. Symptoms include lack of concentration, short attention span, confusion over time, impaired decision making, and denial. Individuals may experience emotional outbursts, resistance to stimuli, and a stunned feeling. Over two years, these symptoms may come and go and often intensify around the anniversary of the loss (Figure 16-1).

Phase 2: Searching and Yearning

During this phase individuals feel empty and seek accountability, often blaming themselves, a spouse, or even a health-care giver for the loss. They will ask questions in an attempt to test what is real. They typically are restless and impatient. They may experience weight fluctuations and harbor feelings of resentment and bitterness as well as guilt and anger. This phase can occur from the second week and intensify between about 9 and 18 months. Again, there may be a peak in symptoms on the anniversary of the loss (Figure 16-2).

Phase 3: Disorientation and Disorganization

This phase can be a time of maximum strain on relationships. The individual is moving out of the testing mode into accepting the reality of the loss. This phase may not lose intensity until the end of the seventh month, often extending into the ninth month. During this time the individual may experience a decline in social support, as

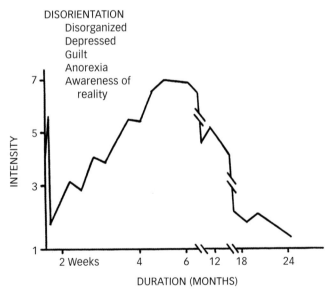

Figure 16-3. *Graph showing the intensity of characteristics of disorientation during the two years following the death of a loved one. Reprinted with permission from Davidson GW:* Understanding Mourning. *Minneapolis, Augsburg Fortress, 1984.*

many people feel that the person should be "getting over it" and on with life. Symptoms include social withdrawal, depression, forgetfulness, guilt, anorexia, and sickness or nausea (Figure 16-3). Phases 2 and 3 are critical times for sonographers dealing with patients who have experienced a miscarriage or fetal demise, since these phases can coincide with the time when delivery was due had the pregnancy progressed to term.

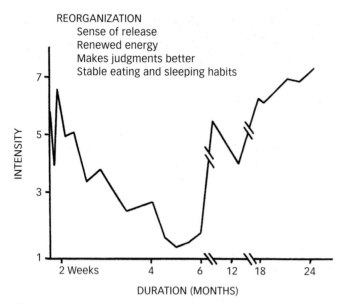

REORGANIZATION
Sense of release
Renewed energy
Makes judgments better
Stable eating and sleeping habits

Figure 16-4. *Graph showing the intensity of characteristics of reorganization during the two years following the death of a loved one. Reprinted with permission from Davidson GW:* Understanding Mourning. *Minneapolis, Augsburg Fortress, 1984.*

Phase 4: Reorganization and Resolution

Between 18 and 24 months after the loss, most individuals begin to feel a sense of release and renewed energy. Sleeping and eating patterns revert to normal, self-esteem increases, and the will to make plans for the future returns. The pain associated with the memory of the loss decreases markedly, and the individual is able to laugh and smile without difficulty (Figure 16-4).

GRIEF SUPPORT

While sonography practitioners are not grief counselors, understanding some basic guidelines for grief counselors is essential for most healthcare providers, including sonographers. In supporting a patient with whom you have ongoing contact, you may have to make a two-year commitment. There are some basic rules for grief support (Box 16-2). This section will survey those rules; the next two sections, "Applying Theory to Everyday Practice" and "Case Studies," will consider how you as a practitioner are most likely to apply them in a clinical context.

Know Your Patient

First, unless you know a patient's personal history, it can be difficult to know where that individual is in the grieving process. Therefore it is important for healthcare providers to try to gain historical information on their patients so they can offer helpful assistance rather than add insult to their patients' pain. Reviewing the patient's

Box 16-2.   Rules of grief support.

1. Recognize that there is no time line.
2. Become a good listener.
3. Be genuine and natural.
4. Do not be judgmental.

history will provide insight into the stage of bereavement that individual may be experiencing. Collecting adequate clinical data is essential not only to making the correct diagnosis but also to understanding a patient's behavior and your conversations with that person when you are trying to provide comfort appropriate to the person's bereavement phase.

Listen

Another rule is to admit your helplessness (you did not experience the loss) and become a good listener. This rule may be the hardest to follow. Do not ask one question after another without a break, and do not give false reassurances. We tend to want to find and express our concern with comforting words; however, silence is often the most effective way to deliver comfort. Silence allows the griever a chance to vent. The griever needs to tell his or her story, often many times. A person going through bereavement may repeatedly recall every aspect of the final days, including how he or she learned of the grave news and how sensitive or insensitive the caregivers appeared. Telling the story helps the griever to accept the reality.

Reciting your own grief experiences is not helpful; there are never words that will solve the unsolvable. You cannot diminish another's pain by telling your own story or that of another—especially if you think your own story is worse or more tragic; such attempts to divert a grieving individual from pain both diminish that pain and deny the process that will eventually lead to some resolution. The important thing to remember is that you do not have to provide the griever with a solution, only permission and the opportunity to grieve. In the context of your role as a healthcare provider, ask what you can do to help, and respect the requests the griever may make in return.

Be Sincere

Healthcare providers should be genuine and natural. Behavior that is insincere or exaggerated will be obvious, and trying to be cheerful to mitigate the reality of death is destructive. If the patient has been told and is aware that there is a problem, be with the person and let him or her know you are concerned. Do not attempt to say something positive about the loss. Simply ask what the patient needs and try to meet those needs. You do not need to be strong for that person by hiding your own pain if it is genuine; displaying authentic (but controlled) feelings can validate the griever's loss. Touch can be powerful for those who are comfortable with it in the appropriate context and assuming compliance with regulations: A pat on the arm or a hug will send a strong message that you care. Let your patient know that it is okay to cry. Tears are good, and crying relieves tension.

Withhold Judgment

Never judge another's grief. Each person has his or her own personality, coping skills, culture, and traditions. Never tell someone that he or she "should" be feeling better by now. The healing process is slow for most people, and the duration of the process for one person should not be compared to that of another. Cultural differences can affect the way an individual reacts to loss. For example, in Brazil when a child dies it is often believed that the child willed his death; perhaps this belief helps the survivors cope and relieves the need to assign blame for the death. In Bali many believe that grief must be kept under control; otherwise the griever becomes a target for evil spirits and thus is at risk for health problems. Latins are often overtly emotive. Eastern Europeans tend to be stoic and to repress their feelings. Although these cultural differences should never be expanded into stereotypes, the healthcare provider should call on cultural sensitivity while remaining aware of individual differences.

Photos

Sometimes parents will request what may seem morbid, such as asking to see and hold an aborted fetus or to take with them a picture of their anomalous baby. What is normal for you may not be normal for another, so judge not. Box 16-3 lists some reasons photographing an infant who has died can be important to the surviving parents. A picture may provide the only tangible and lasting evidence of the baby's life while allowing the parents to confront the reality of the death. A picture shows parents what the baby actually looked like; they do not have to rely on imagination or impressions they developed while in a state of shock and numbness. Moreover, the fantasy of a fetus in pain can often become much more disturbing than the reality depicted in a photographic or ultrasound image.

Box 16-3. Reasons for photographing a dead fetus or infant.

1. A picture reaffirms the existence of the baby's life.
2. The image allows parents to confront the reality of the death.
3. A picture may be the only tangible memento of the baby.
4. Parents who have a tangible image do not have to rely on imagination to remind them of what the baby looked like.

Closure Activities

Closure activities sometimes help with the healing process. Some people may choose to write letters to the deceased, allowing them to say the things they felt did not get said during life or the viable pregnancy. Keeping a journal can provide the same type of comfort by allowing one to write about memories stirred by the loss. Many make donations to charitable organizations in honor of the deceased or plant a tree, shrub, or flower as a more permanent memorial. Hosting a ceremony that will allow people to share their grief by talking, crying, and even laughing together over stories, pictures, and memories is an excellent way to begin to bring closure to a loss.

APPLYING THEORY TO EVERYDAY PRACTICE

Ultrasound practitioners are not grief counselors or therapists. Nevertheless, especially in obstetrics and gynecology, they participate in situations involving grief. They should therefore take CME grief counseling instruction when possible and be prepared to refer patients to licensed clinical therapists or psychiatrists.

Learning About Your Patient

How can this knowledge be applied to everyday practice? After all, we interact with patients for only a short time during the examination.

One way to improve our sensitivity to a patient's grief is to learn that patient's history. This is quite easy with inpatients, because their charts document their histories. Review reasons for surgical procedures and check pregnancy history. Know why your patient is having the sonogram and ask questions to understand her awareness of her status.

When an outpatient is referred for testing, the request should indicate the reason for the sonogram and suggest any history leading up to it. In these cases, be sensitive to the mood of the patient as you prepare for and perform the examination.

Preparing to Receive Your Patient

Prepare to receive your patient by typing his or her name into your character generator prior to the patient's arrival. Complete any preliminary paperwork so that you can focus on the patient once that person is in your presence. Be confident and thorough in your explanation of what you will do. If departmental policy does not allow patients to view the monitor during the examination or forbids you to offer an explanation of what you are seeing during the examination, this is a good time to let the patient know that policy. Make eye contact with the patient; face the person, and smile.

Speaking with Care

Be conscious of the tone in your voice and your body language. You may think you are being professional by acting serious and aloof, but patients may perceive such a manner as cold and uncaring. Your verbal communication should be informative and honest, but be careful not to give medical or legal advice unless you are a doctor or lawyer. Do not make value statements or use euphemisms when answering questions.

The way tone of voice and inflection affect meaning can be illustrated in a single sentence, "I didn't say she was pregnant." Emphasis on different words can change the meaning of the sentence:

"I didn't *say* she was pregnant" suggests that you might have conveyed that she was pregnant in writing or an email but not verbally.

"I didn't say *she* was pregnant" suggests that someone else may be pregnant.

"I didn't say she was *pregnant*" suggests that she may be in another state or condition.

Tone, cadence, and emphasis speak volumes. We need to be careful about not only what we say but also how we say it.

Avoiding Mistakes

If you perform a large volume of gynecologic and obstetric studies in your department, it is not recommended that you display pictures of your children or wear badges

Box 16-4.	Things healthcare providers should not say.

1. It was early in your pregnancy and the fetus was not really a baby yet.
2. The fetus was just a blob of tissue or cells.
3. It is just a miscarriage.
4. You can always have another child.
5. At least you have other children.
6. You are lucky that you can get pregnant.
7. It is not as if you had cancer or AIDS.
8. There was probably something wrong with it anyway.
9. It is better that it happened now rather than later.
10. You have an angel in heaven.
11. It is God's will.

or pins with accolades such as "World's Greatest Mom." These items may be disturbing to an infertility patient or one who may be experiencing a pregnancy loss. Likewise, it also is best not to initiate conversations about your personal life or family. If a patient asks if you have children, answer politely but do not elaborate.

Patients experiencing a problem pregnancy come to your department for the "moment of truth." They experience sonography as a time when they are facing what may be a difficult reality. If a patient receives bad news about her pregnancy, she will begin the shock and numbness phase of bereavement. In an attempt to comfort and reassure her, we may make remarks that are insensitive and inappropriate. Comments to avoid include the following (see also Box 16-4):

- It's not really a baby yet … just a blob of tissue or cells.
- It's just a miscarriage.

Such statements may not be intended to belittle the patient's experience but will suggest to her that what she is feeling is wrong or ridiculous.

Comments that suggest to the patient that she should feel fortunate about the fact that she has fertility are also inappropriate and include these:

- You are young and you can always have another child.
- At least you have other children.
- You are lucky you can get pregnant; some people never can and have to adopt.

Some practitioners may be tempted to describe a worst-case scenario in an attempt to console the patient, which also should be avoided:

- It's not like you have cancer or AIDS.
- It's better that it happened now rather than later because there was probably something wrong with the baby anyway.

Another poor tactic is to give the patient a reason to question her faith, blaming the incident on God:

- Everything happens for the best. It is God's will.
- You should feel special: You have an angel in heaven.

It is never a good idea to get into a discussion about religion, especially when emotions are running high. Although you may mean well, these remarks are hurtful. Couples often begin to make plans for the future the moment they learn of a pregnancy. They begin to decide on names, choose schools, and look forward to activities such as T-ball and ballet lessons. When they learn that the pregnancy has failed, those dreams and plans are shattered. We cannot fix their problem and nothing we say will make them feel better. The best thing we can say is a simple "I'm sorry," which acknowledges their grief, validates their feelings, and does not detract from the enormous impact of the event on their lives. Let them know that you are there for them and ask if there is anything you can do, such as phoning someone. This is especially important if your patient is an outpatient and is alone for the appointment and examination. Informing her that her baby is dead or defective and sending her out to drive a car back to her doctor's office or home can be dangerous when she is in a stunned state. Patients who have had these experiences have often related that they do not remember how they got to their next destination. Patients in shock are therefore a danger to themselves and others when behind the wheel of an automobile.

Confronting the Issue of Time

It can be hard to spend an appropriate amount of time with a patient who is beginning the grief process when your schedule is busy and other patients are waiting. However, in these situations patients need time before they are sent on their way. If you cannot allow the patient to compose herself in your examination room, escort her to another room away from other patients and provide her with a damp cloth, tissues, and a cup of water. Try not to leave her alone but, if you must, check on her frequently.

Answering Questions and Saying the Right Thing

Reassure your patient that there is nothing she could have done to change the outcome and that neither she nor her partner is to blame. At the same time, do not make comments that suggest that she and her husband or their baby received inadequate care or that they should have sought care sooner. They already have doubt and feelings of guilt. Be prepared to answer whatever questions you can. For those you cannot answer, find someone who can, preferably a physician. Patients who are receiving bad news need to speak with a doctor before they leave and should not be sent away without learning the results of the examination. Although departmental protocol will determine the approach to relaying test results, it is very unfair to the patient when a sonologist refuses to speak with her, especially when she knows of her problem and knows that your study will provide the answer, good or bad. If the sonologist does not want to be the bearer of bad news, the referring clinician or another qualified person familiar with the case should be called to speak with the patient before she leaves.

Including the Father and Family

If the father is in attendance, do not forget about him. This tragedy is his too. Offer him support and let him know that he does not have to bear the entire emotional burden or be the "strong one." Encourage him to hold his partner's hand and comfort her, and then give them a few private moments.

Departmental protocols vary with regard to allowing family members in the room with the patient during the examination. However, when there is a loss, give family members, especially the father, an opportunity to view the monitor if they wish. This may be the only visible evidence of their baby that they will see. Take pictures if the parents want tangible evidence of the pregnancy. Some patients, afraid of how they may appear, will not ask. You can gently let them know that pictures are available and that those pictures will remain available in your file if they later decide that they want them. It is not uncommon for parents to request images after they have absorbed the initial shock of the news. Again, the sonogram may be the only tangible evidence that this baby existed.

It is also helpful to keep a list of support groups, such as Resolve Through Sharing, for patients who do not have a good support system through friends and family. Your care and concern will be remembered and appreciated.

What Grieving Persons Must Know

There are seven things that all grieving persons must know (Box 16-5):

1. *You are loved even when you are a confused mess.* Let patients know that you understand and want to be with them even if they are not the best company at the time. Just knowing that someone cares provides some comfort.

2. *Crying is a gift.* Bottling emotions inside can only endanger the health of those in grief. Crying allows emotions to flow freely and relieves physical tension. Let those receiving bad news know that it is okay to cry.

3. *Almost every thought, feeling, and behavior is normal in grief.* The healthcare provider must be watchful for signs of severe depression. Although feeling confused and crazy is normal for those in grief, thinking about suicide is not. Encourage grievers to talk and express themselves.

4. *You are not alone.* Make yourself available when the patient in grief needs to talk. Too many times, people try to avoid unpleasantness by being absent. This adds to the griever's pain and results in a secondary loss: the loss of human empathy when it is needed most.

5. *Most people are uncomfortable with grieving people.* You can explain why some people may distance themselves from the griever or why sometimes hurtful comments are made. Some people will try to be unusually joyful or chatter about nonsensical things to avoid talking about the incident causing the grief, thinking they are helping. Others, as noted above, may relate their own grief experiences. These approaches can add to the griever's confusion. As that person's healthcare provider, you can help your patient understand others' reactions so he or she can prepare to deal with them.

6. *You will survive no matter how bad you feel.* Be careful not to overemphasize this point or leave the impression that a time line for feeling normal is anticipated; simply stating the point should be sufficient.

7. *It takes as long as it takes.* Again, do not put time constraints on grief. Let the griever know that you are there to share the pain and that sharing will make it bearable. Your willingness to support the patient in your capacity as a healthcare provider, for however long it takes, will help to ease the burden of grief and shorten its duration.

Box 16-5.   Things grieving persons should know.

1. You are loved even when you are a confused mess.
2. Crying is a gift.
3. Almost every thought, feeling, or behavior is normal.
4. You are not alone.
5. Most people are uncomfortable with grieving people.
6. You will survive no matter how bad you feel.
7. It takes as long as it takes.

If we can make our patients understand these things, we will have played a significant role in the healing process. The sonography examination will become part of what will be viewed as a positive experience because of the compassion showed during a difficult time and the tangible memory you were able to offer by way of the sonographic image.

CASE STUDIES

The following actual cases demonstrate clinical situations in which the practitioner may need to call upon some grief counseling skills.

Case 1

A 26-year-old female, G-2, P-1, is scheduled to have a repeat cesarean section. By good menstrual dates she is 8 weeks, and the sonogram is performed to confirm her dates and expected delivery by cesarean (EDC). She has had no complaints or discomfort. At 8 weeks' gestation, the sac should occupy one-half of the uterine cavity and a viable fetus should be identifiable. By 10 weeks the sac normally occupies all of the uterine cavity and the fetus is typically well defined, showing upper and lower extremities.

Figure 16-5, a longitudinal scan of the uterus, demonstrates an intrauterine gestational sac filling the entire uterine cavity but showing no evidence of a fetal pole. No adnexal abnormalities are defined. The image demonstrates a large empty sac filling the uterine cavity. In this patient it most likely represents a missed abortion—demise of the pregnancy with failure to expel that has been missed clinically. In most cases a spontaneous abortion is the eventual result, but it may take up to 6 weeks for expulsion to occur. If spontaneous expulsion does not occur, the patient will have to undergo a dilation and curettage procedure.

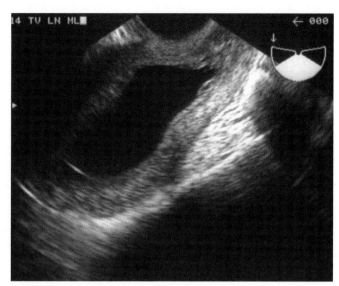

Figure 16-5. *Longitudinal image of a large intrauterine gestational sac that shows no yolk sac or embryo/fetal parts.*

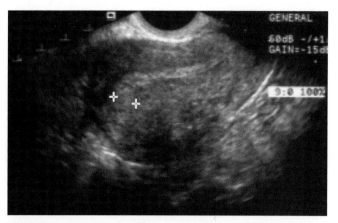

Figure 16-6. *Longitudinal image showing a thick endometrium (calipers) but no evidence of an intrauterine gestational sac.*

Case 2

A 20-year-old female, G-1, P-0, presents with vaginal bleeding and left lower quadrant pain. By menstrual dates she is 9 weeks. We were to rule out a threatened abortion as opposed to an ectopic pregnancy.

Figure 16-6 is a longitudinal view through the uterus; Figure 16-7 is a transverse scan through the right adnexa. The uterine cavity shows decidualization of the endometrium but no evidence of an intrauterine gestational sac. Figure 16-7 reveals an adnexal mass with a tubal ring containing a fetal pole, indicated by the arrow. Positive cardiac activity is identified. These findings are classic for an ectopic pregnancy.

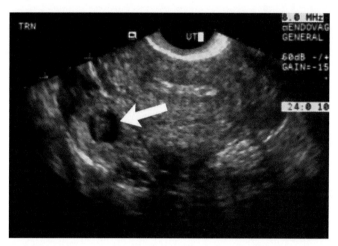

Figure 16-7. *Transverse image showing the empty uterus with a saclike structure in the right adnexa containing a fetal pole (arrow).*

Case 3

Figures 16-8 and 16-9 are from a patient presenting with a positive pregnancy and an episode of severe pelvic pain that has lessened over the weekend. She is seen on the following Monday morning, quite pale and weak. Although she indicates that her pain is gone, she complains of extreme fatigue. Figure 16-8 reveals an empty uterus with a large complex mass in the cul-de-sac. Figure 16-9, a transverse view through the uterus, demonstrates the complex mass extending into the cul-de-sac and along the iliopsoas margin on the left. Further investigation reveals free fluid in Morison's pouch in the right upper quadrant. Surgery is immediately performed and a ruptured ectopic pregnancy is confirmed, as suspected. Apparently her pain was lessened by the rupture of the fallopian tube; however, she bled profusely internally.

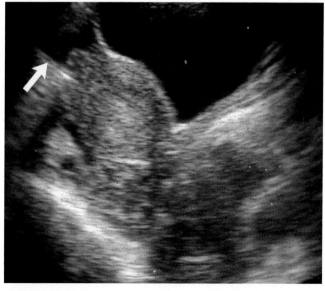

Figure 16-8. *Longitudinal image of an empty uterus with complex material in the cul-de-sac and fluid noted superior to the uterine fundus (arrow).*

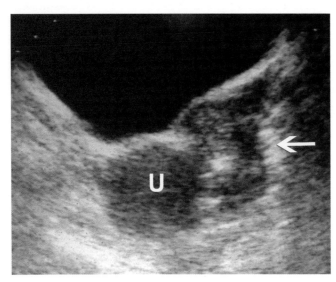

Figure 16-9. *Transverse image showing the mass extending along the left iliopsoas margin (arrow). U = uterus.*

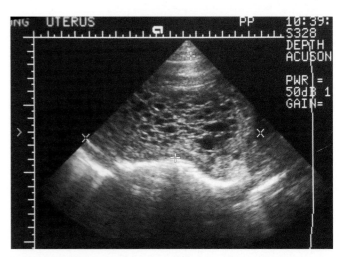

Figure 16-10. *Longitudinal image showing uterus filled with hydropic molar tissue.*

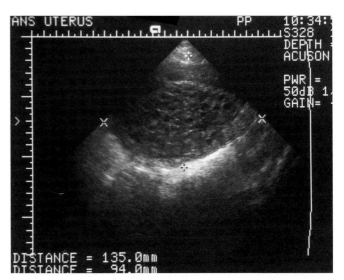

Figure 16-11. *Transverse image showing uterus filled with hydropic molar tissue.*

Ectopic pregnancies are common and potentially life-threatening. A number of conditions may predispose patients to an ectopic pregnancy. Anything that creates tubal obstruction can be a cause. Pelvic inflammatory disease due to one or more of the many sexually transmitted diseases is among the more common causes. Intrauterine contraceptive devices inhibit implantation in the endometrium, so the blastocyst may implant elsewhere. Tubal operations can cause adhesions, and exposure to diethylstilbestrol (DES) may result in tubal abnormalities, including the inability to propel the fertilized egg through the tube. Most patients fail to show the defined gestational sac with a viable embryo or fetus outside the empty uterus. Many simply show an empty uterus with an adnexal mass and/or free fluid. It is imperative that the sonographer know menstrual dates and that the patient has tested positive for pregnancy. A quantitative beta human chorionic gonadotropin (hCG) test can be correlated with ultrasound findings for a more definitive diagnosis. Patients who have had a previous ectopic pregnancy have a 10% chance of having recurrent ectopic pregnancies, and a high percentage may never achieve pregnancy again.

Case 4

A 19-year-old female, G-1, P-0, presents large for gestational age (LGA), bleeding and with no fetal heart tones. By good menstrual dates she is 12–13 weeks. We are to rule out twins and confirm viability as well as placental location. Figures 16-10 and 16-11 show longitudinal and transverse views through her uterus. It is enlarged and filled with tissue containing many small cystic regions.

This presentation is typical of a **molar pregnancy**. With a mole, the embryo usually dies early in the pregnancy and is reabsorbed. Rather than being spontaneously expelled, the placenta remains to grow and become hydropic—hence the numerous cysts seen within the tissue. Most molar pregnancies involve benign hydatidiform moles, but they can be invasive (chorioadenoma destruens) or even metastatic (choriocarcinoma). The rapidly growing trophoblastic tissue may cause hyperstimulation of the ovaries, resulting in bilateral theca-lutein cysts. This hyperstimulation also causes patients to present with hyperemesis gravidarum (excessive nausea and vomiting to

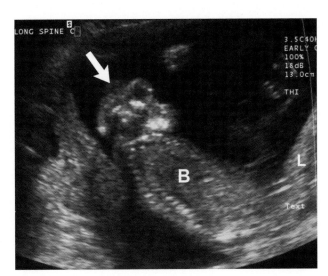

Figure 16-12. *Image showing long axis of the fetus with anencephaly (arrow). B = body, L = leg.*

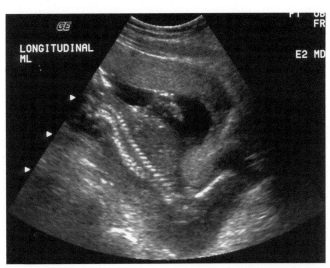

Figure 16-13. *Demise of a second or third trimester pregnancy can be especially hard, since the patient has already begun maternal fetal bonding and can actually feel movement.*

the point of dehydration). Other unusual clinical findings include first trimester pregnancy-induced hypertension (PIH) and extremely high hCG levels. See Chapter 3 for additional information on molar pregnancy.

Case 5

A patient is referred because the clinician cannot hear fetal heart tones. The patient is in her late second trimester. The patient presents LGA and has been feeling excessive movement. The request asks to rule out a multiple gestation. The patient is anxious and excited to learn if she has one or two babies. Instead, anencephaly with polyhydramnios is discovered.

Figure 16-12 demonstrates the fatal anomaly, anencephaly, a severe neural tube defect in which there is little or no brain or cranium. There may be a brain stem or partial brain stem, but it is exposed. Although anencephalic fetuses are viable in utero, death is inevitable. Neural tube defects are often associated with polyhydramnios because the fetal swallowing mechanism is affected, inhibiting the normal circulation of fluid through the fetus. Anencephalic fetuses are often hyperactive. The excess amniotic fluid creates more space in which the fetus can move, and the exposed brain stem is irritated by the amniotic fluid, agitating the fetus. These babies usually die shortly after delivery if not in utero. Anencephaly is thought to be associated with folic acid deficiency and folic acid antagonists such as methotrexate and aminopterin. Folic acid is found in several foods, such as green beans, broccoli,

spinach, citrus fruits, liver, eggs, and yogurt. Other conditions that may predispose a fetus to neural tube defects include maternal diabetes and hyperthermia.

Comments

The patients in Cases 1–4 came to the ultrasound laboratory hoping to learn that their babies were well. First trimester bleeding is a common occurrence. There are many sonographic findings that indicate that a first trimester pregnancy may be abnormal, including a low implantation, poor decidual reaction around the gestational sac, a sac that is too small or large for its contents, the absence of contents inside the sac, and an irregular sac shape. The secondary yolk sac itself may provide clues as well. The yolk sac should be perfectly round and measure not more than 6 mm or less than 2 mm. Any deviation from the norm should make one suspicious.

Losses during the first trimester are not uncommon. However, they do not receive the same degree of attention from family and friends as do other types of death. Many patients begin to make long-term plans once they learn they are pregnant. Their many other hopes and dreams are lost with the failed pregnancy, and we need to be sensitive to those emotions during their time of crisis as well as later.

Demise of a second or third trimester pregnancy can be especially hard, since the patient can actually feel movement and has already begun maternal fetal bonding (Figure 16-13). In Case 5, the patient was feeling her baby's movement and came to the examination excitedly anticipating the possibility of twins. Instead she was told her only baby was severely deformed and would not live. Knowledge of this fact can bring on the grieving process before the death actually occurs.

Sonographers must remain aware that patients watch our every move and expression for signs of encouragement or concern. We must be sure to follow protocols consistently so we do not give information before we intend to. I had a patient who was classified as a habitual aborter, and I had scanned her over several failed pregnancies. Finally, she succeeded in carrying one to term. By then she was well aware of my routine. When her friend became pregnant and experienced some bleeding, she came to my department for her ultrasound examination. She immediately told me that my patient had informed her that I would show her the screen and baby's heartbeat if everything was normal. If not, I would leave to show the pictures to the radiologist before anyone spoke to her. I realized then that I was not being consistent in how I interacted with my patients.

REFERENCES

Chez RA: Acute grief and mourning: one obstetrician's experience. Obstet Gynecol 85:1059–1061, 1995.

Davidson GW: *Understanding Mourning: A Guide for Those Who Grieve.* Minneapolis, Augsburg, 1984.

Goldbach KR, Dunn DS, Toedter LJ, et al: The effects of gestational age and gender on grief after pregnancy. Amer J Orthopsychiatry 6:461–467, 1991.

Kübler-Ross E: *On Children and Death.* New York, Scribner, 1997.

Kübler-Ross E: *On Death and Dying.* New York, Macmillan, 1969.

Layne LL: Motherhood lost: cultural dimensions of miscarriage and stillbirth in America. Women and Health 16:69–97, 1990.

Lister MK, Lovell SM: Healing together: helping couples cope with miscarriage, stillbirth or early infant loss. Bereavement 10:12–13, 1990.

University of Wisconsin–La Crosse, Center for Death Education and Bioethics. *Illness, Crisis and Loss—Multidisciplinary Linkages*, Volume 2, Number 1. Philadelphia, Charles Press, 1992.

York CR, Stichler J: Cultural grief expressions following infant death. Dimens Crit Care Nurs 4:120–127, 1985.

SELF-ASSESSMENT EXERCISES

Questions

1. When a person's activities become limited by an illness or disability that also limits his or her circle of friends, that person is experiencing what kind of death?

    A. Physiologic

    B. Biologic

    C. Psychological

    D. Social

    E. Sociopathologic

2. When life support equipment must be employed, the patient is experiencing what kind of death?

    A. Physiologic

    B. Biologic

    C. Psychological

    D. Social

    E. Sociopathologic

3. Any event that changes the way things have been is called:

    A. Loss

    B. Death

    C. Bereavement

    D. Mourning

    E. Misfortune

4. Signs and symptoms associated with mourning are referred to as:

   A. Grief

   B. Bereavement

   C. Psychological death

   D. Resolution

   E. Melancholy

5. The process of resolving the conflicts associated with loss is called:

   A. Grief

   B. Bereavement

   C. Mourning

   D. Searching and yearning

   E. Depression

6. Of the following statements, which is *not* true of loss?

   A. Loss is associated only with a death of someone or something loved.

   B. Loss is an event while grief is how it makes you feel.

   C. There is no set time frame for someone to overcome a loss.

   D. Loss can be described in terms of time.

   E. Divorce is considered a type of loss.

7. For most individuals, the patterns of mourning occur in four phases and usually take how many months to complete?

   A. 6

   B. 9

   C. 12

   D. 18

   E. 24

8. All of the following are good rules to follow when supporting someone grieving, *except*:

   A. Don't rush someone to "get over" being sad.

   B. Listen more than you talk.

   C. Try to be upbeat and always cheerful and encourage the griever to be the same.

   D. Let the griever cry.

   E. Ask what you can do for the griever.

9. Which statement is *not* true of mourning?

   A. There is a soothing side to mourning.

   B. There is a painful side to mourning.

   C. Mourning is a process that may be associated with any type of loss.

   D. People of different ethnicities may mourn differently.

   E. Mourning and bereavement are synonymous.

10. Which of the following is a myth regarding grief?

    A. Children and adults grieve differently.

    B. Young children should be protected from death and grief.

    C. Grief should be shared.

    D. Almost any feeling associated with grief is normal.

    E. Grief can cause physical symptoms.

Answers

See Appendix F on page 618 for answers and explanations.

Frequently Referenced Measurements

The following tables list some of the most common measurements to which practitioners of obstetric and gynecologic ultrasound must refer in daily practice. These tables of standard measurements are arranged in the order in which they are first cited in the text.

Table 1.	Normal uterine dimensions and volumes by pediatric age.				
Age	Length (cm) (Mean ± SD)	AP Corpus (cm) (Mean ± SD)	AP Cervis (cm) (Mean ± SD)	Transverse Corpus (cm) (Mean)	Volume (ml) (Mean ± SD)
≤ 8 weeks	2.5 ± 5.0	0.25	—	1.0	—
2–7 years	3.3 ± 0.4	0.7 ± 0.2	0.8 ± 0.2	1.7	2.0 ± 1.2
8 years	3.6 ± 0.7	0.9 ± 0.3	0.8 ± 0.2	1.8	3.1 ± 1.5
9 years	3.7 ± 0.4	1.0 ± 0.3	0.9 ± 0.2	1.9	3.7 ± 1.6
10 years	4.0 ± 0.8	1.3 ± 0.5	1.1 ± 0.3	2.4	6.5 ± 3.8
11 years	4.2 ± 0.5	1.3 ± 0.3	1.1 ± 0.3	2.3	6.7 ± 2.9
12 years	5.4 ± 0.8	1.7 ± 0.5	1.4 ± 0.5	3.4	16.2 ± 9.2
13 years	5.4 ± 1.1	1.6 ± 0.4	1.5 ± 0.2	2.9	13.2 ± 5.6

SD = standard deviation. Transverse width is calculated backward from the volume by using length and AP corpus dimensions (that is, volume is divided by length × AP corpus × 0.523).

Reprinted with permission from Goldberg B: *Atlas of Ultrasound Measurements*. Philadelphia, Elsevier, 1990. Table 19-6, p. 214. Data from Orsini LF, Salardi S, Pila C, et al: Pelvic organs in premenarcheal girls: real-time ultrasonography. Radiology 153:113–116, 1984.

Table 2.   Normal uterine dimensions of young nulliparous postpubertal girls.

Age (Years)	Length (cm)		AP Dimension (cm)		Transverse Width (cm)	
	Mean	Range	Mean	Range	Mean	Range
12–20	6.1	4.5–8.7	2.5	1.6–3.0	—	—

Reprinted with permission from Goldberg B: *Atlas of Ultrasound Measurements*. Philadelphia, Elsevier, 1990. Data from Sample WF, Lippe BM, Cyepes MT: Gray-scale ultrasonography of the normal female pelvis, Radiology 125:477–483, 1977; Ivarsson SA, Nilsson KO, Persson PH: Ultrasonography of the pelvic organs in prepubertal and postpubertal girls, Arch Dis Child 58:352–354, 1983; and Colle M, Calabet A, Sanciaume C, et al: Contribution of pelvic ultrasonography (PUS) to endocrine investigations in girls, Pediatr Res 18:113, 1984.

Table 3.   Normal anatomic uterine dimensions in adult women according to age.

Age Range (Years)	Length (cm) (Mean ± SD)	AP Dimension (cm) (Mean ± SD)	Transverse Width (cm) (Mean ± SD)
20–29	9.2 ± 1.6	4.1 ± 0.8	5.5 ± 0.8
30–39	9.4 ± 1.5	4.1 ± 1.5	5.7 ± 1.5
40–49	9.5 ± 1.1	4.2 ± 1.1	5.8 ± 1.1
50–59	8.1 ± 1.8	3.2 ± 1.2	5.0 ± 1.2
60+	8.0 ± 1.9	2.8 ± 0.8	4.5 ± 0.8

SD = standard deviation.

Reprinted with permission from Goldberg B: *Atlas of Ultrasound Measurements*. Philadelphia, Elsevier, 1990. Adapted from Langlois PL: The size of the normal uterus. J Reprod Med 4:221–226, 1970.

Table 4.   Normal anatomic uterine dimensions in adult premenopausal women according to parity.

Parity	Length (cm) (Mean ± SD)	AP Dimension (cm) (Mean ± SD)	Transverse Width (cm) (Mean ± SD)
0	7.7 ± 1.1	2.9 ± 1.1	4.7 ± 0.8
1	8.8 ± 1.5	3.5 ± 1.0	5.0 ± 1.0
2–3	9.2 ± 1.3	3.9 ± 1.3	5.6 ± 1.3
4–5	9.4 ± 1.1	4.2 ± 1.1	5.8 ± 1.1
5+	9.7 ± 1.1	4.2 ± 1.1	5.9 ± 1.1

SD = standard deviation.

Reprinted with permission from Goldberg B: *Atlas of Ultrasound Measurements*. Philadelphia, Elsevier, 1990. Adapted from Langlois PL: The size of the normal uterus. J Reprod Med 4:221–226, 1970.

Table 5. Normal ovarian volumes by pediatric age.

Pediatric Category	Pediatric Age	Volume (ml)
Neonatal	≤ 6 weeks	0.18 (average)
Infancy	6 weeks–2 years	≤ 1.0
Early childhood	2–8 years	0.9 ± 0.3
Late childhood	9 years	2.0 ± 0.8
	10 years	2.2 ± 0.7
	11 years	2.5 ± 1.3
	12 years	3.8 ± 1.4
	13 years	4.2 ± 2.3
	13–14 years	4.1 ± 3.0

Reprinted with permission from Goldberg B: *Atlas of Ultrasound Measurement.* St. Louis, Mosby, pp 196–221, 1990.

Table 7. Approximate mean ovarian volumes in normal postmenopausal women by age.

Age Range (Years)	Mean Ovarian Volume (ml)
40–44	7.9
45–49	6.8
50–54	4.8 ± 2.8
55–59	3.4
60–64	2.7
65–69	1.9 ± 2.0
70+	1.0

Approximate mean ovarian volumes interpolated from Andolf et al.

Reprinted with permission from Goldberg B: *Atlas of Ultrasound Measurements.* Philadelphia, Elsevier, 1990. Adapted from Andolf E, Jergensen C, Svalenius E, et al: Acta Obstet Gynecol Scand 66:387–389, 1987.

Table 6. Normal ovarian volumes in adult premenopausal women.

Maternal Age (Years)	Parity	Mean Volume (ml)	Range (ml)
13–20	Nulliparous	4.0	1.8–5.7
20–45	Mixed (parous and nulliparous)	7.0 ± 4.2	1.4–24.4

Reprinted with permission from Goldberg B: *Atlas of Ultrasound Measurements.* Philadelphia, Elsevier, 1990.

Table 8. Premenopausal ovarian volumes.

Age	Mean (ml)	Upper Limit (ml)	Number of Patients
0–3 months	1.0	3.6	77
4–12 months	1.0	2.7	77
13–24 months	0.7	1.7	77
Premenarche (2–13 years)	0.75 ± 0.41 4.18 ± 2.30	—	101
Premenarche (3–15 years)	3.0 ± 2.3	9.1	32
Menstruating	9.8 ± 5.8	21.9	866 ovaries
Premenopausal	6.8	18.0	406

0.523 × length × width × height.

Reprinted with permission from Callen P: *Ultrasonography in Obstetrics and Gynecology*, 4th edition. Philadelphia, Saunders, 2000, p 861, table 31-1.

Table 9. Nomogram of the transverse cerebellar diameter according to percentile distribution.

Gestational Age (Weeks)	Cerebellum Diameter (mm) Percentile				
	10th	25th	50th	75th	90th
15	10	12	14	15	16
16	14	16	16	16	17
17	16	17	17	18	18
18	17	18	18	19	19
19	18	18	19	19	22
20	18	19	20	20	22
21	19	20	22	23	24
22	21	23	23	24	24
23	22	23	24	25	26
24	22	24	25	27	28
25	23	21.5	28	28	29
26	25	28	29	30	32
27	26	28.5	30	31	32
28	27	30	31	32	34
29	29	32	34	36	38
30	31	32	35	37	40
31	32	35	38	39	43
32	33	36	38	40	42
33	32	36	40	43	44
34	33	38	40	41	44
35	31	37	40.5	43	47
36	36	29	43	52	55
37	37	37	45	52	55
38	40	40	48.5	52	55
39	52	52	52	55	55

Reprinted with permission from Goldstein I, Reece A, Pilu G, et al: Cerebellar measurements with ultrasonography in the evaluation of fetal growth and development. Am J Obstet Gynecol 156:1065, 1987.

Table 10.   Percentile values for fetal abdominal circumference.

Menstrual (Weeks)	Abdominal Circumference (cm)				
	3rd	10th	50th	90th	97th
14	6.4	6.7	7.3	7.9	8.3
15	7.5	7.9	8.6	9.3	9.7
16	8.6	9.1	9.9	10.7	11.2
17	9.7	10.3	11.2	12.1	12.7
18	10.9	11.5	12.5	13.5	14.1
19	11.9	12.6	13.7	14.8	15.5
20	13.1	13.8	15.0	16.3	17.0
21	14.1	14.9	16.2	17.6	18.3
22	15.1	16.0	17.4	18.8	19.7
23	16.1	17.0	18.5	20.0	20.9
24	17.1	18.1	19.7	21.3	22.3
25	18.1	19.1	20.8	22.5	23.5
26	19.1	20.1	21.9	23.7	24.8
27	20.0	21.1	23.0	24.9	26.0
28	20.9	22.0	24.0	26.0	27.1
29	21.8	23.0	25.1	27.2	28.4
30	22.7	23.9	26.1	28.3	29.5
31	23.6	24.9	27.1	29.4	30.6
32	24.5	25.8	28.1	30.4	31.8
33	25.3	26.7	29.1	31.5	32.9
34	26.1	27.5	30.0	32.5	33.9
35	26.9	28.3	30.9	33.5	34.9
36	27.7	29.2	31.8	34.4	35.9
37	28.5	30.0	32.7	35.4	37.0
38	29.2	30.8	33.6	36.4	38.0
39	29.9	31.6	34.4	37.3	38.9
40	30.7	32.4	35.3	38.2	39.9

Reprinted with permission from Hadlock FP, Deter RL, Harrist RB, et al: Estimating fetal age: computer-assisted analysis of multiple fetal growth parameters. Radiology 152:497, 1984.

Table 11.   Mean renal lengths for various gestational ages.

Menstrual Age (Weeks)	Mean Length (cm)	SD	95% CI	N
18	2.2	0.3	1.6–2.8	14
19	2.3	0.4	1.5–3.1	23
20	2.6	0.4	1.8–3.4	22
21	2.7	0.3	2.1–3.2	20
22	2.7	0.3	2.0–3.4	18
23	3.0	0.4	2.2–3.7	13
24	3.1	0.6	1.9–4.4	13
25	3.3	0.4	2.5–4.2	9
26	3.4	0.4	2.4–4.4	9
27	3.5	0.4	2.7–4.4	15
28	3.4	0.4	2.6–4.2	19
29	3.6	0.7	2.3–4.8	12
30	3.8	0.4	2.9–4.6	24
31	3.7	0.5	2.8–4.6	23
32	4.1	0.5	3.1–5.1	23
33	4.0	0.3	3.3–4.7	28
34	4.2	0.4	3.3–5.0	36
35	4.2	0.5	3.2–5.2	17
36	4.2	0.4	3.3–5.0	36
37	4.2	0.4	3.3–5.1	40
38	4.4	0.6	3.2–5.6	32
39	4.2	0.3	3.5–4.8	17
40	4.3	0.5	3.2–5.3	10
41	4.5	0.3	3.9–5.1	4

SD = standard deviation; CI = confidence interval.

Reprinted with permission from Cohen HL, Cooper J, Eisenberg P, et al: Normal length of fetal kidneys: sonographic study in 397 obstetric patients. Am J Roentgenol 157:545–548, 1991.

Table 12. Percentile values for fetal head circumference.

Menstrual (Weeks)	Head Circumference (cm)				
	3rd	10th	50th	90th	97th
14	8.8	9.1	9.7	10.3	10.6
15	10.0	10.4	11.0	11.6	12.0
16	11.3	11.7	12.4	13.1	13.5
17	12.6	13.0	13.8	14.6	15.0
18	13.7	14.2	15.1	16.0	16.5
19	14.9	15.5	16.4	17.4	17.9
20	16.1	16.7	17.7	18.7	19.3
21	17.2	17.8	18.9	20.0	20.6
22	18.3	18.9	20.1	21.3	21.9
23	19.4	20.1	21.3	22.5	23.2
24	20.4	21.1	22.4	23.7	24.3
25	21.4	22.2	23.5	24.9	25.6
26	22.4	23.2	24.6	26.0	26.8
27	23.3	24.1	25.6	27.1	27.9
28	24.2	25.1	26.6	28.1	29.1
29	25.0	25.9	27.5	29.1	30.0
30	25.8	26.8	28.4	30.0	31.0
31	26.7	27.6	29.3	31.0	31.9
32	27.4	28.4	30.1	31.8	32.8
33	28.0	29.0	30.8	32.6	33.6
34	28.7	29.7	31.5	33.3	34.3
35	29.3	30.4	32.2	34.1	35.1
36	29.9	30.9	32.8	34.7	35.8
37	30.3	31.4	33.3	35.2	36.3
38	30.8	31.9	33.8	35.8	36.8
39	31.1	32.2	34.2	36.2	37.3
40	31.5	32.6	34.6	36.6	37.7

Reprinted with permission from Hadlock FP, Deter RL, Harrist RB, et al: Estimating fetal age: computer-assisted analysis of multiple fetal growth parameters. Radiology 152:497, 1984.

Table 13. Percentile values for fetal femur length.

Menstrual Weeks	Femur Length (cm)				
	3rd	10th	50th	90th	97th
14	1.2	1.3	1.4	1.5	1.6
15	1.5	1.6	1.7	1.9	1.9
16	1.7	1.8	2.0	2.2	2.3
17	2.1	2.2	2.4	2.6	2.7
18	2.3	2.5	2.7	2.9	3.1
19	2.6	2.7	3.0	3.3	3.4
20	2.8	3.0	3.3	3.6	3.8
21	3.0	3.2	3.5	3.8	4.0
22	3.3	3.5	3.8	4.1	4.3
23	3.5	3.7	4.1	4.5	4.7
24	3.8	4.0	4.4	4.8	5.0
25	4.0	4.2	4.6	5.0	5.2
26	4.2	4.5	4.9	5.3	5.6
27	4.4	4.6	5.1	5.6	5.8
28	4.6	4.9	5.4	5.9	6.2
29	4.8	5.1	5.6	6.1	6.4
30	5.0	5.3	5.8	6.3	6.6
31	5.2	5.5	6.0	6.5	6.8
32	5.3	5.6	6.2	6.8	7.1
33	5.5	5.8	6.4	7.0	7.3
34	5.7	6.0	6.6	7.2	7.5
35	5.9	6.2	6.8	7.4	7.8
36	6.0	6.4	7.0	7.6	8.0
37	6.2	6.6	7.2	7.9	8.2
38	6.4	6.7	7.4	8.1	8.4
39	6.5	6.8	7.5	8.2	8.6
40	6.6	7.0	7.7	8.4	8.8

Reprinted with permission from Hadlock FP, Deter RL, Harrist RB, et al: Estimating fetal age: computer-assisted analysis of multiple fetal growth parameters. Radiology 152:497, 1984.

Table 14. Multiple fetal parameters in the assessment of gestational age.*

Mean Gestational Age (Weeks)	Mean Biparietal Diameter (mm)	Mean Head Circumference (mm)	Mean Abdominal Circumference (mm)	Mean Femur Length (mm)
12.0	17	68	46	7
12.5	19	75	53	9
13.0	21	82	60	11
13.5	23	89	67	12
14.0	25	97	73	14
14.5	27	104	80	16
15.0	29	110	86	17
15.5	31	117	93	19
16.0	32	124	99	20
16.5	34	131	106	22
17.0	36	138	112	24
17.5	38	144	119	25
18.0	39	151	125	27
18.5	41	158	131	28
19.0	43	164	137	30
19.5	45	170	144	31
20.0	46	177	150	33
20.5	48	183	156	34
21.0	50	189	162	35
21.5	51	195	168	37
22.0	53	201	174	38
22.5	55	207	179	40
23.0	56	213	185	41
23.5	58	219	191	42
24.0	59	224	197	44
24.5	61	230	202	45
25.0	62	235	208	46
25.5	64	241	213	47
26.0	65	246	219	49
26.5	67	251	224	50

(Continued on the next page . . .)

Table 14.   Multiple fetal parameters in the assessment of gestational age, continued.*

Mean Gestational Age (Weeks)	Mean Biparietal Diameter (mm)	Mean Head Circumference (mm)	Mean Abdominal Circumference (mm)	Mean Femur Length (mm)
27.0	68	256	230	51
27.5	69	261	235	52
28.0	71	266	240	54
28.5	72	271	246	55
29.0	73	275	251	56
29.5	75	280	256	57
30.0	76	284	261	58
30.5	77	288	266	59
31.0	78	293	271	60
31.5	79	297	276	61
32.0	81	301	281	62
32.5	82	304	286	63
33.0	83	308	291	64
33.5	84	312	295	65
34.0	85	315	300	66
34.5	86	318	305	67
35.0	87	322	309	68
35.5	88	325	314	69
36.0	89	328	318	70
36.5	89	330	323	71
37.0	90	333	327	72
37.5	91	335	332	73
38.0	92	338	336	74
38.5	92	340	340	74
39.0	93	342	344	75
39.5	94	344	348	76
40.0	94	346	353	77

*Instructions: Take the mean measurements of the four parameters—biparietal diameter, head circumference, abdominal circumference, femur length. Find mean gestational ages of each, add them together, and divide by 4.

Reprinted with permission from Hadlock FP, Deter RL, Harrist RB, et al: Estimating fetal age: computer-assisted analysis of multiple fetal growth parameters. Radiology 152:497, 1984.

Table 15. Amniotic fluid index values in normal pregnancy.

Week	Amniotic Fluid Index Percentile Values (mm)				
	2.5th	5th	50th	95th	97.5th
16	73	79	121	185	201
17	77	83	127	194	211
18	80	97	133	202	220
19	83	90	137	207	225
20	86	93	141	212	230
21	88	95	143	214	233
22	89	97	145	216	235
23	90	98	146	218	237
24	90	98	147	219	238
25	89	97	147	221	240
26	89	97	147	223	242
27	85	95	146	226	245
28	86	94	146	228	249
29	84	92	145	231	254
30	82	90	145	234	258
31	79	88	144	238	263
32	77	86	144	242	269
33	74	83	143	245	274
34	72	81	142	248	278
35	70	79	140	249	279
36	68	77	138	249	279
37	66	75	135	244	275
38	65	73	132	239	269
39	64	72	127	226	255
40	63	71	123	214	240
41	63	70	116	194	216
42	63	69	110	175	192

Reprinted with permission from Moore TR, Cayle JE: The amniotic fluid index in normal human pregnancy. Am J Obstet Gynecol 162:1168, 1990.

Table 16.   Normal percentile ranges for nasal bone lengths (mm) by specific menstrual age.

Gestational Age (Weeks)	Subjects (N = 3537)	Percentile Values				
		2.5th	5th	50th	95th	97.5th
11	16	1.3	1.4	2.3	3.3	3.4
12	54	1.7	1.8	2.8	4.2	4.3
13	59	2.2	2.3	3.1	4.6	4.8
14	82	2.2	2.5	3.8	5.3	5.7
15	103	2.8	3.0	4.3	5.7	6.0
16	134	3.2	3.4	4.7	6.2	6.2
17	203	3.7	4.0	5.3	6.6	6.9
18	252	4.0	4.3	5.7	7.0	7.3
19	388	4.6	5.0	6.3	7.9	8.2
20	440	5.0	5.2	6.7	8.3	8.6
21	322	5.1	5.6	7.1	9.0	9.3
22	208	5.6	5.8	7.5	9.3	10.2
23	157	6.0	6.4	7.9	9.6	9.9
24	121	6.6	6.8	9.3	10.0	10.3
25	123	6.3	6.5	8.5	10.7	10.8
26	96	6.8	7.4	8.9	10.9	11.3
27	80	7.0	7.5	9.2	11.3	11.6
28	103	7.2	7.6	9.8	12.1	13.4
29	95	7.2	7.7	9.8	11.8	12.3
30	104	7.3	7.9	10.0	12.6	13.2
31	92	7.9	8.2	10.4	12.6	13.2
32	66	8.1	8.6	10.5	13.6	13.7
33	54	8.6	8.7	10.8	12.8	13.0
34	41	9.0	9.1	10.9	12.8	13.5
35	37	7.5	8.5	11.0	14.1	15.0
36	40	7.3	7.8	10.8	12.8	13.6
37	36	8.4	8.7	11.4	14.5	15.0
38	13	9.2	9.3	11.7	15.7	16.6
39	12	9.1	9.2	10.9	14.0	14.8
40	6	10.3	10.4	12.1	14.5	14.7

Reprinted with permission from Sonek JD, McKenna D, Webb D, et al: Nasal bone length throughout gestation: normal ranges based on 3537 fetal ultrasound measurements. Ultrasound Obstet Gynecol 21:152–155, 2003.

| Table 17. | Mean fetal binocular distance with standard deviations and 5th, 50th, and 95th percentiles for gestational age. | | | | | | |

Gestational Age (Weeks)	Number of Exams	Mean BOD (cm)	SD (cm)	Percentile		
				5th	50th	95th
14	19	1.91	0.25	1.60	1.90	2.30
15	20	2.15	0.25	1.70	2.10	2.35
16	20	2.24	0.24	1.71	2.31	2.69
17	20	2.55	0.21	2.10	2.51	2.80
18	22	2.78	0.27	2.30	2.81	3.24
19	20	2.97	0.25	2.56	3.00	3.53
20	21	3.07	0.21	2.70	3.10	3.54
21	22	3.29	0.23	2.85	3.25	3.74
22	20	3.46	0.19	3.02	3.50	3.80
23	20	3.67	0.22	3.21	3.66	4.01
24	21	3.77	0.27	3.48	3.75	4.27
25	22	4.03	0.23	3.60	4.06	4.40
26	19	4.16	0.21	3.82	4.15	4.58
27	20	4.33	0.24	3.95	4.31	4.75
28	20	4.49	0.22	4.10	4.52	5.03
29	22	4.67	0.24	4.30	4.61	5.19
30	21	4.76	0.21	4.41	4.79	5.23
31	21	4.98	0.26	4.50	5.04	5.40
32	22	5.05	0.20	4.71	5.12	5.40
33	20	5.17	0.23	4.73	5.20	5.63
34	21	5.39	0.26	4.85	5.41	5.82
35	22	5.46	0.23	4.95	5.60	6.05
36	19	5.56	0.24	5.02	5.62	5.95
37	20	5.65	0.27	5.09	5.70	6.10
38	20	5.81	0.28	5.31	5.80	6.24
39	20	5.82	0.27	5.32	5.90	6.29
40	21	5.95	0.27	5.40	6.00	6.40

BOD = binocular distance; SD = standard deviation.

Reprinted with permission from Tongsong T, Wanapitrak C, Jesadapornchai S, et al: Fetal binocular distance as a predictor of menstrual age. Int J Gynaecol Obstet 38:87–91, 1992.

Table 18.   Values for the fetal orbital diameter (mm).

Menstrual Age (Weeks)	N	Mean	95% CI	Percentile				
				10th	25th	50th	75th	90th
14	10	5.2	4.8–5.7	4.5	5.0	5.3	5.7	5.7
15	26	6.1	5.9–6.3	5.4	5.5	6.2	6.5	6.7
16	25	6.6	6.3–6.9	5.8	6.2	6.5	7.0	7.6
17–18	19	7.3	6.7–7.8	6.2	6.5	6.7	9.0	9.0
19–20	23	9.8	9.3–10.2	8.6	9.0	10.0	10.1	11.3
21	19	10.5	10.0–10.9	9.4	9.9	10.0	11.0	12.0
22	26	10.4	10.0–10.7	9.5	9.6	10.5	11.0	11.3
23	21	10.7	10.4–11.1	9.6	10.0	10.5	11.4	11.5
24	10	11.6	11.3–11.8	10.7	11.0	11.5	12.0	12.5
25	13	11.2	11.4–12.4	10.3	11.0	12.2	12.5	12.8
26	16	12.7	12.0–13.4	11.0	11.0	12.7	13.8	14.5
27	14	13.0	12.4–13.5	11.9	12.0	12.9	13.4	14.8
28	21	13.0	12.7–13.3	12.1	12.0	13.1	13.3	14.1
29	23	13.9	13.4–14.4	12.6	13.0	13.7	14.6	15.7
30–31	24	14.2	13.8–14.5	13.3	13.0	13.9	14.7	15.4
32–33	24	14.4	13.7–15.1	12.2	13.0	14.1	14.8	17.5
34–36	26	15.8	15.4–16.2	14.6	15.0	15.7	16.5	16.9

CI = confidence interval.

Reprinted with permission from Goldstein I, Tamir A, Zimmer EZ, et al: Growth of the fetal orbit and lens in normal pregnancies. Ultrasound Obstet Gynecol 12:175–179, 1998.

Table 19. Mean mandibular measurements (mm) with fitted 2nd, 50th, and 97th percentiles from 12 to 28 weeks' menstrual age (exact weeks).

Gestational Age (Weeks)	Percentile		
	2nd	50th	97th
12	6.3	8.0	9.7
13	8.2	10.2	12.3
14	10.0	12.4	14.7
15	11.7	14.4	17.2
16	13.4	16.4	19.5
17	15.0	18.4	21.8
18	16.5	20.2	24.0
19	18.0	22.1	26.2
20	19.4	23.9	28.3
21	20.8	25.6	30.4
22	22.2	27.3	32.4
23	23.5	28.9	34.4
24	24.8	30.6	36.4
25	26.0	32.2	38.3
26	27.3	33.7	40.2
27	28.4	35.2	42.1
28	29.6	36.7	43.9

Reprinted with permission from Chitty LS, Campbell S, Altman DG: Measurement of the fetal mandible—feasibility and construction of a percentile chart. Prenat Diagn 13:749–756, 1993.

Table 20.   Nomogram of fetal ear length (mm) according to percentile distribution.

Gestational Age (Weeks)	Number of Fetuses	5%	10%	50%	90%	95%
15	34	6.7	7.0	8.5	10.4	10.4
16	464	8.2	8.5	10.0	11.2	11.6
17	387	8.6	9.0	10.6	12.3	12.9
18	258	9.0	9.8	11.7	13.7	14.3
19	248	10.6	11.2	12.9	15.1	15.5
20	217	11.5	12.3	14.3	16.4	17.3
21	142	12.2	13.2	15.3	17.4	18.1
22	101	13.2	14.2	16.7	18.6	18.9
23	68	14.0	14.9	18.1	20.6	21.6
24	44	15.3	15.8	19.7	21.9	22.3
25	39	15.7	16.8	21.4	24.2	24.5
26	37	16.6	16.8	21.2	23.8	24.2
27	29	19.4	19.6	22.5	26.4	27.8
28	28	17.6	19.9	24.4	30.1	31.9
29	43	18.7	20.0	25.3	28.2	28.5
30	22	18.3	20.7	25.1	27.9	31.6
31	41	21.4	21.9	26.7	29.8	31.2
32	40	25.3	25.8	28.1	31.1	33.0
33	53	21.4	23.5	28.6	32.4	32.9
34	48	22.7	26.9	29.2	33.3	34.0
35	57	23.0	26.7	31.2	33.7	35.0
36	47	23.9	27.5	31.1	33.3	34.5
37	63	27.3	28.1	31.9	35.6	36.4
38	34	24.8	25.6	32.2	36.9	38.7
39	23	26.2	27.7	33.3	36.2	37.5
40	16	28.1	29.3	32.6	35.7	37.6

Reprinted with permission from Chitkara U, Lee L, El-Sayed YY, et al: Ultrasonographic ear length measurement in normal second- and third-trimester fetuses. Am J Obstet Gynecol 183:230–234, 2000.

Table 21.   Fetal thoracic circumference measurements (cm).

Gestational Age (Weeks)	N	Predictive Percentiles								
		2.5th	5th	10th	25th	50th	75th	90th	95th	97.5th
16	6	5.9	6.4	7.0	8.0	9.1	10.3	11.3	11.9	12.4
17	22	6.8	7.3	7.9	8.9	10.0	11.2	12.2	12.8	13.3
18	31	7.7	8.2	8.8	9.8	11.0	12.1	13.1	13.7	14.2
19	21	8.6	9.1	9.7	10.7	11.9	13.0	14.0	14.6	15.1
20	20	9.5	10.0	10.6	11.7	12.8	13.9	15.0	15.5	16.0
21	30	10.4	11.0	11.6	12.6	13.7	14.8	15.8	16.4	16.9
22	18	11.3	11.9	12.5	13.5	14.6	15.7	16.7	17.3	17.8
23	21	12.2	12.8	13.4	14.4	15.5	16.6	17.6	18.2	18.8
24	27	13.2	13.7	14.3	15.3	16.4	17.5	18.5	19.1	19.7
25	20	14.1	14.6	15.2	16.2	17.3	18.4	19.4	20.0	20.6
26	25	15.0	15.5	16.1	17.1	18.2	19.3	20.3	21.0	21.5
27	24	15.9	16.4	17.0	18.0	19.1	20.2	21.3	21.9	22.4
28	24	16.8	17.3	17.9	18.9	20.0	21.2	22.2	22.8	23.3
29	24	17.7	18.2	18.8	19.8	21.0	22.1	23.1	23.7	24.2
30	27	18.6	19.1	19.7	20.7	21.9	23.0	24.0	24.6	25.1
31	24	19.5	20.0	20.6	21.6	22.8	23.9	24.9	25.5	26.0
32	28	20.4	20.9	21.5	22.6	23.7	24.8	25.8	26.4	26.9
33	27	21.3	21.8	22.5	23.5	24.6	25.7	26.7	27.3	27.8
34	25	22.2	22.8	23.4	24.4	25.5	26.6	27.6	28.2	28.7
35	20	23.1	23.7	24.3	25.3	26.4	27.5	28.5	29.1	29.6
36	23	24.0	24.6	25.2	26.2	27.3	28.4	29.4	30.0	30.6
37	22	24.9	25.5	26.1	27.1	28.2	29.3	30.3	30.9	31.5
38	21	25.9	26.4	27.0	28.0	29.1	30.2	31.2	31.9	32.4
39	7	26.8	27.3	27.9	28.9	30.0	31.1	32.2	32.8	33.3
40	6	27.7	28.2	28.8	29.8	30.9	32.1	33.1	33.7	34.2

Reprinted with permission from Chitkara U, Rosenberg J, Chervenak FA, et al: Prenatal sonographic assessment of the fetal thorax: normal values. Am J Obstet Gynecol 156:1069, 1987.

Table 22. Ultrasound measurement of the fetal liver from 20 weeks' menstrual age to term.

Menstrual Age (Weeks)	Number of Measurements	Arithmetic Mean (mm)	Standard Deviation (± 2 mm)
20	8	27.3	6.4
21	2	28.0	1.5
22	4	30.6	6.7
23	13	30.9	4.5
24	10	32.9	6.7
25	14	33.6	5.3
26	10	35.7	6.3
27	20	36.6	3.3
28	14	38.4	4.0
29	13	39.1	5.0
30	10	38.7	5.0
31	13	39.6	5.7
32	11	42.7	7.5
33	14	43.8	6.6
34	11	44.8	7.1
35	14	47.8	9.1
36	10	49.0	8.4
37	10	52.0	6.8
38	12	52.9	4.2
39	5	55.4	6.7
40	1	59.0	—
41	2	49.3	2.4

Reprinted with permission from Vintzileos AM, Neckles S, Campbell WA, et al: Fetal liver ultrasound measurements during normal pregnancy. Obstet Gynecol 66:477–480, 1985.

Table 23. Percentile values and means for splenic circumference.

Menstrual Age (Weeks)	Circumference (mm) 5th Percentile	Mean	95th Percentile
18	2.3	3.5	4.7
19	2.7	3.9	5.1
20	3.3	4.5	5.7
21	3.5	4.7	5.9
22	4.1	5.3	6.5
23	4.5	5.7	6.9
24	4.9	6.1	7.2
25	5.3	6.4	7.7
26	5.5	6.7	7.9
27	5.9	7.1	8.3
28	6.2	7.4	8.6
29	6.5	7.7	8.9
30	6.9	8.1	9.3
31	7.3	8.5	9.7
32	7.7	8.9	10.1
33	8.1	9.3	10.5
34	8.6	9.8	11.0
35	9.1	10.3	11.5
36	9.7	10.9	12.1
37	10.4	11.6	12.8
38	11.1	12.3	13.4
39	11.8	13.0	14.2
40	12.7	13.8	15.1

Reprinted with permission from Schmidt W, Yarkoni S, Jeanty P, et al: Sonographic measurements of the fetal spleen: clinical implications. J Ultrasound Med 4:667–672, 1985.

Table 24. Size of the fetal adrenal glands (mm).

Measurement	Fetal Age (Weeks) 20–25	26–29	30–35	36–40
Mean length (AP)	10	13	16	19
Range	7–12	12–17	14–18	16–24
Mean thickness	3	5	5	6
Range	2–5	2–8	3–7	4–9

Modified from Jeanty P, Chervenak F, Grannum P, et al: Normal ultrasonic size and characterics of the fetal adrenal glands. Prenat Diagn 4:21–28, 1984.

Table 25. Lumen diameters (mm) of small bowel and colon at various menstrual ages.

Menstrual Age (Weeks)	N	Small Bowel Lumen Size Average	Largest
> 40	9	4.4	6
35–40	44	3.7	8
30–35	36	2.9	6
25–30	44	1.8	3
20–25	44	1.4	2
15–20	34	1.2	2
10–15	32	1.0	1

Menstrual Age (Weeks)	N	Colon Lumen Size Average	Largest
> 40	9	18.7	28
35–40	44	16.8	26
30–35	36	11.4	16
25–30	44	8.0	13
20–25	44	4.4	6
15–20	34	3.6	5
10–15	32	1.5	2

Reprinted with permission from Parulekar SG: Sonography of normal fetal bowel. J Ultrasound Med 10:211–220, 1991.

Table 26. Descending colon and rectal diameters according to gestational age.

Gestational Age (Weeks)	N	Mean	95% CI	Mean	95% CI
19–20	10	3.52	0.79–6.26	3.64	1.45–5.82
21	16	3.59	0.86–6.32	3.79	1.61–5.97
22	28	3.69	0.96–6.41	3.95	1.78–6.13
23	29	3.82	1.09–6.54	4.14	1.97–6.31
24	29	3.98	1.26–6.7	4.34	2.17–6.52
25	29	4.18	1.46–6.9	4.57	2.40–60.74
26	13	4.43	1.70–7.15	4.82	2.64–6.99
27	7	4.71	1.99–7.43	5.08	2.91–7.26
28	7	5.04	2.32–7.76	5.68	3.20–7.55
29	7	5.42	2.69–8.14	5.69	3.52–7.87
30	8	5.84	3.12–8.57	6.04	3.86–8.21
31	10	6.32	3.60–9.05	6.41	4.23–8.58
32	11	6.86	4.13–9.58	6.80	4.63–8.98
33	17	7.45	4.72–10.17	7.23	5.05–9.40
34	14	8.10	5.37–10.82	7.68	5.51–9.85
35	29	8.81	6.09–11.53	8.17	5.99–10.34
36	32	9.59	6.87–12.31	8.68	6.51–10.85
37	18	10.44	7.71–13.16	9.23	7.06–11.40
38	26	11.35	8.63–14.08	9.81	7.64–11.98
39	17	12.34	9.61–15.07	10.43	8.25–12.61
40	22	13.40	10.66–16.15	11.08	8.89–13.26

CI = confidence interval.

Reprinted with permission from Zalel Y, Perlitz Y, Gamzu R, et al: In-utero development of the fetal colon and rectum: sonographic evaluation. Ultrasound Obstet Gynecol 21:161–164, 2003.

Table 27. Length of fetal long bones (mm).

Week	Humerus Percentile			Ulna Percentile			Radius Percentile			Femur Percentile			Tibia Percentile			Fibula Percentile		
	5th	50th	95th	5th	50th	95th	5th	50th	95th	5th	50th	95th	5th	50th	95th	5th	50th	95th
11	—	6	—	—	5	—	—	5	—	—	6	—	—	4	—	—	2	—
12	3	9	10	—	8	—	—	7	—	—	9	—	—	7	—	—	5	—
13	5	13	20	3	11	18	—	10	—	6	12	19	4	10	17	—	8	—
14	5	16	20	4	13	17	8	13	12	5	15	19	2	13	19	6	11	10
15	11	18	26	10	16	22	12	15	19	11	19	26	5	16	27	10	14	18
16	12	21	25	8	19	24	9	18	21	13	22	24	7	19	25	6	17	22
17	19	24	29	11	21	32	11	20	29	20	25	29	15	22	29	7	19	31
18	18	27	30	13	24	30	14	22	26	19	28	31	14	24	35	10	22	28
19	22	29	36	20	26	32	20	24	29	23	31	38	19	27	35	18	24	30
20	23	32	36	21	29	32	21	27	28	22	33	39	19	29	39	18	27	30
21	28	34	40	25	31	36	25	29	32	27	36	45	24	32	39	24	29	34
22	28	36	40	24	33	37	24	31	34	29	39	44	25	34	39	21	31	37
23	32	38	45	27	35	43	26	32	39	35	41	48	30	36	43	23	33	44
24	31	41	46	29	37	41	27	34	38	34	44	49	28	39	45	26	35	41
25	35	43	51	34	39	44	31	36	40	38	46	54	31	41	50	33	37	42
26	36	45	49	34	41	44	30	37	41	39	49	53	33	43	49	32	39	43
27	42	46	51	37	43	48	33	39	45	45	51	57	39	45	51	35	41	47
28	41	48	52	37	44	48	33	40	45	45	53	57	38	47	52	36	43	47
29	44	50	56	40	46	51	36	42	47	49	56	62	40	49	57	40	45	50
30	44	52	56	38	47	54	34	43	49	49	58	67	41	51	56	38	47	52
31	47	53	59	39	49	59	34	44	53	53	60	67	46	52	58	40	48	57
32	47	55	59	40	50	58	37	45	51	53	62	67	46	54	59	40	50	56
33	50	56	62	43	52	60	41	46	51	56	64	71	49	56	62	43	51	59
34	50	57	62	44	53	59	39	47	53	57	65	70	47	57	64	46	52	56
35	52	58	65	47	54	61	38	48	57	61	67	73	48	59	69	51	54	57
36	53	60	63	47	55	61	41	48	54	61	69	74	49	60	68	51	55	56
37	57	61	64	49	56	62	41	49	53	64	71	77	52	61	71	55	56	58
38	55	61	66	48	57	63	45	49	53	62	72	79	54	62	69	54	57	59
39	56	62	69	49	57	66	46	50	54	64	74	83	58	64	69	55	58	62
40	56	63	69	50	58	65	46	50	54	66	75	81	58	65	69	54	59	62

Reprinted with permission from Jeanty P: Fetal limb biometry (letter). Radiology 147:602, 1983.

Table 28. Gestational age predicted by rib length.

Rib Length (cm)	Gestational Age (Weeks)		
	−2SD	Mean	+2SD
1.50	7.2	11.8	16.5
1.75	8.4	13.1	17.7
2.00	9.7	14.4	19.0
2.25	10.6	15.2	19.9
2.50	11.7	16.3	21.0
2.75	12.8	17.4	22.0
3.00	13.8	18.5	23.1
3.25	14.9	19.5	24.2
3.50	16.0	20.7	25.3
3.75	17.2	21.8	26.4
4.00	18.2	22.9	27.5
4.25	19.3	23.9	28.6
4.50	20.4	25.1	29.7
4.75	21.7	26.3	30.9
5.00	22.6	27.2	31.8
5.25	23.6	28.3	32.9
5.50	24.8	29.4	34.0
5.75	25.9	30.6	35.2
6.00	26.9	31.6	36.2
6.25	28.1	32.7	37.3
6.50	29.2	33.8	38.5
6.75	30.3	34.9	39.6
7.00	31.2	35.8	40.5
7.25	32.5	37.1	41.7
7.50	33.4	38.0	42.6
8.00	35.5	40.2	44.8

SD = standard deviation.

Reprinted with permission from Abuhamad AZ, Sedule-Murphy SJ, Kolm P, et al: Prenatal ultrasonographic fetal rib length measurement: correlation with gestational age. Ultrasound Obstet Gynecol 7:193–196, 1996.

Table 29. Menstrual age predicted by scapular length.

Scapular Length (cm)	Menstrual Age (Weeks + Days)		
	−2SD	Mean	+2SD
0.7	7 + 3	11 + 5	15 ~ 6
0.8	8 + 3	12 + 5	16 + 6
0.9	9 + 3	13 + 5	17 + 6
1.0	10 + 3	14 + 4	18 + 6
1.1	11 + 3	15 + 4	19 + 6
1.2	12 + 3	16 + 4	20 + 6
1.3	13 + 3	17 + 4	21 + 6
1.4	14 + 3	18 + 4	22 + 6
1.5	15 + 2	19 + 4	23 + 5
1.6	16 + 2	20 + 4	24 + 5
1.7	17 + 2	21 + 4	25 + 5
1.8	18 + 2	22 + 4	26 + 5
1.9	19 + 2	23 + 4	27 + 5
2.0	20 + 2	24 + 3	28 + 5
2.1	21 + 2	25 + 3	29 + 5
2.2	22 + 2	26 + 3	30 + 5
2.3	23 + 2	27 + 3	31 + 5
2.4	24 + 2	28 + 3	32 + 5
2.5	25 + 2	29 + 3	33 + 4
2.6	26 + 1	30 + 3	34 + 4
2.7	27 + 1	31 + 3	35 ~ 4
2.8	28 + 1	32 + 3	36 + 4
2.9	29 + 1	33 + 3	37 + 4
3.0	30 + 1	34 + 2	38 + 4
3.1	31 + 1	35 + 2	39 + 4
3.2	32 + 1	36 + 2	40 + 4
3.3	33 + 1	37 + 2	41 + 4
3.4	34 + 1	38 + 2	42 + 4
3.5	35 + 0	39 + 2	43 + 3
3.6	36 + 0	40 + 2	44 + 3
3.7	37 + 0	41 + 2	45 + 3
3.8	38 + 0	42 + 2	46 + 3

SD = standard deviation; mean ± 2SD calculated on basis of regression equation.

Reprinted with permission from Sherer DM, Plessinger MA, Allen TA: Fetal scapular length in the ultrasonographic assessment of gestational age. J Ultrasound Med 13:523–528, 1994.

Table 30.   Percentile values of menstrual age as obtained from clavicle length.

Clavicle Length (mm)	Menstrual Age (Weeks + Days)			Clavicle Length (mm)	Menstrual Age (Weeks + Days)		
	5th	50th	95th		5th	50th	95th
11	8 + 3	13 + 6	17 + 2	29	23 + 2	28 + 5	32 + 1
12	9 + 1	14 + 4	18 + 1	30	24 + 0	29 + 4	34 + 0
13	10 + 0	14 + 3	19 + 6	31	25 + 6	29 + 2	34 + 6
14	11 + 6	15 + 2	20 + 5	32	26 + 5	30 + 1	35 + 4
15	12 + 5	16 + 1	21 + 4	33	27 + 4	31 + 0	35 + 3
16	12 + 3	18 + 0	21 + 3	34	27 + 3	32 + 6	36 + 2
17	13 + 2	18 + 5	22 + 2	35	28 + 1	33 + 5	37 + 1
18	14 + 1	19 + 4	23 + 0	36	29 + 0	33 + 3	39 + 0
19	16 + 0	19 + 3	24 + 6	37	30 + 6	34 + 2	39 + 5
20	16 + 6	20 + 2	25 + 5	38	31 + 5	35 + 1	40 + 4
21	17 + 4	21 + 1	26 + 4	39	32 + 4	37 + 0	40 + 3
22	17 + 3	22 + 6	26 + 2	40	32 + 2	37 + 6	41 + 2
23	18 + 2	23 + 5	27 + 1	41	33 + 1	38 + 4	42 + 0
24	19 + 1	24 + 4	28 + 0	42	35 + 0	38 + 3	43 + 6
25	21 + 0	24 + 3	29 + 6	43	35 + 6	39 + 2	44 + 5
26	21 + 5	25 + 1	30 + 5	44	36 + 5	40 + 1	45 + 4
27	22 + 4	26 + 0	30 + 3	45	36 + 3	41 + 6	45 + 3
28	22 + 3	27 + 6	31 + 2				

Reprinted with permission from Yarkoni S, Schmidt W, Jeanty P, et al: Clavicular measurement: a new biometric parameter for fetal evaluation. J Ultrasound Med 4:467–470, p 469, table 4, 1985.

Table 31.   Percentile values of fetal foot length by menstrual age.

Menstrual Age (Weeks)	N	CV (%)	Fetal Foot Length (cm)				
			5th	10th	50th	90th	95th
15	18	12.7	1.4	1.5	1.8	2.2	2.3
16	146	10.4	1.6	1.7	2.1	2.5	2.6
17	375	9.7	1.9	2.0	2.4	2.8	2.9
18	613	9.8	2.2	2.3	2.7	3.1	3.2
19	1160	8.9	2.5	2.6	3.0	3.3	3.4
20	929	9.3	2.8	2.9	3.2	3.6	3.7
21	552	8.5	3.1	3.2	3.5	3.9	4.0
22	360	8.9	3.4	3.5	3.9	4.2	4.3
23	222	8.1	3.7	3.8	4.2	4.6	4.7
24	177	7.0	4.0	4.1	4.5	4.9	5.0
25	125	7.1	4.3	4.4	4.8	5.1	5.2
26	123	7.0	4.6	4.7	5.1	5.4	5.5
27	108	6.3	4.8	4.9	5.3	5.7	5.8
28	74	5.47	5.1	5.2	5.6	5.9	6.0
29	66	6.2	5.3	5.4	5.8	6.2	6.3
30	65	5.2	5.6	5.7	6.1	6.4	6.5
31	62	5.7	5.8	5.9	6.3	6.7	6.8
32	65	5.3	6.0	6.1	6.5	6.9	7.0
33	39	4.4	6.3	6.4	6.8	7.1	7.2
34	37	6.8	6.5	6.6	7.0	7.4	7.5
35	24	6.2	6.8	6.9	7.3	7.6	7.7
36	15	5.5	7.0	7.1	7.5	7.9	8.0
37	17	5.3	7.3	7.4	7.7	8.1	8.2

CV = coefficient of variation; N = number of fetuses; percentiles are smoothed.

Reprinted with permission from Meirowitz NB, Ananth CV, Smulian JC, et al: Foot length in fetuses with abnormal growth. J Ultrasound Med 19:201–205, 2000.

Table 32.	Comparison of mean postpartum and ultrasonographic foot length with Streeter's pathologic data (1920).		
Gestational Age (Weeks)	Streeter's Data (mm)	Ultrasonographic Foot Length (mm)	Postpartum Foot Length (mm)
11	7	8	—
12	9	9	—
12	11	10	—
14	14	16	—
15	17	16	—
16	20	21	—
17	23	24	—
18	27	27	—
19	31	28	—
20	33	33	33
21	35	35	—
22	40	38	—
23	42	42	—
24	45	44	—
25	48	47	48
26	50	51	—
27	53	54	52
28	55	58	—
29	57	57	57
30	59	61	60
31	61	62	60
32	63	63	66
33	65	67	68
34	68	68	71
35	71	71	72
36	74	74	74
37	77	75	78
38	79	78	78
39	81	78	80
40	83	82	81
41	—	—	82
42	—	—	82
43	—	—	84

In 1920, Streeter described pathologic specimens in Streeter GL: Weight, sitting height, head size, foot length and menstrual age of the human embryo. Contrib Embryol Carnegie Inst 11:143, 1920.

Reprinted with permission from Mercer BM, Sklar S, Shariatmadar A, et al: Fetal foot length as a predictor of gestational age. Am J Obstet Gynecol 156:350, 1987.

Table 33.   Normal fetal body ratios (22 to 40 weeks).

Menstrual Week	Cephalic Index (SD = 4.4)*	Femur/BPD × 100 (SD = 5.0)†	Femur/HC × 100 (SD = 1.1)‡	Femur/AC × 100 (SD = 1.3)§
22	78.3	77.4	18.6	21.6
23	78.3	77.6	18.8	21.7
24	78.3	77.8	19.0	21.7
25	78.3	78.0	19.2	21.8
26	78.3	78.2	19.4	21.8
27	78.3	78.4	19.6	21.9
28	78.3	78.6	19.8	21.9
29	78.3	78.8	20.0	21.9
30	78.3	79.0	20.3	22.0
31	78.3	79.2	20.5	22.0
32	78.3	79.4	20.7	22.1
33	78.3	79.6	20.9	22.1
34	78.3	79.8	21.1	22.2
35	78.3	80.0	21.4	22.2
36	78.3	80.2	21.6	22.2
37	78.3	80.4	21.8	22.3
38	78.3	80.6	22.0	22.3
39	78.3	80.8	22.2	22.3
40	78.3	81.0	22.4	22.4

BPD = biparietal diameter; HC = head circumference; AC = abdominal circumference; SD = standard deviation.

*Data from Hadlock FP, Deter RL, Carpenter RJ, et al: The effect of head shape on the accuracy of BPD in estimating fetal gestational age. AJR 137:83, 1981.

†Data from Hohler CW, Quetel TA: The relationship between fetal femur length and biparietal diameter in the last half of pregnancy. Am J Obstet Gynecol 141:759, 1981.

‡Data from Hadlock FP, Harrist RB, Shah YP, et al: The use of femur length/head circumference relation in obstetrical sonography. J Ultrasound Med 3:439, 1984.

§Data from Hadlock FP, Deter RL, Harrist RB, et al: A date-independent predictor of intrauterine growth retardation: femur length/abdominal circumference ratio. AJR 141:979, 1983.

Table 34.   Comparison of fetal parameters in LGA and AGA fetuses.

Parameter	AGA Group (Mean ± SD)	LGA Group (Mean ± SD)	P Value
BPD (cm)	9.2 ± 0.4	9.6 ± 0.4	< 0.0001
HC (cm)	33.7 ± 1.1	35.2 ± 1.3	< 0.0001
AC (cm)	33.6 ± 1.6	37.4 ± 1.3	< 0.0001
FL (cm)	7.4 ± 0.4	7.6 ± 0.3	< 0.0001
HC/AC	1.0 ± 0.05	0.94 ± 0.04	< 0.0001
FL/AC*	22.0 ± 1.0	20.5 ± 1.0	< 0.0001

AGA = appropriate for gestational age; LGA = large for gestational age; BPD = biparietal diameter; HC = head circumference; AC = abdominal circumference; FL = femur length; SD = standard deviation.

*FL/AC expressed as FL/AC × 100.

Reprinted with permission from Hadlock FP, Harrist RB, Fearneyhough TC, et al: Use of femur length/abdominal circumference ratio in detecting the macrosomic fetus. Radiology 154:503, 1985.

Table 35.   Estimates of fetal weight (g) based on abdominal circumference and femur length.

Femur Length (cm)	Abdominal Circumference (cm)													
	20.0	20.5	21.0	21.5	22.0	22.5	23.0	23.5	24.0	24.5	25.0	25.5	26.0	26.5
4.0	663	691	720	751	783	816	851	887	925	964	1006	1048	1093	1139
4.1	680	709	738	769	802	836	871	907	946	986	1027	1070	1115	1162
4.2	697	726	757	788	821	855	891	928	967	1007	1049	1093	1138	1186
4.3	715	745	776	808	841	875	912	949	988	1029	1071	1116	1162	1209
4.4	734	764	795	827	861	896	933	971	1010	1051	1094	1139	1185	1234
4.5	753	783	815	847	882	917	954	993	1033	1074	1118	1163	1210	1259
4.6	772	803	835	868	903	939	976	1015	1056	1098	1142	1187	1235	1284
4.7	792	823	856	889	924	961	999	1038	1079	1122	1166	1212	1260	1310
4.8	812	844	877	911	947	984	1022	1062	1103	1146	1191	1237	1286	1336
4.9	833	865	899	933	969	1007	1046	1086	1128	1171	1216	1263	1312	1363
5.0	855	887	921	956	993	1031	1070	1111	1153	1197	1243	1290	1339	1390
5.1	877	910	944	980	1016	1055	1095	1136	1179	1223	1269	1317	1367	1418
5.2	899	933	967	1004	1041	1080	1120	1162	1205	1250	1296	1344	1395	1447
5.3	922	956	992	1028	1066	1105	1146	1188	1232	1277	1324	1373	1423	1476
5.4	946	981	1016	1053	1091	1131	1172	1215	1259	1305	1352	1401	1452	1505
5.5	971	1005	1041	1079	1118	1158	1199	1242	1287	1333	1381	1431	1482	1535
5.6	995	1031	1067	1105	1144	1185	1227	1271	1316	1362	1411	1461	1513	1566
5.7	1021	1057	1094	1132	1172	1213	1255	1299	1345	1392	1441	1491	1544	1598
5.8	1047	1084	1121	1160	1200	1242	1285	1329	1375	1422	1472	1523	1575	1630
5.9	1074	1111	1149	1188	1229	1271	1314	1359	1406	1454	1503	1555	1608	1663
6.0	1102	1139	1178	1217	1258	1301	1345	1390	1437	1485	1535	1587	1641	1696
6.1	1130	1168	1207	1247	1289	1331	1376	1421	1469	1518	1568	1620	1674	1730
6.2	1160	1198	1237	1278	1319	1363	1408	1454	1501	1551	1602	1654	1709	1765
6.3	1189	1228	1268	1309	1351	1395	1440	1487	1535	1585	1636	1689	1744	1800
6.4	1220	1259	1299	1341	1384	1428	1473	1520	1569	1619	1671	1724	1779	1836
6.5	1251	1291	1332	1373	1417	1461	1507	1555	1604	1655	1707	1760	1816	1873
6.6	1284	1324	1365	1407	1451	1496	1542	1590	1640	1691	1743	1797	1853	1911
6.7	1317	1357	1399	1441	1486	1531	1578	1626	1676	1728	1780	1835	1891	1949
6.8	1351	1391	1433	1477	1521	1567	1615	1663	1713	1765	1819	1873	1930	1988
6.9	1385	1427	1469	1513	1558	1604	1652	1701	1752	1804	1857	1913	1970	2028
7.0	1421	1463	1506	1550	1595	1642	1690	1740	1791	1843	1897	1953	2010	2069
7.1	1458	1500	1543	1588	1633	1681	1729	1779	1830	1883	1938	1994	2051	2110
7.2	1495	1538	1581	1626	1673	1720	1769	1819	1871	1924	1979	2035	2093	2153
7.3	1534	1577	1621	1666	1713	1761	1810	1861	1913	1966	2021	2078	2136	2196
7.4	1573	1616	1661	1707	1754	1802	1852	1903	1955	2009	2065	2122	2180	2240
7.5	1614	1657	1702	1749	1796	1845	1895	1946	1999	2053	2109	2166	2225	2285
7.6	1655	1699	1745	1791	1839	1888	1939	1990	2043	2098	2154	2211	2270	2331
7.7	1698	1742	1788	1835	1883	1933	1983	2035	2089	2144	2200	2258	2317	2378
7.8	1741	1786	1833	1880	1928	1978	2029	2082	2135	2191	2247	2305	2365	2426
7.9	1786	1832	1878	1926	1975	2025	2076	2129	2183	2238	2295	2353	2413	2474
8.0	1832	1878	1925	1973	2022	2073	2124	2177	2232	2287	2344	2403	2463	2524
8.1	1879	1926	1973	2021	2071	2121	2173	2227	2281	2337	2394	2453	2513	2575
8.2	1928	1974	2022	2070	2120	2171	2224	2277	2332	2388	2446	2504	2565	2626
8.3	1978	2024	2072	2121	2171	2223	2275	2329	2384	2440	2498	2557	2617	2679

(Continued on the next page . . .)

Table 35. Estimates of fetal weight (g) based on abdominal circumference and femur length, continued.

Femur Length (cm)	Abdominal Circumference (cm)													
	27.0	27.5	28.0	28.5	29.0	29.5	30.0	30.5	31.0	31.5	32.0	32.5	33.0	33.5
4.0	1188	1239	1291	1346	1403	1463	1525	1590	1658	1729	1802	1879	1959	2042
4.1	1211	1262	1315	1371	1429	1489	1551	1617	1685	1756	1830	1907	1987	2071
4.2	1235	1287	1340	1396	1454	1515	1578	1644	1712	1783	1858	1935	2016	2100
4.3	1259	1311	1365	1422	1480	1541	1605	1671	1740	1812	1886	1964	2045	2129
4.4	1284	1336	1391	1448	1507	1568	1632	1699	1768	1840	1915	1993	2075	2159
4.5	1309	1362	1417	1474	1534	1596	1660	1727	1797	1869	1944	2023	2105	2189
4.6	1335	1388	1444	1501	1561	1623	1688	1756	1826	1898	1974	2053	2135	2220
4.7	1361	1415	1471	1529	1589	1652	1717	1785	1855	1928	2004	2084	2166	2251
4.8	1388	1442	1498	1557	1618	1681	1746	1814	1885	1959	2035	2115	2197	2283
4.9	1415	1470	1527	1585	1647	1710	1776	1845	1916	1990	2066	2146	2229	2315
5.0	1443	1498	1555	1615	1676	1740	1806	1875	1947	2021	2098	2178	2261	2347
5.1	1471	1527	1584	1644	1706	1770	1837	1906	1978	2053	2130	2210	2294	2380
5.2	1500	1556	1614	1674	1737	1801	1868	1938	2010	2085	2163	2243	2327	2413
5.3	1530	1586	1645	1704	1768	1833	1900	1970	2043	2118	2196	2277	2360	2447
5.4	1560	1617	1675	1736	1799	1865	1933	2003	2076	2151	2229	2311	2395	2482
5.5	1591	1648	1707	1768	1832	1897	1966	2036	2109	2185	2264	2345	2429	2516
5.6	1622	1679	1739	1801	1864	1931	1999	2070	2143	2220	2298	2380	2464	2552
5.7	1654	1712	1772	1834	1898	1964	2033	2104	2178	2254	2333	2415	2500	2587
5.8	1686	1744	1805	1867	1932	1999	2068	2139	2213	2290	2369	2451	2536	2624
5.9	1719	1778	1839	1902	1966	2034	2103	2175	2249	2326	2405	2488	2573	2660
6.0	1753	1812	1873	1936	2002	2069	2139	2211	2286	2363	2442	2525	2610	2698
6.1	1788	1847	1908	1972	2038	2105	2175	2248	2323	2400	2480	2562	2647	2736
6.2	1823	1882	1944	2008	2074	2142	2212	2285	2360	2438	2518	2600	2686	2774
6.3	1858	1919	1981	2045	2111	2180	2250	2323	2398	2476	2556	2639	2725	2813
6.4	1895	1956	2018	2082	2149	2218	2289	2362	2437	2515	2595	2678	2764	2852
6.5	1932	1993	2056	2121	2188	2256	2328	2401	2477	2555	2635	2718	2804	2892
6.6	1970	2031	2094	2160	2227	2296	2367	2441	2517	2595	2675	2759	2844	2933
6.7	2009	2070	2134	2199	2267	2336	2408	2481	2557	2636	2716	2800	2885	2974
6.8	2048	2110	2171	2240	2307	2377	2449	2523	2599	2677	2758	2841	2927	3016
6.9	2089	2151	2215	2281	2348	2418	2490	2564	2641	2719	2800	2884	2969	3058
7.0	2130	2192	2256	2322	2391	2461	2533	2607	2683	2762	2843	2927	3012	3101
7.1	2171	2234	2299	2365	2433	2504	2576	2650	2727	2806	2887	2970	3056	3144
7.2	2214	2277	2342	2408	2477	2547	2620	2694	2771	2850	2931	3014	3100	3188
7.3	2258	2321	2386	2453	2521	2592	2665	2739	2816	2895	2976	3059	3145	3233
7.4	2302	2365	2431	2498	2566	2637	2710	2785	2861	2940	3021	3105	3190	3278
7.5	2347	2411	2476	2543	2612	2683	2756	2831	2908	2987	3068	3151	3236	3324
7.6	2393	2457	2523	2590	2659	2730	2803	2878	2955	3034	3115	3198	3283	3371
7.7	2440	2504	2570	2638	2707	2778	2851	2926	3003	3081	3162	3245	3331	3418
7.8	2488	2553	2618	2686	2755	2827	2899	2974	3051	3130	3211	3294	3379	3466
7.9	2537	2602	2668	2735	2805	2876	2949	3024	3100	3179	3260	3343	3427	3514
8.0	2587	2652	2718	2785	2855	2926	2999	3074	3151	3229	3310	3392	3477	3564
8.1	2638	2702	2769	2837	2906	2977	3050	3125	3202	3280	3360	3443	3527	3614
8.2	2690	2754	2821	2889	2958	3029	3102	3177	3253	3332	3412	3494	3578	3664
8.3	2743	2807	2874	2942	3011	3082	3155	3230	3306	3384	3464	3546	3630	3716

Table 35.   (Continued from previous page.)

Femur Length (cm)	Abdominal Circumference (cm)												
	34.0	34.5	35.0	35.5	36.0	36.5	37.0	37.5	38.0	38.5	39.0	39.5	40.0
4.0	2129	2220	2314	2413	2515	2622	2734	2850	2972	3098	3230	3367	3511
4.1	2158	2249	2344	2442	2545	2652	2764	2880	3002	3128	3260	3397	3540
4.2	2187	2279	2373	2472	2575	2683	2794	2911	3032	3159	3290	3427	3570
4.3	2217	2308	2404	2503	2606	2713	2825	2942	3063	3189	3321	3458	3600
4.4	2247	2339	2434	2533	2637	2744	2856	2973	3094	3220	3352	3488	3630
4.5	2278	2370	2465	2565	2668	2776	2888	3004	3125	3251	3383	3519	3661
4.6	2309	2401	2497	2596	2700	2807	2919	3036	3157	3283	3414	3550	3692
4.7	2340	2432	2528	2628	2732	2840	2952	3068	3189	3315	3446	3582	3723
4.8	2372	2464	2560	2660	2764	2872	2984	3100	3221	3347	3478	3613	3754
4.9	2404	2497	2593	2693	2797	2905	3017	3133	3254	3380	3510	3645	3786
5.0	2437	2530	2626	2726	2830	2938	3050	3166	3287	3412	3542	3677	3818
5.1	2470	2563	2659	2760	2864	2972	3084	3200	3320	3445	3575	3710	3850
5.2	2503	2597	2693	2794	2898	3006	3117	3234	3354	3479	3608	3743	3882
5.3	2537	2631	2728	2828	2932	3040	3152	3268	3388	3513	3642	3776	3915
5.4	2572	2665	2762	2863	2967	3075	3186	3302	3422	3547	3676	3809	3948
5.5	2607	2700	2797	2898	3002	3110	3221	3337	3457	3581	3710	3843	3981
5.6	2642	2736	2833	2933	3038	3145	3257	3372	3492	3616	3744	3877	4015
5.7	2678	2772	2869	2970	3074	3181	3293	3408	3527	3651	3779	3911	4048
5.8	2714	2808	2905	3006	3110	3218	3329	3444	3563	3686	3814	3946	4082
5.9	2751	2845	2942	3043	3147	3254	3366	3480	3599	3722	3849	3981	4117
6.0	2789	2883	2980	3080	3184	3292	3403	3517	3636	3758	3885	4016	4151
6.1	2827	2921	3018	3118	3222	3329	3440	3554	3673	3795	3921	4052	4186
6.2	2865	2959	3056	3157	3260	3367	3478	3592	3710	3832	3957	4087	4222
6.3	2904	2998	3095	3195	3299	3406	3516	3630	3747	3869	3994	4124	4257
6.4	2943	3037	3134	3235	3338	3445	3555	3668	3785	3906	4031	4160	4293
6.5	2983	3077	3174	3274	3378	3484	3594	3707	3824	3944	4069	4197	4329
6.6	3024	3118	3215	3315	3418	3524	3633	3746	3863	3983	4106	4234	4366
6.7	3065	3159	3256	3355	3458	3564	3673	3786	3902	4021	4144	4271	4402
6.8	3107	3200	3297	3397	3499	3605	3714	3826	3941	4060	4183	4309	4439
6.9	3149	3242	3339	3438	3541	3646	3754	3866	3981	4100	4222	4347	4477
7.0	3192	3285	3381	3481	3583	3688	3796	3907	4022	4140	4261	4386	4514
7.1	3235	3328	3424	3523	3625	3730	3838	3948	4062	4180	4300	4425	4552
7.2	3279	3372	3468	3567	3668	3772	3880	3990	4104	4220	4340	4464	4591
7.3	3323	3416	3512	3610	3712	3816	3922	4032	4145	4261	4381	4503	4629
7.4	3369	3461	3557	3655	3756	3859	3966	4075	4187	4303	4421	4543	4668
7.5	3414	3507	3602	3700	3800	3903	4009	4118	4230	4344	4462	4583	4708
7.6	3461	3553	3648	3745	3845	3948	4053	4161	4272	4387	4504	4624	4747
7.7	3508	3600	3694	3791	3891	3993	4098	4205	4316	4429	4545	4665	4787
7.8	3555	3647	3741	3838	3937	4039	4143	4250	4360	4472	4588	4706	4827
7.9	3604	3695	3789	3885	3984	4085	4188	4295	4404	4515	4630	4748	4868
8.0	3653	3744	3837	3933	4031	4131	4234	4340	4448	4559	4673	4790	4909
8.1	3702	3793	3886	3981	4079	4179	4281	4386	4493	4604	4716	4832	4950
8.2	3752	3843	3935	4030	4127	4226	4328	4432	4539	4648	4760	4875	4992
8.3	3803	3893	3985	4080	4176	4275	4376	4479	4585	4693	4804	4918	5034

Reprinted with permission from Hadlock FP, Harrist RB, Carpenter RJ, et al: Sonographic estimation of fetal weight. Radiology 150:535, 1984.

Table 36.   Mean twin and singleton fetal biparietal diameter for 27 to 37 weeks' menstrual age.

Menstrual Age (Weeks)	N	Mean Twin		Singleton BPD (cm)	P Value (Student's t-Test)
		BPD (cm)	SD (cm)		
27	20	6.9	0.4	6.9	0.999
28	20	7.4	0.4	7.2	0.057
29	22	7.4	0.4	7.4	0.919
30	26	7.4	0.5	7.6	0.028
31	18	7.8	0.5	7.9	0.466
32	20	7.9	0.4	8.1	0.028
33	24	8.1	0.4	8.3	0.047
34	16	8.2	0.3	8.5	0.002
35	18	8.4	0.4	8.7	0.006
36	14	8.5	0.3	8.9	0.005
37	6	8.5	0.3	9.1	0.003

BPD = biparietal diameter; SD = standard deviation.

Reprinted with permission from Grumbach K, Coleman BG, Arger PH, et al: Twin and singleton growth patterns compared using US. Radiology 158:237–241, 1986.

Table 37.   Mean twin and singleton fetal femur length for 27 to 37 menstrual weeks.

Menstrual Age (Weeks)	N	Mean Twin		Mean Singleton FFL (cm)	P Value (Student's t-Test)
		FFL (cm)	SD (cm)		
27	10	5.1	0.3	5.0	0.99
28	8	5.7	0.2	5.4	0.60
29	4	5.2	0.3	5.6	0.60
30	16	5.9	0.4	5.8	0.12
31	8	5.9	0.6	6.0	0.44
32	10	6.3	0.5	6.3	0.99
33	10	6.4	0.5	6.5	0.68
34	10	6.6	0.3	6.7	0.62
35	8	6.9	0.3	6.9	0.22
36	8	6.9	0.3	7.1	0.24
37	4	7.2	0.3	7.3	0.62

FFL = fetal femur length; SD = standard deviation.

Reprinted with permission from Grumbach K, Coleman BG, Arger PH, et al: Twin and singleton growth patterns compared using US. Radiology 158:237–241, 1986.

Table 38. Mean twin and singleton abdominal circumference (AC) for 27 to 37 menstrual weeks.

| Menstrual Age (Weeks) | N | Mean Twin | | Mean Singleton AC (cm) | P Value (Student's t-Test) |
		AC (cm)	SD (cm)		
27	12	23.6	1.7	22.7	0.07
28	19	23.9	2.7	23.8	0.68
29	12	24.9	2.5	24.9	0.56
30	18	25.3	1.9	26.0	0.11
31	12	26.9	1.9	27.1	0.68
32	18	27.2	1.8	28.2	0.035
33	14	27.1	2.1	29.3	0.002
34	14	28.9	1.9	30.4	0.012
35	14	29.6	1.7	31.5	0.001
36	10	29.8	1.6	32.6	0.001
37	8	29.2	2.6	33.7	0.009

AC = abdominal circumference; SD = standard deviation.

Reprinted with permission from Grumbach K, Coleman BG, Arger PH, et al: Twin and singleton growth patterns compared using US. Radiology 158:237–241, 1986.

Table 39. Mean values for abdominal circumference in twins (mm).

Menstrual age:	Ong*	Kuno*	Grumbach*
24	197.9	183	—
26	224.7	202	—
28	237.7	219	239
30	259.1	235	253
32	280.7	250	272
34	295.8	264	289
36	311.0	277	298

Study characteristics:

N	884	52	103
Study	Cross-sectional	Longitudinal	Longitudinal
Country	Scotland	Japan	USA

*Complete references appear in original.

Reprinted with permission from Grumbach K, Coleman BG, Arger PH, et al: Twin and singleton growth patterns compared using US. Radiology 158:237–241, 1986.

Table 40. Mean values for femur length in twins (mm).

Menstrual age:	Ong*	Kuno*	Grumbach*
24	197.9	183	—
24	43.1	40	—
26	48.1	45	—
28	51.8	49	57
30	57.1	53	59
32	60.7	56	63
34	65.6	59	66
36	68.2	62	69
38	70.6	64	—

Study characteristics:

N	884	52	103
Study	Cross-sectional	Longitudinal	Longitudinal
Country	Scotland	Japan	USA

*Complete references appear in original.

Reprinted with permission from Grumbach K, Coleman BG, Arger PH, et al: Twin and singleton growth patterns compared using US. Radiology 158:237–241, 1986.

Table 41.   Fetal measurements in twin gestations.

Gestational Age (Weeks)	Biparietal Diameter		Abdominal Circumference	
	Predicted Mean	*Range from 5th to 95th Percentile*	*Predicted Mean*	*Range from 5th to 95th Percentile*
27	69	61–78	236	202–273
28	74	66–82	239	185–293
29	74	66–82	249	199–299
30	74	64–84	253	215–291
31	78	68–88	269	231–307
32	79	71–87	272	236–308
33	81	73–89	271	229–313
34	82	76–88	289	251–327
35	84	76–92	296	262–330
36	85	79–91	298	266–330
37	85	79–91	292	240–344

Data obtained on 103 twin parts.

Reprinted with permission from Goldberg B, Kurtz A: *Atlas of Ultrasound Measurements*. St. Louis, Mosby, 1990. Data from Grumbach K, Coleman BG, Arger PH, et al: Twin and singleton growth patterns compared using US. Radiology 158:237–241, 1986.

Table 42. Estimated fetal weight (grams) in twin pregnancies.

Gestational Age (Weeks)	Percentile				
	5th	25th	50th	75th	95th
16	132	141	154	189	207
17	173	194	215	239	249
18	214	248	276	289	291
19	223	253	300	333	412
20	232	259	324	378	534
21	275	355	432	482	705
22	319	452	540	586	876
23	347	497	598	684	880
24	376	543	656	783	885
25	549	677	793	916	1118
26	722	812	931	1049	1352
27	755	978	1087	1193	1563
28	789	1145	1244	1337	1774
29	900	1266	1395	1509	1883
30	1101	1387	1546	1682	1992
31	1198	1532	1693	1875	2392
32	1385	1677	1840	2068	2793
33	1491	1771	2032	2334	3000
34	1597	1866	2224	2601	3208
35	1703	2093	2427	2716	3336
36	1809	2321	2631	2832	3465
37	2239	2540	2824	3035	3679
38	2669	2760	3017	3239	3894

Weight calculated from formula by Shepard MJ, Richards VA, Berkowitz RL, et al: An evaluation of two equations for predicting fetal weight by ultrasound, Am J Obstet Gynecol 142:42–54, 1982.

Reprinted with permission from Goldberg B, Kurtz A: *Atlas of Ultrasound Measurements*. St. Louis, Mosby, 1990. Data from Yarkoni S, Reece EA, Holfor T, et al: Obstet Gynecol 69:626–639, 1987.

			Bicerebellar	**Humerus**		**Tibia**	**Fibula**	
Weeks	**BPD**	**HC**	**Diameter**	**Length**	**FL**	**Length**	**Length**	**AC**
16	3.5	12.8	1.5	2.1	2.0	1.7	1.6	10.7
17	3.9	14.1	1.6	2.3	2.3	2.0	1.9	11.9
18	4.2	15.3	1.7	2.6	2.6	2.3	2.2	13.1
19	4.5	16.5	1.9	2.8	2.9	2.5	2.4	14.2
20	4.8	17.6	2.0	3.1	3.2	2.8	2.7	15.3
21	5.1	18.7	2.2	3.3	3.5	3.1	2.9	16.4
22	5.4	19.8	2.3	3.5	3.7	3.3	3.2	17.4
23	5.7	20.8	2.5	3.7	4.0	3.5	3.4	18.4
24	6.0	21.8	2.6	3.9	4.2	3.7	3.6	19.4
25	6.2	22.7	2.7	4.1	4.4	3.9	3.7	20.3
26	6.5	23.6	2.8	4.2	4.6	4.1	3.9	21.2
27	6.7	24.5	3.0	4.4	4.8	4.2	4.1	22.1
28	6.9	25.3	3.1	4.6	5.0	4.4	4.2	22.9
29	7.1	26.1	3.2	4.7	5.2	4.5	4.3	23.7
30	7.3	26.8	3.4	4.8	5.4	4.7	4.4	24.5
31	7.5	27.5	3.5	4.9	5.5	4.8	4.6	25.2
32	7.7	28.1	3.6	5.0	5.7	4.9	4.6	25.9
33	7.8	28.7	3.8	5.1	5.8	4.9	4.7	26.6
34	8.0	29.2	3.9	5.2	5.9	5.0	4.8	27.2
35	8.1	29.7	4.0	5.2	6.0	5.1	4.8	27.8

Table 43.   Growth parameters in triplets generated from regression equations.

BPD = biparietal diameter; HC = head circumference; FL = femur length; AC = abdominal circumference.

Reprinted with permission from Rodis JF, Arky L, Egan JF, et al: Comprehensive fetal ultrasonographic growth measurements in triplet gestations. Am J Obstet Gynecol 181:1128, 1999.

Table 44.   Selected medications and reported associated malformations.*

Drug	Malformation
Acetazolamide	Sacrococcygeal teratoma
Acylovir	CDH, neural tube defect, cleft lip, clubfoot, transposition
Alprazolam	Umbilical hernia, clubfoot
Albuterol	Cleft palate, cranioschisis, cardiovascular defect, spina bifida, polydactyly, fetal tachycardia
Amantadine	Cardiac defects
Aminopterin	Neural tube defects, hydrocephalus, limb shortening, cleft lip/palate, clubfoot
p-Aminosalicylic acid	Ear deformity, limb deformity, hypospadias
Amiodarone	IUGR, ventricular septal defect, micrognathia
Amitriptyline	Limb reduction, micrognathia, hypospadias, cleft palate, thanatophoric dysplasia
Ampicillin	Transposition of the great vessels
Amobarbital	Anencephaly, cardiac defects, limb deformity, cleft lip/palate, polydactyly, genitourinary defects, clubfoot
Amphetamine	Cerebral injury in neonates
Aspirin	Intracranial hemorrhage, IUGR
Atenolol	Hypospadias, cardiovascular defects
Atropine	Polydactyly, limb reduction
Azatadine	Oral cleft, limb reduction
Baclofen	Spina bifida
Belladonna	Eye/ear malformations, hypospadias
Benztropine	Cardiovascular defects
Bromides	Polydactyly, gastrointestinal anomalies, clubfoot, IUGR
Busulfan	IUGR, cleft palate, neural tube defects
Captopril	Second-trimester hypocalvaria, oligohydramnios, renal dysfunction
Carbamazepine	Neural tube defects, cardiac defects
Carisoprodol	Oral clefts
Cephalexin	Cardiovascular defects, oral clefts
Cephradine	Cardiovascular defects
Chlorambucil	Renal agenesis, cardiac defects
Chlordiazepoxide	Microcephaly, duodenal atresia, cardiac defects
Chloroquine	Wilms tumor, hemihypertrophy, tetralogy of Fallot
Chlorothiazide	Fetal bradycardia
Chlorpheniramine	Polydactyly, gastrointestinal defects, hydrocephalus
Chlorpromazine	Mirocephaly, syndactyly
Chlorpropamide	Microcephaly, hand anomalies
Ciprofloxacin	Hypospadias, cerebellar hypoplasia, cardiovascular defect, femoral aplasia
Clarithromycin	Craniofacial abnormalities, absent clavicles, spina bifida, cleft lip, pulmonary hypoplasia, coloboma, heart anomaly, choanal atresia, retardation (mental and somatic), genital and ear anomalies (CHARGE) association
Clomiphene	Microcephaly, neural tube defects, cleft lip/palate, cardiac defects, syndactyly, clubfoot, hypospadias
Clonazepam	Cardiovascular defects
Clorazepate	Bifid foot, absent scrotum, short femur, absent fibula, absent metacarpal bones, renal agenesis
Cloxacillin	Cardiovascular defects

(Continued on the next page . . .)

Table 44.   Selected medications and reported associated malformations, continued.*

Drug	Malformation
Cocaine	Spontaneous abortion, placental abruption, cardiac defects, urinary tract and limb abnormalities, bowel atresias, IUGR
Codeine	Pulmonary and genitourinary defects, hydrocephalus, cleft lip/palate
Colchicine	Cardiac malformation, syndactyly, cleft palate
Cortisone	Cataracts, cyclopia, VSD, coarctation of the aorta, clubfoot, cleft lip, gastroschisis
Coumarin derivatives	Spontaneous abortion, IUGR, neural tube defects (open and closed) (dorsal midline dysplasia), cardiac defects, scoliosis, limb hypoplasia, cleft palate
Cyclophosphamide	Cleft palate, hand abnormalities, cardiac defects, IUGR
Cyclosporine	Limb hypoplasia, agenesis of the corpus callosum, anencephaly, IUGR
Cyproheptadine	Cleft lip/palate, hypospadias
Cytarabine	Hand abnormalities (lobster claw deformity), lower limb defects, neural tube defects, cardiac defects
Dacarbazine	Limb reduction defects, cleft palate, encephalocele
Danazol	Ambiguous genitalia
Daunorubicin	IUGR
Dexfenfluramine	Hand malformation, anencephaly, vertebral abnormality
Diazepam	Cleft lip/palate, cardiac defects
Dicyclomine	Polydactyly
Dilantin	Microcephaly, hypertelorism, cleft lip/palate, hypoplasia of distal phalanges, short neck, broad nasal ridge
Diltiazem	Cardiovascular defects
Dimenhydrinate	Cardiovascular defects
Diphenhydramine	Cleft lip/palate, genitourinary defects, clubfoot, cardiac defects
Disulfiram	Clubfoot, vertebral defects, anal atresia, cardiac anomalies, tracheo-esophageal fistula with esophageal atresia, renal anomalies, limb anomalies (VACTERL) syndrome, phocomelia
Doxepin	Oral clefts, polydactyly
Droperidol	Hydrocephalus, cerebral hypoplasia
Enalapril	Hypocalvaria, renal defects
Ephedrine	Clubfoot
Ethanol (alcohol)	IUGR, microphthalmia, micrognathia, microcephaly, hypoplastic maxilla, cardiac defects, genitourinary defects, radioulnar synostosis, Klippel-Feil anomaly, diaphragmatic hernia
Ethoheptazine	Umbilical hernia, hip dislocation
Ethotoin	Cleft lip/palate, patent ductus arteriosus
Ethosuximide	Cleft lip/palate, hydrocephalus, patent ductus arteriosus, spontaneous hemorrhage in the neonate
Etretinate	Neural tube defects, facial dysmorphia, multiple synostoses, syndactylies, limb reduction
Fluconazole	Craniosynostosis, cleft palate, limb shortening
Fluorouracil	Radial aplasia, pulmonary hypoplasia, esophageal and duodenal atresia, cloacal malformation
Fluphenazine	Ocular hypertelorism, cleft lip/palate, imperforate anus
Furosemide	Hypospadias
Griseofulvin	Conjoined twins
Haloperidol	Limb reduction, aortic valve defect
Heparin	Cardiovascular defects

(Continued on the next page . . .)

Table 44.   (Continued from previous page.)

Drug	Malformation
Heroin	IUGR, multiple and varied congenital malformations
Hydroxyprogesterone	Spina bifida, anencephaly, tetralogy of Fallot, truncus arteriosus, VSD
Hydroxyzine	Oral clefts
Hyoscyamine	Polydactyly, limb reduction
Ibuprofen	Oligohydramnios, premature closure of patent ductus arteriosus
Imipramine	Diaphragmatic hernia, cleft palate, exencephaly, renal cystic dysplasia, amelia
Indomethacin	Oliogohydramnios, premature closure of patent ductus arteriosus, phocomelia, penile agenesis
Isoetharine	Clubfoot
Isotretinoin	Hydrocephalus, neural tube defects, microphthalmia, microcephaly, cardiac defects, limb abnormalities, cleft palate
Itraconazole	Limb defect
Ketoconazole	Limb defect
Ketrolac	Constriction of the ductus arteriosus, fetal renal impairment
Levothyroxine	Cardiac defects, polydactyly
Lindane	Hypospadias
Lisinopril	Hypocalvaria, polydactyly, oligohydramnios
Lithium	Cardiac defects (Ebstein anomaly, VSD, coarctation, mitral atresia), neural tube defects
Lovastatin	Aortic hypoplasia, VSD, anal atresia, renal dysplasia, radial aplasia
Lysergic acid diethylamide	IUGR, limb reduction, neural tube defects, cardiac defects
Marijuana	IUGR, facial anomalies
Mechlorethamine	IUGR, oligodactyly, malformed kidneys
Medroxyprogesterone	Cardiovascular defect
Meclizine	Eye and ear defects, hypoplastic heart, respiratory defects
Mefenamic acid	Constriction of the ductus arteriosus
Melphalan	IUGR
Meprobamate	Cardiac defects, omphalocele, joint abnormalities
Mercaptopurine	Cleft palate, microphthalmia, IUGR
Metaproterenol	Polydactyly
Methimazole	Patent urachus
Methotrexate	IUGR, hypertelorism, dextroposition of the heart, absent digits, absence of frontal bone
Methotrimeprazine	Hydrocephalus, cardiac defects
Metronidazole	Spontaneous abortion; limb, cardiac, urinary, and facial abnormalities
Mifepristone	Sirenomelia, caudal regression syndrome
Minoxidil	Omphalocele, clinodactyly, cardiac defects (VSD and transposition)
Misoprostol	Limb defects, hypocalvaria, cleft lip, clubfoot, gastroschisis
Norethindrone	Neural tube defects, hydrocephalus
Norethynodrel	Cardiac defects, hypospadias
Nortriptyline	Limb reduction
Ofloxacin	Myelomeningocele, hydrocephalus, hypospadias
Omeprazole	Anencephaly, hydranencephaly, clubfoot
Oxazepam	Neural tube defects, IUGR
Paramethadione	Spontaneous abortions, IUGR, cardiac defects
Penicillamine	Hydrocephalus, flexion deformities, perforated bowel

(Continued on the next page . . .)

Table 44.   Selected medications and reported associated malformations, continued.*

Drug	Malformation
Pentoxifylline	Cardiac defects
Phenacetin	Craniosynostosis and atresia, musculoskeletal and urinary tract defects
Phenobarbital	Cardiovascular defects
Phensuximide	Ambiguous genitalia
Phenylephrine	Eye and ear abnormalities, syndactyly, clubfoot, musculoskeletal defects
Phenylpropanolamine	Eye and ear abnormalities, polydactyly, hypospadias
Phenytoin	Microcephaly, hypertelorism, cleft lip/palate, hypoplasia of distal phalanges, short neck, broad nasal ridge
Podophyllum	Limb reduction
Procarbazine	IUGR, cardiac defects, oligodactyly, malformed kidneys
Prochlorperazine	Cleft palate/micrognathia, cardiac defects, skeletal defects
Propoxyphene	Limb abnormalities, omphalocele, micrognathia, clubfoot, microcephaly
Quinacrine	Renal agenesis, neural tube defects
Quinine	Neural tube defects, hydrocephalus, limb defects, facial defects, cardiac defects, urogenital abnormalities, vertebral abnormality, gastrointestinal anomaly
Reserpine	Microcephaly, hydronephrosis
Retinoic acid	Hydrocephalus, neural tube defects, microphthalmia, microcephaly, cardiac defects, limb abnormalities, cleft palate
Rifampin	Anencephaly, hydrocephalus, limb malformation
Sodium iodide	Ablation of fetal thyroid gland
Sulfasalazine	Cleft lip/palate, hydrocephalus, cardiac defects, urinary tract abnormalities
Sulfonamides	Limb hypoplasia, urinary tract abnormalities
Sumatriptan	Phocomelia, tibial aplasia, clubfoot, cleft palate
Tamoxifen	Ambiguous genitalia
Tazarotene	Reduced skeletal ossification, hydrocephaly, spina bifida, cardiac defects
Temazepam	Oral clefts
Terfenadine	Polydactyly
Tetracycline	Hypospadias, limb hypoplasia
Thioguanine	Absent digits
Tolbutamide	Syndactyly, cardiac defects, clubfoot
Trifluoperazine	Phocomelia, transposition of the great vessels
Trimethadione	IUGR, microcephaly, cleft lip/palate, cardiac defects, malformed hand, clubfoot, ambiguous genitalia, esophageal atresia, tracheoesophageal fistula
Trimethoprim	Cardiovascular defects
Valproic acid	Neural tube defects, cardiac defects, facial dysmorphism, hypertelorism, protruding eyes, micrognathia, hydrocephalus, cleft lip/palate, microcephaly, limb reduction, scoliosis, renal hypoplasia, duodenal atresia, hand deformity
Zidovudine	Renal agenesis, microphthalmus, polydactyly, cleft lip/palate, clubfoot, VSD

CDH = congenital diaphragmatic hernia; IUGR = intrauterine growth restriction; VSD = ventricular septal defect.

*This list represents selected medications and their possible associations with fetal structural abnormalities. Many of the listed associations are based on isolated case reports that have appeared in the medical literature for which the association is unproven or in animal studies where the dosage of medication far exceeded the normal clinical amount normally used. It is likely that in many cases the reported association was coincidental to, rather than resultant from, the medication. **This list is not intended for patient counseling regarding the likelihood of fetal malformations or abnormalities.** The table should be used by the sonologist/sonographer as a guide for evaluating specific organ systems in addition to a thorough sonographic examination. In all cases of suspected teratogenetic effects, a reproductive geneticist or teratologist and the drug manufacturer should be consulted.

Modified from Briggs GG, Freeman RK, Yaffe SJ: *Drugs in Pregnancy and Lactation*, 7th ed. Philadelphia, Lippincott Williams & Wilkins, 2005. Reprinted by permission.

AIUM Practice Guidelines

Publisher's note: As elsewhere in this book, the AIUM standards are reprinted with the kind permission of the American Institute of Ultrasound in Medicine (AIUM). These standards are the most current as of press time. Because standards are periodically updated, you should visit www.aium.org for the most recent versions of practice guidelines in specialties related to obstetrics and gynecology, where acknowledgments and references also appear.

About the Guidelines

The American Institute of Ultrasound in Medicine (AIUM) is a multidisciplinary association dedicated to advancing the safe and effective use of ultrasound in medicine through professional and public education, research, development of guidelines, and accreditation. To promote this mission, the AIUM is pleased to publish, in conjunction with the American College of Radiology (ACR) and the American College of Obstetricians and Gynecologists (ACOG), these AIUM Practice Guidelines for the Performance of Obstetric Ultrasound Examinations. We are indebted to the many volunteers who con-tributed their time, knowledge, and energy to bringing this document to completion.

The AIUM represents the entire range of clinical and basic science interests in medical diagnostic ultrasound, and, with hundreds of volunteers, the AIUM has pro-moted the safe and effective use of ultrasound in clinical medicine for more than 50 years. This document and oth-ers like it will continue to advance this mission.

Practice guidelines of the AIUM are intended to provide the medical ultrasound community with guidelines for the performance and recording of high-quality ultra-sound examinations. The guidelines reflect what the AIUM considers the minimum criteria for a complete examination in each area but are not intended to establish a legal standard of care. AIUM-accredited practices are expected to generally follow the guidelines with recogni-tion that deviations from these guidelines will be needed in some cases, depending on patient needs and available equipment. Practices are encouraged to go beyond the guidelines to provide additional service and information as needed.

AIUM PRACTICE GUIDELINE FOR THE PERFORMANCE OF OBSTETRIC ULTRASOUND EXAMINATIONS

I. Introduction

The clinical aspects of this guideline (Classification of Fetal Sonographic Examinations, Specifications of the Examination, Equipment Specifications, and Fetal Safety) were revised collaboratively by the American Institute of Ultrasound in Medicine (AIUM), the American College of Radiology (ACR), and the American College of Obstetricians and Gynecologists (ACOG). Recommendations for personnel qualifications, written request for the examination, procedure documentation, and quality control vary among these organizations and are addressed by each separately.

This guideline has been developed for use by practitioners performing obstetric sonographic studies. Fetal ultrasound should be performed only when there is a valid medical reason, and the lowest possible ultrasonic exposure settings should be used to gain the necessary diagnostic information. A limited examination may be performed in clinical emergencies or for a limited purpose such as evaluation of fetal or embryonic cardiac activity, fetal position, or amniotic fluid volume. A limited follow-up examination may be appropriate for reevaluation of fetal size or interval growth or to reevaluate abnormalities previously noted if a complete prior examination is on record.

While this guideline describes the key elements of standard sonographic examinations in the first trimester and second and third trimesters, a more detailed anatomic examination of the fetus may be necessary in some cases, such as when an abnormality is found or suspected on the standard examination or in pregnancies at high risk for fetal anomalies. In some cases, other specialized examinations may be necessary as well.

While it is not possible to detect all structural congenital anomalies with diagnostic ultrasound, adherence to the following guidelines will maximize the possibility of detecting many fetal abnormalities.

II. Classification of Fetal Sonographic Examinations

A. First-Trimester Ultrasound Examination

A standard obstetric sonogram in the first trimester includes evaluation of the presence, size, location, and number of gestational sac(s). The gestational sac is examined for the presence of a yolk sac and embryo/fetus. When an embryo/fetus is detected, it should be measured and cardiac activity recorded by a 2-dimensional video clip or M-mode imaging. Use of spectral Doppler imaging is discouraged. The uterus, cervix, adnexa, and cul-de-sac region should be examined.

B. Standard Second- or Third-Trimester Examination

A standard obstetric sonogram in the second or third trimester includes an evaluation of fetal presentation, amniotic fluid volume, cardiac activity, placental position, fetal biometry, and fetal number, plus an anatomic survey. The maternal cervix and adnexa should be examined as clinically appropriate when technically feasible.

C. Limited Examination

A limited examination is performed when a specific question requires investigation. For example, in most routine nonemergency cases, a limited examination could be performed to confirm fetal heart activity in a bleeding patient or to verify fetal presentation in a laboring patient. In most cases, limited sonographic examinations are appropriate only when a prior complete examination is on record.

D. Specialized Examinations

A detailed anatomic examination is performed when an anomaly is suspected on the basis of history, biochemical abnormalities, or the results of either the limited or standard scan. Other specialized examinations might include fetal Doppler sonography, biophysical profile, a fetal echocardiogram, or additional biometric measurements.

III. Qualifications and Responsibilities of Personnel

See the AIUM Official Statement *Training Guidelines for Physicians Who Evaluate and Interpret Diagnostic Ultrasound Examinations and the AIUM Standards and Guidelines for the Accreditation of Ultrasound Practices.*

IV. Written Request for the Examination

The written or electronic request for an ultrasound examination should provide sufficient information to allow for the appropriate performance and interpretation of the examination.

The request for the examination must be originated by a physician or other appropriately licensed health care provider or under their direction. The accompanying clinical information should be provided by a physician or other appropriate health care provider familiar with the patient's clinical situation and should be consistent with relevant legal and local health care facility requirements.

V. Specifications of the Examination

A. First-Trimester Ultrasound Examination

1. Indications

   Indications for first trimester[1] sonography include but are not limited to:

   a. Confirmation of the presence of an intrauterine pregnancy.

   b. Evaluation of a suspected ectopic pregnancy.

   c. Defining the cause of vaginal bleeding.

   d. Evaluation of pelvic pain.

   e. Estimation of gestational (menstrual[2]) age.

   f. Diagnosis or evaluation of multiple gestations.

   g. Confirmation of cardiac activity.

   h. Imaging as an adjunct to chorionic villus sampling, embryo transfer, and localization and removal of an intrauterine device.

   i. Assessing for certain fetal anomalies, such as anenecephaly, in high-risk patients.

   j. Evaluation of maternal pelvic masses and/or uterine abnormalities.

   k. Measuring the nuchal translucency (NT) when part of a screening program for fetal aneuploidy.

   l. Evaluation of a suspected hydatidiform mole.

   Comment

   A limited examination may be performed to evaluate interval growth, estimate amniotic fluid volume, evaluate the cervix, and assess the presence of cardiac activity.

2. Imaging Parameters

   Comment

   Scanning in the first trimester may be performed either transabdominally or transvaginally. If a transabdominal examination is not definitive, a transvaginal scan or transperineal scan should be performed whenever possible.

   a. The uterus, including the cervix, and adnexa should be evaluated for the presence of a gestational sac. If a gestational sac is seen, its location should be documented. The gestational sac should be evaluated for the presence or absence of a yolk sac or embryo, and the crown-rump length should be recorded, when possible.

   Comment

   A definitive diagnosis of intrauterine pregnancy can be made when an intrauterine gestational sac containing a yolk sac or embryo/fetus with cardiac activity is visualized. A small, eccentric intrauterine fluid collection with an echogenic rim can be seen before the yolk sac and embryo are detectable in a very early intrauterine pregnancy. In the absence of sonographic signs of ectopic pregnancy, the fluid collection is highly likely to represent an intrauterine gestational sac. In this circumstance, the intradecidual sign may be helpful. Follow-up sonography and/or serial determination of maternal serum human chorionic gonadotropin levels are/is appropriate in pregnancies of undetermined location to avoid inappropriate intervention in a potentially viable early pregnancy.

   The crown-rump length is a more accurate indicator of gestational (menstrual) age than is mean gestational sac diameter. However, the mean gestational sac diameter may be recorded when an embryo is not identified.

   Caution should be used in making the presumptive diagnosis of a gestational sac in the absence of a definite embryo or yolk sac. Without these findings, an intrauterine fluid collection could represent a pseudogestational sac associated with an ectopic pregnancy.

   b. Presence or absence of cardiac activity should be reported.

   Comment

   With transvaginal scans, cardiac motion is usually observed when the embryo is 2 mm or greater in length. If an embryo less than 7 mm in length is seen without cardiac activity, a subsequent scan in 1 week is recommended to ensure that the pregnancy is nonviable.

---

[1]For the purpose of this document, first trimester represents 1 week to 13 weeks 6 days.

[2]For the purpose of this document, the terms "gestational" and "menstrual" age are considered equivalent.

c. Fetal number should be documented.

Comment

Amnionicity and chorionicity should be documented for all multiple gestations when possible.

d. Embryonic/fetal anatomy appropriate for the first trimester should be assessed.

e. The nuchal region should be imaged, and abnormalities such as cystic hygroma should be documented.

Comment

For those patients desiring to assess their individual risk of fetal aneuploidy, a very specific measurement of the NT during a specific age interval is necessary (as determined by the laboratory used). See the section entitled Guidelines for NT Measurement. Nuchal translucency measurements should be used (in conjunction with serum biochemistry) to determine the risk for having a fetus with aneuploidy or other anatomic abnormalities such as heart defects. In this setting, it is important that the practitioner measure the NT according to established guidelines for measurement. A quality assessment program is recommended to ensure that false-positive and -negative results are kept to a minimum.

f. The uterus including the cervix, adnexal structures, and cul-de-sac should be evaluated. Abnormalities should be imaged and documented.

Comment

The presence, location, appearance, and size of adnexal masses should be documented. The presence and number of leiomyomata should be documented. The measurements of the largest or any potentially clinically significant leiomyomata should be documented. The cul-de-sac should be evaluated for the presence or absence of fluid. Uterine anomalies should be documented.

B. *Second- and Third-Trimester Ultrasound Examination*

1. Indications

Indications for second- and third-trimester sonography, include but are not limited to:

a. Screening for fetal anomalies.

b. Evaluation of fetal anatomy.

Guidelines for NT Measurement

i.   The margins of the NT edges must be clear enough for proper placement of the calipers.

ii. The fetus must be in the midsagittal plane.

iii. The image must be magnified so that it is filled by the fetal head, neck, and upper thorax.

iv. The fetal neck must be in a neutral position, not flexed and not hyperextended.

v.   The amnion must be seen as separate from the NT line.

vi. The (+) calipers on the ultrasound must be used to perform the NT measurement.

vii. Electronic calipers must be placed on the inner borders of the nuchal line space with none of the horizontal crossbar itself protruding into the space.

viii. The calipers must be placed perpendicular to the long axis of the fetus.

ix. The measurement must be obtained at the widest space of the NT.

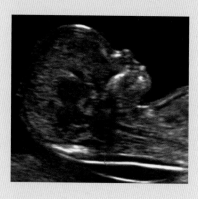

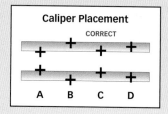

c. Estimation of gestational (menstrual) age.

d. Evaluation of fetal growth.

e. Evaluation of vaginal bleeding.

f. Evaluation of abdominal or pelvic pain.

g. Evaluation of cervical insufficiency.

h. Determination of fetal presentation.

i. Evaluation of suspected multiple gestation.

j. Adjunct to amniocentesis or other procedure.

k. Evaluation of a significant discrepancy between uterine size and clinical dates.

l. Evaluation of a pelvic mass.

m. Evaluation of a suspected hydatidiform mole.

n. Adjunct to cervical cerclage placement.

o. Suspected ectopic pregnancy.

p. Suspected fetal death.

q. Suspected uterine abnormalities.

r. Evaluation of fetal well-being.

s. Suspected amniotic fluid abnormalities.

t. Suspected placental abruption.

u. Adjunct to external cephalic version.

v. Evaluation of a premature rupture of membranes and/or premature labor.

w. Evaluation of abnormal biochemical markers.

x. Follow-up evaluation of a fetal anomaly.

y. Follow-up evaluation of placental location for suspected placenta previa.

z. History of previous congenital anomaly.

aa. Evaluation of fetal condition in late registrants for prenatal care.

bb. Assessment for findings that may increase the risk for aneuploidy.

Comment

In certain clinical circumstances, a more detailed examination of fetal anatomy may be indicated.

2. Imaging Parameters for a Standard Fetal Examination

a. Fetal cardiac activity, fetal number, and presentation should be documented.

Comment

An abnormal heart rate and/or rhythm should be documented. Multiple gestations require the docu-mentation of additional information: chorionicity, amnionicity, comparison of fetal sizes, estimation of amniotic fluid volume (increased, decreased, or normal) in each gestational sac, and fetal genitalia (when visualized).

b. A qualitative or semiquantitative estimate of amniotic fluid volume should be documented.

Comment

Although it is acceptable for experienced examiners to qualitatively estimate amniotic fluid volume, semiquantitative methods have also been described for this purpose (eg, amniotic fluid index, single deepest pocket, 2-diameter pocket).

c. The placental location, appearance, and relationship to the internal cervical os should be documented. The umbilical cord should be imaged, and the number of vessels in the cord documented. The placental cord insertion site should be documented when technically possible.

Comment

It is recognized that apparent placental position early in pregnancy may not correlate well with its location at the time of delivery.

Transabdominal, transperineal, or transvaginal views may be helpful in visualizing the internal cervical os and its relationship to the placenta.

Transvaginal or transperineal ultrasound may be considered if the cervix appears shortened or cannot be adequately visualized during the transabdominal sonogram. A velamentous (also called membranous) placental cord insertion that crosses the internal os of the cervix is vasa previa, a condition that has a high risk of fetal mortality if not diagnosed before labor.

d. Gestational (menstrual) age assessment.

First-trimester crown-rump measurement is the most accurate means for sonographic dating of pregnancy. Beyond this period, a variety of sonographic parameters such as biparietal diameter, abdominal circumference, and femoral diaphysis length can be used to estimate gestational (menstrual) age. The variability of gestational (menstrual) age estimation, however, increases with advancing pregnancy. Significant discrepancies between gestational (menstrual) age and fetal measurements may suggest the possibility of a fetal growth abnormality, intrauterine growth restriction, or macrosomia.

Comment

The pregnancy should not be redated after an accurate earlier scan has been performed and is available for comparison.

i.   Biparietal diameter is measured at the level of the thalami and cavum septi pellucidi or columns of the fornix. The cerebellar hemispheres should not be visible in this scanning plane. The measurement is taken from the outer edge of the proximal skull to the inner edge of the distal skull.

Comment

The head shape may be flattened (dolichocephaly) or rounded (brachycephaly) as a normal variant. Under these circumstances, certain variants of normal fetal head development may make measurement of the head circumference more reliable than biparietal diameter for estimating gestational (menstrual) age.

ii. Head circumference is measured at the same level as the biparietal diameter, around the outer perimeter of the calvarium. This measurement is not affected by head shape.

iii. Femoral diaphysis length can be reliably used after 14 weeks' gestational (menstrual) age. The long axis of the femoral shaft is most accurately measured with the beam of insonation being perpendicular to the shaft, excluding the distal femoral epiphysis.

iv. Abdominal circumference or average abdominal diameter should be determined at the skin line on a true transverse view at the level of the junction of the umbilical vein, portal sinus, and fetal stomach when visible.

Comment

Abdominal circumference or average abdominal diameter measurement is used with other biometric parameters to estimate fetal weight and may allow detection of intrauterine growth restriction or macrosomia.

e. Fetal weight estimation.

Fetal weight can be estimated by obtaining measurements such as the biparietal diameter, head circumference, abdominal circumference or average abdominal diameter, and femoral diaphysis length. Results from various prediction models can be compared to fetal weight percentiles from published nomograms.

Comment

If previous studies have been performed, appropriateness of growth should also be documented. Scans for growth evaluation can typically be performed at least 2 to 4 weeks apart. A shorter scan interval may result in confusion as to whether measurement changes are truly due to growth as opposed to variations in the technique itself.

Currently, even the best fetal weight prediction methods can yield errors as high as ±15%. This variability can be influenced by factors such as the nature of the patient population, the number and types of anatomic parameters being measured, technical factors that affect the resolution of ultrasound images, and the weight range being studied.

f. Maternal anatomy.

Evaluation of the uterus, adnexal structures, and cervix should be performed when appropriate. If the cervix cannot be visualized, a transperineal or transvaginal scan may be considered when evaluation of the cervix is needed.

Comment

This will allow recognition of incidental findings of potential clinical significance. The presence, location, and size of adnexal masses and the presence of at least the largest and potentially clinically significant leiomyomata should be documented. It is not always possible to image the normal maternal ovaries during the second and third trimesters.

g. Fetal anatomic survey.

Fetal anatomy, as described in this document, may be adequately assessed by ultrasound after approximately 18 weeks' gestational (menstrual) age. It may be possible to document normal structures before this time, although some structures can be difficult to visualize due to fetal size, position, movement, abdominal scars, and increased maternal abdominal wall thickness. A second- or third-trimester scan may pose technical limitations for an anatomic evaluation due to imaging artifacts from acoustic shadowing. When this occurs, the report of the sonographic examination should document the nature of this technical limitation. A follow-up examination may be helpful.

The following areas of assessment represent the minimal elements of a standard examination of fetal anatomy. A more detailed fetal anatomic examination may be necessary if an abnormality or suspected abnormality is found on the standard examination.

    i.   Head, face, and neck

       Lateral cerebral ventricles

       Choroid plexus

       Midline falx

       Cavum septi pellucidi

       Cerebellum

       Cisterna magna

       Upper lip

Comment

A measurement of the nuchal fold may be helpful during a specific age interval to assess the risk of aneuploidy.

   ii.   Chest;

       Heart

       Four-chamber view

       Left ventricular outflow tract

       Right ventricular outflow tract

  iii.   Abdomen;

       Stomach (presence, size, and situs)

       Kidneys

       Urinary bladder

       Umbilical cord insertion site into the fetal abdomen

       Umbilical cord vessel number

   iv.   Spine;

       Cervical, thoracic, lumbar, and sacral spine

    v.   Extremities;

       Legs and arms

   vi.   Sex;

       In multiple gestations and when medically indicated.

VI. Documentation

Adequate documentation is essential for high-quality patient care. There should be a permanent record of the ultrasound examination and its interpretation. Images of all appropriate areas, both normal and abnormal, should be recorded. Variations from normal size should be accompanied by measurements. Images should be labeled with the patient identification, facility identification, examination date, and side (right or left) of the anatomic site imaged. An official interpretation (final report) of the ultrasound findings should be included in the patient's medical record. Retention of the ultrasound examination should be consistent both with clinical needs and with relevant legal and local health care facility requirements.

Reporting should be in accordance with the *AIUM Practice Guideline for Documentation of an Ultrasound Examination.*

VII. Equipment Specifications

These studies should be conducted with real-time scanners, using a transabdominal and/or transvaginal approach. A transducer of appropriate frequency should be used. Real-time sonography is necessary to confirm the presence of fetal life through observation of cardiac activity and active movement.

The choice of transducer frequency is a tradeoff between beam penetration and resolution. With modern equipment, 3- to 5-MHz abdominal transducers allow sufficient penetration in most patients while providing adequate resolution. A lower-frequency transducer may be needed to provide adequate penetration for abdominal imaging in an obese patient. During early pregnancy, a 5-MHz abdominal transducer or a 5- to 10-MHz or greater vaginal transducer may provide superior resolution while still allowing adequate penetration.

VIII. Fetal Safety

Diagnostic ultrasound studies of the fetus are generally considered safe during pregnancy. This diagnostic procedure should be performed only when there is a valid medical indication, and the lowest possible ultrasonic exposure setting should be used to gain the necessary diagnostic information under the ALARA (as low as reasonably achievable) principle.

A thermal index for soft tissue (Tis) should be used at earlier than 10 weeks' gestation, and a thermal index for bone (Tib) should be used at 10 weeks' gestation or later when bone ossification is evident. In keeping with the ALARA principle, M-mode imaging should be used instead of spectral Doppler imaging to document embryonic/fetal heart rate.

The promotion, selling, or leasing of ultrasound equipment for making "keepsake fetal videos" is considered by the US Food and Drug Administration to be an unapproved use of a medical device. Use of a diagnostic ultrasound system for these purposes, without a physician's order, may be in violation of state laws or regulations.

IX. Quality Control and Improvement, Safety, Infection Control, and Patient Education

Policies and procedures related to quality control, patient education, infection control, and safety should be developed and implemented in accordance with the *AIUM Standards and Guidelines for the Accreditation of Ultrasound Practices.*

Equipment performance monitoring should be in accordance with the *AIUM Standards and Guidelines for the Accreditation of Ultrasound Practices.*

X. ALARA Principle

The potential benefits and risks of each examination should be considered. The ALARA principle should be observed when adjusting controls that affect the acoustic output and by considering transducer dwell times. Further details on ALARA may be found in the AIUM publication *Medical Ultrasound Safety*, Second Edition.

AIUM PRACTICE GUIDELINE FOR THE PERFORMANCE OF PELVIC ULTRASOUND EXAMINATIONS

I. Introduction

The clinical aspects contained in specific sections of this guideline (Introduction, Indications, Specifications of the Examination, and Equipment Specifications) were developed collaboratively by the American Institute of Ultrasound in Medicine (AIUM), the American College of Radiology (ACR), the American College of Obstetricians and Gynecologists (ACOG), and the Society of

Radiologists in Ultrasound (SRU). Recommendations for physician requirements, the written request for the examination, documentation, and quality control vary among these organizations and are addressed by each separately.

This guideline has been developed to assist physicians performing sonographic studies of the female pelvis. Ultrasound examinations of the female pelvis should be performed only when there is a valid medical reason, and the lowest possible ultrasonic exposure settings should be used to gain the necessary diagnostic information. In some cases, additional or specialized examinations may be necessary. While it is not possible to detect every abnormality, adherence to the following guideline will maximize the probability of detecting most abnormalities.

II. Indications

Indications for pelvic sonography include but are not limited to the following:

1. Pelvic pain;
2. Dysmenorrhea (painful menses);
3. Amenorrhea;
4. Menorrhagia (excessive menstrual bleeding);
5. Metrorrhagia (irregular uterine bleeding);
6. Menometrorrhagia (excessive irregular bleeding);
7. Follow-up of a previously detected abnormality;
8. Evaluation, monitoring, and/or treatment of infertility patients;
9. Delayed menses, precocious puberty, or vaginal bleeding in a prepubertal child;
10. Postmenopausal bleeding;
11. Abnormal or technically limited pelvic examination;
12. Signs or symptoms of pelvic infection;
13. Further characterization of a pelvic abnormality noted on another imaging study;
14. Evaluation of congenital anomalies;
15. Excessive bleeding, pain, or signs of infection after pelvic surgery, delivery, or abortion;
16. Localization of a intrauterine contraceptive device;
17. Screening for malignancy in patients at increased risk;
18. Urinary incontinence or pelvic organ prolapse; and
19. Guidance for interventional or surgical procedures.

III. Qualifications of Personnel

See www.aium.org for AIUM Official Statements including *Standards and Guidelines for the Accreditation of Ultrasound Practices* and relevant Physician Training Guidelines.

IV. Written Request for the Examination

The written or electronic request for an ultrasound examination should provide sufficient information to allow for the appropriate performance and interpretation of the examination.

The request for the examination must be originated by a physician or other appropriately licensed health care provider or under their direction. The accompanying clinical information should be provided by a physician or other appropriate health care provider familiar with the patient's clinical situation and should be consistent with relevant legal and local health care facility requirements.

V. Specifications of the Examination

This section details the examination to be performed for each organ and anatomic region in the female pelvis. All relevant structures should be identified by a transabdominal and/or transvaginal approach. In some cases, both will be needed. A transrectal or transperineal approach may be useful in patients who are not candidates for introduction of a vaginal probe and in assessing the patient with pelvic organ prolapse.

A. General Pelvic Preparation

For a complete transabdominal pelvic sonogram, the patient's bladder should, in general, be distended adequately to displace the small bowel from the field of view. Occasionally, overdistention of the bladder may compromise the evaluation. When this occurs, imaging may be repeated after the patient partially empties the bladder.

For a transvaginal sonogram, the urinary bladder is preferably empty. The patient, the sonographer, or the physician may introduce the vaginal transducer, preferably under real-time monitoring. Consideration of having a chaperone present should be in accordance with local policies.

B. Uterus

The vagina and uterus provide anatomic landmarks that can be used as reference points for the other pelvic structures, whether normal or abnormal. In examining the uterus, the following should be evaluated: (1) the uterine size, shape, and orientation; (2) the endometrium; (3) the myometrium; and (4) the cervix. The vagina may be imaged as a landmark for the cervix and lower uterine segment.

Overall uterine length is evaluated in the long axis from the fundus to the cervix (to the external os, if it can be identified). The depth of the uterus (anteroposterior dimension) is measured in the same long-axis view from its anterior to posterior walls, perpendicular to the length. The maximum width is measured in the transaxial or coronal view. If volume measurements of the uterine corpus are performed, the cervical component should be excluded from the uterine length measurement.

Abnormalities of the uterus should be documented. The myometrium and cervix should be evaluated for contour changes, echogenicity, masses, and cysts. Masses that may require follow-up or intervention should be measured in at least 2 dimensions, acknowledging that it is not usually necessary to measure all fibroids.

The endometrium should be analyzed for thickness, focal abnormalities, and the presence of fluid or masses in the endometrial cavity. The endometrium should be measured on a midline sagittal image, including anterior and posterior portions of the basal endometrium and excluding the adjacent hypoechoic myometrium and any endometrial fluid. Assessment of the endometrium should allow for variations expected with phases of the menstrual cycle and with hormonal supplementation. If the endometrium is difficult to image in its entirety or poorly defined, this should be reported. Sonohysterography may be a useful adjunct for evaluating the patient with abnormal or dysfunctional uterine bleeding or to further clarify an abnormally thickened endometrium. If the patient has an intrauterine contraceptive device, its location should be documented. (See the *AIUM Practice Guideline for the Performance of Sonohysterography.*)

When available, the addition of a reconstructed coronal view of the uterus from a 3-dimensional volume may be useful.

C. Adnexa Including Ovaries and Fallopian Tubes

When evaluating the adnexa, an attempt should be made to identify the ovaries first since they can serve as a major point of reference for assessing the presence of adnexal pathology. Ovarian size may be determined by measuring the ovary in 3 dimensions (width, length, and depth), on views obtained in 2 orthogonal planes. Any ovarian abnormalities should be documented. The ovaries may not be identifiable in some females. This occurs most frequently prior to puberty, after menopause, or in the presence of a large leiomyomatous uterus. The normal fallopian tubes are not commonly identified. The adnexal region should be surveyed for abnormalities, particularly masses and dilated tubular structures.

If an adnexal abnormality is noted, its relationship to the ovaries and uterus should be assessed. The size and sonographic characteristics of adnexal masses should be documented.

Spectral, color, and/or power Doppler ultrasound may be useful for evaluating the vascular characteristics of pelvic lesions.

D. Cul-de-sac

The cul-de-sac and bowel posterior to the uterus may not be clearly defined. This area should be evaluated for the presence of free fluid or a mass. If a mass is detected, its size, position, shape, sonographic characteristics, and relationship to the ovaries and uterus should be documented. Differentiation of normal loops of bowel from a mass may be difficult if only a transabdominal examination is performed. A transvaginal examination may be helpful to distinguish a suspected mass from fluid and feces within the normal rectosigmoid colon.

VI. Documentation

Adequate documentation is essential for high-quality patient care. There should be a permanent record of the ultrasound examination and its interpretation. Images of all appropriate areas, both normal and abnormal, should be recorded. Variations from normal size should be accompanied by measurements. Images should be labeled with the patient identification, facility identification, examination date, and side (right or left) of the anatomic site imaged. An official interpretation (final report) of the ultrasound findings should be included in the patient's medical record. Retention of the ultrasound examination should be consistent both with clinical needs and with relevant legal and local health care facility requirements.

Reporting should be in accordance with the *AIUM Practice Guideline for Documentation of an Ultrasound Examination.*

VII. Equipment Specifications

The sonographic examination of the female pelvis should be conducted with a real-time scanner, preferably using sector, curved linear, and/or endovaginal transducers. The transducer or scanner should be adjusted to operate at the highest clinically appropriate frequency, realizing that there is a trade-off between resolution and beam penetration. With modern equipment, studies performed from the anterior abdominal wall can usually use frequencies of 3.5 MHz or higher, while scans performed from the vagina should use frequencies of 5 MHz or higher.

VIII. Quality Control and Improvement, Safety, Infection Control, and Patient Education

Policies and procedures related to quality control, patient education, infection control, and safety should be developed and implemented in accordance with the *AIUM Standards and Guidelines for the Accreditation of Ultrasound Practices.*

Equipment performance monitoring should be in accordance with the *AIUM Standards and Guidelines for the Accreditation of Ultrasound Practices.*

IX. As Low as Reasonably Achievable Principle

The potential benefits and risks of each examination should be considered. The as low as reasonably achievable (ALARA) principle should be observed when adjusting controls that affect the acoustic output and by considering transducer dwell times. Further details on ALARA may be found in the AIUM publication *Medical Ultrasound Safety, Second Edition.*

AIUM PRACTICE GUIDELINE FOR THE PERFORMANCE OF SONOHYSTEROGRAPHY

Guideline developed in collaboration with the American College of Radiology, the American College of Obstetricians and Gynecologists, and the Society of Radiologists in Ultrasound

I. Introduction

The clinical aspects contained in specific sections of this guideline (Introduction, Indications and Contraindications, Specifications for Individual Examinations, and

Equipment Specifications) were developed collaboratively by the American Institute of Ultrasound in Medicine (AIUM), the American College of Radiology (ACR), the American College of Obstetricians and Gynecologists (ACOG), and the Society of Radiologists in Ultrasound (SRU). Recommendations for physician qualifications, written request for the examination, procedure documentation, and quality control may vary among the 4 organizations and are addressed by each separately.

This guideline has been developed to assist qualified physicians performing sonohysterography. Properly performed sonohysterography can provide information about the uterus, endometrium, and fallopian tubes. Additional studies may be necessary for complete diagnosis. Adherence to the following guideline will maximize the diagnostic benefit of sonohysterography.

Sonohysterography is the evaluation of the endometrial cavity using the transcervical injection of sterile fluid. Various terms such as saline infusion sonohysterography and simply sonohysterography have been used to describe this technique. The primary goal of sonohysterography is to visualize the endometrial cavity in more detail than is possible with routine endovaginal sonography. Sonohysterography can also be used to assess tubal patency.

II. Indications and Contraindications

A. Indications

Indications include but are not limited to evaluation of:

1. Abnormal uterine bleeding;
2. Uterine cavity, especially with regard to uterine myomas, polyps, and synechiae;
3. Abnormalities detected on endovaginal sonography, including focal or diffuse endometrial or intracavitary abnormalities;
4. Congenital abnormalities of the uterus;
5. Infertility; and
6. Recurrent pregnancy loss.

B. Contraindications

Sonohysterography should not be performed in a woman who is pregnant or who could be pregnant. This is usually avoided by scheduling the examination in the follicular phase of the menstrual cycle, after menstrual flow has essentially ceased but before the patient has ovulated. In a patient with regular cycles, sonohysterography should not in most cases be performed later than the 10th day of the menstrual cycle. Sonohysterography should not be performed in patients with a pelvic infection or unexplained pelvic tenderness, which could be due to pelvic inflammatory disease. Active vaginal bleeding is not a contraindication to the procedure but may make the interpretation more challenging.

III. Qualifications and Responsibilities of the Physician

See the *AIUM Official Statement Training Guidelines for Physicians Who Evaluate and Interpret Diagnostic Ultrasound Examinations and the AIUM Standards and Guidelines for the Accreditation of Ultrasound Practices.*

IV. Written Request for the Examination

The written or electronic request for an ultrasound examination should provide sufficient information to allow for the appropriate performance and interpretation of the examination.

The request for the examination must be originated by a physician or other appropriately licensed health care provider or under the provider's direction. The accompanying clinical information should be provided by a physician or other appropriate health care provider familiar with the patient's clinical situation and should be consistent with relevant legal and local health care facility requirements.

V. Specifications for Individual Examinations

A. Patient Preparation

Pelvic organ tenderness should be assessed during the preliminary endovaginal sonogram. If adnexal tenderness or pain suspicious for an active pelvic infection is found before fluid infusion, the examination should be deferred until after an appropriate course of treatment. In the presence of nontender hydrosalpinges, consideration may be given to administering antibiotics at the time of the examination; in this case, it is prudent to discuss the antibiotic regimen with the referring physician. A pregnancy test is advised when clinically indicated. Patients should be questioned about a latex allergy before use of a latex sheath. The optimal time to perform this test in a menstruating woman is after the bleeding ends but before ovulation.

B. Procedure

Preliminary endovaginal sonography with measurements of the endometrium and evaluation of the uterus, ovaries, and pelvic free fluid should be performed before sonohysterography. A speculum is used to allow visualization of the cervix. The presence of unusual pain, lesions, or purulent vaginal or cervical discharge may require rescheduling the procedure pending further evaluation. Before insertion, the catheter should be flushed with sterile fluid to avoid introducing air during the study. After cleansing the external os, the cervical canal and/or uterine cavity should be catheterized using aseptic technique, and appropriate sterile fluid should be instilled slowly by means of manual injection under real-time sonographic imaging. Imaging should include real-time scanning of the endometrial and cervical canal.

C. Contrast Agent

Appropriate sterile fluid such as normal saline or water should be used for sonohysterography.

D. Images

Precatheterization images should be obtained and recorded, in at least 2 planes, to show normal and abnormal findings. These images should include the thickest bilayer endometrial measurement on a sagittal image when possible.

Once the uterine cavity is filled with fluid, a complete survey of the uterine cavity should be performed and representative images obtained to document normal and abnormal findings. If a balloon catheter is used for the examination, images should be obtained at the end of the procedure with the balloon deflated to fully evaluate the endometrial cavity, particularly the cervical canal and lower portion of the endometrial cavity.

Additional techniques such as color Doppler and 3-dimensional imaging may be helpful in evaluating both normal and abnormal findings.

VI. Documentation

Adequate documentation is essential for high-quality patient care. There should be a permanent record of the ultrasound examination and its interpretation. Images of all appropriate areas, both normal and abnormal, should be recorded. Variations from normal size should be accompanied by measurements. Images should be labeled with the patient identification, facility identification, examination date, and side (right or left) of the anatomic site imaged. An official interpretation (final report) of the ultrasound findings should be included in the patient's medical record. Retention of the ultrasound examination should be consistent both with clinical needs and with relevant legal and local health care facility requirements.

Reporting should be in accordance with the *AIUM Practice Guideline for Documentation of an Ultrasound Examination.*

VII. Equipment Specifications

Sonohysterography is usually conducted with a high-frequency endovaginal transducer. In cases of an enlarged uterus, additional transabdominal images during infusion may be required to fully evaluate the endometrium. The transducer should be adjusted to operate at the highest clinically appropriate frequency under the ALARA (as low as reasonably achievable) principle.

VIII. Quality Control and Improvement, Safety, Infection Control, and Patient Education

Policies and procedures related to quality control, patient education, infection control, and safety should be developed and implemented in accordance with the *AIUM Standards and Guidelines for the Accreditation of Ultrasound Practices.*

Equipment performance monitoring should be in accordance with the *AIUM Standards and Guidelines for the Accreditation of Ultrasound Practices.*

IX. ALARA Principle

The potential benefits and risks of each examination should be considered. The ALARA (as low as reasonably achievable) principle should be observed when adjusting controls that affect the acoustic output and by considering transducer dwell times. Further details on ALARA may be found in the AIUM publication *Medical Ultrasound Safety, Second Edition.*

AIUM PRACTICE GUIDELINE FOR ULTRASONOGRAPHY IN REPRODUCTIVE MEDICINE

Prepared in collaboration with the American Institute of Ultrasound in Medicine (AIUM) and the Society for Reproductive Endocrinology and Infertility (SREI), an affiliate of the American Society of Reproductive Medicine (ASRM)

Ultrasound Examination of the Female Pelvis for Infertility and Reproductive Medicine

The following are proposed guidelines for ultrasound evaluation of the female pelvis. The document consists of 2 parts:

Part I: Equipment and Documentation Guidelines

Part II: Guidelines for Performance of the Ultrasound Examination of the Female Pelvis for Infertility and Reproductive Medicine

This guideline has been developed to provide assistance to practitioners performing ultrasound studies of the female pelvis. In some cases, additional and/or specialized examinations may be necessary. While it is not possible to detect every abnormality, adherence to the following will maximize the probability of detecting most of the abnormalities that occur.

This guideline includes excerpts from various previously published guidelines of the AIUM. The latest versions of all AIUM guidelines are available at www.aium.org.

Part I: Equipment and Documentation Guidelines

Equipment

The sonographic examination of the female pelvis should be conducted with a real-time scanner, with the availability of multiple types of transducers. The transducer or scanner should be adjusted to operate at the highest clinically appropriate frequency, realizing that there is a trade-off between resolution and beam penetration. With modern equipment, studies performed from the anterior abdominal wall can usually use frequencies of 3.5 MHz or higher, while scans performed from the vagina should use frequencies of 5 MHz or higher.

Care of the Equipment

All probes should be cleaned after each patient examination. Transvaginal probes should be covered by a protective sheath prior to insertion. Patients should be questioned about latex allergy prior to use of a latex sheath. Following each examination, the sheath should be disposed, and the probe washed, dried, and appropriately disinfected (see section below: "Guidelines for Cleaning and Preparing Endocavitary Ultrasound Transducers Between Patients"). The type of antimicrobial solution and the methodology for disinfection depend on manufacturer and infectious disease recommendations.

Documentation

Adequate documentation is essential for high-quality patient care. A permanent record of the ultrasound examination and its interpretation should be kept by the facility performing the study. Images of all appropriate areas, both normal and abnormal, should be recorded. Variations from normal size should be accompanied by measurements. Images are to be appropriately labeled with the examination date, facility name, patient identification, and image orientation and/or organ imaged when appropriate. A report of the ultrasound findings should be included in the patient's medical record. Urgent or clinically important unexpected results should be communicated verbally to any referring and/or treating physician and this communication documented in the report. Retention of the permanent record of the ultrasound examination should be consistent both with clinical needs and with the relevant legal and local health care facility requirements.

Part II: Guidelines for Performance of the Ultrasound Examination of the Female Pelvis for Infertility and Reproductive Medicine

The following guidelines describe the examination to be performed for each organ and anatomic region in the female pelvis. Whenever possible, all relevant structures should be identified by the vaginal approach. When a transvaginal scan fails to image all areas needed for diagnosis, a transabdominal scan should be performed. In some cases, both a transabdominal and a transvaginal scan may be needed.

General Pelvic Preparation

For a pelvic sonogram performed transabdominally, the patient's urinary bladder should, in general, be distended adequately to displace the small bowel and its contained gas from the field of view. Occasionally, overdistension of the bladder may compromise evaluation. When this occurs, imaging may be repeated after the patient partially empties her bladder.

For a transvaginal sonogram, the urinary bladder is preferably empty. The patient, the sonographer, or the physician may introduce the transvaginal transducer, preferably under real-time monitoring. Transvaginal sonography is a specialized form of a pelvic examination. Therefore, policies applied locally regarding chaperone or patient privacy issues during a pelvic examination should also be applied during a transvaginal ultrasound examination.

Uterus

The vagina and the uterus provide anatomic landmarks that can be used as reference points when evaluating the pelvic structures. In evaluating the uterus, the following should be documented: (1) uterine size, shape, and orientation; (2) the endometrium; (3) the myometrium; and (4) the cervix. The vagina may be imaged as a landmark for the cervix and lower uterine segment. Uterine length is evaluated on a long axis view as the distance from the fundus to the cervix. The anteroposterior (AP) diameter of the uterus is measured in the same long axis view from its anterior to posterior walls, perpendicular to its long axis. The transverse diameter is measured from the transaxial or coronal view, perpendicular to the long axis of the uterus. If volume measurements of the uterine corpus are performed, the cervical component should be excluded from the uterine measurement.

Abnormalities of the uterus should be documented. The endometrium should be analyzed for thickness, focal abnormalities, and the presence of fluid or masses in the endometrial cavity. Assessment of the endometrium should allow for variations expected with phases of the menstrual cycle and with hormonal supplementation. The endometrial thickness measurement should include both layers, measured anterior to posterior, in the sagittal plane. Any fluid within the endometrial cavity should be excluded from this measurement. If the endometrial echo is difficult to image or ill-defined, a comment should be added to the report.

The myometrium and cervix should be evaluated for contour changes, echogenicity, and masses. Masses, if identified, should be measured in at least 2 dimensions and their locations recorded.

Adnexa (Ovaries and Fallopian Tubes)

When evaluating the adnexa, an attempt should be made to identify the ovaries first since they can serve as a major point of reference for assessing the presence of adnexal pathology. Although their location is variable, the ovaries are most often situated anterior to the internal iliac (hypogastric) vessels, lateral to the uterus, and superficial to the obturator internus muscle. The ovaries should be measured, and ovarian abnormalities should be documented. Ovarian size can be determined by measuring the ovary in 3 dimensions on views obtained in 2 orthogonal planes. It is recognized that the ovaries may not be identifiable in some women. This occurs most frequently after menopause or in patients with a large leiomyomatous uterus.

The normal fallopian tubes are not commonly identified. This region should be surveyed for abnormalities, particularly dilated tubular structures.

If an adnexal mass is noted, its relationship to the uterus and the ovaries, if separately visualized, should be documented. Its size, echogenicity, and internal characteristics (cystic, solid, or complex) should be determined. Doppler ultrasound may be useful in select cases to identify the vascular nature of pelvic structures.

Cul-de-sac

The cul-de-sac and bowel posterior to the uterus may not be clearly defined. This area should be evaluated for the presence of free fluid or masses. When free fluid is detected, its echogenicity should be assessed. If a mass is detected, its size, position, shape, echogenicity, internal characteristics (cystic, solid, or complex), and relationship to the ovaries and uterus should be documented. Identification of peristalsis can be helpful in distinguishing a loop of bowel from a pelvic mass. In the absence of peristalsis, differentiation of normal loops of bowel from a mass may be difficult. A transvaginal examination may be helpful to distinguish a suspected mass from fluid and feces within the normal rectosigmoid. An ultrasound water enema study or a repeat examination after a cleansing enema may also help to distinguish a suspected mass from bowel.

Limited Examination

In some circumstances, a limited pelvic ultrasound examination is appropriate, especially when monitoring ovarian stimulation (e.g., an ovarian folliculogram study or determining endometrial qualities prior to cryopreserved embryo transfer). A comprehensive exam should have previously been performed in the preceding 4 to 6 months to rule out other gynecologic pathology. The limited exam can be restricted to the organ or measurements of interest. In the case of an ovarian folliculogram, the following should be documented: ovarian follicle number in each ovary, endometrial thickness, and endometrial morphologic appearance. In addition, follicular diameters in 2 dimensions for each follicle above 10 mm should be recorded. A single recorded value representing the mean of 2 diameter measurements performed at right angles is also acceptable. Given that these patients will have had a full pelvic exam at the appropriate interval prior to initiating therapy, for infertility patients undergoing limited folliculogram studies, permanent recorded images should be obtained as indicated. Pertinent clinical information should be recorded in the patient record.

Ultrasound-Guided Procedures

A. Follicle Puncture: Ultrasound-assisted (transvaginal or transabdominal) follicle puncture for retrieving eggs for in vitro fertilization (IVF) is appropriate in the following circumstances:

1. The patient has undergone comprehensive sonographic evaluation of the pelvis within 4 to 6 months prior to the start of hormonal stimulation of the ovaries.

2. Real-time continuous guidance is available, and the image demonstrates a safe approach for the needle path.

3. The ovaries can be brought in close proximity to the ultrasound transducer, thus avoiding the puncture of vital structures (e.g., bowel and blood vessels).

B. Cyst Aspiration: Ultrasound-assisted (transvaginal or transabdominal) ovarian cyst puncture and aspiration is appropriate in patients who have been diagnosed with a persistent ovarian cyst and who meet the following criteria:

1. Failed resolution of the cyst following observation and/or hormonal manipulation.

2. The cyst is unilocular and thin-walled without internal excrescences or septations.

3. Real-time continuous guidance is available, and the image demonstrates a safe approach for the needle path.

4. The cyst can be brought in close proximity to the ultrasound transducer, thus avoiding the puncture of vital structures (e.g., bowel and blood vessels).

C. Embryo Transfer: Ultrasound-assisted embryo transfer is appropriate in patients undergoing a "fresh" IVF cycle or following embryo cryopreservation or embryo/egg donation. If an abdominal ultrasound examination is performed, the bladder should be full to facilitate visualization of the endometrium and the transfer catheter.

Qualifications and Responsibilities of the Physician

Physicians who perform or supervise ultrasound-guided follicular aspiration or embryo transfer should be skilled in pelvic ultrasonography and appropriate placement of catheters and ultrasound-guided needle placement. They should understand the indications, limitations, and possible complications of the procedure. Physicians should have training, experience, and demonstrated competence in gynecologic ultrasonography and treatment procedures. Physicians are responsible for the documentation of the examination, quality control, and patient safety. Urgent or clinically important unexpected results should be communicated verbally to any referring and/or treating physician and this communication documented in the report.

Ultrasound Examination of the Female Pelvis in the First 10 Weeks (Embryonic Period) of Pregnancy

Introduction

This portion of the guideline has been developed for use by practitioners performing sonographic studies only during the first 10 menstrual weeks of pregnancy. Such sonography should be performed only when there is a valid medical reason, and the lowest possible ultrasonic exposure settings should be used to gain the necessary diagnostic information. A limited examination may be performed in clinical emergencies or in specific clinical scenarios, such as evaluation of fetal or embryonic cardiac activity. A limited follow-up examination may be appropriate if a complete prior examination is on record. While this guideline describes the key elements of standard sonographic examinations in the first 10 weeks of pregnancy, in some cases, other specialized examinations may be necessary as well.

Specifications of the Examination

1. Indications

A sonographic examination can be of benefit in many circumstances in the embryonic period of pregnancy, including but not limited to the following indications:

a. To confirm the presence of an intrauterine pregnancy.

b. To evaluate a suspected ectopic pregnancy.

c. To define the cause of vaginal bleeding.

d. To evaluate pelvic pain.

e. To date the pregnancy.

f. To diagnose or evaluate multiple gestations.

g. To confirm cardiac activity.

h. To evaluate maternal pelvic masses and/or uterine abnormalities.

i. To evaluate a suspected hydatidiform mole.

Comment

A limited examination may be performed to assess the presence of cardiac activity.

2. Imaging Parameters

Overall Comment

Scanning in the first 10 weeks of pregnancy may be performed either transabdominally or transvaginally, although transvaginal scanning is preferred. Patients should be questioned about latex allergy prior to use of a latex sheath.

a. The uterus, including the cervix, and adnexa should be evaluated for the presence of a gestational sac. If a gestational sac is seen, its location should be documented. The gestational sac should be evaluated for the presence or absence of a yolk sac or embryo, and the embryonic size should be measured and recorded, when possible.

Comment

Embryonic size is a more accurate indicator of gestational (menstrual) age than is mean gestational sac diameter. However, the mean gestational sac diameter may be measured and recorded when an embryo is not identified. Caution should be used in making the presumptive diagnosis of a gestational sac in the absence of a definite embryo or yolk sac. Without these findings, an intrauterine fluid collection could represent a pseudo-gestational sac associated with an ectopic pregnancy.

b. Presence or absence of cardiac activity should be reported.

Comment

With transvaginal scans, cardiac motion is usually observed when the embryo is 5 mm or greater in length. If an embryo less than 5 mm in length is seen without

cardiac activity, a subsequent scan at a later time may be needed to document cardiac activity. If possible, the M-mode function of the scanner should be used to document cardiac activity.

c. Embryonic number should be reported.

Comment

Amnionicity and chorionicity should be documented for all multiple pregnancies when possible.

d. Evaluation of the uterus, adnexal structures, and cul-de-sac should be performed.

Comment

The presence, location, and size of adnexal masses should be recorded. The presence of leiomyomata should be recorded, and measurements of the largest or any potentially clinically significant leiomyomata should be recorded. The cul-de-sac should be scanned for the presence or absence of fluid.

3. Equipment Specifications

These studies should be conducted with real-time scanners, using a transabdominal and/or a transvaginal approach. A transducer of appropriate frequency should be used.

Comment

Real-time sonography is necessary to confirm the presence of cardiac activity. A transvaginal scanning approach is preferred for this indication.

4. Fetal Safety

Diagnostic ultrasound studies of the fetus are generally considered to be safe during pregnancy. This diagnostic procedure should be performed only when there is a valid medical indication, and the lowest possible ultrasonic exposure setting should be used to gain the necessary diagnostic information under the as low as reasonably achievable (ALARA) principle.

The promotion, selling, or leasing of ultrasound equipment for making "keepsake fetal videos" is considered by the US Food and Drug Administration (FDA) to be an unapproved use of a medical device. Use of a diagnostic ultrasound system for these purposes, without a physician's order, may be in violation of state laws or regulations.

Sonohysterography in Reproductive Medicine and Infertility

Introduction

This portion of the guideline has been developed to provide assistance to qualified physicians performing sonohysterography. Properly performed sonohysterography can provide information about the uterus and the endometrium. Additional studies may be necessary for complete diagnosis. However, adherence to the following standard will maximize the diagnostic benefit of sonohysterography.

Definition

Sonohysterography consists of sonographic imaging of the uterus and uterocervical cavity, using real-time sonography during injection of sterile fluid (saline or water) into the uterine cavity.

Goal

The goal of sonohysterography is to visualize the endometrial cavity in more detail than is possible with routine transvaginal sonography.

Indications and Contraindications

The most common indication for sonohysterography is abnormal uterine bleeding in both premenopausal and postmenopausal women. Other indications include but are not limited to:

A. Indications

1. Infertility and habitual abortion.
2. Congenital abnormalities and/or anatomic variants of the uterine cavity.
3. Preoperative and postoperative evaluation of the uterine cavity, especially with regard to uterine myomas, polyps, and cysts.
4. Suspected uterine cavity synechiae.
5. Further evaluation of suspected abnormalities seen on transvaginal sonography, including focal or diffuse endometrial thickening or debris.
6. Inadequate imaging of the endometrium by transvaginal sonography.
7. Screening evaluation of the uterine cavity prior to fertility treatment(s) using assisted reproductive technologies.

B. Contraindications

Sonohysterography should not be performed in a woman who is pregnant or who could be pregnant. This is usually avoided by scheduling the examination in the follicular phase of the menstrual cycle, after menstrual flow has essentially ceased, but before the patient has ovulated. In a patient with regular cycles, sonohysterography should not in most cases be performed later than the 10th day of the menstrual cycle. Sonohysterography should not be performed in patients with a pelvic infection or unexplained pelvic tenderness, which may be due to chronic pelvic inflammatory disease. Pelvic organ tenderness should be assessed during the preliminary transvaginal sonogram. Active vaginal bleeding is not a contraindication to the procedure but may make the interpretation more challenging.

Qualifications and Responsibilities of the Physician

Physicians who perform or supervise diagnostic sonohysterography should be skilled in pelvic ultrasonography and appropriate placement of catheters. They should understand the indications, limitations, and possible complications of the procedure. Physicians should have training, experience, and demonstrated competence in gynecologic ultrasonography and sonohysterography. Physicians are responsible for the documentation of the examination, quality control, and patient safety. Urgent or clinically important unexpected results should be communicated verbally to any referring and/or treating physician and this communication documented in the report.

Specifications of the Examination

A. Patient Preparation

The referring physician may elect to prescribe prophylactic antibiotics if patients routinely take these for other invasive procedures. If painful, dilated, and/or obstructed fallopian tubes are found prior to fluid infusion, and the patient is not taking prophylactic antibiotics, the examination should be delayed until treatment can be administered. In the presence of nontender hydrosalpinges, consideration may be given to administering antibiotics at the time of the examination. A pregnancy test is advised when clinically indicated. Patients should be questioned about latex allergy prior to use of a latex sheath.

B. Procedure

Preliminary routine transvaginal sonography with measurements of the endometrium and evaluation of the uterus and the ovaries should be performed prior to sonohysterography. A speculum is used to allow visualization of the cervix. The presence of unusual pain, lesions, or purulent vaginal or cervical discharge may require rescheduling the procedure pending further evaluation. After cleansing the external os, the cervical canal and/or uterine cavity should be catheterized using aseptic technique, and appropriate sterile fluid should be instilled slowly by means of manual injection under real-time sonographic imaging. Imaging should include real-time scanning of the endometrial and cervical canals.

For infertility patients, tubal patency may be determined during sonohysterography by using the following methods: During the preliminary sonogram, the posterior cul-de-sac and pelvis should be evaluated for the presence of free fluid. If none is present before injection of fluid and it is present after fluid injection, then one can state that at least 1 tube is patent. Additionally, contrast material or a small amount of air injected with the fluid may be used with concurrent real-time sonographic imaging of the cornua, adnexae, and cul-de-sac to assess tubal patency. This can facilitate assessing patency of each fallopian tube.

C. Distension Media

Appropriate sterile fluid such as normal saline or water should be used for sonohysterography.

D. Images

Appropriate images, in at least 2 planes, using a high-frequency transvaginal ultrasound probe should be produced and recorded to demonstrate normal and abnormal findings. Pre-catherization images should be obtained, including the thickest bilayer endometrial measurement on a sagittal image.

Once the uterine cavity is filled with fluid, representative images with a complete survey of the uterine cavity are obtained as necessary for diagnostic evaluation. If a balloon catheter is used for the examination, images should be obtained at the end of the procedure with the balloon deflated to fully evaluate the endometrial cavity and particularly the cervical canal and the lower uterine segment.

E. Equipment Specifications

Sonohysterography is usually conducted with a transvaginal transducer. In cases of an enlarged uterus, additional transabdominal images during infusion may be required to fully evaluate the endometrium. The transducer should be adjusted to operate at the highest clinically appropriate frequency under the ALARA principle.

Training Guidelines for Physicians Who Evaluate and Interpret Diagnostic Ultrasound Examinations

Adapted from the AIUM Official Statement *Training Guidelines for Physicians Who Evaluate and Interpret Diagnostic Ultrasound Examinations*, ©2008 by the American Institute of Ultrasound in Medicine.

Physicians who evaluate and interpret diagnostic ultrasound examinations should be licensed medical practitioners who have a thorough understanding of the indication and guidelines for ultrasound examinations as well as familiarity with the basic physical principles and limitations of the technology of ultrasound imaging. They should be familiar with alternative and complementary imaging and diagnostic procedures and should be capable of correlating the results of these other procedures with the ultrasound examination findings. They should have an understanding of ultrasound technology and instrumentation, ultrasound power output, equipment calibration, and safety. Physicians responsible for ultrasound examinations should be able to demonstrate familiarity with the anatomy, physiology, and pathophysiology of those organs or anatomic areas that are being examined. These physicians should provide evidence of training and requisite competence needed to successfully perform and interpret diagnostic ultrasound examinations in the area(s) they practice. The training should include methods of documentation and reporting of ultrasound studies. Physicians performing diagnostic ultrasound examinations should meet at least one of the following:

1. Completion of an approved residency program, fellowship, or postgraduate training that includes the equivalent of at least 3 months of diagnostic ultrasound

training in the area(s) they practice under the supervision of a qualified physician(s),* during which the trainees will have evidence of being involved with the performance, evaluation, and interpretation of at least 300** sonograms.

2. In the absence of formal fellowship or postgraduate training or residency training, documentation of clinical experience could be acceptable providing the following could be demonstrated:

   a. Evidence of 100 *AMA PRA Category 1 Credits*™ dedicated to diagnostic ultrasound in the area(s) they practice, and

   b. Evidence of being involved with the performance, evaluation, and interpretation of the images of at least 300** sonograms within a 3-year period. It is expected that in most circumstances, examinations will be under the supervision of a qualified physician(s)*. These sonograms should be in the area(s) they are practicing.

Cases presented as preselected, limited image sets, such as in lectures, case conferences, and teaching files, are excluded. The ability to analyze a full image set, determining its completeness and the adequacy of image quality, and performing the diagnostic process, distinguishing normal from abnormal, is considered a primary goal of the training experience.

Guidelines for Cleaning and Preparing Endocavitary Ultrasound Transducers Between Patients

Adapted from the AIUM Official Statement *Guidelines for Cleaning and Preparing Endocavitary Ultrasound Transducers Between Patients*, ©2003 by the American Institute of Ultrasound in Medicine.

The purpose of this document is to provide guidance regarding the cleaning and disinfection of transvaginal ultrasound probes.

*A qualified physician is one who, at minimum, meets the criteria defined above in this document.

**Three hundred cases were selected as a minimum number needed to gain experience and proficiency with ultrasonography as a diagnostic modality. This is necessary to develop technical skills, to appreciate the practical applications of basic physics as it affects image quality and artifact formation, and to acquire an experience base for understanding the range of normal and recognizing deviations from normal.

All sterilization/disinfection represents a statistical reduction in the number of microbes present on a surface. Meticulous cleaning of the instrument is the essential key to an initial reduction of the microbial/organic load by at least 99%. This cleaning is followed by a disinfecting procedure to ensure a high degree of protection from infectious disease transmission, even if a disposable barrier covers the instrument during use.

Medical instruments fall into different categories with respect to potential for infection transmission. The most critical level of instruments is that which is intended to penetrate skin or mucous membranes. These require sterilization. Less critical instruments (often called "semi-critical" instruments) that simply come into contact with mucous membranes such as fiber-optic endoscopes require high-level disinfection rather than sterilization.

Although endocavitary ultrasound probes might be considered even less critical instruments because they are routinely protected by single-use disposable probe covers, leakage rates of 0.9% to 2% for condoms and 8% to 81% for commercial probe covers have been observed in recent studies. For maximum safety, one should therefore perform high-level disinfection of the probe between each use and use a probe cover or condom as an aid to keeping the probe clean.

There are 4 generally recognized categories of disinfection and sterilization. Sterilization is the complete elimination of all forms or microbial life, including spores and viruses. Disinfection, the selective removal of microbial life, is divided into 3 classes:

High-Level Disinfection: Destruction/removal of all microorganisms except bacterial spores.

Mid-Level Disinfection: Inactivation of *Mycobacterium tuberculosis*, bacteria, most viruses, and most fungi and some bacterial spores.

Low-Level Disinfection: Destruction of most bacteria, some viruses, and some fungi. Low-level disinfection will not necessarily inactivate *M tuberculosis* or bacterial spores.

The following specific recommendations are made for the use of endocavitary ultrasound transducers. Users should also review the Centers for Disease Control and Prevention (CDC) document on sterilization and disinfection of medical devices to be certain that their procedures conform to the CDC principles for disinfection of patient care equipment.

1. Cleaning: After removal of the probe cover, use running water to remove any residual gel or debris from the probe. Use a damp gauze pad or other soft cloth and a small amount of mild nonabrasive liquid soap (household dishwashing liquid is ideal) to thoroughly cleanse the transducer. Consider the use of a small brush especially for crevices and areas of angulation depending on the design of your particular transducer. Rinse the transducer thoroughly with running water, and then dry the transducer with a soft cloth or paper towel.

2. Disinfection: Cleaning with a detergent/water solution as described above is important as the first step in proper disinfection since chemical disinfectants act more rapidly on clean surfaces. However, the additional use of a high-level liquid disinfectant will ensure further statistical reduction in the microbial load. Because of the potential disruption of the barrier sheath, additional high-level disinfection with chemical agents is necessary. Examples of such high-level disinfectants include but are not limited to

   a. 2.4% to 3.2% glutaraldehyde products (a variety of available proprietary products, including Cidex, Metricide, and Procide).

   b. Non-glutaraldehyde agents, including Cidex OPA (*o*-phthalaldehyde) and Cidex PA (hydrogen peroxide and peroxyacetic acid).

   c. 7.5% hydrogen peroxide solution.

   d. Common household bleach (5.25% sodium hypochlorite) diluted to yield 500 parts per million chlorine (10 cc in 1 L of tap water). This agent is effective but generally not recommended by probe manufacturers because it can damage metal and plastic parts.

   Other agents such as quaternary ammonium compounds are not considered high-level disinfectants and should not be used. Isopropanol is not a high-level disinfectant when used as a wipe, and probe manufacturers generally do not recommend soaking probes in the liquid.

   The FDA has published a list of approved sterilants and high-level disinfectants for reprocessing reusable medical and dental devices. That list can be consulted to identify agents that may be useful for probe disinfection.

   Practitioners should consult the labels of proprietary products for specific instructions. They should also consult instrument manufacturers regarding compatibility of these agents with probes. Many of the chemical disinfectants are potentially toxic, and many require adequate precautions such as proper ventilation, personal protective devices (gloves, face/eye protection, etc) and thorough rinsing before reuse of the probe.

3. Probe Covers: The transducer should be covered with a barrier. If the barriers used are condoms, these should be non-lubricated and non-medicated. Practitioners should be aware that condoms have been shown to be less prone to leakage than commercial probe covers and have a 6-fold enhanced acceptable quality level (AQL) when compared to standard examination gloves. They have an AQL equal to that of surgical gloves. Users should be aware of latex sensitivity issues and have available non–latex-containing barriers.

4. Aseptic Technique: For the protection of the patient and the health care worker, all endocavitary examinations should be performed with the operator properly gloved throughout the procedure. Gloves should be used to remove the condom or other barrier from the transducer and to wash the transducer as outlined above. As the barrier (condom) is removed, care should be taken not to contaminate the probe with secretions from the patient. At the completion of the procedure, hands should be thoroughly washed with soap and water.

Note: An obvious disruption in condom integrity does not require modification of this protocol. These guidelines take into account possible probe contamination due to a disruption in the barrier sheath. In summary, routine high-level disinfection of the endocavitary probe between patients plus the use of a probe cover or condom during each examination is required to properly protect patients from infection during endocavitary examinations. For all chemical disinfectants, precautions must be taken to protect workers and patients from the toxicity of the disinfectant.

Clinical Data Sheets

Many practitioners use clinical data sheets to collect specific information related to the exam, including information about other imaging tests. As illustrated in the following samples, these forms should address the patient's physical symptoms as well as laboratory tests, history, and results from other imaging modalities.

Pelvic Ultrasound Worksheet

X-ray Number: _____   Date: _____

Patient Name: _____   Age: _____
Referring Physician: _____
Indication: _____
LMP: _____   G: _____ P: _____ Ab: _____

Pelvic Structures Seen:

Normal   Abnormal
( )   ( )   **Uterus Measurements:**

Long: _____ cm   AP: _____ cm   Trans: _____ cm

Technical Observations: _____
_____

( )   ( )   **Right Ovary Measurements:**

Long: _____ cm   AP: _____ cm   Trans: _____ cm

Technical Observations: _____
_____

( )   ( )   **Left Ovary Measurements:**

Long: _____ cm   AP: _____ cm   Trans: _____ cm

Technical Observations: _____
_____

Technical Observations: _____
_____

Sonographer: _____, RDMS

AMERICAN SOCIETY FOR REPRODUCTIVE MEDICINE
REVISED CLASSIFICATION OF ENDOMETRIOSIS

Patient's Name _____   Date _____

Stage I (Minimal)   - 1–5
Stage II (Mild)   - 6–15
Stage III (Moderate) - 16–40
Stage IV (Severe)   - >40

Laparoscopy _____ Laparotomy _____ Photography _____
Recommended Treatment _____
_____

Total _____   Prognosis _____

PERITONEUM	ENDOMETRIOSIS	< 1cm	1–3cm	> 3cm
	Superficial	1	2	4
	Deep	2	4	6
OVARY	R Superficial	1	2	4
	Deep	4	16	20
	L Superficial	1	2	4
	Deep	4	16	20

	POSTERIOR CULDESAC OBLITERATION	Partial	Complete
		4	40

	ADHESIONS	< 1/3 Enclosure	1/3–2/3 Enclosure	> 2/3 Enclosure
OVARY	R Filmy	1	2	4
	Dense	4	8	16
	L Filmy	1	2	4
	Dense	4	8	16
TUBE	R Filmy	1	2	4
	Dense	4*	8*	16
	L Filmy	1	2	4
	Dense	4*	8*	16

*If the fimbriated end of the fallopian tube is completely enclosed, change the point assignment to 16.
Denote appearance of superficial implant types as red [(R), red, red-pink, flamelike, vesicular blobs, clear vesicles], white [(W), opacifications, peritoneal defects, yellow-brown], or black [(B) black, hemosiderin deposits, blue]. Denote percent of total described as R ___%, W ___% and B ___%. Total should equal 100%.

Additional Endometriosis: _____
_____
_____
_____

Associated Pathology: _____
_____
_____
_____

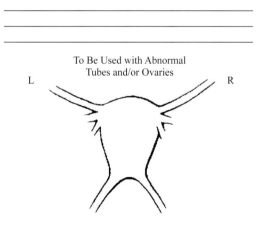

To Be Used with Normal
Tubes and Ovaries

To Be Used with Abnormal
Tubes and/or Ovaries

American Society for Reproductive Medicine *Revised ASRM classification: 1996*

EXAMPLES & GUIDELINES

STAGE I (MINIMAL)

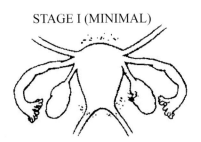

PERITONEUM
  Superficial Endo – 1–3cm +2
R. OVARY
  Superficial Endo – < 1cm +1
  Filmy Adhesions – < 1/3 +1
      TOTAL POINTS 4

STAGE II (MILD)

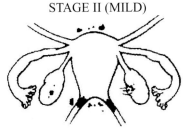

PERITONEUM
  Deep Endo – < 3cm +6
R. OVARY
  Superficial Endo – < 1cm +1
  Filmy Adhesions – < 1/3 +1
L. OVARY
  Superficial Endo – < 1cm +1
      TOTAL POINTS 9

STAGE III (MODERATE)

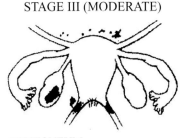

PERITONEUM
  Deep Endo – > 3cm +6
CULDESAC
  Partial Obliteration – +4
L. OVARY
  Deep Endo – 1–3cm +16
      TOTAL POINTS 26

STAGE III (MODERATE)

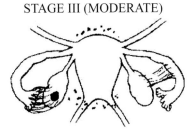

PERITONEUM
  Superficial Endo – > 3cm +4
R. TUBE
  Filmy Adhesions – < 1/3 +1
R. OVARY
  Filmy Adhesions – < 1/3 +1
L. TUBE
  Dense Adhesions – < 1/3 +16*
L. OVARY
  Deep Endo – < 1cm +4
  Dense Adhesions – < 1/3 +4
      TOTAL POINTS 30

STAGE IV (MILD)

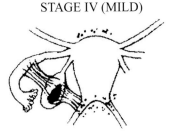

PERITONEUM
  Superficial Endo – > 3cm +4
L. OVARY
  Deep Endo – 1–3cm +32**
  Dense Adhesions – < 1/3 +8**
L. TUBE
  Dense Adhesions – < 1/3 +8**
      TOTAL POINTS 52

*Point assignment changed to 16
**Point assignment doubled

STAGE IV (MODERATE)

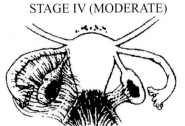

PERITONEUM
  Deep Endo – > 3cm +6
CULDESAC
  Complete Obliteration +40
R. OVARY
  Deep Endo – 1–3cm +16
  Dense Adhesions – < 1/3 +4
L. TUBE
  Dense Adhesions – > 2/3 +16
L. OVARY
  Deep Endo – 1–3cm +16
  Dense Adhesions – > 2/3 +16
      TOTAL POINTS 114

Determination of the stage or degree of endometrial involvement is based on a weighted point system. Distribution of points has been arbitrarily determined and may require further revision or refinement as knowledge of the disease increases.

To ensure complete evaluation, inspection of the pelvis in a clockwise or counterclockwise fashion is encouraged. Number, size and location of endometrial implants, plaques, endometriomas and/or adhesions are noted. For example, five separate 0.5cm superficial implants on the peritoneum (2.5 cm total) would be assigned 2 points. (The surface of the uterus should be considered peritoneum.) The severity of the endometriosis or adhesions should be assigned the highest score only for peritoneum, ovary, tube or culdesac. For example, a 4cm superficial and a 2cm deep implant of the peritoneum should be given a score of 6 (not 8). A 4cm deep endometrioma of the ovary associated with more than 3cm of superficial disease should be scored 20 (not 24).

In those patients with only one adnexa, points applied to disease of the remaining tube and ovary should be multipled by two. **Points assigned may be circled and totaled. Aggregation of points indicates stage of disease (minimal, mild, moderate, or severe).

The presence of endometriosis of the bowel, urinary tract, fallopian tube, vagina, cervix, skin etc., should be documented under "additional endometriosis." Other pathology such as tubal occlusion, leiomyomata, uterine anomaly, etc., should be documented under "associated pathology." All pathology should be depicted as specifically as possible on the sketch of pelvic organs, and means of observation (laparoscopy or laparotomy) should be noted.

Property of the American Society for Reproductive Medicine 1996

For additional supply write to: American Society for Reproductive Medicine,
1209 Montgomery Highway, Birmingham, Alabama 35216

American Society for Reproductive Medicine *Revised ASRM classification: 1996*   *Fertlity and Sterility®*

Chart #_____/

Institute of Ultrasound Diagnostics
Diagnostic Ultrasound Service

Patient #_____/

Patient Name _____ Age _____ Date _____

Referring Physician _____ Initial Exam _____ Repeat _____

Indication _____

G _____ P _____ Ab _____ LMP _____/_____/_____ Clinical EDC _____/_____/_____

Technical Observations _____

_____

_____

Gestation	**Presentation**	**Fetal Biometry**	**Fetal Activity**
( ) Single	( ) Cephalic	CRL	
( ) Twin	( ) Breech	____ mm ____ wks ± _____	Yes No
( ) Other	( ) Transverse	BPD	( ) ( ) Limb
	( ) Oblique	____ mm ____ wks ± _____	( ) ( ) Cardiac
	( ) Variable	HC	( ) ( ) Resp.

Gestation
( ) Single
( ) Twin
( ) Other

Presentation
( ) Cephalic
( ) Breech
( ) Transverse
( ) Oblique
( ) Variable

Amniotic Fluid
( ) Normal
( ) Oligohydramnios
( ) Polyhydramnios

Fetal Biometry
CRL
____ mm ____ wks ± _____
BPD
____ mm ____ wks ± _____
HC
____ mm ____ wks ± _____
AC
____ mm ____ wks ± _____
Femur Length
____ mm ____ wks ± _____

Fetal Activity
Yes No
( ) ( ) Limb
( ) ( ) Cardiac
( ) ( ) Resp.
Amniocentesis
( ) Yes
( ) No

Placenta
( ) Anterior   ( ) Rt
( ) Posterior   ( ) Lt
( ) Fundal
     ( ) Previa
     ( ) Marginal
     ( ) Partial
     ( ) Total

Fetal Anatomy
Yes No
( ) ( ) Kidneys   1   2
( ) ( ) Bladder
( ) ( ) Extremities   1   2   3   4
( ) ( ) Stomach
( ) ( ) Spine

Ultrasound EDC

_____/_____/_____

EFA _____ wks _____ da
EFW _____ grms

Comments _____

Impression _____

Radiologist _____ M.D.

Department of Radiology
Evaluation Form

Name: _____

Date: _____

Fetal Number: _____

History:

G. _____ P. _____ LMP _____ EDC _____

Other: _____

Ultrasound Findings: LMP _____ EDC _____

Measurements:

	mm sac	mm CRL	mm BPD	CI	mm Femur	mm AD#1	mm AD#2	HC	AC	Est. Wt.
Baby A										
Baby B										
Baby C										
Baby D										

Average Weeks:

Baby A _____ Baby B _____ Baby C _____ Baby D _____

Presentation:

	Baby A	Baby B	Baby C	Baby D
Cephalic				
Breech				
Transverse				
Oblique				
Variable				

Amniotic Fluid:

Normal _____ Polyhydramnios _____ Oligohydramnios _____

Placenta Location:

Previa _____ Marginal _____ Partial _____ Total _____

Sonographer: _____

Comments: _____

_____

_____

OB Sheet

X-RAY #_____

Patient Name_____ **Age**_____ **Date**_____

Referring Physician_____ **Initial Exam**_____ **Repeat**_____

Indication_____

_____

GESTATION	**PRESENTATION**	**FETAL ACTIVITY**	**AMNIOTIC FLUID**
( ) Single	( ) Cephalic	**YES NO**	( ) Normal
( ) Twin	( ) Breech	( ) ( ) Limb	( ) Oligohydramnios
( ) Other	( ) Transverse	( ) ( ) Cardiac	( ) Polyhydramnios
	( ) Oblique	( ) ( ) 4 Chamber	AFI _____
	( ) Variable		

PLACENTA   **FETAL ANATOMY**

PLACENTA	FETAL ANATOMY	
( ) Anterior	**YES NO**	**HEART RATE** _____ **BPM**
( ) Posterior	( ) ( ) Kidneys 1 2	
( ) Fundal	( ) ( ) Bladder	
( ) Rt Wrap	( ) ( ) Extremities 1 2 3 4	
( ) Lt Wrap	( ) ( ) Stomach	
( ) Previa	( ) ( ) Spine	
( ) Marginal		
( ) Partial	( ) ( ) Yolk Sac	
( ) Total		

FETAL BIOMETRY   **ULTRASOUND EDC**   **LMP   EDC**

CRL _____ mm _____ wks _____   _____/_____/_____   _____/_____/_____

BPD _____ mm _____ wks _____   EFA _____ wks _____ days _____   EFA _____ wks _____ days _____

HC _____ mm _____ wks _____   EFW_____grams   LMP_____/_____/_____

AC _____ mm _____ wks _____   _____ lbs _____ oz

FL _____ mm _____ wks _____   Last US _____ at _____wks   INTERVAL_____wks

Technical Observations_____

_____

_____

Exam Date: _____

1st TRIMESTER OBSTETRICAL ULTRASOUND
Sonographer's Findings

Gravida: _____   Para: _____   Abortion: _____   Miscarriages: _____ (at Week # _____)

Pre-gestational Diabetes / Gestational Diabetes   Y   N   Hypertension   Y   N   Fertility Therapy   Y   N

Reason for Exam: _____

_____

LMP: _____ / _____ / _____ = _____ wks by dates

Prior Scan: ❑ Y   ❑ N

If Yes, Date of 1st Scan: _____ / _____ / _____

Mean Ultrasound Age (1st Scan) _____ wks + Interval of _____ wks = (Ultrasound Age Today _____ wks)

Gest Sac Size: _____ mm × _____ mm × _____ mm

Avg. Diam: _____ mm = (mean _____ wks) (range _____ to _____ wks)

Borders of the Sac: ❑ Normal   ❑ Abnormal

Yolk Sac Seen?   Y   N

Normal Yolk Sac?   Y   N

Embryo / Fetus Seen?   Y   N

Heart Motion Seen?   Y   N

CRL: _____ mm = (mean _____ wks) (range _____ to _____ wks)

| Uterine Mass: Y   N | Adnexal Mass: Y   N | Cul-de-sac Fluid: Y   N |

Comments: _____

_____

_____

Sonographer: _____

2nd and 3rd Trimester Obstetrical Ultrasound Preliminary Worksheet

NAME: _____ DATE: _____ ID: _____ AGE: _____

HISTORY: _____ TECH: _____

CLINICAL DATES

LMP: _____ - _____ - _____

MA: _____w_____d

EDD: _____ - _____ - _____

DATES BY 1st ULTRASOUND

MA: _____w_____d

EDD: _____ - _____ - _____

DATES BY TODAY'S ULTRASOUND

MA: _____w_____d

EDD: _____ - _____ - _____

TODAY'S MEASUREMENTS

	1	2	Avg (cm)	Avg Weeks
BPD:	____	____	_____	____w____d
HC:	____	____	_____	____w____d
AC:	____	____	_____	____w____d
FL:	____	____	_____	____w____d

FHR: _____bpm

EFW: _____ grams (_____ lbs _____oz)

AFI: _____cm

RATIOS   Normal Range

CI: _____   (_____ – _____)

FL/BPD: _____   (_____ – _____)

FL/BC: _____   (_____ – _____)

FL/AC: _____   (_____ – _____)

BC/AC: _____   (_____ – _____)

FETAL NUMBER: _____

PRESENTATION: _____

PLACENTAL LOC: _____

PLACENTAL GRADE: ___0 ___1 ___2 ___3

FETAL MOVEMENT: _____

THREE VESSEL CORD: _____

CORD INSERTION: _____ nl _____ abn

4 CHAMBER HEART: _____

FETAL STOMACH: _____

FETAL BLADDER: _____

FETAL KIDNEYS: _____

FETAL SPINE: _____

LATERAL VENTRICLES: _____ nl _____ abn

CEREBELLUM: _____ nl _____ abn

CISTERNA MAGNA: _____ nl _____ abn

RT OV: _____

RT ADNEXA: _____

LT OV: _____

LT ADNEXA: _____

UTERUS: _____

CUL-DE-SAC: _____

CERVICAL LENGTH: _____ cm

COMMENTS: _____

_____

_____

_____

Exam Date: _____

2nd & 3rd TRIMESTER OBSTETRICAL ULTRASOUND
Sonographer's Findings

Gravida: _____ Para: _____ Abortion: _____ Miscarriages: _____ (at Week # _____)

Pre-gestational Diabetes / Gestational Diabetes Y N   Hypertension Y N   Pre-term Labor / Pre-term Delivery Y N

LMP: _____ / _____ / _____ = _____ wks by dates

Reason for Exam (prior OB History, Fetal anomalies, etc.): _____

Date of 1st Scan: _____ / _____ / _____

Mean Age at 1st Ultrasound _____ wks + Interval of _____ wks = Ultrasound Age Today _____ wks

---

BPD _____ mm = (mean _____ wks) (range _____ to _____ wks)

CEPH Index   (BPD _____ / FOD _____) × 100 = _____ (normal range 74–83)

BPD _____ mm = (mean _____ wks) (range _____ to _____ wks)

HC _____ mm = (mean _____ wks) (range _____ to _____ wks)

AC _____ mm = (mean _____ wks) (range _____ to _____ wks)

FL _____ mm = (mean _____ wks) (range _____ to _____ wks)

HC: AC _____ ( ) Normal   ( ) Abnormal   FL Proportionate to BPD   Y   N

Fetal Weight: _____ gm ± 15%   Percentile: _____ % for Gestational Age of _____ wks

---

( ) Singleton   ( ) Twin   ( ) Other

Fetal Position: ( ) CEP ( ) BRC ( ) TRV ( ) OBL ( ) VAR

Placenta Position: _____

Previa? Y   N

Cervical Length (endovaginal scan) = _____ mm

Amniotic Fluid ( ) WNL ( ) Volume Decreased ( ) Volume Increased

AFI _____ (Percentile _____ %) or Largest AP Pocket _____ mm

Uterine Mass: Y   N   Adnexal Mass: Y   N

	Visualise	WNL
Lateral Ventricles	Y N	Y N
Cerebellum	Y N	Y N
Cisterna Magna	Y N	Y N
Nuchal Fold	(14–20 wks) _____ mm	
Fetal Heart Rate	_____ BPM	
4-Chamber Heart	Y N	Y N
Outflow Tracts	Y N	Y N
Spine	Y N	Y N
Stomach	Y N	Y N
Kidneys	Y N	Y N
Bladder	Y N	Y N
Cord Insertion	Y N	Y N
3 – VC	Y N	Y N
4 Extremities	Y N	Y N

Date of Last Study: _____ / _____ / _____   Interval Since Last Study _____ wks

Mean GA (today) _____ + Mean GA (last) _____) ÷ 2 = Mean GA _____

BPD (today) _____ mm − BPD* (last) _____ mm = (growth) _____ mm ÷ interval _____ wks = _____ mm/wk

AC (today) _____ mm − AC (last) _____ mm = (growth) _____ mm ÷ interval _____ wks = _____ mm/wk

BPD Percentile _____ %   AC Percentile _____ %

* Use corrected BPD if CI < 74 or > 83)

Umbilical Artery (RI:) (S/D:)	MCA RI:	UA$_{RI}$: MCA$_{RI}$ _____ (normal ratio > 1.1)
( ) Near Fetus ( ) Mid Cord ( ) Near Placenta	Velocity:	( ) Normal ( ) Abnormal

Sonographer: _____

SECOND AND THIRD TRIMESTER STAGE / OBSTETRICAL ULTRASOUND REPORT

PATIENT NAME _____

☐ INITIAL EXAM
☐ REPEAT EXAM

PATIENT I.D. NO. _____

EXAM DATE: ☐☐ ☐☐ ☐☐
MO   DAY   YEAR

LMP DATE: ☐☐ ☐☐ ☐☐
MO   DAY   YEAR

UNKNOWN ☐

SMOKER: ☐ YES   ☐ NO

PATIENT AGE: ☐ YRS   RACE: ☐   HEIGHT: ☐ ft. ☐ in.   WEIGHT: ☐ lbs.

INDICATION CODE NUMBER: ☐

G ☐ P ☐☐☐☐
F P A L

ESTIMATED CLINICAL DATES: ☐ **WEEKS**

DESCRIPTIVE DATA SECTION

THE FETUS

Number: ☐ 1 ☐ 2 ☐ 3
Presentation: ☐ VTX ☐ BREECH
☐ Transverse ☐ Other

Activity: ☐ Heart ☐ Body
☐ Breathing

Gender: ☐ Male ☐ Female
☐ Unknown

PELVIC MASS
☐ None Seen
☐ Present (Describe): _____
_____
_____

THE PLACENTA

Location: ☐ Anterior   ☐ Posterior
☐ R Lateral   ☐ L Lateral

Height: ☐ Fundal   ☐ High
☐ Mid   ☐ Low
☐ Marginal Previa
☐ Partial Previa
☐ Complete Previa

Grade 3: ☐ No   ☐ Yes

UTERUS PATHOLOGY
☐ None Seen
☐ Present (Describe): _____
_____
_____

AMNIOTIC FLUID AMOUNT
☐ Normal
☐ Increased
☐ Decreased

EXAM TECHNICAL QUALITY
☐ Good   ☐ Fair   ☐ Poor

FETAL BLADDER / KIDNEYS
☐ Bladder Only Seen
☐ Kidneys Only Seen
☐ Both Seen
☐ Neither Seen

Abnormal fetal anatomy seen or suspected: ☐ No ☐ Yes (Describe): _____
Second opinion ultrasound consultation planned: ☐ No ☐ Yes

MEASUREMENTS AND CALCULATION SECTION

BPD ☐ cms   OFD ☐ cms   A-PAD ☐ cms   TAD ☐ cms   FEMUR ☐ cms

Head Circumference ☐ cms   Abdominal Circumference ☐ cms

RESULTS AND INTERPRETATION SECTION

ULTRASOUND AGE ESTIMATE

BPD Weeks = ☐
Femur Weeks = ☐
ABD Circ Weeks = ☐
Head Circ Weeks = ☐
Average Estimated
Gestational Age = ☐

ULTRASOUND FETAL WEIGHT ESTIMATE

☐ grams

☐ lbs/oz

RATIOS

Cephalic Index = ☐ %

Femur/BPD = ☐ %

Head Circ/
Abd. Circ = ☐ %

REMARKS: _____

_____

GESTATIONAL AGE
☐ Good Clinical Dates   ☐ Poor Clinical Dates

WEIGHT FOR DATES
☐ AGA   ☐ LGA   ☐ SGA

_____
Signature of Responsible Physician

Twin OB Ultrasound Worksheet

X-RAY #_____   Date _____

Patient Name _____ Age _____

Referring Physician _____ Initial Exam _____ Repeat _____

Indication _____

G_____ P_____ Ab _____ LMP____ / ____ / ____ Clinical EDC____ / ____ / ____

PRESENTATION

Baby	A	B
Cephalic	( )	( )
Breech	( )	( )
Transverse	( )	( )
Oblique	( )	( )
Variable	( )	( )

FETAL ACTIVITY

Baby	A Y	A N	B Y	B N
Limb	( )	( )	( )	( )
Cardiac	( )	( )	( )	( )
4 Chamber Heart	( )	( )	( )	( )
Respirations	( )	( )	( )	( )

AMNIOTIC FLUID

( ) Normal
( ) Oligohydramnios
( ) Polyhydramnios

PLACENTA

( ) Anterior
( ) Posterior
( ) Fundal
( ) Rt Wrap
( ) Lt Wrap
( ) Previa
( ) Marginal
( ) Partial
( ) Total

FETAL ANATOMY

Baby	A Y	A N	B Y	B N
Renals	( )	( )	( )	( )
Bladder	( )	( )	( )	( )
Extremities	1 2 3 4		1 2 3 4	
Stomach	( )	( )	( )	( )
Spine	( )	( )	( )	( )

Draw Fetal Presentation

FETAL BIOMETRY Baby A

CRL _____ mm _____ wks _____
BPD _____ mm _____ wks _____
HC _____ mm _____ wks _____
AC _____ mm _____ wks _____
FL _____ mm _____ wks _____

ULTRASOUND EDC Baby A

_____ / _____ / _____
EFA _____ wks _____ days _____
EFW_____ grams
_____ lbs _____ oz

FETAL BIOMETRY Baby B

CRL _____ mm _____ wks _____
BPD _____ mm _____ wks _____
HC _____ mm _____ wks _____
AC _____ mm _____ wks _____
FL _____ mm _____ wks _____

ULTRASOUND EDC Baby B

_____ / _____ / _____
EFA _____ wks _____ days _____
EFW_____ grams
_____ lbs _____ oz

Comments: _____
_____
_____
_____
_____
_____
_____
_____
_____

Sonographer: _____

Glossary

Editor's note: The terms and concepts defined below, which are explained in the text and discussed in sonographic contexts, are fully defined under both spelled-out and abbreviated versions for the reader's convenience. Chapter numbers appear at the ends of most entries to reference places in this volume where these concepts receive significant discussion; in cases where the term is used in passing throughout the text, chapter references are omitted. Finally, "see also" cross-references direct readers to related terms defined in this glossary.

A

abdominal circumference (**AC**)—The circumference of the fetal abdomen, as measured by most modern instruments but also calculated as the sum of anterior/posterior diameter and abdominal diameter times a correction factor of 1.62 or 1.57 (depending on the authority used). *Chapter 4.*

abdominal ectopic pregnancy—Also known as a tubal pregnancy, a pregnancy in which the fertilized egg is expelled out of the fallopian tube into the pelvic cavity, where it communicates with the abdominal cavity, allowing the zygote to migrate into the abdomen, attach itself to something vascular, and grow. *Chapter 3.*

abducted thumb—An outward-turned thumb, often referred to as the "hitchhiker" thumb, associated with diastrophic dwarfism. *Chapter 11. See also* adducted thumb; diastrophic dwarfism.

abnormal uterine bleeding (**AUB**)—Uterine bleeding that is not part of the normal ovarian cycle, which can result from a variety of conditions, such as endocrine disorders, growths, and medications. *Chapter 2. See also* dysfunctional uterine bleeding.

abortion—Premature expulsion of the embryo or fetus, including the placenta, from the uterus. *Chapter 3.*

- *complete/spontaneous a.*—Emptying of the endometrial cavity before 20 weeks, which is the earliest point that the fetus generally can arrive on its own; hCG levels tend to fall rapidly.

- *elective a.*—Legal, deliberate medical termination of pregnancy.

- *habitual a.*—Three or more consecutive spontaneous pregnancy losses prior to the 20th week of gestation.

- *incomplete a.*—Bleeding and cramping with retention of some of the products of conception.

- *induced or medical a.*—Ingestion of antiprogesterone mifepristone (RU486) to induce abortion.

- *inevitable a.*—Positive pregnancy test with bleeding, cramping, and dilated cervix.

- *missed a.*—Demise of embryo/fetus with failure to expel.

- *threatened a.*—Positive pregnancy test with bleeding and cramping.

abruption placenta—Premature separation of the placenta from the uterine wall; also known as abruptio placentae or placental abruption. *Chapter 5.*

abruptio placentae—Abruption placenta.

abscess—A localized collection of pus. *Chapters 1, 2.*

AC—Abdominal circumference: the circumference of the fetal abdomen, as measured by most modern instruments but also calculated as the sum of anterior/posterior diameter and abdominal diameter times a correction factor of 1.62 or 1.57 (depending on the authority used). *Chapter 4.*

acardia—Congenital absence of the heart. A fetus suffering from acardia may be referred to as an acardiac monster. *Chapter 9.*

acardiac parabiotic twinning—A condition in which one twin has normal circulation but must provide circulation for the other twin; also known as twin reversed arterial perfusion (TRAP) sequence. *Chapter 9.*

acardius acephalus—An acardiac twin exhibiting a lower body and extremities only. *Chapter 9.*

acardius acormus—An acardiac twin exhibiting a head only. *Chapter 9.*

acardius amorphus—An acardiac twin exhibited as a lump of teratomatous tissue. *Chapter 9.*

acardius anceps—An acardiac twin with a head, body, and acetylcholinesterase—the enzyme present in the nervous tissue, muscle, and red blood cells. *Chapter 9.*

accessory ovary—An ectopic ovary located near a normal ovary, attached to it either directly or in the adjacent broad ligament. *Chapter 2. See also* ectopic ovaries.

achondrogenesis—A very rare skeletal dysplasia characterized by extreme short-limbed dwarfism and lack of development of the ribs and other major bone formations. *Chapter 7.*

achondroplasia—The most common genetic disorder of bone growth evident at birth, characterized by short arms and legs and normal torso dimensions. *Chapter 7.*

acoustic window—Any medium (tissue) or structure of the body that transmits sound well. *Chapter 1.*

acquisition artifacts—Artifacts that occur during volume sonography in the imaging process; in obstetrics and gynecology, the most common are motion artifacts, such as sudden fetal movement during a slow acquisition of data. *Chapter 14.*

acrania—The absence of the ossified cranium, with the brain intact and usually well defined. *Chapter 7.*

adducted thumb—A thumb turned inward, toward the palm, associated with aqueductal stenosis. *Chapter 11. See also* abducted thumb; aqueductal stenosis; diastrophic dwarfism.

adenomatous polyp—A polyp that is typically a benign pedunculated or sessile projection of the endometrium, associated with heavy and painful if normal menstrual flow. *Chapter 2.*

adenomyosis—Also referred to as internal endometriosis, a condition in which the endometrium invades and grows into the myometrium. *Chapter 2.*

adnexa—In gynecology, the structures adjacent to or accessories of the uterus, such as the ovaries, fallopian tubes, and ligaments that secure the uterus; also known as adnexa uteri. *Chapters 2, 10, 14.*

adnexal masses—Lumps of tissue in the uterine adnexa (ovaries or fallopian tubes). *Chapter 10.*

adnexal torsion—Twisting of the ovary and sometimes the fallopian tube on the ligament-like structures that support them, cutting off blood flow to these organs. *Chapter 12.*

adult polycystic kidney disease (APKD)—An autosomal dominant polycystic kidney disease also known as Potter type III; it may affect the liver, pancreas, and spleen. *Chapter 8.*

advanced maternal age (AMA)—A maternal age of 35 years or more at delivery. *Chapter 11.*

AFI—Amniotic fluid index: a four-quadrant calculation to assess amniotic fluid volume quantitatively. *Chapter 4.*

AFP—Alpha-fetoprotein: plasma protein produced by the fetal liver, yolk sac, and gastrointestinal tract. *Chapter 11.*

agenesis—Failure to form. *Chapters 2, 4, 7, 8. See also* renal agenesis; uterine agenesis.

agonist—A drug that has an affinity for the cellular receptors of another drug or natural substance that produces the same physiologic effect. *Chapter 13.*

allantoic cyst—A cystic dilatation of the primitive embryonic allantois. *Chapter 5.*

allantois—A membranous outpouching from the caudal wall of the yolk sac that is involved in early blood production, gives rise to the umbilical blood vessels, and contributes to the formation of the urinary bladder, after which it obliterates to form the fibrous cord known as the urachus. *Chapter 3.*

alobar holoprosencephaly—Holoprosencephaly in which the lateral ventricles are fused, forming a large single ventricle that is horseshoe-shaped; the severest form of cleavage failure of the forebrain before 6 weeks' gestation. *Chapter 7. See also* holoprosencephaly; lobar holoprosencephaly; semilobar holoprosencephaly.

alpha-fetoprotein (**AFP**)—Plasma protein produced by the fetal liver, yolk sac, and gastrointestinal tract. *Chapter 11.*

alpha thalassemia—A lethal type of fetal hydrops seen in patients of Asian descent. *Chapter 10. See also* fetal hydrops.

Alzheimer disease—Irreversible senile dementia. *Chapter 11.*

AMA—Advanced maternal age: a maternal age of 35 years or more at delivery. *Chapter 11.*

amenorrhea—Absence or abnormal cessation of the menses. *Chapter 2.*

amniocentesis—A sonography-guided procedure in which a needle is inserted into the uterus through the abdomen and a sample of amniotic fluid is withdrawn for the purpose of fetal genetic testing and determining fetal lung maturity. *Chapters 11, 15.*

amnioinfusion—A sonography-guided invasive technique in which fluid, typically normal saline, is infused into the uterine cavity to improve visualization of the fetus with severe oligohydramnios or anhydramnios. *Chapter 15.*

amnion—The innermost membrane enclosing the developing embryo/fetus. *Chapter 3.*

amnionitis—Inflammation of the amniotic membrane. *Chapter 6.*

amnioreduction—A sonography-guided invasive procedure similar to amniocentesis in which amniotic fluid is removed in order to reduce its volume. *Chapter 15.*

amniotic band—A thin strand of amniotic tissue that develops when the amnion separates from the chorion. It can attach to and wrap around fetal parts, causing strictures, deformities, and amputations. *Chapter 5. See also* amniotic sheets.

amniotic band syndrome—Persistent separation of the amnion from the chorion, whereby the amnion may adhere to fetal parts, impeding movement, becoming entangled or wrapped around fetal structures, and causing deformities and/or disruption of normal development. *Chapters 5, 11.*

amniotic cavity—The slit-like structure that forms during trophoblastic development, when small spaces that appear between the invading trophoblast and the inner cell mass coalesce. *Chapter 3.*

amniotic fluid—The clear, straw-colored, sterile liquid that fills the uterus and surrounds the fetus throughout a pregnancy. *Chapters 4, 7, 8, 10, 11, 15.*

amniotic fluid index (**AFI**)—A four-quadrant calculation to assess amniotic fluid volume quantitatively. *Chapters 4, 8. See also* single deepest pocket method.

amniotic sheets—Synechiae covered over by the amnion and chorion. Amniotic sheets are thicker than amniotic bands, have a free edge that is often globular, and are considered benign. *Chapter 5. See also* amniotic band.

ampulla—A dilated segment of a tubular structure; in gynecology, the longest and widest portion of the fallopian tube. *Chapter 2.*

anasarca—A generalized massive edema. *Chapter 8.*

anastomosis—Interconnectedness of tubular structures; the point at which structures join or are joined surgically. *Chapter 9.*

androblastoma—A solid androgenic ovarian tumor, usually benign; also known as a Sertoli-Leydig tumor. *Chapter 2.*

androgen—Any steroid hormone that promotes male characteristics. *Chapter 2.*

androgenic—Having to do with or producing male traits. *Chapter 2.*

anechoic—Producing no echoes. *Chapter 1.*

anembryonic pregnancy—A pregnancy during which the gestational sac never contained an embryo. *Chapter 3. See also* blighted ovum.

anencephaly—The congenital absence of the brain and cranial vault, with the cerebral hemispheres completely missing or greatly reduced in size. *Chapter 7.*

aneuploidy—A state of having chromosomes in a number that is not an exact multiple of the haploid number. *Chapters 4, 11. See also* haploid number.

angling—Tilting the transducer from side to side; cross-plane motion. *Chapter 1.*

anhydramnios—The absence of amniotic fluid. *Chapter 15.*

annular placenta—A ring-shaped placenta that attaches around the circumference to the myometrium; also known as placenta membranacea. *Chapter 5.*

anomaly—A deviation from normal; an abnormality. *Chapter 1.*

anophthalmia—The congenital absence of the eye. *Chapters 4, 11.*

anorexia—A lack or loss of appetite for food. *Chapter 16.*

anovulation—The absence of ovulation. *Chapters 2, 13.*

antagonist—A drug that binds to a cellular receptor for a hormone, a neurotransmitter, or another drug, blocking the action of that substance without producing any physiologic effect itself. *Chapter 13.*

anteflexed—The position of the uterus when the fundus of the uterus points toward the anterior abdominal wall; when the urinary bladder is empty, the uterus normally is in the anteflexed position with flexion occurring at the cervix. *Chapter 1.*

anterior—Located at or toward the front of the body, often used to indicate the position of one structure in relation to another; near the head of certain embryos. *Chapter 1.*

anterior cul-de-sac—The area between the anterior uterine wall and the posterior bladder; the uterovesical space. *Chapter 2.*

anterior/posterior (AP) plane—The scan plane that divides the body into front and back parts; the coronal plane. *Chapter 1.*

anteverted—The position of the uterus when it is pushed downward as the urinary bladder fills, displacing the surrounding bowel. It remains tilted anteriorly, but the bend at the cervix is unfolded. *Chapter 2.*

antral follicle—A follicle at the final stage in the oocyte development, when the cavity becomes filled with fluid and is sonographically visible. *Chapter 13.*

aortic arch—A prominent arch in the left ventricular outflow tract as it courses superiorly in the fetal thorax and then curves to the right to form the descending aorta. *Chapter 4.*

aortic semilunar valve—A one-way valve with (normally) three crescent-shaped cusps situated where the aorta originates from the left ventricle, preventing backflow of blood into the left ventricle by closing during diastole. *Chapter 4.*

AP—Anteroposterior or anterior/posterior. *Chapter 1.*

Apgar score—An assessment performed five minutes after birth to evaluate five parameters of the newborn: heart rate, respiration, muscle tone, reflexes, and skin color. *Chapter 8.*

APKD—Adult polycystic kidney disease: an autosomal dominant polycystic kidney disease also known as Potter type III; it may affect the liver, pancreas, and spleen. *Chapter 8.*

apposition—Placement or position of adjacent structures or parts so that they can come into contact. *Chapter 5.*

aqueduct of Sylvius—The mesencephalic duct or aqueductus mesencephali, which connects the third and fourth ventricles within the mesencephalon (or midbrain). *Chapter 7.*

aqueductal stenosis—Congenital obstruction of the channel between the third and fourth cerebral ventricles, resulting in enlarged lateral ventricles. *Chapter 7.*

arachnoid cyst—Cerebrospinal fluid–filled sacs lined with arachnoid tissue usually located on the surface of the brain or in the cisterns. *Chapter 7.*

Arnold-Chiari malformation—Chiari's malformation type II, a congenital anomaly almost always associated with spina bifida and hydrocephalus that involves the cerebellum protruding into the cervical spine. *Chapters 4, 7.*

ARPKD—Autosomal recessive polycystic kidney disease. *Chapter 8.*

arrhenoblastoma—A neoplasm (also referred to as an androblastoma or Sertoli-Leydig cell tumor) seen mainly in women in their reproductive years and causing virilism and malignancy in 20% of cases. *Chapter 2.*

arrhythmia—An irregular beating or rhythm of the heart. *Chapter 4.*

ART—Assisted reproductive technology: a variety of techniques including oocyte retrieval/harvesting and transfer of the gametes/zygotes into the uterus or fallopian tubes. *Chapter 13.*

arthrogryposis—A condition characterized by multiple joint contractures. *Chapter 7.*

ascites—An abnormal accumulation of serous fluid within the peritoneal cavity. *Chapters 2, 7.*

ASD—Atrial septal defect: a defect in the wall (septum) separating the right and left atria of the heart. *Chapters 4, 7.*

Asherman syndrome—A condition characterized by amenorrhea and secondary sterility resulting from adhesions and synechiae within the endometrial cavity. *Chapter 2.*

assisted reproductive technology (**ART**)—A variety of techniques including oocyte retrieval/harvesting and transfer of the gametes/zygotes into the uterus or fallopian tubes. *Chapter 13.*

asymmetrical macrosomia—The tendency in diabetic pregnancies for insulin-sensitive tissues to overgrow while non–insulin-sensitive tissues exhibit normal growth. *Chapter 10.*

asynclitism—The obliquity (lack of synclitism or parallelism) of the presenting part of the fetus in relation to the pelvic plane; the presentation of the fetal head at an angle, when the suture lines of the skull are deflected either anteriorly toward the symphysis pubis or posteriorly toward the sacrum. *Chapter 4.*

atrial flutter—An abnormal heart rhythm resulting from the atria of the heart contracting much faster than the ventricles. *Chapter 4.*

atrial septal defect (**ASD**)—A defect in the wall (septum) separating the right and left atria of the heart. *Chapters 4, 7.*

atrial septum—The muscular division between the right and left atria of the heart. *Chapter 4.*

atrioventricular (**AV**) **block**—An arrhythmia in which the atrial rate may be normal but the ventricular rate is often bradycardic. *Chapter 4.*

atrioventricular (**AV**) **valves**—The tricuspid and bicuspid valves, which lie between the atria and the ventricles of the heart and control flow. *Chapter 4.*

atrioventricular canal (**AVC**)—A large hole in the center of the heart that exists where the wall between the upper chambers joins the wall between the lower chambers. *Chapter 7.*

atypical hyperplasia—Abnormal overgrowth of tissue. *Chapter 2.*

AUB—Abnormal uterine bleeding: bleeding not part of the normal ovarian cycle, which can result from a variety of conditions, such as endocrine disorders, growths, and medications. *Chapter 2. See also* dysfunctional uterine bleeding.

autosomal dominant—A genetic pattern indicating a 50% chance of inheritance. *Chapters 8, 11.*

autosomal recessive—A genetic pattern indicating a 25% chance of inheritance. *Chapters 8, 11.*

autosomal recessive polycystic kidney disease (**ARPKD**)—Infantile polycystic kidney disease. *Chapter 8.*

AV block—Atrioventricular block: an arrhythmia in which the atrial rate may be normal but the ventricular rate is often bradycardic. *Chapter 4.*

AV valves—Atrioventricular valves: the tricuspid and bicuspid valves, which lie between the atria and the ventricles of the heart and control flow. *Chapter 4.*

AVC—Atrioventricular canal: a large hole in the center of the heart that exists where the wall between the upper chambers joins the wall between the lower chambers. *Chapter 7.*

B

B-mode diagnostic ultrasound imaging—The two-dimensional gray-scale form of ultrasonography. *Chapter 1.*

banana sign—The displacement and flattening of the cerebellum, making it look like a banana. *Chapter 7.*

BART—An acronym and mnemonic device used to describe blood flow, meaning "blue, away; red, toward" the transducer.

basal body temperature (BBT)—The body's core temperature during rest. *Chapter 13.*

basic scan—The minimum number of images, views, and measurements required to meet the national standard for documentation for an obstetric ultrasound examination. *Chapter 4.*

battledore placenta—A placenta where the umbilical cord inserts at the edge of the placenta. *Chapter 5.*

BBT—Basal body temperature: the body's core temperature during rest. *Chapter 13.*

Beckwith-Wiedemann syndrome—A genetic disorder associated with organomegaly (abnormally large organs) and macroglossia. *Chapter 11.*

benign—Nonmalignant; nonrecurrent; favorable for recovery. *Chapter 1.*

bereavement—Patterns of signs and symptoms associated with mourning. *Chapter 16.*

bicornuate uterus—Malformation of the uterus in which two uterine horns and two endometrial canals appear. *Chapter 2.*

bicuspid valve—A dual-flap valve in the heart that lies between the left atrium and the left ventricle, allowing blood to flow from the left atrium into the left ventricle while preventing backflow; also known as the mitral valve. *Chapter 4.*

Big Mac sign—The term used for the appearance of the fetal labia on sonography, with the buns being the labia and the space between being the patty; also known as the hamburger sign. *Chapter 4.*

bilaminar (embryonic) disc—A cell mass consisting of endoderm and ectoderm. *Chapter 3.*

bilateral renal agenesis (BRA)—Failure of the kidneys to develop, resulting in the fetus's inability to produce urine; also known as classic Potter syndrome. *Chapter 8.*

binocular distance—The distance from the lateral edge of one orbit to the lateral edge of the contralateral orbit; also known as outer orbital distance. *Chapters 4, 11.*

bioeffects—Effects on biologic tissues; in the context of sonography, the effects of ultrasound. *Chapter 12.*

biologic death—The permanent cessation of all life functions. *Chapter 16.*

biophysical profile (BPP)—A profile of the fetus that evaluates fetal well-being using five parameters: fetal heart rate, gross fetal body movements, fetal breathing motion, amniotic fluid level, and fetal tone. *Chapter 8.*

biparietal diameter (BPD)—A measurement of the fetal skull across the widest diameter, from parietal bone to parietal bone. *Chapter 4.*

bipartite placenta—A placenta divided into two relatively equal lobes. *Chapter 5.*

bladder exstrophy—The failure of the lower fetal abdomen to close, allowing the bladder to extend outside the abdomen. *Chapter 7.*

bladder trigone—The posterior aspect of the urinary bladder, where the ureters enter and the urethra exits. *Chapter 2.*

blastocyst—The conceptus in the postmorula stage, consisting of the trophoblast and the inner cell mass. *Chapter 3.*

blastomere—One of the cells produced by cleavage of a fertilized egg. *Chapter 3.*

blighted ovum—A slightly outdated term used to refer to an anembryonic gestation. *Chapter 3. See also* anembryonic pregnancy.

body stalk anomaly—A set of disruptive abnormalities associated with failure of the umbilical cord to develop, including lateral body wall defects involving trunk, spine, and limb anomalies; also known as the limb–body wall complex (LBWC) or VACTERL. *Chapters 5, 7. See also* limb–body wall complex.

bolus—A concentrated mass of material or preparation to be passed through the system. *Chapter 8.*

BPD—Biparietal diameter: a measurement of the fetal skull across the widest diameter, from parietal bone to parietal bone. *Chapter 4.*

BPP—Biophysical profile: a profile of the fetus that evaluates fetal well-being using five parameters: fetal heart rate, gross fetal body movements, fetal breathing motion, amniotic fluid level, and fetal tone. *Chapter 8.*

BRA—Bilateral renal agenesis: failure of the kidneys to develop, resulting in the fetus being unable to produce urine. *Chapter 8.*

brachiocephalic artery—The artery that begins at the aortic arch (first branch) and ends at the bifurcation into the right common carotid and right subclavian arteries. *Chapter 4.*

brachycephaly—A disproportionate shortness of the head, the head being too round; also known as flat head syndrome. *Chapters 4, 11.*

bradycardia—A slow, sluggish heart rate; in the fetus, less than 100 beats per minute. *Chapter 4.*

breech—A fetal position in which the fetal buttocks present at the cervical os. *Chapters 4, 9.*

Brenner tumor—A solid, benign tumor with estrogenic properties. *Chapter 2.*

Breus mole—A large subchorionic hematoma. *Chapter 5.*

broad ligament—A broad, sheet-like structure (actually a fold of peritoneum) attached to each side of the uterus. *Chapter 2.*

C

c-section—Cesarean section: delivery of a fetus by way of incision through the abdominal wall and uterus.

CA-125—Cancer antigen 125: a cancer-screening blood test ordered to help rule out ovarian cancer. *Chapter 2.*

cachexia—A wasting syndrome characterized by the loss of both adipose and musculoskeletal tissue, reflecting profoundly ill health and/or malnutrition. *Chapter 2.*

camptodactyly—The permanent flexion of a finger. *Chapter 11.*

Canavan disease—The spongy deterioration of the central nervous system. *Chapter 11.*

cancer antigen 125 (CA-125)—A cancer-screening blood test ordered to help rule out ovarian cancer. *Chapter 2.*

cardiomegaly—An enlarged heart. *Chapter 7.*

cardiomyopathy—A general diagnostic term used to describe primary myocardial disease; in the context of obstetrics, an enlarged, poorly functioning fetal heart that may be caused by structural defects or flow alterations. *Chapter 7.*

caudal—At or toward the tail. In sonography and medicine, toward the feet or base of the spine. *Chapter 1.*

caudal aplasia/dysplasia sequence—Agenesis of the lower spine or sacrum associated with maternal diabetes

and gastrointestinal/gastrourinary anomalies; also known as caudal regression syndrome. *Chapters 10, 11.*

caudal regression syndrome—Agenesis of the lower spine/sacrum associated with maternal diabetes and gastrointestinal/gastrourinary anomalies; also known as caudal aplasia/dysplasia sequence. *Chapters 10, 11.*

CCAM—Congenital cystic adenomatoid malformation: overgrowth of abnormal lung tissue that may form fluid-filled cysts. There are three types, defined by the amount of fluid-filled cysts in the mass. *Chapter 7.*

CCCT—Clomiphene citrate challenge test: a test to determine whether a patient has a normal ovarian reserve. *Chapter 13.*

cebocephaly—Having a trunk-like nasal structure with a single nostril. *Chapter 11.*

centrum—The body of a vertebra. *Chapter 4.*

cephalic—Pertaining to or in the vicinity of the head. *Chapters 1, 4.*

cephalic index—A calculation performed to determine fetal head shape. *Chapter 4.*

cerclage—A surgical procedure to reinforce the cervix for correction of abnormal cervical competence. *Chapter 6. See also* McDonald purse-string technique; Shirodkar cerclage.

cerebellum—A section of the metencephalon consisting of two lateral hemispheres, separated by the vermis, located posterior in the calvarium. *Chapter 4.*

cerebral peduncles—The ventral (on the underside) half of the midbrain. *Chapter 4.*

cerebral resistivity index (CRI)—A method of evaluating the fetal middle cerebral arteries, calculated on a Doppler spectral waveform obtained from one of the two middle cerebral arteries. *Chapter 12.*

cerebral-umbilical ratio—An indicator of relative resistance between the fetus and the placenta. *Chapter 12.*

cervical—Pertaining to the neck or to the cervix.

cervical canal—The cavity between the internal and external cervical os. *Chapter 6.*

cervical ectopic pregnancy—A pregnancy in a cervical location, with the gestational sac implanted within the endocervical canal. It can be difficult to differentiate from an inevitable abortion. *Chapter 3.*

cervical incompetence—Passive premature cervical dilation, a leading cause of second trimester pregnancy loss. *Chapter 5.*

cervical os—The opening to the cervix, including the internal os, on the uterine side, and the external os, on the vaginal side. *Chapters 2, 6.*

cervical pregnancy—A rare form of ectopic pregnancy in the cervix, occurring in approximately 1 in 8500 deliveries. *Chapter 6.*

cervical vertebrae—The bones of the neck. *Chapter 4.*

cervix—The neck of the uterus. *Chapter 2.*

cesarean section (**c-section**)—Delivery of a fetus by way of incision through the abdominal wall and uterus. *Chapter 4.*

chocolate cyst—A walled-off collection of old blood from bleeding ectopic endometrial tissues; also known as an endometrioma. *Chapter 2.*

cholecystitis—Inflammation of the gallbladder. *Chapter 10.*

chordae tendineae—Complex cords, connected to the posterior surface of the atrioventricular valves, that function to open and close the leaflets. *Chapter 4.*

chorioadenoma destruens—An invasive mole that rarely metastasizes. *Chapter 3.*

chorioangioma—A benign vascular neoplasm of the placenta. *Chapter 5.*

choriocarcinoma—A malignant neoplasm of trophoblastic cells formed by abnormal proliferation of the placental epithelium without production of chorionic villi. *Chapters 3, 12.*

chorion—The outermost part of the fetal membranes, composed of trophoblastic cells lined with mesoderm, from which the placenta develops. *Chapters 3, 5, 9.*

chorion frondosum—The part of the chorion covered by villi; also known as the villous chorion. *Chapter 5.*

chorionic plate—The portion of the chorion related directly to the placenta. *Chapter 5.*

chorionic villi (*sing.* **chorionic villus**)—The numerous branching projections from the external portion of the chorion that provide for exchanges between maternal and fetal blood. *Chapter 5.*

chorionic villus sampling (**CVS**)—The withdrawal of some of the villi from the placenta during the first trimester in order to test for genetic or chromosomal anomalies. *Chapters 11, 15.*

choroid plexus—Vascular fringe-like folds within the ventricles of the brain responsible for the formation of cerebrospinal fluid. *Chapter 4.*

choroid plexus cysts—Cysts, relatively common, that develop in the echogenic choroid plexus in the lateral ventricles. *Chapter 7.*

CIA—Common iliac arteries: the right and left common iliac arteries are the two terminal branches of the abdominal aorta. They arise to the left of the body of the fourth lumbar vertebra and pass inferolaterally for approximately 5 cm before terminating as the internal and external iliac arteries at the level of the pelvic inlet. *Chapter 12. See also* external iliac arteries; iliac arteries; internal iliac arteries.

circle of Willis—A ring of arteries made up of the posterior cerebral arteries, posterior communicating arteries, middle cerebral arteries, and anterior communicating arteries that serves as a safety mechanism for blood flow through the fetal (and later adult) brain. *Chapter 4.*

circummarginate placenta—A placenta in which the membranous chorion does not extend to the edge, creating a flattened ring formed by the attachment of membranes. *Chapter 5.*

circumvallate placenta—A placenta in which the membranous chorion does not extend to the edge, creating a thick and raised ring formed by attachment of membranes. *Chapter 5.*

cisterna magna—A large subarachnoid space in the brain between the caudal part of the cerebellum and the medulla oblongata; also known as the cisterna cerebellomedullaris posterior. *Chapter 4.*

class A diabetes—White's classification for gestational diabetes. *Chapter 10. See also* gestational diabetes.

class B diabetes—White's classification for type 2 diabetes. *Chapter 10. See also* type 2 diabetes.

classic Potter syndrome—Failure of both kidneys to develop, resulting in the fetus's inability to produce urine; also known as bilateral renal agenesis. *Chapter 8.*

cleavage—Cell division. *Chapter 3.*

cleft lip—Separation in the upper lip where the two sides of the lip did not fuse properly during development. *Chapter 11.*

cleft palate—Separation of the roof of the mouth where the two sides of the palate did not fuse properly during development. *Chapter 11.*

clinodactyly—The curving of the fifth finger in toward the fourth finger because of underdevelopment of the middle phalanx of the fifth finger. *Chapter 11.*

cloacal exstrophy—A defect in the lower abdomen with eversion of the fetal bladder (leaving it open to amniotic fluid) and other intestinal anomalies. *Chapter 7.*

Clomid—A brand name for clomiphene citrate. *Chapter 13. See also* clomiphene citrate.

clomiphene citrate (Clomid)—A fertility drug used to stimulate the production of ovarian follicles. *Chapter 13.*

clomiphene citrate challenge test (CCCT)—A test to determine whether a patient has a normal ovarian reserve. *Chapter 13. See also* clomiphene citrate.

Cloquet's canal—The remnants of the hyaloid artery that are suspended in the vitreous humor of the eye and are sometimes seen as floaters. *Chapter 4. See also* hyaloid artery.

clubfoot—A deformity that causes the foot to turn inward toward the midline; also known as talipes equinovarus. *Chapter 11.*

clubhand—A congenital deformity of the hand that can be either radial or ulnar. The radial type (radial aplasia) is more common and is usually associated with other abnormalities, whereas the ulnar type is associated with absence of the ulna but may also be an isolated condition. Also known as talipomanus. *Chapter 11.*

coarctation of the aorta—A congenital heart anomaly in which part of the aorta narrows. *Chapter 7.*

coccygeus muscles—The muscles arising from the ischium and sacrospinous ligaments that are inserted into the coccyx and sacrum; also known as the pubococcygeus muscles. *Chapter 2.*

color Doppler—Conversion of Doppler frequency shifts into colors that are superimposed on a 2D image; also known as color flow imaging. *Chapter 12.*

comet-tail artifact—A sonographic artifact caused by a strong interface in which a thin line of echoes occurs within an essentially echo-free area; a smaller version of a ring-down artifact. *Chapter 1.*

common iliac arteries (CIAs)—The two terminal branches of the abdominal aorta, right and left. They arise to the left of the body near the fourth lumbar vertebra and pass inferolaterally for approximately 5 cm before terminating as the internal and external iliac arteries at the level of the pelvic inlet. *Chapter 12. See also* external iliac arteries; iliac arteries; internal iliac arteries.

complete hydatidiform mole—The most common type of gestational trophoblastic neoplasia, occurring in grape-like clusters of hydropic villi that fill the uterine cavity. *Chapters 3, 12. See also* gestational trophoblastic disorder; hydatidiform mole.

compression—Pressing down or exerting downward pressure. *Chapter 4.*

compression maneuver—Gently pressing down with the transducer to displace bowel gas, compress adipose tissue, or separate structures. *Chapter 1.*

concealed abruption—A hemorrhage confined within the uterine cavity. *Chapter 5.*

conceptual age—The age of the conceptus since the date of fertilization. *Chapter 3.*

conceptus—The fertilized egg, blastocyst, embryo, or fetus. *Chapter 2.*

cone biopsy—The removal of a thin or thick cone-shaped piece of abnormal cervical tissue for laboratory examination. *Chapter 6.*

congenital cystic adenomatoid malformation (CCAM)—Overgrowth of abnormal lung tissue that may form fluid-filled cysts. There are three types, defined by the amount of fluid-filled cysts in the mass. *Chapter 7.*

congenital nephrosis—An autosomal recessive disorder, associated with extremely high levels of maternal serum alpha-fetoprotein, requiring a neonatal kidney transplant if the infant is to survive. *Chapter 11. See also* maternal serum alpha-fetoprotein.

congenital vertical talus—A form of clubfoot, often called rocker bottom foot, that can result from an abnormally short Achilles tendon. The heel is prominent, extending beyond the calf, and the sole of the foot is convex, with the toes pointing upward like a pixie-toe shoe. *Chapter 11.*

conjoined twins—A rare anomaly of monozygotic twinning in which twins are conjoined at some section of the body. *Chapter 9.*

continuous-wave (CW) Doppler ultrasound—An ultrasound technology in which the transducer contains two elements, one that continuously transmits sound and one that continuously receives sound. *Chapter 12. See also* pulsed-wave (PW) Doppler ultrasound.

contralateral—Referring to or situated on the opposite side. *Chapter 8. See also* ipsilateral.

convex linear—A type of transducer in linear array format with a curved scan head; also known as curved linear. *Chapter 1.*

cord prolapse—A complication of delivery that occurs when the umbilical cord drops (prolapses) through the dilated cervix into the vagina prior to the fetus, which during its passage can entrap or compress the cord, cutting off the blood supply to the fetus; a life-threatening event for the fetus. *Chapter 5.*

cordocentesis—A sonography-guided invasive procedure in which a needle is inserted into the umbilical vein to obtain fetal blood for testing purposes; also known as fetal blood sampling or percutaneous umbilical blood sampling (PUBS). *Chapters 11, 15.*

cornual ectopic pregnancy—A pregnancy that occurs where the fallopian tube inserts into the uterus; part of the gestational sac is within the uterus and part is within the fallopian tube. *Chapter 3. See also* ectopic pregnancy.

coronal plane—The scan plane that divides the body into anterior and posterior parts; the anterior/posterior (AP) plane. *Chapter 1.*

corpus—A body.

corpus callosum—The midline structure that overlies the lateral ventricles and carries nerve fibers that connect the right and left hemispheres of the brain; it serves learning and memory functions. *Chapter 7.*

corpus luteum—An empty follicle after it has discharged its ovum. The ruptured follicle produces progesterone, beginning the luteal phase (days 15–28) of menstruation, but if a pregnancy does not occur, the corpus luteum breaks down and disappears. *Chapters 2, 3.*

corpus luteum cyst—A cyst that develops in the empty follicle (corpus luteum) when the follicle fills with fluid or blood. *Chapters 2, 3, 10.*

cos θ—A number associated with a sonographer-controllable variable in the Doppler formula, or the cosine of theta. (A cosine is a number associated with an angle.) Values between 0 and 1 are assigned to angles between 90 and 0 degrees, and as the angle approaches 90, the cosine approaches zero. The calculated Doppler frequency is modified by cos θ. *Chapter 12.*

cotyledon—One of the lobules constituting the maternal side of the placenta and consisting primarily of a rounded mass of villi. *Chapter 5.*

craniopagus—The head-to-head fusion of conjoined twins. *Chapter 9.*

CRI—Cerebral resistivity index: a method of evaluating the fetal middle cerebral arteries, calculated on a Doppler spectral waveform obtained from one of the two middle cerebral arteries. *Chapter 12.*

CRL—Crown-rump length: a measurement used during the first trimester for calculating gestational age. The measurement is taken from the top of the fetal head to the tip of the tail. *Chapter 3.*

cross-plane motion—Holding the transducer in one plane and angling in the opposite direction; also known as angling or tilting. *Chapter 1.*

crossed renal ectopia—Displacement of one kidney to the opposite side, with or without fusion. *Chapter 4.*

crown-rump length (CRL)—A measurement used during the first trimester for calculating gestational age. The measurement is taken from the top of the fetal head to the tip of the tail. *Chapter 3.*

crucial triangle—The lower uterine segment, formed by the cervix, maternal bladder, and sacral prominence. *Chapter 5.*

cryptomenorrhea—A condition in which the symptoms of menstruation are experienced but no external bleeding occurs. *Chapter 2.*

cryptorchidism—A defect of development that results in one or both testes failing to descend into the scrotum. *Chapters 11, 13.*

cubitus valgus—An abnormal outward bending of the forearms. *Chapter 11.*

cumulus oophorus—The small solid mass of follicular cells surrounding the ovum in the vesicular ovarian follicle. *Chapters 2, 13.*

curved linear—A type of transducer in linear array format with a curved scan head; also known as convex linear. *Chapter 1.*

CVS—Chorionic villus sampling: the withdrawal of some of the villi from the placenta during the first trimester in order to test for genetic or chromosomal anomalies. *Chapters 11, 15.*

CW Doppler—Continuous-wave Doppler ultrasound: an ultrasound technology in which the transducer contains two elements, one that continuously transmits sound and one that continuously receives sound. *Chapter 12.*

cyanosis—Blue discoloration of the skin, signifying insufficient oxygen in the blood. *Chapter 8.*

cyclopia—Severe hypotelorism in which the eyes form a single central orbit. *Chapter 11.*

cyllosoma—Another term for limb–body wall complex. *Chapters 5, 7. See also* limb–body wall complex.

cyst—A mass filled with clear, serous fluid. *Chapter 1.*

cystadenocarcinoma—A malignant multiseptated cystic tumors of the ovary, which can grow quite large. *Chapter 2.*

cystadenoma—A benign multiseptated cystic tumor of the ovary, which can grow quite large. *Chapter 2.*

cystic degeneration—The death (necrosis) of tissue in a solid mass that outgrows its blood supply. *Chapter 1.*

cystic fibrosis—A hereditary disorder that involves abnormal thickening of body secretions. *Chapters 7, 11.*

cystic hygromas—Multilocular cysts that form from budding lymphatics, commonly identified in the fetal neck and axilla. *Chapter 7.*

cystic teratoma—A benign tumor that contains tissues from all three fetal layers—endoderm, mesoderm, and ectoderm—and thus can contain nearly all types of tissue, including hormone-producing tissue. *Chapter 2.*

cystocele—A hernial protrusion of the urinary bladder, usually through the vaginal wall. *Chapter 2.*

cytotrophoblast—The inner (cellular) layer of the trophoblast. *Chapter 3.*

D

D&C—Dilation (or dilatation) and curettage. *Chapter 6.*

Dandy-Walker malformation—The absence (agenesis) of the cerebellar vermis, resulting in a dilated fourth ventricle with splaying of the cerebellar hemispheres. Hydrocephalus may be present. *Chapter 7.*

Dandy-Walker variant—Underdevelopment (hypoplasia) of the cerebellar vermis, resulting in the types of changes seen with the Dandy-Walker malformation, but to a lesser degree. *Chapter 7.*

decidua—The inner lining of the uterus; the endometrium. *Chapter 5.*

decidua basalis—The portion of the endometrium in which the implanted ovum rests; the maternal side of the placenta. *Chapters 3, 5.*

decidua capsularis—The part of the endometrium that covers the implanted ovum. *Chapters 3, 5.*

decidua parietalis/vera—The portion of the endometrial lining that is not occupied by the implanted ovum. *Chapters 3, 5.*

decidual septal cysts—Rare cysts that occur in the vicinity between the cotyledons of the placenta. *Chapter 5.*

decidualized endometrium—The thickened, vascularized lining of the uterus that develops after ovulation. *Chapter 3.*

dedicated mechanized volume probe—A probe with a mechanical drive contained within the probe case itself, commonly referred to as a volume probe. *Chapter 14.*

deformation—The distortion of normal structure by some mechanical force, whether intrinsic or extrinsic. *Chapter 11.*

demise—Death. *Chapters 8, 9.*

dermoid—A teratoma that contains only ectodermal tissue, also known as a dermoid cyst (a type of cystic teratoma). *Chapter 2. See also* cystic teratoma; dermoid cyst; dermoid plug; fibroid.

dermoid cyst—A lay term for a cystic teratoma, a mass that is usually benign, commonly found in women age 20 or younger. Also called simply a dermoid, the latter term is more precisely a teratoma that contains only ectodermal tissue. *Chapter 2. See also* cystic teratoma; dermoid.

dermoid plug—A solid protuberance that forms on the interior surface of a cyst and can contain bones, teeth, and matted hair. *Chapter 2.*

DET—Donor embryo transfer: use of a donor egg, which is usually fertilized, with the sperm of the patient's partner, although both sperm and egg can be donated. *Chapter 13.*

Deuel's sign—A halo effect that subcutaneous scalp edema produces on radiography of the fetal head, which has been associated with intrauterine death of the fetus; also known as Deuel's halo sign. *Chapter 8.*

dextrocardia—The abnormal positioning of the heart in the right hemithorax. *Chapter 4.*

dextroposed—Pertaining to a uterus deviated to the right of the midline. *Chapter 2.*

diabetes mellitus—A broad term used to describe a range of metabolic disorders involving the production and release of insulin by the pancreas. *Chapter 10. See also* type 1 diabetes; type 2 diabetes; White's classification.

diamniotic—Developing within separate amniotic cavities. *Chapter 9.*

diaphragmatic hernia—A defect in the fetal diaphragm (usually on the left side) that allows the intra-abdominal contents to travel into the chest cavity, displacing the lungs and heart. *Chapter 7.*

diastole—The rhythmic relaxation and dilatation of the heart chambers, especially the ventricles, during which they fill with blood. *Chapter 4.*

diastolic notch—The appearance of a rapid vertical deflection of the spectral waveform at the beginning of diastole. *Chapter 12.*

diastolic velocity—The speed at which the heart fills with blood after contracting. *Chapter 12. See also* end-diastolic velocity; peak systolic velocity.

diastrophic dwarfism—A rare form of dwarfism that involves short-limb skeletal dysplasia, clubfeet, ear swelling, and progressive spinal deformity and joint contractures, including an abducted, or "hitchhiker," thumb. *Chapter 11. See also* abducted thumb; adducted thumb.

dicephalus—A fetus with two heads. *Chapter 9.*

dichorionic—Having two distinct chorions, as in dizygotic twins. *Chapter 9.*

digital examination—Palpation of the cervix by inserting a finger or fingers through the vagina. *Chapter 6.*

dilation (or **dilatation**) **and curettage** (**D&C**)—A procedure that opens the cervix to allow access to the endometrial cavity. *Chapter 6.*

diploid—Pertaining to the fetus's having two homologous copies of each chromosome, usually one from the mother and one from the father. *See also* haploid number.

discordance (or **discordancy**)—A difference: Pertaining to weight, a difference of more than 500 grams (20%–25%) between twin fetuses; associated with the intrauterine death of the fetus. *Chapter 9.*

disorder—An abnormality of function, categorized as chromosomal, single-gene (Mendelian), multifactorial, or environmental (teratogenic). *Chapter 11.*

disruption—Something extrinsic that affects the normal developmental process. *Chapter 11.*

diverticulum—An outpouching. *Chapter 2.*

dizygotic—Resulting from the fertilization of two separate eggs; pertaining to fraternal twins. *Chapter 9.*

dolichocephaly—Having an unusually long and narrow head shape. *Chapters 4, 9.*

dominant follicle—The follicle that reaches maturity during the menstrual cycle; the Graafian follicle. *Chapter 2.*

donor embryo transfer (**DET**)—Use of a donor egg, which is usually fertilized, with the sperm of the patient's partner, although both sperm and egg can be donated. *Chapter 13.*

Doppler effect—The change in frequency of a (sound) wave perceived by a stationary observer (or ultrasound transducer) as a moving source of sound approaches and then passes the observer. Often likened to the shifting frequency of sound from an approaching train or airplane as it passes the observer, the Doppler effect underlies the application of Doppler ultrasound in the evaluation of moving blood cells. *Chapter 12.*

Doppler frequency—*See* Doppler shift.

Doppler imaging—A noninvasive ultrasound technology used to evaluate blood flow. *Chapter 12.*

Doppler shift—The difference in frequency between the transmitted and the reflected ultrasound whenever ultrasound is reflected from moving tissue.

double bleb sign—A sonographic sign at 5–6 weeks signifying that the amnion has stretched and surrounded the embryo, filling with amniotic fluid. It appears as two small circular structures, one the amnion and the other the secondary yolk sac. *Chapter 3.*

double bubble—The classic sonographic sign indicating duodenal atresia, formed by the normal fluid-filled stomach (first bubble) and the dilated duodenum (second bubble). *Chapter 7.*

double decidual ring—The appearance of the decidualized endometrium surrounding the thick echogenic chorion of the gestational sac. *Chapter 3.*

double decidual sac sign—The sonographic identification of two layers of endometrium covering the gestational sac with a hypoechoic cavity between. *Chapter 5.*

Down syndrome—The chromosomal disorder characterized by a small anteroposteriorly flattened skull, short flat-bridge nose, epicanthal folds, short phalanges, widened spaces between the first and second digits of the hands and feet, and moderate to severe mental retardation; also known as trisomy 21. *Chapters 4, 11.*

dry tap—The inability to withdraw amniotic fluid during an amniocentesis. *Chapter 15.*

DUB—Dysfunctional uterine bleeding: heavy periods or bleeding between periods that usually occurs when the patient is not ovulating and is caused by a hormonal imbalance. *Chapter 2. See also* abnormal uterine bleeding.

Duchenne muscular dystrophy—A childhood form of muscular dystrophy. *Chapter 11.*

ductus arteriosus—The arterial duct, which connects the pulmonary artery to the aortic arch in the fetal heart, allowing most of the blood from the right ventricle to bypass the fetus's fluid-filled lungs. *Chapter 4.*

ductus venosus (DV)—A fetal blood channel that shunts approximately half of the blood flow from the umbilical vein to the inferior vena cava and allows oxygenated blood from the placenta to bypass the liver; together with other shunts in the fetal circulation, it functions to preferentially shunt oxygenated blood to the fetal brain. *Chapter 12.*

duodenal atresia—A complete obliteration of the duodenal lumen of the small intestine, which results in a large stomach and polyhydramnios. *Chapter 7.*

duplex mode imaging—The simultaneous presentation of two types of information—anatomic and physiologic—by B-mode and pulsed-wave (PW) Doppler ultrasound.

duty cycle—The ratio that compares the amount of time the transducer spends sending energy with the time it spends receiving and processing energy.

DV—Ductus venosus: a fetal blood channel that shunts approximately half of the blood flow from the umbilical vein to the inferior vena cava and allows oxygenated blood from the placenta to bypass the liver; together with other shunts in the fetal circulation, it functions to preferentially shunt oxygenated blood to the fetal brain. *Chapter 12.*

dysencephalia splanchnocystica—A condition associated with posterior encephalocele, polydactyly, and polycystic kidneys. *Chapter 11.*

dysfunctional uterine bleeding (DUB)—a heavy period or bleeding between periods that usually occurs when the patient is not ovulating and is caused by a hormonal imbalance. *Chapter 2. See also* abnormal uterine bleeding.

dysgerminoma—A rare malignant ovarian tumor considered the female counterpart of the male seminoma. *Chapter 2.*

dysmenorrhea—Painful menstruation. *Chapter 2.*

dyspareunia—Difficult or painful sexual intercourse. *Chapter 2.*

dysplasia—Any abnormality of development.

E

E/A ratio—The ratio of early (E) to late or atrial (A) ventricular filling velocity.

Eagle-Barrett syndrome—A condition resulting from obstruction of the posterior urethral valves, causing complete dilation of the urinary tract. The bladder becomes so grossly distended that the abdominal musculature does not develop and the baby will have a flabby, wrinkled belly upon decompression of the bladder; also known as prune belly syndrome. *Chapter 11.*

EBF—Erythroblastosis fetalis: a disorder characterized by destruction of fetal red blood cells by the maternal immune system because of an Rh factor. *Chapter 10.*

Ebstein's anomaly—Displacement of one or more of the tricuspid leaflets toward the apex of the right ventricle. *Chapter 7.*

echogenic—Producing many echoes. *Chapter 1.*

echogenic bowel—A fetal bowel that appears as bright or brighter than adjacent bone. *Chapters 4, 11.*

echopenic—Producing relatively few low-level echoes, which results in less bright imaging in that area. *Chapter 1. See also* hypoechoic.

eclampsia—The convulsive stage of pregnancy-induced hypertension. *Chapter 10.*

ectopia cordis—The condition in which the fetal heart protrudes outside the chest through a defect in the sternum and chest wall. *Chapter 7.*

ectopic kidney—Abnormal positioning of the kidney, often in the pelvic cavity. *Chapter 4.*

ectopic ovary—An ovary located in an abnormal anatomic position or arising from abnormal tissue or an abnormal site. *Chapter 2. See also* accessory ovary; supernumerary ovary.

ectopic pregnancy—Any pregnancy that occurs outside the uterus. *Chapter 3.*

ectrodactyly—A congenital defect involving a complete or partial absence of one or more central digits; also known as the lobster claw anomaly. *Chapter 11.*

edema—Accumulation of fluid beneath the skin or within tissue; dropsy, hydrops. *Chapter 10.*

EDV—End-diastolic velocity: the maximum velocity of blood flow at the end of diastole, just before the systolic upstroke. *Chapter 12. See also* diastolic velocity; peak systolic velocity.

Edwards syndrome—A chromosomal disorder associated with early onset of severe growth restriction with deformities of the hands and feet; also known as trisomy 18. *Chapter 11.*

effacement—Obliteration of form or features; when applied to the process of labor, the thinning of the cervix. *Chapter 6.*

EFW—Estimated fetal weight: the fetus's estimated weight calculated according to ultrasound findings of femur length, head circumference, and abdominal circumference. *Chapter 4.*

embryo transfer—Use of a donor egg, which is usually fertilized with the sperm of the patient's partner, although both sperm and egg can be donated. *Chapter 13.*

embryoblast—The embryonic disc. *Chapter 3.*

embryonal rhabdomyosarcoma—A highly malignant tumor arising from striated muscle or embryonic mesenchymal (loosely packed, unspecialized) cells. *Chapter 2.*

embryonic period—Weeks 2–8 postfertilization. *Chapter 3.*

encephalocele—Herniation of a fluid-filled sac through a defect in the fetal cranium that may or may not include brain tissue. *Chapter 7.*

end-diastolic velocity (**EDV**)—The maximum blood-flow velocity at the end of diastole, just before the systolic upstroke. *Chapter 12. See also* diastolic velocity; peak systolic velocity.

endocardial cushion defect—A collection of heart defects including abnormalities of the atrioventricular valves; strongly associated with Down syndrome. *Chapter 7.*

endocrine—Secreting internally; hormone-producing. *Chapter 10.*

endodermal sinus tumor—A highly malignant tumor developing within the germ cells of a fetus; a yolk sac tumor. *Chapter 2.*

endometrial carcinoma—Cancer of the endometrium. *Chapter 2.*

endometrial hyperplasia—Excessive proliferation of the endometrial lining. *Chapter 2.*

endometrial polyp—A benign projection of the endometrium, which can be either pedunculated (supported on a stalk) or sessile (attached at the base without a stalk). *Chapter 2.*

endometrioma—A walled-off collection of old blood from bleeding ectopic endometrial tissues; a chocolate cyst. *Chapter 2.*

endometriosis—The invasion of ectopic, hormone-responsive endometrial tissues into the myometrium, the fallopian tubes, and, through them, extrauterine structures and tissues. *Chapter 2.*

endometritis—Inflammation of the endometrium. *Chapter 2.*

endometrium—The mucous membrane lining the uterus. *Chapter 2.*

endovaginal—Through the vagina; transvaginal. *Chapter 1.*

enhancement artifact—One of the most common kinds of artifacts in imaging the uterus during volume sonography, in which the echogenic endometrium appears to spread beyond the endometrial/myometrial interface, causing the adjacent myometrium to appear artifactually hyperechoic. *Chapter 14.*

enteric duplication cysts—Best described as diverticula, cysts resulting from a rare congenital malformation of the intestinal tract that share at least one layer with the normal intestine, denoted sonographically by the double wall or "muscular rim" sign; also known as gut cysts. *Chapter 7.*

enterocele—A hernia that contains intestine. *Chapter 2.*

epiphysis—The end of a long bone. *Chapter 4.*

erythroblastosis fetalis (**EBF**)—A disorder characterized by destruction of fetal red blood cells by the maternal immune system because of an Rh factor. *Chapter 10.*

estimated fetal weight (**EFW**)—The fetus's estimated weight, calculated according to ultrasound findings of femur length, head circumference, and abdominal circumference. *Chapter 4.*

estradiol—The most potent naturally occurring estrogen in humans. *Chapter 13.*

estrogen—A natural steroid secreted by the ovaries that stimulates the development of female secondary sex characteristics and promotes the growth and maintenance of the female reproductive system. *Chapter 2.*

estrogenic—Capable of producing the female hormone estrogen; also, resulting from estrogen. *Chapter 2.*

exencephaly—The absence of the cranial vault, although brain tissue with identifiable normal structures is present. *Chapter 7.*

exocoelomic membrane—A membrane, arising from the cytotrophoblast, that lines the primary yolk sac. *Chapter 3. See also* cytotrophoblast.

exophthalmia—Hyperextension of the eyeball.

external iliac arteries—The arteries that form off the common iliac arteries, in front of the sacroiliac joint of the pelvis, and descend along the medial border of the psoas major muscles. *Chapter 12. See also* common iliac arteries; iliac arteries; internal iliac arteries.

extracorporeal liver—A liver (sometimes accompanied by bowel) that has herniated into a thin sac composed of peritoneum and amnion. *Chapter 7.*

extraembryonic coelom—A body cavity outside the embryo. *Chapter 3.*

extrinsic—Of external origin. *Chapter 11.*

eyeballing—A method of evaluating the amniotic fluid based on the sonographer's subjective assessment during an examination, which requires experience; any subjective assessment based on sonographic skill and experience. *Chapter 4.*

F

facial/brachial plexus palsies—Paralyses of the fetal face or arm, usually caused by traumatic delivery. *Chapter 10.*

failed pregnancy—Embryonic or fetal demise or anembryonic pregnancy. *Chapter 3.*

fallopian tube—A tube that carries the egg (ovum) from the ovary to the uterus; a woman has two fallopian tubes, one extending from each ovary. *Chapter 2.*

false knots—Complications resulting from an abnormally long umbilical cord in which loops of cord fold on one another. *Chapter 5.*

false pelvis—Pelvic cavity that includes the bowel and extends to the umbilicus; also known as major pelvis. *Chapter 2.*

falx—A fold of dura mater separating the cerebral hemispheres. *Chapter 4.*

FAS—Fetal alcohol syndrome: effects on the fetus that result from alcohol use by the mother during pregnancy; according to the National Library of Medicine, because alcohol easily passes across the placenta to the fetus, no amount of alcohol can be considered "safe" for fetal development. *Chapter 11.*

femoral hypoplasia–unusual facies syndrome—A syndrome associated with diabetic pregnancies that involves hypoplasia of the femur and/or humerus and may include absence of the fibula (which can be identified sonographically) as well as facial anomalies (generally too mild to detect). *Chapter 10.*

femur—The large bone in the thigh. *Chapter 4.*

fetal alcohol syndrome (**FAS**)—Effects on the fetus that result from alcohol use by the mother during pregnancy; according to the National Library of Medicine, because alcohol easily passes across the placenta to the fetus, no amount of alcohol can be considered "safe" for fetal development. *Chapter 11.*

fetal blood sampling—A sonography-guided invasive procedure in which a needle is inserted into the umbilical vein to obtain fetal blood for testing purposes; also known as cordocentesis or percutaneous umbilical blood sampling (PUBS). *Chapters 11, 15.*

fetal demise—Fetal death, which, according to the World Health Organization, is characterized by the fetus or neonate not breathing or showing other signs of life, such as a heartbeat, umbilical cord pulsation, or movement of voluntary muscles. *Chapter 8.*

fetal hydrops—Hydrops in a fetus, causing pleural effusions, abdominal ascites, and gross dermal edema; also known as hydrops fetalis. *Chapters 7, 10.*

fetal parabiotic syndrome—Artery-to-vein anastomosis within the shared placenta of twins, causing a mixing of fetal blood that shunts too much to the recipient twin and not enough to the donor twin. *Chapter 9. See also* twin-to-twin transfusion syndrome.

fetal period—The period 9–40 weeks postfertilization. *Chapter 3.*

fetal tone—A parameter of the biophysical profile of the fetus that measures the extension and flexion of fetal extremities. *Chapter 8.*

fetus in fetu—A small, imperfect fetus (incapable of living on its own) that becomes incorporated into the developing body of another fetus. *Chapter 9. See also* vanishing twin.

fetus papyraceous—A paper-thin fetus that has been flattened by compression against the uterus by another twin. *Chapter 9. See also* vanishing twin.

fibroid—A benign tumor made of muscle and connective tissue found in the uterus. *Chapter 2. See also* leiomyoma; myoma.

fibroma—A benign neoplasm typically seen in postmenopausal patients and rarely associated with hormone production. *Chapter 2.*

fibula—A small lateral bone of the lower leg. *Chapter 4.*

fimbriae (*sing.* **fimbria**)—Finger-like projections within the infundibulum that grab the ovum after ovulation and propel it up into the fallopian tube. The celia within the tube help to propel the zygote through the tube into the uterus. *Chapters 2, 3.*

fimbrial cysts—Small cysts found in the mesosalpinx and around the terminal portion of the fallopian tube. *Chapter 2.*

Fitz-Hugh–Curtis syndrome—Perihepatitis associated with the spread of infection from pelvic inflammatory disease. *Chapter 2.*

five-chamber view—A method of imaging the heart that is similar to the four-chamber view but also includes the aortic valve and left ventricular outflow tract. *Chapter 4. See also* four-chamber view.

FL/AC ratio—The ratio of femur length to abdominal circumference. *Chapter 8.*

flat head syndrome—A disproportionate shortness of the head, the head being too round; also known as brachycephaly. *Chapters 4, 11.*

follicle-stimulating hormone (**FSH**)—A hormone produced by the anterior lobe of the pituitary gland that stimulates the growth of the ovum-containing follicles in the ovary and activates sperm-forming cells. *Chapters 2, 13.*

follicular cyst—A fluid-filled structure that releases the immature egg during ovulation. *Chapter 2.*

folliculogenesis—The growth of follicles in the ovary, stimulated by the hormone FSH. *Chapter 2.*

foramen ovale—An oval-shaped opening in the atrial septum, located between the right and left atria, that serves as a passageway for blood for the fetus. *Chapter 4.*

fornix—A recess formed between the vaginal wall and the vaginal part of the cervix. *Chapter 2.*

four-chamber view—The screening view most widely used to determine fetal heart health. *Chapter 4. See also* five-chamber view.

four-dimensional Doppler—3D color Doppler imaging in real time. *Chapter 12.*

four-dimensional sonography (**4D sonography**)—3D imaging in real time. *Chapter 14.*

four-quadrant amniotic fluid index—A method of evaluating the amniotic fluid in which the uterine cavity is divided into four quadrants and the deepest pocket of fluid in each quadrant is measured after ensuring that the pockets are void of fetal body parts and the umbilical cord. Once the pockets in all quadrants have been measured, they are added together and their sum is used for the measurement. *Chapter 4.*

frontal bossing—An unusually large, protuberant forehead. *Chapter 7.*

FSH—Follicle-stimulating hormone: a hormone produced by the anterior lobe of the pituitary gland that stimulates the growth of the ovum-containing follicles in the ovary and activates sperm-forming cells. *Chapters 2, 13.*

functional midline—The longitudinal image of the uterus that includes vagina, cervix, corpus, fundus, and endometrial canal. *Chapter 2.*

fundus—The bottom or base portion of an organ, opposite its opening. In the case of the uterus, the rounded portion cephalad to the insertion of the fallopian tubes. *Chapter 2.*

funneling—The extension or protrusion of an intact amniotic sac into the dilated endocervical canal. *Chapter 6.*

G

gallstones—Crystalline bodies formed from bile components. *Chapter 7.*

gamete intrafallopian transfer (**GIFT**)—The procedure in which sperm and eggs (ova) are placed within the fallopian tube through a cannula. *Chapter 13.*

Gartner's duct cyst—A cyst found in the vaginal canal. *Chapter 2.*

gastroschisis—Herniation of the intestines through a defect on the side, usually the left side, of the umbilical cord. *Chapter 7.*

gender—Sex. *Chapter 4.*

gestational age—The age of the fetus, calculated from the first day of the last menstrual period; gestational age is always 2 weeks older than the conceptual age; also known as menstrual age. *Chapters 3, 6.*

gestational diabetes—Diabetes whose onset is first recognized during (but not prior to) pregnancy, excluding women who are lactosuric. The occurrence of gestational diabetes is more prevalent in individuals with a family history of diabetes, a history of sugar in the urine, obesity, and a history of glucose intolerance. In White's

classification, gestational diabetes is class A diabetes. *Chapter 10. See also* type 1 diabetes; type 2 diabetes; White's classification.

gestational sac—A rounded or ovoid cystic structure normally found within the endometrial cavity where the developing embryo/fetus is contained. *Chapter 3.*

gestational trophoblastic disorder (**GTD**)—An abnormal proliferation of placenta after embryonic/fetal demise. *Chapters 3, 16. See also* molar pregnancy.

gestational trophoblastic neoplasia/neoplasm (**GTN**)—A form of invasive mole, or fleshy mass, that forms in the uterus upon the abnormal development of a fertilized ovum. Although invasive moles are considered malignant, they rarely metastasize and are considered highly curable. *Chapter 3.*

gestational trophoblastic tumor (**GTT**)—A form of invasive mole, or fleshy mass, that forms in the uterus upon the abnormal development of a fertilized ovum. Although invasive moles are considered malignant, they rarely metastasize and are considered highly curable. *Chapter 3.*

GIFT—Gamete intrafallopian transfer: the procedure in which sperm and eggs (ova) are placed within the fallopian tube through a cannula. *Chapter 13.*

glucose—Simple sugar. *Chapter 10.*

glucose tolerance test—A test of the body's ability to utilize carbohydrates. *Chapter 10.*

glycogen—A polysaccharide that is the chief carbohydrate storage material in animals. *Chapter 10.*

GnRH—Gonadotropin-releasing hormone. *Chapter 2.*

gonadal arteries—Blood vessels that supply oxygenated blood to the ovaries in women and the testes in men. They arise from the abdominal aorta below the renal arteries and do not pass out of the abdominal cavity. *Chapter 12.*

Graafian follicle—In the menstrual cycle, the follicle that reaches maturity; the dominant follicle. *Chapter 2.*

granulosa cell tumors—Also known as theca cell tumors, common and usually benign ovarian tumors that are estrogenic and cause feminizing effects. *Chapter 2.*

Graves' disease—A clinical syndrome characterized by hyperthyroidism in which thyrotoxicosis is associated with diffuse goiter and exophthalmia; characterized by hyperthyroidism. *Chapter 10.*

gray-scale image—A B-mode image that shows strength of echoes by brightness of displayed dots. *Chapter 14.*

great vessels—The outflow tracts of the heart, consisting of the right and left ventricular outflow tracts. *Chapter 4.*

grief—The emotional response to a loss. *Chapter 16.*

GTD—Gestational trophoblastic disorder: an abnormal proliferation of placenta after embryonic/fetal demise. *Chapters 3, 16. See also* molar pregnancy.

GTN—Gestational trophoblastic neoplasia or neoplasm: a form of invasive mole, or fleshy mass, that forms in the uterus upon the abnormal development of a fertilized ovum. Although invasive moles are considered malignant, they rarely metastasize and are considered highly curable. *Chapter 3.*

GTT—Gestational trophoblastic tumor: a form of invasive mole, or fleshy mass, that forms in the uterus upon the abnormal development of a fertilized ovum. Although invasive moles are considered malignant, they rarely metastasize and are considered highly curable. *Chapter 3.*

gut cysts—Best described as diverticula, cysts resulting from a rare congenital malformation of the intestinal tract that share at least one layer with the normal intestine, denoted sonographically by the "double wall" or "muscular rim" sign; also known as enteric duplication cysts. *Chapter 7.*

gynatresia—Occlusion of some part of the female genital tract. *Chapter 2.*

H

Hamburger sign—A term applied to the appearance of the fetal labia on sonography, with the buns being the labia and the space in between being the patty; also known as the Big Mac sign. *Chapter 4.*

haploid number—Half the number of chromosomes normally found in diploid cells of an organism. *Chapter 11. See also* diploid.

HC—Head circumference: one of the two most commonly used measurements for dating pregnancies in the second and third trimesters (the other being biparietal diameter). *Chapter 4. See also* biparietal diameter.

HC/AC ratio—The ratio of head circumference to abdominal circumference. *Chapter 8.*

hCG—Human chorionic gonadotropin: a hormone produced by trophoblastic cells. *Chapters 3, 5, 11.*

hCS—Human chorionic somatomammotropin: a protein essential for the maintenance and growth of a pregnancy. *Chapter 5.*

head circumference (HC)—The circumference of the fetal head, one of the two most commonly used measurements for dating pregnancies in the second and third trimesters (the other being biparietal diameter). The calculation is $HC = 5 (BPD + OFD) \times 1.62$, where BPD is biparietal diameter, OFD is occipital frontal diameter, and 1.62 is the factor used to correct for the typical ellipsoid shape of the fetal head (although some sources give 1.57 as the corrective factor). *Chapter 4. See also* biparietal diameter.

head-sparing—Normal growth of brain but decreased growth of abdomen with asymmetrical intrauterine growth restriction. *Chapter 8.*

HELLP—Hemolysis-elevated liver enzymes and low platelets associated with hypertension. *Chapter 10.*

hematocolpos—Menstrual blood that is retained within a distended vagina. *Chapter 2.*

hematoma—A localized collection of extravasated blood, usually clotted. *Chapters 1, 2.*

hematometra—A collection of retained menstrual blood that fills the uterine cavity. *Chapter 2.*

hematopoiesis—The formation of blood cells. *Chapter 3.*

hematosalpinx—The accumulation of blood within the uterine tube. *Chapter 2.*

hemifacial microsomia—Developmental deficiencies in parts of the face, most commonly the lower half of the face, including ears, mouth, and jaw.

hemimelia—An anomaly of development in which there is complete or partial absence of a long bone, sometimes with the absence of the forearm, hand, lower leg, or foot. *Chapter 7.*

hemivertebra—A congenital malformation of the spine in which only half of a vertebral body develops. *Chapter 14.*

hemodynamics—The movement of blood in and around human soft tissues and organs. *Chapter 12.*

hemolysis—Ruptures of erythrocytes (red blood cells) with release of hemoglobin into the plasma. *Chapter 10.*

hepatoblastoma—A rare malignant liver tumor seen in infants and young children. *Chapter 11.*

heterogeneous—Of mixed, nonuniform quality, composition, or structure. *Chapter 1.*

heterotopic pregnancy—An ectopic pregnancy coexisting with a normal intrauterine pregnancy. *Chapter 3.*

hirsutism—Abnormal hairiness, especially in women. *Chapter 2.*

hockey stick sign—The junction of the umbilical vein and the left branch of the portal vein, which forms the shape of a hockey stick, where the abdominal circumference should be taken; also known as the J sign. *Chapter 4.*

holoprosencephaly—A disorder characterized by the failure of the brain to separate into two hemispheres. Alobar holoprosencephaly is the severest form, semilobar is an intermediate form, and lobar is the least severe form. *Chapter 7. See also* alobar holoprosencephaly; lobar holoprosencephaly; semilobar holoprosencephaly.

Holt-Oram syndrome—An autosomal dominant heart condition associated with skeletal malformation that typically involves an atrial or ventricular septal defect, varying in severity. *Chapter 11.*

homogeneous—Smooth; of uniform quality, composition, or structure. *Chapter 1.*

homozygous achondroplasia—Fatal dwarfism that occurs when both parents carry the achondroplasia gene. *Chapter 7.*

hormone replacement treatment/therapy (**HRT**)—Use of female hormones to treat peri- and postmenopausal symptoms, almost always including an estrogen component and often a progesterone component. *Chapter 12.*

hourglass membranes—Intact fetal membranes prolapsed through the external cervical os. *Chapter 6.*

HRT—Hormone replacement treatment or therapy: use of female hormones to treat peri- and postmenopausal symptoms, almost always including an estrogen component and often a progesterone component. *Chapter 12.*

HSG—Hysterosalpingography: radiographic imaging of the uterus and fallopian tubes, using injection of an opaque material, to examine their shape; also known as uterosalpingography. *Chapter 14.*

human chorionic gonadotropin (**hCG**)—Often called the "pregnancy hormone," a protein produced by trophoblastic cells of the placenta that nourishes the conceptus and is essential for its maintenance and growth. Elevated levels can be detected by blood test about 11 days after conception. *Chapters 3, 5, 11.*

human chorionic somatomammotropin (**hCS**)—A protein, produced by the syncytiotrophoblast during pregnancy, that regulates the mother's carbohydrate and protein metabolism and ensures that the fetus receives glucose for energy and protein for fetal growth. *Chapter 5.*

humerus—The proximal large bone in the upper arm. *Chapter 4.*

hyaline membrane disease—A disorder of newborns, typically born preterm, characterized by the formation of a thin, glassy membrane lining the terminal respiratory passages and causing severe dyspnea and cyanosis. *Chapter 10.*

hyaloid artery—A branch of the ophthalmic artery that aids in the development of the lens in the growing fetus. *Chapter 4.*

hydatidiform mole—A benign, noninvasive, gestational trophoblastic disorder. *Chapters 3, 12. See also* gestational trophoblastic disorder.

hydatids of Morgagni—Cyst-like remnants of the müllerian duct attached to a testis or oviduct. *Chapter 2.*

hydranencephaly—An extreme form of porencephaly in which the cerebral hemispheres form normally but, because of vascular insult, become totally replaced by cerebrospinal fluid. *Chapter 7. See also* porencephaly.

hydrocele—Fluid around the testis. *Chapter 10.*

hydrocephalus—A condition in which the cerebral ventricles are dilated, which in children may occur before closure of the skull. In the fetus, there are two major types of hydrocephalus, communicating and noncommunicating. The former results from an abnormality in the capacity to absorb fluid from the arachnoid space but not obstruction; in the latter, the cause is an obstruction in the ventricular system, most commonly aqueductal stenosis or spina bifida. It can cause an enlarged head with a prominent forehead, brain atrophy, convulsions, and mental deterioration. *Chapter 7.*

hydrocephaly—An abnormal accumulation of cerebrospinal fluid (CSF) in the cranium due to an imbalance between the production and absorption of CSF. *Chapters 3, 7.*

hydrocolpos—An accumulation of fluid in the vagina. *Chapter 7.*

hydrometrocolpos—An accumulation of fluid in the vagina and uterus. *Chapter 7.*

hydronephrosis—Distention of the renal pelvis and calices with urine, usually caused by the obstruction of the collecting system of the kidney. *Chapters 8, 10.*

hydrops—Two or more abnormal serous fluid collections found in body cavities or tissues; edema. *Chapter 10.*

hydrops fetalis—Fetal hydrops, causing pleural effusions, abdominal ascites, and gross dermal edema. *Chapters 7, 10.*

hydrosalpinx—A distention of the fallopian tubes resulting from fluid caused by inflammation, an end stage of pyosalpinx (pus in the fallopian tubes). *Chapter 2.*

hydroureter—A dilated ureter filled with urine. *Chapters 8, 11, 15.*

hymen—The fold of mucous membrane that surrounds or partially covers the external vaginal opening (vaginal introitus). *Chapter 2.*

hyperechoic—Producing bright, high-intensity echoes. *Chapter 1. See also* echogenic.

hyperemesis gravidarum—Excessive nausea and vomiting to the point of dehydration. *Chapter 10.*

hyperglycemia—A high blood sugar level. *Chapter 10.*

hypertelorism—An abnormally increased distance between the eyes. *Chapters 4, 11.*

hypertension—High blood pressure.

hyperthermia—High body temperature that does not result from fever; it may cause neural tube defects, intrauterine death, abortion, or preterm labor. *Chapter 10. See also* pyrexia.

hyperthyroidism—A clinical syndrome in which thyrotoxicosis is associated with diffuse goiter and exophthalmos; Graves' disease. *Chapter 10.*

hypoechoic—Producing relatively few low-level echoes, resulting in less bright imaging. *Chapter 1. See also* echopenic.

hypogastric arteries—The iliac arteries. *Chapters 4, 12. See also* common iliac arteries; external iliac arteries; iliac arteries; internal iliac arteries.

hypoglycemia—Low blood sugar. *Chapter 8.*

hypoplasia—Incomplete development or underdevelopment. *Chapter 7.*

hypoplastic left heart syndrome—Hypoplasia of the left ventricle, resulting in a number of structural anomalies. *Chapter 7.*

hypoplastic ventricle—An underdeveloped ventricle of the heart that usually includes valves and arteries associated with that particular side of the heart. *Chapter 7.*

hypotelorism—Having eyes spaced abnormally close together. *Chapters 4, 11.*

hypotension—Low blood pressure. *Chapter 7.*

hypothalamus—A gland located below the thalamus, just above the brain stem. It links the nervous system to the endocrine system via the pituitary gland. *Chapter 2.*

hypothermia—The inability to maintain normal body temperature. *Chapter 8.*

hypothyroidism—A deficiency of the thyroid gland. *Chapter 10.*

hypoxia—A broad term used to describe diminished availability of oxygen to the body tissues. *Chapters 8, 12.*

hysterosalpingography (**HSG**)—Radiographic imaging of the uterus and fallopian tubes, using injection of an opaque material, to examine their shape; also known as uterosalpingography. *Chapter 14.*

hysteroscopy—An endoscopic procedure used to examine the canal of the cervix and uterus visually. *Chapter 14.*

I

iliac arteries—A group of arteries located in the pelvis, including the common iliac arteries (which form at the end of the descending aorta), the external iliac arteries (which form where the common iliac arteries bifurcate), and the internal iliac arteries (which form where the common iliac arteries bifurcate). *Chapter 12. See also* common iliac arteries; external iliac arteries; internal iliac arteries.

iliopsoas muscles—A group of large strap muscles that form a continuation of the abdominal psoas. *Chapter 2.*

immune hydrops—An accumulation of fluid within fetal compartments associated with an Rh incompatibility between the Rh− mother and the Rh+ fetus. *Chapters 7, 10. See also* Rh isoimmunization.

in-plane motion—Holding the transducer in one spot and angling along the curve or rounded portion of the scan head; also known as rocking. *Chapter 1.*

in vitro fertilization (IVF)—The process of fertilizing egg cells (ova) with sperm outside the womb. *Chapter 13.*

incompetent cervix—A weakened cervix, resulting in preterm cervical dilatation. *Chapters 3, 6.*

indistinct uterus sign—The inability to appreciate the uterine edges sonographically when infection has matted the adjacent structures to the bowel, broad ligament, and uterus. *Chapter 2.*

induced abortion—Ingestion of antiprogesterone mifepristone (RU486) to induce abortion. *Chapter 3.*

infantile polycystic kidney disease (IPKD)—An inherited autosomal recessive disorder that results in the formation of multiple tiny renal cysts and the failure of the fetal kidneys to produce adequate urine. *Chapter 8.*

inferior vena cava (IVC)—The large vein that brings deoxygenated blood from the lower half of the body to the right atrium. *Chapter 4.*

infertility—The inability to achieve pregnancy after one year of unprotected intercourse for women under 35 and six months for those over 35 years old. *Chapters 2, 13.*

inflow tracts—The superior vena cava and inferior vena cava, which are part of the venous system that carries blood toward the heart and deposits it. *Chapter 4.*

infundibulum—Generally any funnel-shaped structure; in the context of female anatomy and gynecology, the part of the fallopian tube located between the fimbriae and the ampulla. *Chapter 2.*

iniencephaly—A cephalic disorder involving extreme retroflexion of the fetal head associated with severe open neural tube defects of the upper spine. *Chapter 7.*

interface—The boundary layer between different types of human tissue that have different acoustic properties; the acoustic interface.

internal endometriosis—Also referred to as adenomyosis, a condition in which the endometrium invades and grows into the myometrium. *Chapter 2.*

internal iliac arteries—The inner branches of the common iliac arteries on both sides of the body. *Chapter 6. See also* common iliac arteries; external iliac arteries; iliac arteries; vaginal arteries.

internal os—The opening of the cervix on the uterine side. *Chapter 5.*

interocular distance (IOD)—The distance between the ocular orbits measured from the innermost aspect of one orbit to the innermost aspect of the other; also known as the inner orbital distance or interorbital distance. *Chapters 4, 11.*

interorbital distance (IOD)—The distance between the ocular orbits measured from the innermost aspect of one orbit to the innermost aspect of the other; also known as the inner orbital distance or interocular distance. *Chapters 4, 11.*

interstitial fallopian tube—The portion of the fallopian tube that inserts into the uterine cornu. *Chapters 2, 3.*

interstitial ectopic pregnancy—A cornual ectopic pregnancy, one that occurs where the fallopian tube inserts into the uterus and in which part of the gestational sac is within the uterus and part is within the fallopian tube. *Chapter 3. See also* ectopic pregnancy.

intracorporeal liver—Referring to a fetus with an omphalocele that contains only bowel, where the liver is located within the fetus. *Chapter 7.*

intraembryonic mesoderm—The middle layer of the three fetal germ layers, which forms during the first eight weeks of gestation. *Chapter 11.*

intramural—Within the wall of an organ; in obstetrics and gynecology, this refers to the myometrium (uterine wall). *Chapter 2.*

intramural fibroid—A fibroid found within the muscle layer of the uterus (myometrium). *Chapter 2. See also* fibroid.

intrauterine contraceptive device (IUCD, IUD)—A contraceptive device that is inserted into the womb. *Chapter 2.*

intrauterine fetal transfusion—A sonography-guided invasive technique used to treat fetal anemia. *Chapter 15.*

intrauterine growth restriction (IUGR)—Fetal growth that is slower than the normal rate; usually defined as present in fetuses whose weight falls below the 10th percentile for age. *Chapters 8, 10.*

intrauterine pregnancy (IUP)—Any pregnancy that takes place within the womb. *Chapter 1.*

intrinsic—Originating entirely within. *Chapter 11.*

invasive mole—A malignant gestational trophoblastic disorder that may or may not metastasize. *Chapters 3, 12.*

IOD—Interorbital (inner orbital or interocular) distance: the distance between the ocular orbits measured from the innermost aspect of one orbit to the innermost aspect of the other. *Chapters 4, 11.*

IPKD—Infantile polycystic kidney disease: an inherited autosomal recessive disorder that results in the formation of multiple tiny renal cysts and the failure of the fetal kidneys to produce adequate urine; also known as autosomal recessive polycystic kidney disease (ARPKD), it has a high rate of perinatal mortality and nearly always leads to hypertension and, for some, fibrotic or cystic liver disease. *Chapter 8.*

ipsilateral—Pertaining to the side of the body that is in question. *Chapter 12. See also* contralateral.

ischemic—Experiencing a decrease in blood supply.

ischiopagus—Pertaining to conjoined twins sharing a common ischium and sacrum. *Chapter 9.*

isoechoic—Having the same echogenicity as surrounding structures. *Chapter 1.*

isthmus—The neck of a structure. *Chapter 2.*

IUCD—Intrauterine contraceptive device: a contraceptive device that is inserted into the womb. *Chapter 2.*

IUD—Intrauterine device: a contraceptive device that is inserted into the womb. *Chapter 2.*

IUGR—Intrauterine growth restriction: fetal growth that is slower than the normal rate, usually defined as present in fetuses whose weight falls below the 10th percentile for age. *Chapters 8, 10.*

IUP—Intrauterine pregnancy: any pregnancy that takes place within the womb. *Chapter 1.*

IVC—Inferior vena cava: the large vein that brings deoxygenated blood from the lower half of the body to the right atrium. *Chapter 4.*

IVF—In vitro fertilization: the process of fertilizing egg cells (ova) with sperm outside the womb. *Chapter 13.*

J

J sign—The junction of the umbilical vein and the left branch of the portal vein, where the abdominal circumference should be taken, which forms a J shape; also known as the hockey stick sign. *Chapter 4.*

jejunal atresia—Obstruction of the fetal bowel at the second level of the small intestine, usually because of an ischemic event. *Chapter 7.*

jiggle test—A method of identifying the sex of a fetus in response to patting on the maternal abdomen: A scrotum will jiggle like gelatin; swollen labia will not jiggle. *Chapter 4.*

K

ketoacidosis—An accumulation of ketone bodies in the blood. *Chapter 10.*

ketone—Any compound containing the carbonyl group and having hydrocarbon groups attached. *Chapter 10.*

kleeblattschädel—The cloverleaf skull deformity, denoting intrauterine synostosis of several or all cranial structures. *Chapter 7.*

Krukenberg tumor—A metastasis from a primary tumor, such as one of the gastrointestinal tract, breast, pancreas, or ovary; these tumors are bilateral. *Chapter 2.*

kyphosis—An exaggerated convex curvature of the spine resulting in a humpback. *Chapter 7.*

L

labium (*pl.* **labia**)—A fleshy border or lip, often referring to the vaginal labia. *Chapter 4.*

lamina (*pl.* **laminae**)—A thin, flat plate or layer. *Chapter 4.*

large for gestational age (**LGA**)—A fetus, typically of a diabetic mother, that may have normal head and brain growth but an abnormally increased rate of growth of the abdominal organs and trunk, resulting in asymmetrical growth noted at 28–32 weeks. Between 10% and 50% show asymmetrical macrosomia, weighing more than 4500 grams at birth; such children are at increased risk for perinatal morbidity and mortality. *Chapter 10. See also* small for gestational age.

last menstrual period (**LMP**)—The menstrual period preceding pregnancy. Gestational (or menstrual) age is calculated from the first day of the mother's last menstrual period rather than from the date of conception. *Chapter 2.*

LBWC—Limb–body wall complex: a set of disruptive abnormalities associated with failure of the umbilical cord to develop, including lateral body wall defects involving the trunk, spine, and limb anomalies; also known as body stalk anomaly or VACTERL. *Chapters 5, 7.*

leading edge to inner edge method—The method of taking fetal head measurements in an axial scanning plane, at the level of the thalamus, the frontal horns, and the cavum septum pellucidum. Head shape should be oval and the measurement should be taken from the outer edge of the parietal bone in the near field of the image to the inner edge of the parietal bone in the far field of the image. Visible skin and hair are not included in the measurement. Also known as the outer edge to inner edge method. *Chapter 4.*

lecithin-to-sphingomyelin (L/S) ratio—The ratio of lecithin to sphingomyelin in amniotic fluid, used to determine fetal lung maturity. *Chapter 10.*

left atrium—The chamber of the heart that receives oxygenated blood from the lungs and pumps it down into the left ventricle, from which it is delivered to the body. *Chapter 4.*

left common carotid artery—The artery that begins at the aortic arch (second branch) and ends at the carotid bifurcation. *Chapter 4.*

left ventricular outflow tract (LVOT)—The ascending aorta. *Chapter 4.*

leiomyoma—A benign tumor made of muscle and connective tissue; a myoma. *Chapter 2. See also* fibroid.

leiomyosarcoma—A sarcoma containing cells of smooth muscle. *Chapter 2.*

lemon sign—The flattening of the frontal head bones of the fetus, sonographically resembling a lemon shape. *Chapter 7.*

leuprolide (Lupron)—A drug used to treat endometriosis, fibroids, and infertility. It inhibits the production of follicle-stimulating hormone and luteinizing hormone by temporarily cutting off the communication between the brain and the pituitary gland. When fertility drugs are added, multiple dominant follicles develop as the drug suppresses the body's normal selection process, which allows for ovulation of only one egg per cycle. *Chapter 2.*

levator ani muscles—The muscles that form the floor of the pelvis. *Chapter 2.*

level I scan—Old terminology for what is now known as the basic scan. *Chapter 4. See also* basic scan.

levocardia—The condition of the heart being on the left (normal) side of the body while related structures are on the wrong side. *Chapter 4.*

levoposed—Pertaining to a uterus deviated to the left of the midline. *Chapter 2.*

LGA—Large for gestational age: a fetus, typically of a diabetic mother, that may have normal head and brain growth but an abnormally increased rate of growth of the abdominal organs and trunk, resulting in asymmetrical growth noted at 28–32 weeks. Between 10% and 50% show asymmetrical macrosomia, weighing more than 4500 grams at birth; such children are at increased risk for perinatal morbidity and mortality. *Chapter 10. See also* small for gestational age.

LH—Luteinizing hormone: a hormone secreted by the anterior lobe of the pituitary gland that stimulates ovulation. *Chapter 2.*

limb–body wall complex (LBWC)—A set of disruptive abnormalities associated with failure of the umbilical cord to develop, including lateral body wall defects involving the trunk, spine, and limb anomalies; also known as body stalk anomaly or VACTERL. *Chapters 5, 7.*

linear array—A rectangularly formatted image produced by a transducer with many small electronically fired elements oriented side by side. *Chapter 1.*

lithopedion—A calcified fetus. *Chapter 9.*

LMP—Last menstrual period: the menstrual period preceding pregnancy. *Chapter 2.*

lobar holoprosencephaly—The mildest form of holoprosencephaly or failure of the brain to separate into two hemispheres, in which the interhemispheric fissure is well developed anteriorly and posteriorly but there is still some fusion of the lateral ventricles and the cavum septum pellucidum is absent. *Chapter 7.*

lobster claw—A congenital defect with minimal manifestations involving a complete or partial absence of one or more central digits of the hand or foot, creating a gap and inward-curving digits reminiscent of a lobster claw; also known as ectrodactyly. *Chapter 11.*

long axis—The axis that divides a structure into right and left sections; also known as the longitudinal plane or sagittal plane. *Chapter 1.*

longitudinal plane—The scan plane that divides the body into right and left sections through the midline; also known as the long axis or sagittal plane. *Chapter 1.*

lordosis—An exaggerated anterior curvature of the spine causing severe swayback. *Chapter 7.*

loss—Any event that deprives a person of some portion of his or her normal daily life. *Chapter 16. See also* physical loss; symbolic loss.

low-lying placenta—A placenta with the placental edge coming within 2 cm of the internal cervical os. *Chapter 5.*

lower uterine segment—The lower portion of the uterus, between the cervix and the body of the uterus. *Chapter 4.*

L/S ratio—The ratio of lecithin to sphingomyelin in amniotic fluid, used to determine fetal lung maturity. *Chapter 10.*

lumbar vertebrae—The five lower back bones, beneath the thoracic vertebrae. *Chapter 4.*

lumbosacral—Pertaining to the distal spine. *Chapter 4.*

Lupron (leuprolide)—A drug used to treat endometriosis, fibroids, and infertility. It inhibits the production of follicle-stimulating hormone and luteinizing hormone by temporarily cutting off the communication between the brain and pituitary gland. When fertility drugs are added, multiple dominant follicles develop as the drug suppresses the body's normal selection process, which allows for ovulation of only one egg per cycle. *Chapter 2.*

luteal phase—The phase of the menstrual cycle that begins at ovulation (days 15–28), when the endometrium is brightest (most echogenic) and thickest, measuring 8–12 mm; also known as the secretory phase. *Chapter 2.*

luteal phase deficiency—An inability of the corpus luteum cyst to produce adequate amounts of progesterone. *Chapters 3, 13.*

luteinizing hormone (LH)—A hormone secreted by the anterior lobe of the pituitary gland that stimulates ovulation. *Chapter 2.*

LVOT—Left ventricular outflow tract: the ascending aorta. *Chapter 4.*

lymphadenopathy—Enlargement of the lymph nodes as a result of infection or malignancy. *Chapter 2.*

lymphangiectasia—Dilation of the lymphatic vessels. *Chapter 11.*

lymphocele—A collection of lymph fluid that can develop anytime there is a disruption of the lymphatic system. It is not an uncommon postoperative complication. *Chapter 2.*

lymphocytes—Lymph cells. *Chapter 2.*

M

maceration—Degeneration and disintegration of tissues. *Chapter 8.*

macroglossia—An enlarged tongue. *Chapter 11.*

macrosomia—A fetal body size greater than 4500 grams. *Chapters 4, 8, 10.*

magnetic resonance imaging (MRI)—An imaging technology that uses magnetic fields and pulses of radio-wave energy to generate images of internal organs and soft tissues. *Chapters 2, 14.*

major pelvis—A pelvic cavity that includes the bowel and extends to the umbilicus; also known as false pelvis. *Chapter 2.*

malignant—Having a tendency to progress in virulence; cancerous. *Chapter 2.*

mandible length (ML)—The length of the lower jaw. *Chapter 4.*

marginal placenta—A placenta in which the placental edge encroaches on but does not cover the internal cervical os. *Chapters 5, 6.*

marginal placenta previa—A form of placenta previa characterized by the encroachment of the placenta into the margin of the internal cervical os. *Chapter 6. See also* placenta previa.

maternal serum alpha-fetoprotein (MSAFP)—Alpha-fetoprotein in a mother's blood during pregnancy. *Chapters 5, 10.*

maternal serum quad screen—A test that determines how much alpha-fetoprotein is present in a mother's blood during pregnancy. *Chapter 10.*

matrix array transducers—Volume probes composed of a very high number of transducer elements, typically 1000–6000. These acquisition systems offer the advantages of fast frame rates, reasonable image spatial resolution, focus on the elevational plane, probes with a small footprint, and simultaneous visualization of two orthogonal planes without loss of resolution; they are, however, expensive, with narrow apertures and limited probe configurations. *Chapter 14.*

maximum-intensity projection—A projection that preferentially displays high-intensity echoes such as bony structures. *Chapter 14.*

McDonald purse-string technique—A cerclage technique used to manage cervical incompetence, in which a suture resembling a purse-string closure is employed; it is as effective as the Shirodkar technique but with significantly less dissection. *Chapter 6. See also* cerclage; Shirodkar cerclage.

MDKD—Multicystic dysplastic kidney disease, in which multiple cysts of varying sizes replace renal tissue during the embryonic stage of development; can be associated with Potter type II. *Chapter 8.*

mean sac diameter (**MSD**)—A measurement calculated from the longitudinal, transverse, and anterior/posterior gestational sac measurements by adding them together and dividing the sum by 3. *Chapter 3.*

mechanical index (**MI**)—Peak rarefaction pressure divided by the square root of the operating frequency; the risk of inertial cavitation has been found to increase proportionally with increasing rarefaction pressure and to decrease by a square-root relationship with increasing frequency. *Chapter 12.*

Meckel syndrome—An autosomal recessive condition associated with posterior encephalocele, polydactyly, and polycystic kidneys. *Chapters 8, 11.*

meconium—Fetal bowel contents. *Chapters 4, 7, 8.*

meconium peritonitis—Inflammation of the peritoneum following exposure to meconium from a ruptured fetal bowel. *Chapter 7.*

median plane—the mid-sagittal plane. *Chapter 3.*

medical termination—Ingestion of antiprogesterone mifepristone (RU486) to induce abortion. *Chapter 3.*

megacystis microcolon malrotation intestinal hyperperistalsis—The female counterpart of prune belly syndrome. *Chapter 11.*

Meigs syndrome—Pelvic ascites and right-sided pleural effusion associated with an ovarian fibroid. *Chapter 2.*

menarche—The onset of menstruation. *Chapter 2.*

Mendelian disorder—A disorder resulting from inheritance of traits from one parent. *Chapter 11.*

meningocele—Herniation of the cerebrospinal fluid–filled, meninges-covered sac through a defect in the neural tube. *Chapter 7.*

menopause—The cessation of menstruation, which occurs naturally in most women in their early fifties or can occur premenopausally as a result of chemotherapies such as tamoxifen therapy. *Chapter 2.*

menorrhagia—Excessive menstruation and/or prolonged periods. *Chapter 2.*

menses—The monthly discharge of blood from the endometrium. *Chapter 2.*

menstrual age—Gestational age, which is calculated from the first day of the last menstrual period before pregnancy and is 2 weeks older than the conceptual age. *Chapter 3.*

menstruation—A cyclic, hormonally generated bleeding and shedding of the endometrial lining that occurs approximately monthly, from menarche to menopause. *Chapter 2.*

mermaid syndrome—A rare anomaly in which the lower fetal limbs are fused; also known as sirenomelia. *Chapters 10, 11.*

mesenteric cyst—A fluid-filled sac arising from the fold of tissue that anchors organs to the back of the abdominal wall. *Chapter 7.*

mesoblastic nephroma—A hamartomatous tumor of the kidney that resembles a Wilms tumor. *Chapter 11.*

mesosalpinx—The part of the uterine broad ligament extending from the ovary to the fallopian tube. *Chapter 2.*

metrorrhagia—Uterine bleeding that occurs at irregular intervals; bleeding between periods. *Chapter 2.*

MI—Mechanical index: peak rarefaction pressure divided by the square root of the operating frequency; the risk of inertial cavitation has been found to increase proportionally with increasing rarefaction pressure and to decrease by a square-root relationship with increasing frequency. *Chapter 12.*

Mickey Mouse sign—The sonographic appearance of the umbilical cord imaged in cross section; the larger umbilical vein resembles the head and the two small arteries are the ears. *Chapter 4.*

microcephaly—An abnormally small head, with a circumference of 2 or more (or 3 or more, depending on the source) standard deviations below the mean for the gestational age. *Chapter 7.*

micrognathia—An abnormally small jaw with recessive chin. *Chapters 4, 11.*

microphthalmia—Abnormally small eyes. *Chapters 4, 11.*

microtia—The condition of having small ears. *Chapter 4.*

middle cerebral artery—One of the three major paired arteries that supply blood to the cerebrum. *Chapters 4, 12.*

mid-sagittal plane—Referring to an imaginary line down the midline that divides a bilaterally a symmetrical animal (e.g., a human patient) into right and left halves; also known as the median plane. *Chapter 3.*

minimum-intensity projection—A projection that preferentially displays low-intensity echoes such as soft tissues or fluid. *Chapter 14.*

minor pelvis—The portion of the pelvic compartment that includes the bladder and pelvic organs (uterus and ovaries); the true pelvis. *Chapter 2.*

mirror-image artifact—A reflection from a curved surface causing an identical image to appear behind the original source on the ultrasound image. *Chapter 1.*

mirror-image twins—Another name for identical twins, characterized by opposite or reversed features. *Chapter 9.*

miscarriage—Spontaneous abortion, or an abortion that occurs naturally rather than by medical intervention. *Chapter 3. See also* abortion.

mitral valve—The dual-cusp valve in the heart that lies between the left atrium and the left ventricle; also known as the bicuspid valve. *Chapter 4.*

mittelschmerz—A German term for the sharp pain or dull cramping some women experience when ovulation occurs. *Chapter 2.*

mixed/complex mass—A mass that has both cystic and solid characteristics. Three common types of complex masses are regularly seen: predominantly cystic, predominantly solid, and those that contain thick fluid. *Chapter 1.*

ML—Mandible length: the length of the lower jaw. *Chapter 4.*

molar pregnancy—Fertilization of a nonviable egg that develops into a partial or complete hydatidiform mole, invasive mole, or possibly malignant cancerous tumor. *Chapters 3, 16. See also* gestational trophoblastic disorder.

monoamniotic—Developing within the same amniotic cavity. *Chapter 9.*

monochorionic—Developing within the same placenta. *Chapter 9.*

monodermal—From one germinal/fetal layer. *Chapter 2.*

monophasic—Pertaining to waveforms representing a continuous forward flow of blood. *Chapter 12.*

monozygotic—Resulting from the fertilization of a single egg; produces identical twins. *Chapter 9.*

morphologic—Pertaining to form and structure, especially those of a particular organism, organ, tissue, or cell.

morula—The stage after fertilization at which cleavage of a fertilized ovum results in a cell mass of 12–16 cells. *Chapter 3.*

mourning—A process that results in resolving the conflicts associated with loss. *Chapter 16.*

MRI—Magnetic resonance imaging: an imaging technology that uses magnetic fields and pulses of radio-wave energy to generate images of internal organs and soft tissues. *Chapters 2, 14.*

MSAFP—Maternal serum alpha-fetoprotein: alpha-fetoprotein in a mother's blood during pregnancy. *Chapters 5, 10.*

MSD—Mean sac diameter: a measurement calculated from the longitudinal, transverse, and anterior/posterior gestational sac measurements by adding them together and dividing the sum by 3. *Chapter 3.*

mucinous—Containing mucin, a thick gelatinous material. *Chapter 2.*

mucinous cystadenocarcinoma—A malignant ovarian tumor filled with a gelatinous material that can grow to the point of rupture. *Chapter 2.*

mucinous cystadenoma—A benign ovarian tumor filled with a gelatinous material. *Chapter 2.*

müllerian ducts—An embryologic tubular structure, of which there are two, each extending along the mesonephros, and in the female the uterus, fallopian tubes, and superior portion of the vagina develop from their fusion (in the male, the prostatic utricle); also known as the paramesonephric ducts. *Chapter 2.*

multicystic dysplastic kidney disease (**MDKD**)—A condition in which multiple cysts of varying sizes replace renal tissue during the embryonic stage of development; can be associated with Potter type II. *Chapter 8.*

multiparous—Having been pregnant multiple times; also, producing more than one offspring at one birth. *Chapters 2, 6.*

multiplanar display—A display method used for volume sonography that simultaneously shows three orthogonal 2D planes—longitudinal, transverse, and coronal—through the volume. *Chapter 14.*

multiplanar imaging—Imaging in several different planes or projections. *Chapter 14.*

myelomeningocele—A herniation of nerve tissue and the cerebrospinal fluid–filled, meninges-covered sac through a defect in the neural tube. *Chapter 7.*

myoma—A benign tumor made of muscle and connective tissue; a leiomyoma. *Chapter 2. See also* fibroid.

myomectomy—The surgical removal of a leiomyoma. *Chapter 2.*

myometrial cysts—Cysts affecting the muscular wall of the uterus (myometrium), between the endometrium and the myometrial border; they have been associated with adenomyosis but are of little clinical significance. *Chapter 2.*

myometrium—The muscular layer or wall of the uterus. *Chapter 2.*

N

nabothian cyst—A cyst-like formation caused by occlusion of the lumina of glands of the mucosa in the uterine cervix. They will distend in response to retained secretions. *Chapter 2.*

neonatal—Pertaining to the period between birth and the twenty-ninth day of life, or to the newborn.

neonate—A newborn. *Chapter 8.*

nephrosis—Any kidney disease, particularly one associated with destructive lesions of the renal tubules. *Chapter 11.*

nephrostomy—The creation of a permanent opening into the renal pelvis. *Chapter 8.*

neural tube—In embryonic development, the structure that ultimately forms the central nervous system. *Chapters 3, 7.*

neural tube defect (**NTD**)—A birth defect of the brain and spinal cord, commonly associated with maternal diabetes. Common NTDs include spina bifida (in which the spinal column does not completely close during the first month of pregnancy, resulting in some lower-extremity paralysis) and anencephaly (which leads to lack of brain development); in the latter case, survival is almost always limited to infancy. *Chapters 7, 10.*

neuroblastoma—A childhood malignant tumor of nervous system origin, usually adrenal Noonan syndrome (the male counterpart of Turner syndrome). *Chapter 11.*

neuropathy—A general term denoting functional disturbances and pathologic changes in the peripheral nervous system. *Chapter 8.*

NIH—Nonimmune hydrops: fetal hydrops that is not related to the immune system. *Chapters 7, 10.*

nonimmune hydrops (**NIH**)—Fetal hydrops that is not related to the immune system. *Chapters 7, 10.*

nonstress test—A test that monitors and records fetal heart rate in response to fetal movement. *Chapters 4, 8.*

Noonan syndrome—A syndrome whose presentation is identical to that of Turner syndrome, except that Noonan syndrome fetuses can be male or female, whereas Turner syndrome fetuses are always female and Noonan carries a greater hereditary risk as an autosomal dominant condition. *Chapter 11.*

notochord—In embryonic development, the structure that forms the origin of the axial skeleton. *Chapter 3.*

NT—Nuchal translucency: an area of thickening seen posterior to the neck in all fetuses; also known as nuchal lucency. *Chapter 4.*

NTD—Neural tube defect: a birth defect of the brain and spinal cord, commonly associated with maternal diabetes. Common NTDs include spina bifida (in which the spinal column does not completely close during the first month of pregnancy, resulting in some lower-extremity paralysis) and anencephaly (which leads to lack of brain development); in the latter case, survival is almost always limited to infancy. *Chapters 6, 10.*

nuchal—Pertaining to the nape or back of the neck. *Chapter 4.*

nuchal cord—An umbilical cord that is wrapped around the fetal neck. *Chapters 4, 5.*

nuchal fold—The skin from the occipital bone of the fetal cranium to the outer edge of the fetal skin. *Chapters 4, 11.*

nuchal translucency (NT)—An area of thickening seen posterior to the neck in all fetuses; also known as nuchal lucency. *Chapters 4, 11.*

nulliparous—Never having given birth to a viable child. *Chapter 2.*

Nyquist limit—The maximum frequency shift that can be accurately interpreted in a pulsed-Doppler ultrasound unit. *Chapter 12.*

O

oblique lie—A cross between any two of the following fetal positions: cephalic, transverse, and breech. *Chapter 4.*

oblique plane—Any scan plane that is not longitudinal, coronal (anterior/posterior), or transverse. *Chapter 1.*

obturator internus—A muscle group that marks the lateral pelvic sidewalls. *Chapter 2.*

occlusion—A blockage.

OD—Orbital diameter: the distance across one orbit (eyeball). *Chapter 4.*

oligohydramnios—The condition of having too little amniotic fluid. *Chapters 4, 8.*

oligohydramnios sequence—Five conditions: bilateral renal agenesis (classic Potter), autosomal recessive polycystic kidney disease (Potter type I), hereditary renal adysplasia (Potter type II), autosomal dominant polycystic kidney disease (Potter type III), and multicystic dysplasia of the kidneys due to long-term obstruction (Potter type IV). Also known as Potter syndrome or Potter sequence.

oligomenorrhea—Light menses. *Chapter 2.*

omental cysts—Cysts found within the greater and lesser omenta, either single simple unilocular cysts or multiple and complex cysts, ranging in size from a few millimeters to 40 cm. *Chapter 7.*

omphalocele—The herniation of abdominal viscera into the base of the umbilical cord. *Chapter 7.*

omphalomesenteric duct—A structure connecting the yolk sac to the embryo; also known as the vitelline duct. *Chapters 3, 5.*

omphalomesenteric duct cyst—A cyst involving the yolk of an ovum; a vitelline duct cyst. *Chapter 5.*

omphalopagus—The fusion of abdomen to abdomen in conjoined twins. *Chapter 9.*

oocyte—A developing ovum or egg. *Chapter 2.*

OOD—The outer orbital distance: the distance from the lateral edge of one orbit to the lateral edge of the contralateral orbit; also known as binocular distance. *Chapters 4, 11.*

orbital diameter (OD)—The diameter of one fetal orbit (eyeball). *Chapter 4.*

organogenesis—The origin or development of organs. *Chapter 11.*

ossification—The formation of or conversion to bone. *Chapter 4.*

osteogenesis imperfecta—A group of genetic bone diseases that affect collagen in connective tissue in the body and result in brittle bones that may fracture in utero. *Chapter 7.*

outer edge to inner edge method—The method of taking fetal head measurements in an axial scanning plane, at the level of the thalamus, the frontal horns, and the cavum septum pellucidum. Head shape should be oval and the measurement should be taken from the outer edge of the parietal bone in the near field of the image to the inner edge of the parietal bone in the far field of the image. Also known as the leading edge to inner edge method. *Chapter 4.*

outer orbital distance (OOD)—The distance from the lateral edge of one orbit to the lateral edge of the contralateral orbit; also known as binocular distance. *Chapters 4, 11.*

outflow tracts—The great vessels of the heart, consisting of the right and left ventricular outflow tracts. *Chapter 4.*

ovarian arteries—Blood vessels that supply oxygenated blood to the ovaries. They arise from the abdominal aorta below the renal artery and do not pass out of the abdominal cavity. Also known as gonadal arteries. *Chapter 12.*

ovarian carcinoma—Cancer in the ovary. *Chapter 2.*

ovarian cyst—A fluid-filled sac arising from and located in the ovary. *Chapters 2, 7.*

ovarian drilling—A treatment for polycystic ovarian disease in which a laser or electrosurgical needle is used to puncture the ovary several times. *Chapter 13.*

ovarian hyperstimulation—Overstimulation of the ovary to produce follicles, a common complication arising from use of fertility medications. *Chapter 13.*

ovarian reserve—The number of a woman's remaining eggs and therefore her fertility potential. *Chapter 13.*

ovarian torsion—Twisting of the ovaries, which can cause obstruction of the arterial supply, lymphatics, and venous drainage. *Chapters 2, 10.*

ovary—An endocrine organ that contains approximately 100,000 ova (eggs), which are depleted across a woman's fertile lifetime. A woman has two ovaries, connected to the uterus by the fallopian tubes. *Chapter 2.*

oviducts—The fallopian tubes. A woman has two fallopian tubes, each leading from one of the ovaries to the uterus, and alternately down which an ovum (egg) travels during each menstrual cycle. Also known as uterine tubes or salpinges. *Chapter 2.*

ovulation—Discharge of a mature ovum from the ovary. *Chapter 2.*

ovulation induction—A fertility technique used to stimulate the ovaries into releasing more than one egg. *Chapter 2.*

ovum (*pl.* **ova**)—A female reproductive cell (egg), which becomes a zygote after fertilization. *Chapter 2.*

P

PAC—Premature atrial contraction: a contraction of the heart in which the atrium beats too soon, resulting in the sensation of the heart skipping a beat. *Chapter 4.*

papillary muscles—Muscles that limit the movements of the mitral and tricuspid valves, bracing the valves against high pressure and preventing regurgitation of ventricular blood back into the atrial cavities. *Chapter 4.*

paraovarian—Around the ovary. *Chapter 2.*

paraovarian cyst—A unilocular cyst located in the broad ligament. *Chapter 2.*

parity—Number of live-born children. *Chapter 2.*

partial mole—A benign hydatidiform mole that results from the fertilization of a single egg by two sperm cells. *Chapter 3.*

partial placenta previa—A form of placenta previa in which there is partial occlusion of the internal cervical os by the placenta. *Chapter 6. See also* placenta previa.

parvovirus—One of a group of very small, morphologically similar, ether-resistant DNA viruses. *Chapter 10.*

Patau syndrome—A suite of conditions, resulting from a chromosomal abnormality, that most often results in fetal death. Fetuses present with a rounded head shape and flattening of the frontal bones. Also known as trisomy 13. *Chapter 11. See also* lemon sign; trisomy 13.

patent ductus arteriosus—An arterial duct that fails to close after birth. The baby often becomes cyanotic (a blue baby) as a result of a decreased oxygen supply in the bloodstream. *Chapter 4. See also* ductus arteriosus.

PCOS—Polycystic ovarian disease: an endocrine disorder, or more correctly syndrome or complex of symptoms, most often seen in women in their teens and 20s, that causes excessive androgen secretion to inhibit maturation of the ovarian follicles. Symptoms include a high ratio of luteinizing hormone to follicle-stimulating hormone, high serum testosterone and aldosterone, obesity, infertility, and hirsutism. *Chapter 2.*

peak systolic velocity (**PSV**)—The maximum flow state used in calculating the degree of vascular resistance and pulsatility. PSV increases with the narrowing of an artery and thus is useful in grading carotid stenosis. *Chapter 12. See also* diastolic velocity; end-diastolic velocity.

pedunculated—Extending from a stalk or pedicle. *Chapter 2.*

pedunculated fibroid—A fibroid extending from a stalk (pedicle), which allows movement and thus makes it difficult to identify sonographically. *Chapter 2. See also* fibroid.

pelvic congestion—Engorged veins in adnexal regions. *Chapter 2.*

pelvic girdle—The group of irregular, ring-shaped pelvic bones creating the pelvic cavity; it connects to the femur and spinal cord. *Chapter 2.*

pelvic inflammatory disease (**PID**)—Infection of the fallopian tubes, usually involving the ovaries and surrounding peritoneum. *Chapter 2.*

pelvic kidney—A kidney that, during development, fails to rise from its lower lumbar location to its normal position above the level of the waistline. *Chapter 2.*

pentalogy of Cantrell—A syndrome associated with anterior chest and abdominal wall defects. *Chapter 11.*

percutaneous umbilical blood sampling (**PUBS**)—A sonography-guided invasive procedure in which a needle is inserted into the umbilical vein to obtain fetal blood for testing purposes; also known as cordocentesis or fetal blood sampling. *Chapters 11, 15.*

perihepatitis—Inflammation around the liver. *Chapter 2.*

perimetrium—The outer serous layer of the uterus. *Chapter 2.*

periovulatory phase—The midmenstrual cycle, when the endometrium becomes edematous and begins to thicken. *Chapter 2.*

peritoneum—The serous membrane that lines the abdominal cavity and its contents. *Chapter 2.*

pessary—An instrument placed in the vagina to support a prolapsed uterus or rectum; also an instrument used as a contraceptive device. *Chapter 2.*

phased array format—A format in which the transducer transmits and receives sound in the same manner as other array transducers but the image shape is that of a sector scan (triangular) because of the circular alignment of the piezoelectric elements. *Chapter 1.*

phenotype—The outward visible expression of the hereditary constitution of an organism.

philtrum—The vertical groove in the middle of the upper lip. *Chapter 11.*

physical loss—A type of loss that affects a person's physical abilities, such as the loss imposed by cancer's effect on a young woman's fertility. *Chapter 16. See also* loss; symbolic loss.

physiologic death—Cessation of function of vital organs. *Chapter 16.*

physiologic herniation—Rapid growth around 9–10 weeks' gestation, causing the intestines to be pushed outside the body cavity until involution occurs at 11–12 weeks. *Chapter 3.*

PI—Pulsatility index: peak systole minus diastole divided by the mean (time average maximal velocity). *Chapter 12.*

PID—Pelvic inflammatory disease: infection of the fallopian tubes, usually involving the ovaries and surrounding peritoneum. *Chapter 2.*

PIH—Pregnancy-induced hypertension: elevated blood pressure that occurs during pregnancy only. *Chapter 10.*

piriformis muscles—The gray, ovoid muscles arising from the front of the sacrum, moving out of the pelvis through the greater sciatic foramen and entering the upper border of the femur (the greater trochanter). *Chapter 2.*

pitting edema—Edema in which pressure leaves a persistent depression in the tissues. *Chapter 10.*

pituitary gland—The endocrine organ that produces various hormonal secretions directly or indirectly, controlling or affecting most basic body functions. *Chapter 2.*

placenta—The temporary organ that connects the fetus to the mother's uterus during pregnancy. *Chapter 3.*

placenta accreta—The place where the placental villi penetrate the decidua but do not invade the myometrium. *Chapter 5.*

placenta extrachorialis—A placenta whose membranous chorion does not extend to the edge, forming a ring that may be complete or partial. *Chapter 5.*

placenta increta—A placenta whose placental villi penetrate into myometrium but not serosa. *Chapter 5.*

placenta membranacea—A ring-shaped placenta that attaches around the circumference to the myometrium; also known as an annular placenta. *Chapter 5.*

placenta percreta—A placenta whose placental villi penetrate through the myometrium and serosa, which may result in a uterine rupture. *Chapter 5.*

placenta previa—A placenta that partially or entirely covers over the internal cervical os; it often occurs in the second or third trimester. *Chapter 5.*

placental abruption—The premature separation of the placenta from the uterine wall; also known as abruptio placentae or abruption placenta. *Chapter 5.*

placental grading—The classification of placental maturity based on sonographically observable changes. *Chapter 5.*

placental infarction—A condition resulting in the death of some placental tissue as the result of an obstruction of circulation. *Chapter 5.*

placental migration—A misnomer associated with placenta previa; it describes the changes in the architecture of the uterus that cause the placenta to appear to migrate. *Chapter 6.*

placental retraction—A previously reported low placenta that changes position as a result of uterine growth. *Chapter 5.*

placental site trophoblastic tumor (**PSTT**)—A form of invasive mole, or fleshy mass, that forms in the uterus upon the abnormal development of a fertilized ovum. Although invasive moles are considered malignant, they rarely metastasize and are considered highly curable. *Chapter 3.*

pleural effusion—Excess fluid between the two membranes that envelop the lungs. *Chapter 7.*

polar body twinning—The formation of half-identical twins, a phenomenon that occurs when the egg splits before fertilization. Each half is then fertilized by different sperm cells. *Chapter 9.*

polarity—The positive/negative value that correlates with direction of flow. *Chapter 12.*

polycystic ovarian disease (**PCOS**)—An endocrine disorder, or more correctly syndrome or complex of symptoms, most often seen in women in their teens and 20s, that causes excessive androgen secretion to inhibit maturation of the ovarian follicles. Symptoms include a high ratio of luteinizing hormone to follicle-stimulating hormone, high serum testosterone and aldosterone, obesity, infertility, and hirsutism. *Chapter 2.*

polycythemia—The overproduction of red blood cells. *Chapter 8.*

polydactyly—The presence of extra fingers or toes. *Chapter 11.*

polyhydramnios—The presence of too much amniotic fluid. *Chapters 4, 7, 9, 10.*

polyp—Any growth or mass extending from a mucous membrane. *Chapter 2.*

polyuria—Excessive urination. *Chapters 7, 10.*

porencephaly—A process in which normal brain tissue is destroyed and replaced by a cystic lesion usually communicating with the cerebral ventricles. *Chapter 7. See also* hydranencephaly.

posterior—Located at or toward the back of the body, often used to indicate the position of one structure in relation to another. *Chapter 1.*

posterior cul-de-sac—A blind pouch that lies between the posterior uterus and the rectum; also known as the pouch of Douglas or the rectouterine space. *Chapter 2.*

posterior enhancement—Through-transmission; the increased brightness of echoes behind a fluid-filled structure. *Chapter 1.*

posterior urethral valve (**PUV**)—A condition, either unilateral or bilateral, in which the male urethra develops tissue projections extending from the back of the posterior into the urethral canal, causing urinary tract obstruction. *Chapter 8.*

postnatal—After birth.

Potter sequence—*See* Potter syndrome.

Potter syndrome—Used to denote five conditions: bilateral renal agenesis (classic Potter), autosomal recessive polycystic kidney disease (Potter type I), hereditary renal adysplasia (Potter type II), autosomal dominant polycystic kidney disease (Potter type III), and multicystic dysplasia of the kidneys due to long-term obstruction (Potter type IV). Also known as oligohydramnios sequence.

Potter type I—A condition causing multiple tiny renal cysts; infantile polycystic kidney disease (IPKD). *Chapter 8.*

Potter type II—A condition that occurs when one fetal kidney is underdeveloped (hypoplastic) and the other is absent (renal agenesis), hypoplastic, or malformed (dysplastic, including multicystic). *Chapter 8.*

Potter type III—Autosomal dominant polycystic kidney disease (ADPKD), rarely seen in utero; also known as adult polycystic kidney disease (APKD). *Chapter 8.*

Potter type IV—Multicystic dysplasia of the kidneys due to long-term obstruction to the fetal kidneys or ureters. *Chapter 8.*

pouch of Douglas—A blind pouch that lies between the posterior uterus and the rectum; the posterior cul-de-sac or rectouterine space. *Chapter 2.*

power Doppler—A Doppler imaging technology in which overall Doppler energy is displayed as color without regard to directionality; color Doppler energy. *Chapters 12, 14.*

PPROM—Preterm premature rupture of membranes: rupturing of the cervical membranes prior to 38 weeks' gestation. *Chapter 8.*

pre-eclampsia—A pathologic condition that usually occurs late in pregnancy, associated with maternal edema, proteinuria, and hypertension. *Chapter 10.*

pre-embryonic period—The period from fertilization through the end of the second week following fertilization. *Chapter 3.*

pregnancy-induced hypertension (**PIH**)—Elevated blood pressure that occurs during pregnancy only. *Chapter 10.*

premature atrial contraction (**PAC**)—A contraction of the heart in which the atrium beats too soon, resulting in the sensation of the heart skipping a beat. *Chapter 4.*

premature rupture of membranes (**PROM**)—Rupturing of the cervical membranes after 37 weeks' gestation but before the onset of labor. *Chapter 8.*

premature ventricular contraction (**PVC**)—A contraction of the heart in which the ventricles beat too soon; one of the most common types of arrhythmias that occur in a fetus. *Chapter 4.*

prenatal—Before birth.

preterm birth (**PTB**)—Birth occurring before the 37th week of gestation; also known as premature birth. *Chapter 6.*

preterm labor (**PTL**)—Labor occurring before the 37th or 38th week of gestation; also known as premature labor. *Chapter 6.*

preterm premature rupture of membranes (**PPROM**)—Rupturing of the cervical membranes prior to 38 weeks' gestation. *Chapter 8.*

primary yolk sac—The structure that gives rise to the intestines and germ cells but degenerates before sonographic evidence of pregnancy. *Chapter 3.*

primiparous—Pertaining to a first pregnancy. *Chapter 6.*

primitive streak—A structure in embryonic development that forms near the caudal end of the embryonic disc and gives rise to mesenchymal cells. *Chapter 3.*

proboscis—A trunk-like appendage with either one or two openings, usually associated with a missing nose (arhina) and located above the orbital area. It is a feature of holoprosencephaly. *Chapter 11.*

progesterone—The hormone, produced by the corpus luteum cyst, that initiates the secretory phase of the ovarian cycle. *Chapter 2.*

proliferative phase—Regrowth of the endometrium in response to estrogen released by ovarian follicles at the end of menses, when the endometrium has completely sloughed off; the endometrial stripe is thin, measuring 3–6 mm in diameter. *Chapter 2.*

PROM—Premature rupture of membranes: rupturing of the cervical membranes after 37 weeks' gestation but before the onset of labor. *Chapter 8.*

prone—Lying face downward.

propagation velocity artifact—A change in sound velocity as the sound waves pass through tissues of varying densities and stiffness causes misregistration of information. *Chapter 1.*

prophylactic—Treatment intended to ward off disease or an event.

prostaglandins—A group of naturally occurring, chemically related, long-chain hydroxyl fatty acids that affect the contractility of the uterus and other smooth muscle tissues. *Chapter 10.*

proteinuria—An excess of serum proteins in the urine. *Chapter 10.*

prune belly syndrome—A condition resulting from obstruction of the posterior urethral valves, causing complete dilation of the urinary tract. The bladder becomes so grossly distended that the abdominal musculature does not develop and the baby will have a flabby, wrinkled belly upon decompression of the bladder. Also known as Eagle-Barrett syndrome. *Chapter 11.*

pseudocyesis—False pregnancy. *Chapter 3.*

pseudomyxoma peritoni—A rare condition in which a mucinous cystadenocarcinoma ruptures and spills a jelly-like substance into the abdominal cavity. *Chapter 2.*

pseudosac—A false sac; the appearance given when there is fluid in the endometrial cavity and the endometrium is brightly decidualized (in the luteal or secretory phase). *Chapter 3.*

PSTT—Placental site trophoblastic tumor: a form of invasive mole. *Chapter 3.*

PSV—Peak systolic velocity: the maximum flow state used in calculating the degree of resistance and pulsatility.

PSV increases with the narrowing of an artery and thus is useful in grading carotid stenosis. *Chapter 12. See also* diastolic velocity; end-diastolic velocity.

psychological death—Personality changes associated with coming to terms with an affliction. *Chapter 16.*

PTB—Preterm birth: birth occurring before the 37th week of gestation; also known as premature birth. *Chapter 6.*

PTL—Preterm labor: labor occurring before the 37th or 38th week of gestation; also known as premature labor. *Chapter 6.*

pubococcygeus muscles—The muscles arising from the ischium and sacrospinous ligaments that are inserted into the coccyx and sacrum; also known as the coccygeus muscles. *Chapter 2.*

PUBS—Percutaneous umbilical blood sampling: a sonography-guided invasive procedure in which a needle is inserted into the umbilical vein to obtain fetal blood for testing purposes; also known as cordocentesis or fetal blood sampling. *Chapters 11, 15.*

pulmonary artery—An artery that delivers deoxygenated blood to the lungs to pick up necessary oxygen to deliver to the entire body. *Chapter 4. See also* right ventricular outflow tract.

pulmonary hypoplasia—Underdevelopment of the fetal lungs. *Chapter 8.*

pulmonary semilunar valve—A valve that controls blood flow from the right ventricle of the heart into the pulmonary artery. *Chapter 4.*

pulmonary sequestration—An extra or accessory lobe of the lung. *Chapter 7.*

pulsatility index (PI)—Peak systole minus diastole divided by the mean (time average maximal velocity). *Chapter 12.*

pulsed-wave (PW) Doppler ultrasound—A type of Doppler ultrasound technology that transmits a short-duration burst of sound into the region to be examined. The Doppler-shifted signals are processed from a limited depth range. The depth range is determined by a sample gate whose position and size usually can be selected by the instrument operator. *Chapter 12. See also* continuous-wave (CW) Doppler ultrasound.

PUV—Posterior urethral valve: a process in which the male urethra develops tissue projections extending from the back of the posterior into the urethral canal, causing urinary tract obstruction. *Chapter 8.*

PVC—Premature ventricular contraction: a contraction of the heart in which the ventricles beat too soon; one of the most common types of arrhythmias that occur in a fetus. *Chapter 4.*

PW ultrasound—Pulsed-wave Doppler ultrasound: an ultrasonography technology in which one transducer element cyclically transmits and receives. *Chapter 12.*

pyelonephritis—A bacterial kidney infection. *Chapter 10.*

pyeloureteral—Pertaining to the renal pelvis and ureter. *Chapter 8.*

pygopagus—In conjoined twins, the state of being joined dorsally at the buttocks and sacrum, facing away from each other. *Chapter 9.*

pyometra—An accumulation of pus within the uterus. *Chapter 2.*

pyosalpinx—A distended fallopian tube filled with pus. *Chapter 2. See also* hydrosalpinx.

pyrexia—High body temperature that results from fever; in a pregnant woman, the condition may cause neural tube defects, intrauterine death, abortion, or preterm labor. *Chapter 10. See also* hyperthermia.

Q

quickening—A first notice of fetal movement, occurring at 15–20 weeks' gestational age. *Chapter 8.*

R

rachischisis—An open neural tube defect that involves much of the spinal column, which is open like a ditch and covered by skin or meninges. *Chapter 7.*

radial aplasia—The absence of the radius. *Chapter 11.*

radius—The smaller bone in the forearm that is on the thumb side. *Chapters 4, 11.*

real-time imaging—Continuously and rapidly updated imaging that creates a moving picture. *Chapters 12, 14.*

real-time volume sonography—A form of volume sonography used to guide procedures, such as egg retrievals and cyst aspirations, allowing greater accuracy. *Chapter 14. See also* volume sonography.

rectouterine space—The blind pouch that lies between the posterior uterus and the rectum; also known as the posterior cul-de-sac or pouch of Douglas. *Chapter 2.*

rectus sheath—Tissue encasing the abdominal wall muscles. *Chapter 2.*

refraction—The deviation of the sound beam caused by a rounded or curved surface. *Chapter 1.*

region of interest (ROI) box—An area that marks the size of a color Doppler image. *Chapter 14.*

renal agenesis—The failure of the kidneys to develop. Kidneys can be absent unilaterally or bilaterally. Bilateral renal agenesis is also known as classic Potter syndrome. *Chapters 4, 8.*

rendering artifacts—Artifacts, unique to volume sonography, arising when imaging data (e.g., a portion of a structure such as the fetal lip) is removed from a rendered image. Editing artifacts can make normal structures appear abnormal, leading to a misdiagnosis. *Chapter 14.*

resistivity index (RI)—A measure of an organ's resistance to perfusion, calculated as follows: peak systole minus diastole divided by peak systole. *Chapter 12.*

resolution—The amount of detail that an image displays. *Chapter 2.*

retroflexed—The position of a uterus that bends posteriorly at the cervix or fundus. *Chapters 1, 2.*

retrognathia—A recessed chin due to posterior displacement of the mandible. *Chapter 4.*

retroverted—The position of a uterus that is tilted posteriorly. *Chapter 2.*

reverberation artifact—An artifact caused by sound waves bouncing back and forth between two strong (highly reflective) interfaces. *Chapter 1.*

Rh blood group—An antigen system that describes blood types as Rh+ or Rh− depending on whether the Rh factor (the Rh antigen) is present. *Chapter 10.*

Rh isoimmunization—The development in a mother of antibodies against a blood-incompatible fetus, resulting in destruction of the fetal red blood cells. *Chapters 7, 10. See also* immune hydrops.

rhabdomyosarcoma—A malignant tumor generated within muscle tissue. *Chapter 2.*

rhombencephalon—The primitive hindbrain. *Chapter 3.*

RI—Resistivity index: a measure of an organ's resistance to perfusion, calculated as follows: peak systole minus diastole divided by peak systole. *Chapter 12.*

right common carotid artery—The artery that begins at the innominate bifurcation and ends at the carotid bifurcation. *Chapter 4.*

right ventricle—The chamber of the heart that receives blood from the right atrium and pumps it to the main pulmonary artery. *Chapter 4.*

right ventricular outflow tract (RVOT)—The outflow tract from the right ventricle that delivers deoxygenated blood to the lungs. *Chapter 4. See also* pulmonary artery.

ring-down artifact—An extreme form of reverberation in which the ultrasound hits a strong interface and bounces back and forth between the strong interface and the transducer, causing numerous parallel lines shaped like a tornado; a larger version of a comet-tail artifact. *Chapter 1.*

Robert's sign—A radiologic/sonographic indication of fetal demise pertaining to identification of intra-abdominal/thoracic gas in the fetus. *Chapter 8.*

rocker bottom foot—A congenital vertical talus: a form of clubfoot that can result from an abnormally short Achilles tendon. The heel is prominent, extending beyond the calf, and the sole of the foot is convex, with the toes pointing upward like a pixie-toe shoe. *Chapter 11.*

rocking—Holding the transducer in one spot and tilting it along the curve or rounded portion of the scan head; also known as in-plane motion. *Chapter 1.*

ROI—Region of interest. *Chapter 14.*

rotating—Twisting the transducer in a circular motion while holding it in one spot. *Chapter 1.*

RVOT—Right ventricular outflow tract: the outflow tract from the right ventricle that delivers deoxygenated blood to the lungs. *Chapter 4. See also* pulmonary artery.

S

sacrococcygeal teratoma—A tumor composed of the three primary layers of fetal cells—endoderm, mesoderm, and ectoderm—usually located near the fetal coccyx. It is classified according to the percentage of the tumor that is inside and outside the fetus. *Chapter 7.*

sacrum—The large triangular bone at the base of the spine between the two hip bones. *Chapter 4.*

sagittal plane—The scan plane that divides the body into right and left sections through the midline; also known as the long axis or longitudinal plane. *Chapter 1.*

saline—Salty; often used to refer to saline solution. *Chapter 2.*

saline infusion sonohysterography (**SIS**)—An imaging technique used to evaluate the endometrium and endometrial cavity of the uterus by injecting saline into the endometrial cavity, then imaging with transvaginal sonography. *Chapter 2.*

salpinges (*sing.* **salpinx**)—The fallopian tubes; also known as uterine tubes or oviducts. *Chapter 2.*

salpingitis—Inflammation of the fallopian tubes. *Chapter 2.*

sample volume—A clearly defined area within which Doppler characteristics are measured. *Chapter 12.*

sandal gap toe—*See* Sandal toe.

sandal toe—The condition of the large toe being widely spaced away from the others; when detected sonographically in the fetus, it raises concerns over the presence of other anomalies that might indicate Down or another syndrome; also known as a sandal gap toe. *Chapter 11.*

sarcoma botryoides—Embryonal rhabdomyosarcoma arising in the submucosal tissue, usually the upper vagina, cervix, or neck of the bladder in young children and infants. *Chapter 2.*

schizencephaly—A developmental disorder of the fetal brain with abnormal clefting of the cerebral hemispheres. *Chapter 7.*

scoliosis—A sideways curvature of the spine. *Chapter 7.*

S/D ratio—The ratio of systolic to diastolic blood flow. *Chapter 12.*

secondary yolk sac—The sac responsible for hematopoiesis and transfer of nutrients during a pregnancy; it arises as the primary yolk sac regresses. *Chapter 3.*

secretory phase—The phase in the menstrual cycle that begins at ovulation (days 15–28), when the endometrium is brightest (most echogenic) and thickest, measuring 8–12 mm; also known as the luteal phase. *Chapter 2.*

sector format—A triangular or pie-shaped image produced by a transducer with a small footprint. *Chapter 1.*

selective reduction—The deliberate medical termination of one or more fetuses of a multifetal pregnancy of three or more fetuses in order to give the remaining fetus(es) the best chance of developing normally and progressing to term. *Chapter 13.*

semilobar holoprosencephaly—Like alobar holoprosencephaly, a form of holoprosencephaly showing fused thalami and a single monoventricle, but unlike the alobar form, one with partially developed occipital horns and falx. The cavum septum pellucidum is absent. There is decreased brain matter, and the prognosis is poor. *Chapter 7. See also* alobar holoprosencephaly; holoprosencephaly; lobar holoprosencephaly.

semilunar (**SL**) **valves**—The valves of the heart that control the outward flow of blood from the heart through the pulmonary and aortic arteries. *Chapter 4.*

sensitivity zone—The region common to the transmitted beam and the focused depth of the receiving transducer. *Chapter 12.*

seroma—A collection of clear serous fluid. *Chapter 2.*

Serophene—A brand name for clomiphene citrate. *Chapter 13. See also* clomiphene citrate.

serous—Thin, watery. *Chapter 2.*

serous cystadenocarcinoma—A malignant ovarian tumor filled with clear, watery fluid; the most common form of ovarian malignancy. *Chapter 2.*

serous cystadenoma—A benign ovarian tumor filled with a clear, watery fluid. *Chapter 2.*

Sertoli-Leydig cell tumor—A solid androgenic ovarian tumor, usually benign; also known as an androblastoma. *Chapter 2.*

SGA—Small for gestational age: a characteristic of a fetus whose weight falls below the 10th percentile for age, leading to concern over intrauterine growth restriction. *Chapter 8. See also* large for gestational age.

shadowing—A lack of sound transmission, causing a blank spot on the image. *Chapter 1.*

Shirodkar cerclage—The placement of a submucosal band at the internal cervical os to manage cervical incompetence, developed by Dr. V. N. Shirodkar in 1955. *Chapter 6. See also* cerclage; McDonald purse-string technique.

short axis—The axis that divides a structure into superior and inferior sections; also known as the transverse plane. *Chapter 4.*

short umbilical cord syndrome—Another term for limb–body wall complex. *Chapters 5, 7. See also* limb–body wall complex.

sickle cell anemia—A severe chronic hereditary blood disorder in which the abnormal shape of red blood cells leads to vascular obstruction. *Chapter 7.*

side lobe artifact—A secondary, off-axis concentration of energy not parallel to the beam axis. *Chapter 1.*

single deepest pocket method—A method used to obtain the amniotic fluid index (AFI). *Chapter 4. See also* amniotic fluid index.

single umbilical artery (**SUA**)—The absence of an umbilical artery; a two-vessel cord. *Chapter 5.*

single ventricle—A cardiac anomaly in which the lateral ventricles are fused into one large ventricle. *Chapter 7.*

single-puncture method—A technique for performing an amniocentesis on twins in which only one needle insertion is required, reducing risk. The site is determined by the position of the separating membrane; after the first specimen has been obtained, the needle is simply advanced through the membrane into the second sac, from which fluid is aspirated. *Chapter 15.*

sirenomelia—A rare anomaly in which the lower limbs are fused; also known as mermaid syndrome. *Chapters 10, 11.*

SIS—Saline infusion sonohysterography: an imaging technique used to evaluate the endometrium and endometrial cavity of the uterus by injecting saline into the endometrial cavity, then imaging with transvaginal sonography. *Chapter 2.*

situs inversus—A condition in which the organs of the thorax and/or abdomen are arranged in a reversed position; also known as situs transversus. *Chapter 4.*

situs solitus—The normal arrangement of the fetal heart, stomach, liver, spleen, and gallbladder; also known as normal situs. *Chapter 4.*

situs transversus—A condition in which the organs of the thorax and/or abdomen are arranged in a reversed position; also known as situs inversus. *Chapter 4.*

SL valves—Semilunar valves: the valves of the heart that control the outward flow of blood from the heart through the pulmonary and aortic arteries. *Chapter 4.*

slice-thickness artifact—An artifact resulting from a three-dimensional anatomic slice compressed into two dimensions, superimposing tissues and creating artifactual echoes that result in diagnostic ambiguity. *Chapter 1.*

sliding—Moving the transducer from one place to another. *Chapter 1.*

slough—To shed or eliminate; the endometrium is sloughed at the end of the menstrual cycle. *Chapter 2.*

small for gestational age (**SGA**)—A characteristic of a fetus whose weight falls below the 10th percentile for age, leading to concern over intrauterine growth restriction. *Chapter 8. See also* large for gestational age.

smooth chorion—The nonvillous part of the chorion. *Chapter 5.*

social death—A death resulting from an illness or handicap that causes one's circle of friends and social activity to decrease. *Chapter 16.*

solid mass—A mass with ill-defined or irregular borders containing multiple internal echoes. *Chapter 1.*

sonohysterography—An sonographic examination technique in which fluid is injected through the cervix into the uterus, permitting detailed simultaneous evaluation of the uterine cavity, the endometrial lining, and the myometrium. *Chapter 14. See also* saline infusion sonohysterography.

sonologist—A physician (M.D.) who is responsible for interpreting sonographic images. *Chapter 3.*

sonolucent—Pertaining to the sonographic appearance of a fluid-filled structure. *Chapter 1.*

space of Retzius—A space that lies between the anterior bladder wall and the pubic bone. *Chapter 2.*

Spalding's sign—A radiologic/sonographic indication of fetal demise pertaining to visualization of collapse and overlapping of cranial bones. *Chapter 8.*

spectral waveform—Waveforms created in real-time fashion, where the velocity of blood in a clearly defined area is acquired and displayed over a period of time. *Chapter 12.*

speculum—An instrument used for opening or distending a bodily orifice or cavity, such as the vagina, to permit visual inspection. *Chapter 2.*

spina bifida—An incomplete closure or development of the embryonic neural tube, causing defects in the spinal cord and bones. *Chapter 7.*

spina bifida aperta—Open spina bifida that involves membranes and nerves of the spine. *Chapter 7.*

spina bifida cystica—Spina bifida in which both meningoceles and myelomeningoceles are present. *Chapter 7.*

spina bifida occulta—Closed spina bifida, usually diagnosed by radiography, which may include some minimal nerve involvement if skin changes or a patch of hair is present over the defect. *Chapter 7.*

spinal dysraphism—Spina bifida involving incomplete closure of the raphe; all forms of spina bifida fall under this description. *Chapter 7.*

spiral arteries—Maternal vessels located in the base of the placenta; when they develop abnormally, spiral arteries can restrict blood flow to the intervillous space. *Chapter 12.*

split-image artifact—Refraction of sound as it travels through abdominal muscles and produces a duplicate image beside the original reflector. *Chapter 1.*

Stein-Leventhal syndrome—A condition associated with polycystic ovary disease in which the patient presents with hirsutism, obesity, and amenorrhea. *Chapter 2.*

stenosis—A narrowing of a canal or passageway.

stent—An intraluminal support device for tubular structures.

stillborn—Born dead.

strawberry head—A rounded head shape with flattening of the frontal bones, a marker for Edwards syndrome (trisomy 18). *Chapter 11. See also* Edwards syndrome; trisomy 18.

struma ovarii—A rare ovarian tumor made up primarily of thyroid tissue. *Chapter 2.*

stuck twin syndrome—An extreme example of twin-to-twin transfusion in which one twin is growth-restricted within a severely oligohydramniotic sac pressed up against the uterine wall by the larger hydropic twin within a polyhydramniotic sac. The smaller twin appears "stuck" to the wall of the uterus; also known as twin oligohydramnios/polyhydramnios sequence (TOPS). *Chapter 9. See also* fetal parabiotic syndrome; twin-to-twin transfusion syndrome.

SUA—Single umbilical artery: the absence of an umbilical artery; a two-vessel cord. *Chapter 5.*

subchorionic hematoma—A small detached area filled with blood that is left behind when the chorion does not fuse completely with the decidua parietalis. *Chapter 5.*

subcostal—Deep to the ribs.

submucosal—Under the endometrium. *Chapter 2.*

submucosal fibroid—A fibroid that develops underneath the endometrium and may cause endometrial displacement or obliteration. *Chapter 2. See also* fibroid.

submucosal leiomyoma—A benign tumor located below the endometrium that may cause irregular menstrual bleeding. *Chapter 2.*

subserous/subserosal—Under the perimetrium. *Chapter 2.*

subserous/subserosal fibroid—A fibroid that typically develops outside the uterus or in the outer uterine wall, often without symptoms, although these fibroids can cause pain, pressure, abdominal swelling, and—if located near the ovaries—interference with transport of the ovum to the fallopian tube. *Chapter 2. See also* fibroid; perimetrium.

succenturiate placenta—A placenta with a smaller accessory lobe attached to the main lobe. *Chapter 5.*

superior vena cava (SVC)—The large vein that brings deoxygenated blood from the upper half of the body to the right atrium. *Chapter 4.*

supernumerary ovary—An ectopic ovary located away from the normal ovary and not connected to it. *Chapter 2. See also* ectopic ovaries.

supine—Lying face upward. *Chapters 1, 10.*

supine hypotensive syndrome—Fetal compression of the maternal inferior vena cava, decreasing maternal circulation to the point at which the patient begins to faint. *Chapter 10.*

surface rendering—A technology used to image soft surface tissues such as the fetal face. *Chapter 14.*

SVC—Superior vena cava: the large vein that brings deoxygenated blood from the upper half of the body to the right atrium. *Chapter 4.*

symbolic loss—A loss of independence, control, identity, self-esteem, or intimacy, often attendant to and compounding a physical loss. *Chapter 16. See also* loss; physical loss.

symphysis pubis—A line of the union of the bodies of the pelvic bones in the median plane. *Chapter 1.*

syncytiotrophoblast—The outer layer of the trophoblast. *Chapters 3, 5.*

syndactyly—The fusion of two or more digits. *Chapter 11.*

syndrome—Two or more characteristics associated with a specific disorder or process. *Chapter 11.*

synechia (*pl.* **synechiae**)—An adhesion within the endometrial cavity; also known as Asherman syndrome. *Chapters 2, 5.*

systole—The rhythmic contraction of the heart chambers, especially the ventricles, during which they pump blood outward through the aorta and pulmonary artery into the body's circulatory system. *Chapter 4.*

systolic-to-diastolic (S/D) ratio—A measurement of the umbilical cord artery that compares the systolic with the diastolic flow and identifies the amount of resistance in the placental vasculature. *Chapter 12.*

systolic velocity—The speed at which the left ventricle contracts after filling with blood, forcing the blood into the aorta and pulmonary artery. *Chapter 12.*

T

tachycardia—An abnormally fast heart rate. *Chapter 4.*

talipes equinovarus—A deformity that causes the foot to turn inward toward the midline; also known as clubfoot. *Chapter 11.*

talipomanus—A congenital deformity of the hand that can be either radial or ulnar. The radial type (radial aplasia) is more common and usually associated with other abnormalities, while the ulnar type is associated with absence of the ulna but may also be an isolated condition. Also known as clubhand. *Chapter 11.*

talus—The highest of the tarsal bones, which with the tibia and fibula articulates to form the ankle joint. *Chapter 11.*

tamoxifen—A nonsteroidal oral antiestrogen used in palliative treatment of breast cancer in postmenopausal women. *Chapter 2.*

tampon—A pack, pad, or plug made of cotton, sponge, or other material used for control of hemorrhage or absorption of secretions. *Chapter 2.*

targeted scan—Images in addition to those acquired during a basic scan that focus on a suspected anomaly; these images are not routinely included during a basic scan. *Chapter 4.*

Tay-Sachs disease—A common ganglioside storage disease inherited in an autosomal recessive fashion primarily by northeast European Jews. *Chapter 11.*

tenaculum—A hook-like surgical instrument used for grasping and holding. *Chapter 2.*

teratogen—An agent that causes defects in a developing embryo. *Chapter 11.*

teratoma—A neoplasm containing tissues from all three fetal layers: endoderm, mesoderm, and ectoderm. *Chapters 2, 7.*

TES—Twin embolization syndrome: a condition in which clots and debris from a dead twin migrate to a surviving twin, obstructing blood supply and causing organ infarction of central nervous system, genitourinary, and gastrointestinal structures; sometimes known as thrombotic emboli syndrome. *Chapter 9.*

tetralogy of Fallot—A cardiac defect consisting of four main features: a ventricular septal defect, an overriding aorta, pulmonary stenosis, and hypertrophy of the right ventricle (not usually appreciated until after birth). *Chapter 7.*

TGA—Transposition of the great arteries: a cardiac defect in which the aorta abnormally connects to the right ventricle and the pulmonary artery abnormally connects to the left ventricle. *Chapters 4, 7.*

TGV—Transposition of the great vessels: a cardiac defect in which the aorta abnormally connects to the right ventricle and the pulmonary artery abnormally connects to the left ventricle. *Chapters 4, 7.*

thalami—Two large, ovoid structures composed of gray matter and situated at the base of the cerebrum. *Chapter 4.*

thalassemia—A heterogeneous group of hereditary hemolytic anemias marked by a decreased rate of synthesis of one or more hemoglobin polypeptide chains. *Chapters 10, 11.*

thanatophoric dysplasia—The most common lethal skeletal dysplasia, characterized by extremely short long bones (femurs may be curved like a telephone receiver), thoracic dysplasia, small vertebral bodies, and sometimes a cloverleaf skull. *Chapter 7.*

theca cell tumors—An ovarian tumor similar to a fibroid that contains lipoid areas and is derived from theca cells. *Chapter 2. See also* granulosa cell tumors.

theca-lutein cyst—Bilaterally hyperstimulated ovaries; the ovaries become hyperstimulated and present as big, multiseptated cystic masses on both sides. *Chapters 2, 10.*

thecoma—A benign neoplasm that is typically seen in postmenopausal patients and is estrogenic. *Chapter 2.*

thermal index (**TI**)—A predictive value; the ratio of power used to that required to produce a temperature rise of 1 degree Celsius. The temperature rise is dependent on tissue type and is particularly dependent on the presence of bone. The subindices are the thermal index in soft tissue (TIS), the thermal index in bone (TIB), and the thermal index in the cranium (TIC). *Chapter 12.*

thickened nuchal fold—A thickening of tissue at the back of the fetus's neck, suggestive of Down syndrome. *Chapter 11.*

thoracic—Pertaining to the chest. *Chapter 4.*

thoracic vertebrae—The 12 bones of the spine between the cervical (neck) bones and the lumbar (lower back) bones. *Chapter 4.*

thoracoabdominal syndrome—A syndrome associated with anterior chest and abdominal wall defects; also known as pentalogy of Cantrell. *Chapter 11.*

thoracopagus—The most common form of conjoined twins, fused at the thorax. *Chapter 9.*

three-dimensional Doppler—Volume information that is acquired in 3D. *Chapter 12.*

three-dimensional sonography (**3D sonography**)—Imaging in three planes—longitudinal, transverse, and coronal—which allows for seeing depth. *Chapter 14.*

TI—Thermal index: a predictive value; the ratio of power used to that required to produce a temperature rise of 1 degree Celsius. The temperature rise is dependent on tissue type and is particularly dependent on the presence of

bone. The subindices are the thermal index in soft tissue (TIS), the thermal index in bone (TIB), and the thermal index in the cranium (TIC). *Chapter 12.*

tibia—The inner and larger bone of the lower leg. *Chapter 4.*

tilting—The angling of the transducer from side to side in a cross-plane motion. *Chapter 1.*

tip of the iceberg sign—A sign associated with a teratoma/dermoid cyst where calcifications and matted hair absorb the sound so that tissue and structures behind the material are in an acoustic shadow and cannot be seen sonographically, making it impossible to appreciate the true size and extent of the mass. *Chapter 2.*

TOA—Tubo-ovarian abscess: infection of the fallopian tube and ovary. *Chapter 2.*

TOPS—Twin oligohydramnios/polyhydramnios sequence: the result of twin-to-twin transfusion, in which one twin is growth-restricted within a severely oligohydramniotic sac, pressed up against the uterine wall by the larger hydropic twin within a polyhydramniotic sac; also known as stuck twin syndrome. *Chapter 9.*

TORCH infections—Infections associated with toxoplasmosis, rubella, cytomegalovirus, and herpes. *Chapter 2.*

total parenteral hyperalimentation—Nutrition provided by way of needle or catheter triple marker screening. *Chapter 11.*

total placenta previa—A form of placenta previa in which the internal cervical os is completely covered by placenta. *Chapter 6.*

trabeculae—Fibromuscular support bands. *Chapter 4.*

transabdominal—Through the abdominal wall. *Chapters 1, 6, 14.*

transcrestal plane—Transverse plane at the level of the top of the pelvic bones. *Chapter 1.*

translabial—Across the labia minora. *Chapter 6.*

transperineal—Across the tissue between the vagina and rectum. *Chapter 6.*

transposition of the great arteries (**TGA**)—Transposition of the great vessels: a cardiac defect in which the aorta abnormally connects to the right ventricle and the pulmonary artery abnormally connects to the left ventricle. *Chapters 4, 7.*

transposition of the great vessels (**TGV**)—A cardiac defect in which the aorta abnormally connects to the right ventricle and the pulmonary artery abnormally connects to the left ventricle. *Chapters 4, 7.*

transvaginal—Through the vagina; endovaginal. *Chapters 1, 6.*

transverse lie—A fetal position in which the fetus presents shoulder-first, lying horizontally across the mother's abdomen. *Chapter 9.*

transverse plane—A scan plane that divides the body through an imaginary horizontal line across the waistline into superior and inferior sections; also known as the short axis. *Chapter 1.*

transvesical—Through the (usually full) urinary bladder. *Chapter 1.*

TRAP—Twin reversed arterial perfusion sequence: a condition in which one twin has normal circulation but also has to provide circulation for the other twin; also known as acardiac parabiotic twinning. *Chapter 9.*

tricuspid atresia—The absence or abnormal formation of the tricuspid valve. *Chapter 7.*

tricuspid valve—The valve in the heart between the right atrium and ventricle; it pumps blood from the right atrium to the right ventricle while preventing backflow. *Chapter 4.*

trigone—A triangle or triangular area.

trilaminar disc—An embryonic cell mass consisting of endoderm, mesoderm, and ectoderm. *Chapter 3.*

triple marker screening—A screening test for chromosomal anomalies that measures levels of human chorionic gonadotropin, estriol, and alpha-fetoprotein. *Chapter 11.*

triplex system—Also known as tri-mode or triplex mode imaging, an ultrasound imaging mode that simultaneously presents of three types of information: B-mode, pulsed-wave (PW) Doppler, and color Doppler. *Chapter 12.*

triploid pregnancy—Gestation having triple the haploid number of chromosomes. *Chapter 3.*

triploidy—Having triple the haploid number of chromosomes. *Chapter 11.*

trisomy—The presence of an additional (third) chromosome of one type in an otherwise diploid (two-chromosome) cell. *Chapter 11.*

trisomy 13—A usually fatal chromosomal abnormality characterized by rounded head shape with flattening of the frontal bones; also known as Patau syndrome. *Chapter 11. See also* lemon sign.

trisomy 18—Associated with early onset of severe growth restriction with deformities of the hands and feet; also known as Edwards syndrome. *Chapter 11. See also* strawberry head.

trisomy 21—A chromosomal disorder characterized by a small, anteroposteriorly flattened skull, short flat-bridge nose, epicanthal folds, short phalanges, widened spaces between the first and second digits of the hands and feet, and moderate to severe mental retardation; also known as Down syndrome. *Chapters 4, 11.*

trophoblast—Peripheral cells of the blastocyst that attach the fertilized ovum to the uterus and become the placenta. *Chapter 3.*

trophoblastic—Pertaining to the placenta. *Chapter 3.*

trophotropism—Placental growth toward areas of greatest blood supply, resulting in atrophy of areas of lesser perfusion; placental retraction. *Chapter 5.*

true cyst—A cyst of the umbilical cord that is made up of remnants of early embryonic structures and has an epithelial lining. *Chapter 5.*

true knots—A complication resulting from an abnormally long umbilical cord in which actual knots exist in the cord. *Chapter 5.*

true pelvis—The portion of the pelvic compartment that includes the bladder and pelvic organs (uterus and ovaries); also known as the minor pelvis. *Chapter 2.*

truncus arteriosus—An artery connected with the fetal heart developing into the aortic and pulmonary arches. *Chapter 7.*

TTTS—Twin-to-twin transfusion syndrome: a complication of monozygotic twinning in which twins share a single placenta and an artery-to-vein anastomosis shunts blood from one twin to the other, causing growth restriction in the donor twin and hydrops in the recipient. *Chapter 9. See also* fetal parabiotic syndrome.

tubal abortion—Abdominal ectopic pregnancy: abortion resulting from a tubal pregnancy, in which the fertilized egg is expelled out of the fallopian tube into the pelvic cavity, where it communicates with the abdominal cavity, allowing the zygote to migrate into the abdomen, attach itself to a vascular structure, and grow. *Chapter 3.*

tubal ring—A rounded fluid collection surrounded by a thick echogenic ring seen in the adnexa consistent with a tubal ectopic pregnancy. *Chapter 3.*

tubo-ovarian abscess (TOA)—An infection of the fallopian tube and ovary. *Chapter 2.*

Turner syndrome—A condition affecting females in which one of the sex chromosomes (XO) is absent; also known as XO syndrome. *Chapter 11.*

turtle sign—A term applied to describe the fetal scrotum (appearing as the turtle's back) and the penis (turtle's neck and head). *Chapter 4.*

twin embolization syndrome (TES)—A condition in which clots and debris from a dead twin migrate to a surviving twin, obstructing blood supply and causing organ infarction of central nervous system, genitourinary, and gastrointestinal structures; sometimes known as thrombotic emboli syndrome. *Chapter 9.*

twin oligohydramnios/polyhydramnios sequence (TOPS)—A result of twin-to-twin transfusion in which one twin is growth-restricted within a severely oligohydramniotic sac pressed up against the uterine wall by the larger hydropic twin within a polyhydramniotic sac; stuck twin syndrome. *Chapter 9. See also* fetal parabiotic syndrome; twin-to-twin transfusion syndrome.

twin peak sign—Also known as the lambda or chorionic peak sign, this sign refers to chorionic villi that grow into the potential interchorionic space for a short distance beyond where the membranes meet; there is no potential space if there is only one chorion/placenta. The twin peak sign can also suggest dichorionicity, but it is not 100% reliable. *Chapter 9.*

twin reversed arterial perfusion (TRAP) sequence—A condition in which one twin has normal circulation but also has to provide circulation for the other twin; acardiac parabiotic twinning. *Chapter 9.*

twin-to-twin transfusion syndrome (TTTS)—A complication of monozygotic twinning in which twins share a single placenta and an artery-to-vein anastomosis shunts blood from one twin to the other, causing growth restriction in the donor twin and hydrops in the recipient. *Chapter 9. See also* fetal parabiotic syndrome.

two-vessel cord—The absence of an umbilical artery; also known as single umbilical artery (SUA). *Chapter 5.*

type 1 diabetes—The condition in which the pancreas has ceased insulin production; patients experience juvenile onset of diabetes and are insulin-dependent. In White's classification, type 1 diabetics can be further classified as classes C–T. *Chapter 10. See also* gestational diabetes; type 2 diabetes; White's classification.

type 2 diabetes—The condition in which the pancreas produces insufficient amounts of insulin; patients typically experience adult onset of the disease, although its association with obesity has increasingly led to diagnoses in children and young adults as well. In White's classification, this form is class B. *Chapter 10. See also* gestational diabetes; type 1 diabetes; White's classification.

U

uE3—Unconjugated estriol, serum levels of which provide a sensitive indication of fetal well-being and placental function. *Chapter 11.*

ulna—The longer bone in the forearm on the side of the little finger. *Chapter 4.*

umbilical artery—A paired artery (with one for each half of the body) that is found in the abdominal and pelvic regions. In the fetus, it extends into the umbilical cord. *Chapters 5, 12.*

umbilical artery resistivity index (URI)—A measure of resistivity calculated from a spectral waveform obtained from the umbilical artery. *Chapter 12.*

umbilical cord—The stalk that connects the trophoblast to the embryonic disc. *Chapters 3, 4, 5.*

umbilical vein—A vein present during fetal development that carries oxygenated blood from the placenta to the growing fetus. *Chapter 12.*

umbilical venous thrombosis—Torsion, knotting, or compression of the umbilical cord, preventing normal perfusion and commonly resulting in fetal demise. *Chapter 5.*

umbilicus—A depressed scar marking the site of entry of the umbilical cord into the fetus; the naval. *Chapter 2.*

unconjugated estriol (uE3)—A hormone whose serum levels in a pregnant woman provide a sensitive indication of fetal well-being and placental function. *Chapter 11.*

unicornuate uterus—A uterus with only one fully developed müllerian duct. *Chapter 2.*

uniplex mode imaging—The presentation of one type of information: pulsed-wave (PW) vs. B-mode. *Chapter 12.*

unusual facies syndrome—*See* Femoral hypoplasia–unusual facies syndrome.

UPJ—Ureteropelvic junction: the junction of the ureter and the renal pelvis. *Chapter 8.*

urachal cyst—A cyst that forms in the canal connecting the fetal bladder to the allantois, a structure that is normally obliterated during fetal development. *Chapter 7.*

urachus—The connecting tube within the embryo/fetus that runs from the superior bladder to the umbilicus (allantois). *Chapter 3.*

ureterocele—A ballooning of the lower end of the ureter into the bladder. *Chapter 2.*

ureteropelvic junction (**UPJ**)—The junction of the ureter and the renal pelvis. *Chapter 8.*

ureteropelvic junction (**UPJ**) **obstruction**—A simple stricture, narrowing of the ureter, or other obstruction at the junction of the ureter and the renal pelvis. *Chapter 8.*

ureterovesical junction (**UVJ**) **obstruction**—An obstruction that is usually associated with primary megaureter and rarely with a distal ureteral stricture or valve. *Chapter 8.*

URI—Umbilical artery resistivity index: a measure of resistivity calculated from a spectral waveform obtained from the umbilical artery. *Chapter 12.*

urinary tract disorder—An obstruction or infection of the urinary tract, common during pregnancy. *Chapter 10.*

urinoma—A collection of urine. *Chapter 8.*

uterine adnexa—Uterine appendages, including the ovaries and fallopian tubes. *Chapter 2.*

uterine agenesis—The absence of the uterus above the vagina. *Chapter 2.*

uterine artery—The artery that attaches to the upper third of the cervix and continues its course upward along the lateral aspect of the uterus; it supplies blood to the uterus. *Chapter 12.*

uterine cornu—The point where the uterus meets the uterine tubes; the uterine horn. *Chapter 2.*

uterine flexion—The displacement of the uterus, in which the organ is bent so far anteriorly or posteriorly that an acute angle forms between the fundus and the cervix. *Chapter 2.*

uterine isthmus—The neck of the uterus or lower uterine segment. *Chapter 6.*

uterine prolapse—Downward displacement of the uterus. *Chapter 2.*

uterine sound—An instrument used to measure uterine depth or the distance between the cervix and the uterine fundus. *Chapter 2.*

uterine tubes—The fallopian tubes; also known as oviducts or salpinges. *Chapter 2.*

uterosalpingography—Radiographic imaging of the uterus and fallopian tubes, using injection of an opaque material, to examine their shape; also known as hysterosalpingography. *Chapter 14.*

uterovesical space—The area between the anterior uterine wall and the posterior bladder; the anterior cul-de-sac. *Chapter 2.*

uterus—The major female reproductive organ. *Chapter 2.*

UVJ—Ureterovesical junction. *Chapter 8.*

V

VACTERL—A syndrome with vertebral, anal, cardiac, tracheoesophogeal, renal, and limb abnormalities; a body stalk anomaly or limb–body wall complex (LBWC). *Chapter 7.*

vagina—The fibromuscular tubular tract leading from the uterus to the exterior of the body. *Chapter 2.*

vaginal arteries—The branches of the internal iliac artery that provide blood for the vagina and the base of the bladder and the rectum. *Chapter 12.*

Valsalva maneuver—Having the patient bear down on the abdominal muscles as if the patient were having a bowel movement. *Chapter 12.*

vanishing twin—A first trimester complication in which one twin dies early in the pregnancy and becomes reabsorbed, resulting in a singleton at birth. *Chapter 9. See also* fetus in fetu; fetus papyraceous.

varicocele—Varicose veins of the spermatic cord, responsible for male infertility. *Chapter 13.*

vasa previa—An umbilical cord presenting at internal cervical os, associated with high fetal mortality due to hemorrhage at the time of labor and birth. *Chapter 5.*

vein of Galen aneurysm—An arteriovenous (AV) malformation in which blood shunts from cerebral arteries into a dilated vein of Galen. *Chapter 7.*

velamentous insertion—The insertion of the cord into membranes rather than the placental mass. *Chapter 5.*

velocimetry—The measurement of blood flow velocities in the middle cerebral artery. *Chapter 12.*

ventricular septal defect (**VSD**)—A defect in the wall that separates the right and left ventricles of the heart. *Chapters 4, 7.*

ventricular septum—The wall in the heart that divides the left and right ventricles. *Chapter 4.*

ventriculomegaly—Enlargement of the ventricles in the fetal brain. *Chapter 7.*

vernix—A cheesy film of fetal skin cells and hair that shed into the amniotic fluid and remain on the fetus at birth. *Chapter 4.*

vertex—The normal cephalic fetal position, in which the fetus presents with the top of the head.

vesicoureteral—Pertaining to the bladder and ureter. *Chapter 8.*

vesicoureteral reflux—A backwash of urine caused by malfunctioning muscles at the junction of ureter and bladder. *Chapter 8.*

villous chorion—The part of the chorion covered by villi; the chorion frondosum. *Chapter 5.*

vitelline duct—The structure connecting the yolk sac to the embryo; the omphalomesenteric duct. *Chapters 3, 5.*

vitelline duct cyst—A cyst involving the yolk sac of an ovum; also known as the omphalomesenteric duct cyst. *Chapter 5.*

volume probe—A probe with a mechanical drive contained within the probe case itself; also referred to as a dedicated mechanized volume probe. *Chapter 14.*

volume sonography—Three-dimensional (as opposed to two-dimensional) ultrasonography. Planes that are inaccessible to conventional two-dimensional ultrasonography are calculated from a volume data set and displayed as 3D imagery. *Chapter 14.*

volume sonohysterography—A technique of sonohysterography with a dedicated volume ultrasound system, similar to conventional sonohysterography. *Chapter 14.*

voxel—A volumetric picture element in a grid representing a three-dimensional value, processed by computer from a two-dimensional slice. *Chapter 14.*

VSD—Ventricular septal defect: a defect in the wall that separates the right and left ventricles of the heart. *Chapters 4, 7.*

W

wedge resection—A surgical procedure that decreases the amount of androgen-producing ovarian tissue of a polycystic ovary in order to increase the chances for fertility. *Chapters 2, 13.*

Wharton's jelly—The mucus around the vessels of the umbilical cord. *Chapters 4, 5.*

White's classification—A system for classifying the impact of gestational diabetes on the child based on the research of Priscilla White. Class A denotes the highest probability of fetal survival, with no insulin and minor dietary regulation; B, onset at age 20 or later with less than 10 years' duration before pregnancy; C, onset between 10 and 19 years of age, with minimal vascular disease; D, onset before age 20 with 20 or more years' duration and moderate to advanced vascular disease; E, same as class D and with calcification of the pelvic vessels; F, with nephritis added; G, with many organ failures; H, with cardiomyopathy; R, with active retinitis; and T, requiring renal transplant. *Chapter 10. See also* gestational diabetes; type 1 diabetes; type 2 diabetes.

Willis, circle of—A ring of arteries made up of the posterior cerebral arteries, posterior communicating arteries, middle cerebral arteries, and anterior communicating arteries that serves as a safety mechanism for blood flow through the fetal (and later adult) brain. *Chapter 4.*

Wilms tumor—A highly malignant childhood tumor of the kidney. *Chapter 11.*

X

xiphopagus—The fusion of the anterior abdominal wall to the umbilicus. *Chapter 9.*

XO syndrome—A condition affecting females in which one of the sex chromosomes (XO) is absent; also known as Turner syndrome. *Chapter 11.*

Y

yolk sac—A membranous sac attached to the embryo's midgut by a tube (the yolk stalk), providing early nourishment and blood formation; refers first to the primary and then to the secondary yolk sac. *Chapter 3.*

yolk sac tumor—A highly malignant tumor developing within the germ cells of a fetus; also known as an endodermal sinus tumor. *Chapter 2.*

yolk stalk—The tube that connects the embryo to the yolk sac during early stages of pregnancy. *Chapter 5.*

Z

ZIFT—Zygote intrafallopian tube transfer: the placement of an embryo or zygote within the fallopian tube via an endovaginal guided cannula. *Chapter 13.*

zygomatic arches—The cheek bones. *Chapter 4.*

zygosity—The number of eggs fertilized. *Chapter 9.*

zygote—The fertilized ovum. *Chapter 3.*

zygote intrafallopian transfer (ZIFT)—The placement of an embryo or zygote within the fallopian tube via an endovaginal guided cannula. *Chapter 13.*

Application for CME Credit

Ultrasound in Obstetrics and Gynecology: A Practitioner's Guide

INTRODUCTION

Ultrasound in Obstetrics and Gynecology: A Practitioner's Guide is a continuing medical educational (CME) activity approved for 15 hours of credit by the Society of Diagnostic Medical Sonography and may be used by more than one person (see *Note* below).

Who May Apply for CME Credit

This credit may be applied as follows:

- Sonographers and technologists may apply these hours toward the CME requirements of ARDMS, ARRT, and/or CCI, as well as to the CME requirements of ICAVL for technologists and sonographers in ICAVL-accredited facilities.

- Physicians may apply a certain maximum number of SDMS-approved credit hours toward the CME requirements of ICAVL for accreditation of diagnostic facilities. (Be sure to confirm current requirements with the pertinent organizations.) Physicians who are registered sonographers or technologists may apply all of these hours toward the CME requirements of the

ARDMS, ARRT, and/or CCI. SDMS-approved credit is not applicable toward the AMA Physician's Recognition Award.

If you have any questions about CME requirements that affect you, please contact the responsible organization directly for current information. CME requirements can and sometimes do change.

OBJECTIVES OF THE ACTIVITY

Upon completion of this educational activity, you will be able to:

1. Explain how, when, and why ultrasonography is applied in the practice of obstetrics and gynecology.

2. Describe how the female pelvic anatomy is imaged in two dimensions.

3. Describe how, when, and why gynecologic and fetal measurements are made.

4. Describe normal and abnormal prenatal development from conception through the three trimesters of pregnancy.

5. Describe the diseases, disorders, complications, and coexisting disorders of the female reproductive system, pregnancy, and antepartum and postpartum fetus.

6. Differentiate normal from abnormal obstetric and gynecologic sonographic findings and explain the correlations between these findings and pertinent laboratory, imaging, and biophysical studies.

7. Explain the differences between the basic and targeted scans during the second and third trimesters, listing the images required to document each and identifying the indications for a targeted scan.

8. List the maternal and fetal complications associated with maternal disorders during pregnancy and discuss how sonography plays a role in their diagnosis, monitoring, and treatment.

9. Discuss the sonographic tests performed to identify a fertility problem and the techniques of ultrasonography used in fertility assistance.

10. Explain the therapeutic and diagnostic capabilities of amniocentesis, cordocentesis, amnioreduction, amnioinfusion, fetal blood sampling, intrauterine fetal transfusion, and minimally invasive ultrasound-guided surgery.

HOW TO OBTAIN CME CREDIT

To apply for credit, please do all of the following:

1. Read and study the book and complete the interactive exercises it contains.

2. Make copies of the applicant information page, evaluation questionnaire (you grade us!), and answer sheet.

3. Make copies of the completed forms and quiz for your records and then return the originals (i.e., the photocopied forms with your original writing) to the following address:

Davies Publishing, Inc.
Attn: CME Coordinator
32 South Raymond Avenue, Suite 4
Pasadena, California 91105-1961

You may also fax us the applicable pages and pay by credit card. Our fax number is 626-792-5308. You may call us with your credit card, expiration date, and 3- or 4-digit security code or include it with the fax. We grade quizzes within 24 hours of receipt and will email and mail your certificate. Questions? Please call us at 626-792-3046.

4. If more than one person will be applying for credit, be sure to photocopy the applicant information, evaluation form, and CME quiz so that you always have the original on hand for use.

NOTE

The original purchaser of this CME activity is entitled to submit this CME application for an administrative fee of $39.50. Please enclose a check payable to Davies Publishing Inc. with your application. Others may also submit applications for CME credits by completing the activity as explained above and enclosing an administrative fee of $49.50. The CME administrative fee helps to defray the cost of processing, evaluating, and maintaining a record of your application and the credit you earn. Fees may change without notice. For the current fee, call us at 626-792-3046, e-mail us at **cme@DaviesPublishing.com**, or write to us at the aforementioned address. We will be happy to help!

Ultrasound in Obstetrics and Gynecology: A Practitioner's Guide

APPLICANT INFORMATION

Name _____   Date of birth _____

Current credentials _____

Home address _____

City/State/Zip _____

Telephone _____   email address _____

ARDMS # _____   ARRT # _____   SDMS # _____   CCI # _____

Credit Card # _____   Expiration date _____   Security code _____

❏ I purchased this book myself.   ❏ I borrowed the book.

Signature certifying your completion of the activity _____

EVALUATION—YOU GRADE US!

Please let us know what you think of *Ultrasound in Obstetrics and Gynecology: A Practitioner's Guide*. Participating in this quality survey is a requirement for CME applicants, and it benefits future readers by ensuring that current readers are satisfied and, if not, that their comments and opinions are heard and taken into account. Your opinions count!

1. Why did you purchase *Ultrasound in Obstetrics and Gynecology: A Practitioner's Guide*? (Check primary reason.)

   ❏ REGISTRY REVIEW   ❏ COURSE TEXT
   ❏ CLINICAL REFERENCE   ❏ CME ACTIVITY

2. Have you used *Ultrasound in Obstetrics and Gynecology: A Practitioner's Guide* for other reasons, too? (Check all that apply.)

   ❏ REGISTRY REVIEW   ❏ COURSE ACTIVITY
   ❏ CLINICAL REFERENCE   ❏ CME ACTIVITY

3. To what extent did *Ultrasound in Obstetrics and Gynecology: A Practitioner's Guide* meet its stated objectives and your needs? (Check one.)

   ❏ GREATLY   ❏ MODERATELY
   ❏ MINIMALLY   ❏ INSIGNIFICANTLY

4. The content of *Ultrasound in Obstetrics and Gynecology: A Practitioner's Guide* was (check one):

   ❏ Just right   ❏ Too basic
   ❏ Too advanced

5. The quality of the questions and explanations was mainly (check one):

   ❏ EXCELLENT   ❏ GOOD
   ❏ FAIR   ❏ POOR

6. The manner in which *Ultrasound in Obstetrics and Gynecology: A Practitioner's Guide* presents the material is mainly (check one):

   ❏ EXCELLENT   ❏ GOOD
   ❏ FAIR   ❏ POOR

7. If you used this book to prepare for the registry exam, did you also use other materials or take any exam-preparation courses?

   ❏ NO   ❏ YES (PLEASE SPECIFY WHAT MATERIALS AND COURSES)

   _____

   _____

   _____

8. If you used this book for a course, please name the course, the instructor's name, the name of the school or program, and any other textbooks you may have used:

   COURSE/INSTRUCTOR/SCHOOL OR PROGRAM: _____

   _____

   _____

   _____

   OTHER TEXTBOOKS: _____

   _____

   _____

   _____

9. What did you like best about *Ultrasound in Obstetrics and Gynecology: A Practitioner's Guide?*

   _____

   _____

   _____

   _____

10. What did you like least about *Ultrasound in Obstetrics and Gynecology: A Practitioner's Guide?*

   _____

   _____

   _____

   _____

11. If you used *Ultrasound in Obstetrics and Gynecology: A Practitioner's Guide* to prepare for the ARDMS exam in OB/GYN, did you pass?

   ❏ YES   ❏ No   ❏ HAVEN'T YET TAKEN IT

12. May we quote any of your comments in our catalogs or promotional material?

   ❏ YES   ❏ No   ❏ FURTHER COMMENT . . .

   _____

   _____

   _____

   _____

   _____

   _____

   _____

   _____

   _____

   _____

   _____

   _____

   _____

   _____

Ultrasound in Obstetrics and Gynecology: A Practitioner's Guide

ANSWER SHEET

Circle the correct answer below and return this sheet to Davies Publishing Inc. Passing criterion is 70%. Applicant may have no more than 3 attempts to pass.

1. A B C D E	39. A B C D E	77. A B C D E	114. A B C D E
2. A B C D E	40. A B C D E	78. A B C D E	115. A B C D E
3. A B C D E	41. A B C D E	79. A B C D E	116. A B C D E
4. A B C D E	42. A B C D E	80. A B C D E	117. A B C D E
5. A B C D E	43. A B C D E	81. A B C D E	118. A B C D E
6. A B C D E	44. A B C D E	82. A B C D E	119. A B C D E
7. A B C D E	45. A B C D E	83. A B C D E	120. A B C D E
8. A B C D E	46. A B C D E	84. A B C D E	121. A B C D E
9. A B C D E	47. A B C D E	85. A B C D E	122. A B C D E
10. A B C D E	48. A B C D E	86. A B C D E	123. A B C D E
11. A B C D E	49. A B C D E	87. A B C D E	124. A B C D E
12. A B C D E	50. A B C D E	88. A B C D E	125. A B C D E
13. A B C D E	51. A B C D E	89. A B C D E	126. A B C D E
14. A B C D E	52. A B C D E	90. A B C D E	127. A B C D E
15. A B C D E	53. A B C D E	91. A B C D E	128. A B C D E
16. A B C D E	54. A B C D E	92. A B C D E	129. A B C D E
17. A B C D E	55. A B C D E	93. A B C D E	130. A B C D E
18. A B C D E	56. A B C D E	94. A B C D E	131. A B C D E
19. A B C D E	57. A B C D E	95. A B C D E	132. A B C D E
20. A B C D E	58. A B C D E	96. A B C D E	133. A B C D E
21. A B C D E	59. A B C D E	97. A B C D E	134. A B C D E
22. A B C D E	60. A B C D E	98. A B C D E	135. A B C D E
23. A B C D E	61. A B C D E	99. A B C D E	136. A B C D E
24. A B C D E	62. A B C D E	100. A B C D E	137. A B C D E
25. A B C D E	63. A B C D E	101. A B C D E	138. A B C D E
26. A B C D E	64. A B C D E	102. A B C D E	139. A B C D E
27. A B C D E	65. A B C D E	103. A B C D E	140. A B C D E
28. A B C D E	66. A B C D E	104. A B C D E	141. A B C D E
29. A B C D E	67. A B C D E	105. A B C D E	142. A B C D E
30. A B C D E	68. A B C D E	106. A B C D E	143. A B C D E
31. A B C D E	69. A B C D E	107. A B C D E	144. A B C D E
32. A B C D E	70. A B C D E	108. A B C D E	145. A B C D E
33. A B C D E	71. A B C D E	109. A B C D E	146. A B C D E
34. A B C D E	72. A B C D E	110. A B C D E	147. A B C D E
35. A B C D E	73. A B C D E	111. A B C D E	148. A B C D E
36. A B C D E	74. A B C D E	112. A B C D E	149. A B C D E
37. A B C D E	75. A B C D E	113. A B C D E	150. A B C D E
38. A B C D E	76. A B C D E		

Ultrasound in Obstetrics and Gynecology: A Practitioner's Guide

CME QUIZ

Please answer the following questions after you have completed the CME activity. There is one *best* answer for each question. Circle it on the answer sheet that appears on the previous page.

1. Which group of muscles forms the floor of the pelvis?
   A. Obturator internus
   B. Piriformis
   C. Coccygeus
   D. Levator ani
   E. Iliopsoas

2. What type of transducer produces a rectangular format?
   A. Sector
   B. Phased array
   C. Linear
   D. Mechanical
   E. Curved linear

3. For which of the following conditions would use of a fetal shunt be indicated?
   A. Duodenal atresia
   B. Polycystic kidneys
   C. Hydranencephaly
   D. Pleural effusion
   E. All of the above

4. A fetus small for gestational age is most commonly associated with:
   A. Maternal exposure to radiation
   B. Intrauterine infection
   C. Incorrect dates
   D. Maternal alcohol use
   E. Maternal cigarette smoking

5. Hypoplasia of the middle phalanx of the fifth finger results in:
   A. Adactyly
   B. Polydactyly
   C. Clinodactyly
   D. Syndactyly
   E. C and D

6. Which of the following would lead you to suspect infantile polycystic kidneys?
   A. Kidneys abnormally small in appearance
   B. Kidneys with hyperechoic appearance
   C. Appearance of absent kidneys
   D. Kidneys with hypoechoic appearance
   E. Kidneys with irregular or distorted appearance

7. Which condition would *not* be associated with a thick, hydropic placenta?
   A. TORCH infections
   B. Gestational diabetes
   C. Intrauterine growth restriction
   D. Fetal hydrops
   E. Triploidy

8. The alobar, semilobar, and lobar forms are three types of:
   A. Holoprosencephaly
   B. Diaphragmatic hernia
   C. Congenital cystic adenomatoid malformation
   D. Spina bifida
   E. Encephalocele

9. Posterior urethral valves are *not*:
   A. Associated with oligohydramnios
   B. A cause of unilateral hydronephrosis
   C. A cause of bilateral hydronephrosis
   D. A cause of urinary tract dilation
   E. Usually fatal

10. When should every pregnant patient be evaluated for diabetes?

    A. Between 16 and 20 weeks

    B. Between 28 and 32 weeks

    C. Between 20 and 24 weeks

    D. Between 24 and 28 weeks

    E. Between 34 and 36 weeks

11. The compression maneuver for scanning is *not* used to:

    A. Elicit tissue response

    B. Test the patient's tolerance for discomfort

    C. Compress fat

    D. Displace bowel gas

    E. Determine cystic from solid

12. In gynecologic and obstetric ultrasound, which artifact is most common?

    A. Editing

    B. Acquisition

    C. Motion

    D. Rendering

13. The normal uterine position for most women, when the urinary bladder is empty, is:

    A. Retroverted

    B. Retroflexed

    C. Levoposed

    D. Anteverted

    E. Anteflexed

14. An ectopic pregnancy is most often located in the:

    A. Cervix

    B. Ampullary portion of the fallopian tube

    C. Abdomen

    D. Cornual portion of the fallopian tube

    E. Ovary

15. A diamniotic/monochorionic pregnancy is suggested by a separating membrane that measures:

    A. < 4 mm

    B. > 4 mm

    C. < 2 mm

    D. 1 cm

    E. > 2 mm

16. Amnioreduction is *not* indicated for:

    A. Twin-to-twin transfusion syndrome associated with monochorionicity

    B. Maternal discomfort resulting from polyhydramnios

    C. Maternal difficulty breathing resulting from polyhydramnios

    D. Fetal hydrops associated with Rh sensitization

    E. Maternal insomnia caused by polyhydramnios

17. In a transabdominal, longitudinal image, the feet of the patient are toward:

    A. The bottom of the image

    B. The left side of the image

    C. The right side of the image

    D. Depends on whether patient is supine or prone.

    E. The top of the image

18. All of the following statements about 3D/4D imaging are true *except*:

    A. You should use the lowest frame rate possible.

    B. You should use the slowest acquisition speed.

    C. The field of view should be the narrowest possible.

    D. The overall field of view should be the shallowest possible.

19. Normally physiologic herniation of the fetal midgut resolves by which gestational age?

    A. 8 weeks

    B. 12 weeks

    C. 4 weeks

    D. 10 weeks

    E. 6 weeks

20. Ovarian teratomas (commonly called dermoids) usually are *not*:

    A. Monodermal

    B. Malignant

    C. Composed of fetal tissues

    D. More common in young adults

    E. Bilateral

21. Amniocentesis should be performed with:

    A. A 20-gauge needle

    B. An 8-gauge needle

    C. A 22-gauge needle

    D. A 16-gauge needle

    E. A needle of any size

22. Which of the following Doppler ultrasound studies will *not* help predict fetal growth restriction?

    A. Internal iliac artery Doppler

    B. Fetal cerebral artery Doppler

    C. Umbilical artery Doppler

    D. Uterine artery Doppler

23. A normal fetal nuchal fold should not measure more than:

    A. 4 mm

    B. 2 mm

    C. 3 mm

    D. 6 mm

    E. 5 mm

24. On sonography, pulmonary sequestration can resemble:

    A. Microcystic adenomatoid malformation

    B. Pericardial effusion

    C. Left-sided diaphragmatic hernia

    D. Macrocystic adenomatoid malformation

    E. Right-sided diaphragmatic hernia

25. Which of the following is indicated by an increase in basal body temperature?

    A. Fertilization has occurred.

    B. Fertilization is certain.

    C. Ovulation has occurred.

    D. Ovulation will occur in 48 hours.

    E. The patient has an infection.

26. The combination of hydrops in one fetal twin and small for gestational age in the other suggests:

    A. Intrauterine growth restriction

    B. Acardiac parabiotic twinning

    C. Twin reversed arterial perfusion sequence

    D. Twin-to-twin transfusion syndrome

    E. Twin embolization syndrome

27. Which structure within the gestational sac is the first that can be imaged with sonography?

    A. Secondary yolk sac

    B. Primary yolk sac

    C. Vitelline duct

    D. Amnion

    E. Embryonic disc

28. The cervix is best measured by means of:

    A. Transabdominal sonography

    B. Digital examination

    C. Translabial sonography

    D. Transperineal sonography

    E. Transvaginal sonography

29. What is the name for the maternal surface of the placenta?

    A. Decidual reaction

    B. Decidua parietalis

    C. Decidua vera

    D. Decidua capsularis

    E. Decidua basalis

30. All of the following findings suggest fetal demise *except*:

    A. Spalding's sign

    B. Negative fetal heart tones

    C. Absence of fetal motion

    D. Increased fundal height

    E. Decreased fundal height

31. The term denoting a short, wide, and very round fetal head shape is:

A. Microcephaly

B. Brachycephaly

C. Macrocephaly

D. Exencephaly

E. Dolichocephaly

32. Which of these characteristics of multiple gestations is the most difficult to define sonographically?

A. Gender

B. Zygosity

C. Twin presentation

D. Amnionicity

E. Chorionicity

33. Percutaneous umbilical blood sampling is indicated for which of the following?

A. Evaluation for fetal infection

B. Rapid karyotyping

C. Evaluation for fetal thrombocytopenia

D. Evaluation of fetal anemia

E. All of the above

34. A fetal transfusion should be stopped when:

A. Blood streaming is seen in the umbilical vein

B. The fetus is moving

C. Tachycardia is noted in the fetus

D. Bradycardia is noted in the fetus

E. Fetal respiration begins

35. What should you do if a patient presents with supine hypotensive syndrome?

A. Consult the referring clinician.

B. Roll her into a left lateral decubitus position.

C. Rule out fetal anomalies by performing a targeted scan.

D. Take vital signs.

E. Immediately send the patient to the emergency room.

36. Which of the following measurements at 5–10 weeks suggests an abnormal secondary yolk sac?

A. < 5 mm

B. < 2 mm

C. < 6 mm

D. > 3 mm

E. < 4 mm

37. Nuchal fold thickness is measured at the level of the:

A. Thalami

B. Cerebellum

C. Falx

D. Third ventricle

E. Cerebral ventricles

38. Which of the following symptoms would make you suspect a missed abortion?

A. A fetus large for gestational age

B. Bleeding with cramping

C. Abdominal pain with or without bleeding

D. Hyperemesis gravidarum

E. There are no definitive symptoms associated with a missed abortion.

39. Which of the following statements is most often correct for ovarian tumors?

A. Most are malignant.

B. Most occur premenopausally.

C. Most are solid.

D. Most are benign.

E. Most are androgenic.

40. Where should you place the spectral range gate (sample volume) when conducting a Doppler study of the uterine artery?

A. Mid-vessel, with strongest color signal

B. Near the cervix

C. Near the origin of the uterine artery at the internal iliac artery

D. Anywhere along the course of the uterine artery

41. On which day of the menstrual cycle are the levels of estradiol and follicle-stimulating hormone lowest?

A. Day 4

B. Day 2

C. Day 15

D. Day 28

E. Day 3

42. The growth asymmetry associated with a large-for-gestational-age fetus is usually recognized at:

A. 16–20 weeks

B. 34–36 weeks

C. 20–24 weeks

D. 24–28 weeks

E. 28–32 weeks

43. Amniotic fluid does *not*:

A. Support fetal lung development

B. Absorb shock from abrupt motion

C. Support the musculoskeletal system's normal development

D. Nourish the fetus

E. Regulate fetal temperature

44. A nabothian cyst is found in the:

A. Vagina

B. Endometrium

C. Broad ligament

D. Ovary

E. Cervix

45. At the 12–16-cell stage, the fertilized egg is called a:

A. Zygote

B. Blastocyst

C. Blastomere

D. Morula

E. Ovum

46. During labor, which process is associated with the obliteration of the cervix?

A. Funneling

B. Effacement

C. Atrophy

D. Engorgement

E. Degeneration

47. Which are the primary vessels that deliver blood to the pelvic organs?

A. Spermatic arteries

B. Gonadal arteries

C. Internal iliac arteries

D. External iliac arteries

48. A cerclage procedure would *not* be indicated for which condition?

A. Preterm labor

B. Placenta previa

C. Multiple gestations

D. Incompetent cervix

E. Habitual abortion

49. The appearance of multiple joint contractures should make one suspect:

A. Arthrogryposis

B. Osteogenesis imperfecta

C. Thanatophoric dwarfism

D. Achondrogenesis

E. Cubitus varus

50. The pelvic mass that can be missed because it resembles the urinary bladder is the:

A. Hemorrhagic corpus luteum cyst

B. Theca-lutein cyst

C. Cystadenoma

D. Benign cystic teratoma

E. Paraovarian cyst

51. Which procedure involves the introduction of radiopaque dye into the uterus and fallopian tubes for x-ray visualization?

A. Sonohysterography

B. Endoscopy

C. Hysterography

D. Hysteroscopy

E. Laparoscopy

52. The best time to perform chorionic villus sampling (CVS) is at:

    A. 16–18 weeks

    B. 10–12 weeks

    C. 4–6 weeks

    D. 20 weeks or later

    E. 14–16 weeks

53. The amniotic fluid index serves the following function:

    A. It is part of the basic guidelines for performing obstetric sonograms.

    B. It is a method for performing an amniocentesis.

    C. It is a means of calculating amniotic fluid qualitatively.

    D. It is a means of calculating amniotic fluid quantitatively.

    E. It is not reliable as a method for evaluating the level of amniotic fluid.

54. Which images are *not* required to meet the guidelines for the basic scan?

    A. All four fetal extremities

    B. Fetal hands and feet

    C. Umbilical cord insertion into the fetal abdomen

    D. Three-vessel cord

    E. Four-chamber view of the heart

55. Although individuals vary, most will complete the four phases of mourning within:

    A. 9 months

    B. 24 months

    C. 12 months

    D. 18 months

    E. 5 years

56. The valve imaged between the left atrium and left ventricle of the fetal heart is the:

    A. Foramen ovale

    B. Pulmonary

    C. Aortic

    D. Mitral

    E. Tricuspid

57. Assisted reproductive technology can be associated with an increased risk of:

    A. Ectopic pregnancy

    B. Uterine rupture

    C. Endometriosis

    D. Pelvic inflammatory disease

    E. Ovarian cancer

58. Fetal blood transfusion is rarely successful before how many weeks' gestation?

    A. 22 weeks

    B. 26 weeks

    C. 18 weeks

    D. 24 weeks

    E. 20 weeks

59. Which of the following conditions is associated with the double bubble sign?

    A. Patent urachus

    B. Duodenal atresia

    C. Choledochal cyst

    D. Bilateral hydroceles

    E. Meconium peritonitis

60. Diastolic runoff into a distal vascular bed is best indicated by the:

    A. Resistivity index

    B. Pulsatility index

    C. S/D ratio

    D. End-diastolic velocity

61. The examiner can eliminate a split-image artifact by:

    A. Instructing the patient to take and hold a deep breath.

    B. Changing the transducer's focus.

    C. Changing the transducer's frequency.

    D. Administering an enema to the patient.

    E. Scanning from a different projection.

62. Which is the most common ovarian tumor among patients 20 years of age and younger?

    A. Dysgerminoma

    B. Cystic teratoma

    C. Fibroma

    D. Brenner tumor

    E. Cystadenoma

63. Alobar holoprosencephaly is often associated with:

    A. Down syndrome

    B. Triploidy

    C. Patau syndrome

    D. Aneuploidy

    E. Edwards syndrome

64. Which statement is true of 3D imaging?

    A. Volume sonography is used primarily in the specialties of cardiology and obstetrics.

    B. Anomalies that cannot be seen with 2D images are well demonstrated with 3D.

    C. Because fetal skin and subcutaneous tissues are not developed enough to visualize, 3D imaging is useful in the first trimester.

    D. Motion artifacts make it impossible to evaluate the fetal heart with 3D/4D.

65. Dizygotic twins are not:

    A. Considered identical twins

    B. Always diamniotic

    C. The most common type of twins

    D. Chromosomally different

    E. Always dichorionic

66. All of the following statements about fetal hydronephrosis are true *except*:

    A. It affects females less frequently than males.

    B. It is the most common fetal renal abnormality.

    C. By the third trimester the AP diameter of the renal pelvis should be greater than 10 mm.

    D. The ends of the calyces are rounded.

    E. The ratio of the renal pelvis AP diameter to the kidney diameter should be less than 50%.

67. A placenta with two equal lobes connected by vessels is a:

    A. Lobar placenta

    B. Circumvallate placenta

    C. Bipartite placenta

    D. Succenturiate lobe

    E. Membranous placenta

68. In volume sonography, the best method for demonstrating bony structures is:

    A. Surface rendering

    B. Multiplanar viewing

    C. Maximum-intensity projections

    D. Minimum-intensity projections

69. By which gestational age have the amnion and chorion usually fused?

    A. Week 10

    B. Week 14

    C. Week 6

    D. Week 12

    E. Week 8

70. A common characteristic of multicystic dysplastic kidneys is that they are usually:

    A. Unilateral and nonfunctional

    B. Unilateral but functional

    C. Located in the pelvic region

    D. Bilateral but functional

    E. Bilateral and nonfunctional

71. Where can the right ventricle, pulmonary semilunar valve, pulmonary artery, and right atrium be demonstrated?

    A. Aortic arch

    B. Right ventricular outflow tract

    C. Four-chamber view

    D. Five-chamber view

    E. Left ventricular outflow tract

72. At what gestational age is an embryo termed a *fetus*?
    A. 4 weeks
    B. 12 weeks
    C. 6 weeks
    D. 8 weeks
    E. 10 weeks

73. Fetal teratomas are usually located in the:
    A. Neck
    B. Sacrococcygeal region
    C. Mediastinum
    D. Axilla
    E. Face

74. With no evidence of a dilated ureter or bladder, the most likely diagnosis for a fetal kidney with dilation of the renal pelvis would be:
    A. Obstruction at the ureteropelvic junction
    B. Obstruction at the mid-ureteral junction
    C. Renal hypoplasia
    D. Obstruction at the ureterovesical junction
    E. Posterior urethral valves

75. The placenta's primary functions include all of the following *except*:
    A. To protect the fetus from infection
    B. To support the exchange of gases
    C. To transfer antibodies and hormones from the mother to the fetus
    D. To excrete waste through the maternal system
    E. To nourish the fetus

76. For a pregnant woman, blood pressure is considered high if it exceeds:
    A. 110/60 mmHg
    B. 140/90 mmHg
    C. 120/80 mmHg
    D. 135/85 mmHg
    E. 150/100 mmHg

77. Cervical length during pregnancy would be considered abnormal if it measures less than:
    A. 3 cm
    B. 5 cm
    C. 1 cm
    D. 2 cm
    E. 4 cm

78. The most common tumor of placental origin is consider to be the:
    A. Angioma
    B. Hemangioma
    C. Chorioangioma
    D. Angiomyoma
    E. Angiosarcoma

79. Which of the following fetal anomalies is most specifically associated with diabetes mellitus?
    A. Amniotic band syndrome
    B. Caudal regression syndrome
    C. Femoral hypoplasia–unusual facies syndrome
    D. Potter syndrome
    E. Prune belly syndrome

80. A FIRP (First International Reference Preparation) hCG level of 4000 can be expressed in the 2nd IS (Second International Standard) as approximately:
    A. 4000
    B. 8000
    C. 1000
    D. 6000
    E. 2000

81. In an endovaginal, longitudinal image, the patient's feet point toward which part of the image?
    A. Top
    B. Right side
    C. Bottom
    D. Left side
    E. Depends on the patient's position, supine or prone

82. With which of the following is asymmetrical growth restriction usually *not* associated?
    A. Low fetal weight
    B. SGA
    C. Oligohydramnios
    D. Anomalies
    E. Decreased mental capacity

83. At term, the maximum thickness of the placenta of a gestational diabetic should not exceed:
    A. 5–6 cm
    B. 3–4 cm
    C. 4–5 cm
    D. 7–8 cm
    E. 1–2 cm

84. A low level of alpha-fetoprotein in maternal blood could suggest any of the following *except*:
    A. Placental abnormalities
    B. Blighted ovum
    C. Fetal demise
    D. Congenital nephrosis
    E. Down syndrome

85. By approximately what amount does the hematocrit decrease daily in cases of fetal transfusion for fetal anemia?
    A. 2%
    B. 5%
    C. 3%
    D. 4%
    E. 1%

86. Which type of maternal diabetes is most likely to result in severe abnormalities in the fetus?
    A. Type 1 diabetes
    B. Class A diabetes
    C. Gestational diabetes
    D. Borderline diabetes
    E. Type 2 diabetes

87. The term *rhizomelia* denotes shortening of:
    A. The distal end of a limb
    B. The proximal segment of a limb
    C. The distal segment of a limb
    D. The middle segment of a limb
    E. An entire limb

88. In cases of fetal demise, maceration usually becomes sonographically apparent how long afterward?
    A. 24 hours
    B. 12 hours
    C. 1 month
    D. 4 days
    E. 10–14 days

89. In volume sonography, the name for the individual volume elements that create a volume data set obtained from 2D slices for rendering in 3D is:
    A. Frames
    B. Voxels
    C. Pixels
    D. RAM
    E. Bit maps

90. Which distance from the internal cervical os must the placental edge be in order to be considered in a satisfactory position?
    A. 1.5 cm
    B. 2.5 cm
    C. 2.0 cm
    D. 0.5 cm
    E. 1.0 cm

91. Which cardiac abnormality is least likely to be imaged in the four-chamber view of the heart?
    A. An endocardial cushion defect
    B. A ventricular septal defect
    C. Cardiomyopathy
    D. Transposition of the great vessels
    E. Ebstein's anomaly

92. What happens to the functional cervical length as the uterine cervix begins to dilate?

A. It gets shorter.

B. It is unchanged.

C. It becomes more echogenic.

D. It becomes ill defined.

E. It gets longer.

93. All of the following suggest a simple cyst *except*:

A. Poor through-transmission

B. Well-defined outline

C. Refractive edge shadows

D. Posterior enhancement

E. Lack of internal echoes

94. Amnionicity refers to the number of:

A. Ova

B. Placentas

C. Cords

D. Fetuses

E. Sacs

95. The likelihood that an autosomal recessive disorder will be passed to the fetus is:

A. 0%

B. 100%

C. 50%

D. 25%

E. 75%

96. An intrauterine contraceptive device can be associated with all but which of the following complications?

A. Ovarian hyperstimulation

B. Pelvic inflammatory disease

C. Ectopic pregnancy

D. Uterine perforation

E. Menorrhagia

97. At normal term, the placenta should not measure more than:

A. 2–3 cm

B. 4–5 cm

C. 3–4 cm

D. 5–6 cm

E. 1–2 cm

98. Which of the following terms denotes the condition in which the placenta invades the myometrium and penetrates the serosa?

A. Placenta previa

B. Placenta percreta

C. Placental abruption

D. Placenta increta

E. Placenta accreta

99. In a patient with an anteflexed uterus, where does the endometrium point in a sagittal endovaginal image?

A. Right lower corner

B. Left upper corner

C. Left lower corner

D. Middle of the image

E. Right upper corner

100. Which of the following is the most common of the neural tube defects?

A. Hydrocephalus

B. Anencephaly

C. Myelomeningocele

D. Encephalocele

E. Spina bifida

101. Amniocentesis can be associated with all of the following complications *except*:

A. Rupture of membranes

B. Preterm labor

C. Fetal demise

D. Bleeding and cramping

E. Pre-eclampsia

102. Blood-filled masses show less posterior enhancement than those containing pus because:

    A. Blood contains protein and absorbs more sound

    B. Red blood cells refract sound

    C. Blood is thicker than pus

    D. A and B

    E. A and C

103. Amnioinfusion can facilitate all but which of the following?

    A. Amniocentesis

    B. Placing a shunt for bladder outlet obstruction

    C. Fetal lung maturity

    D. Testing for premature rupture of membranes

    E. Visualizing fetal anatomy in cases of oligohydramnios

104. Which of these statements is *not* true with regard to placental circulation?

    A. Deoxygenated blood leaves the fetus by way of the umbilical vein.

    B. The spiral arteries demonstrate low-pressure flow throughout pregnancy.

    C. The umbilical vein provides oxygenated blood to the fetus while the arteries return deoxygenated blood.

    D. Fetal and maternal blood do not mix during pregnancy.

    E. Inadequate blood flow to the uterus can result in fetal hypoxia and intrauterine growth restriction.

105. Which condition is associated with the stuck twin syndrome?

    A. Twin reversed arterial perfusion

    B. Twin-to-twin transfusion syndrome

    C. Vanishing twin syndrome

    D. Conjoined twins

    E. Twin peak

106. All but which of the following structures can be measured for menstrual age?

    A. Cisterna magna

    B. Foot

    C. Cerebellum

    D. Clavicle

    E. Ocular diameters

107. A thin endometrium is characteristic of the following menstrual stage:

    A. Early proliferative

    B. Secretory

    C. Periovulatory

    D. Late proliferative

    E. Preovulatory

108. Acardia is caused by:

    A. Conjoined twins

    B. Twin-to-twin transfusion syndrome

    C. Twin embolization syndrome

    D. Twin reversed arterial perfusion sequence

    E. Stuck twin syndrome

109. Turner syndrome is often associated with:

    A. Omphaloceles

    B. Macroglossia

    C. Cystic hygromas

    D. Sacrococcygeal teratomas

    E. Spina bifida

110. Which laboratory test determines maternal glycemic control?

    A. SMA-12

    B. MSAFP

    C. CEA

    D. HgBA1C

    E. Beta-hCG

111. Which of the following conditions is generally considered incompatible with life?

    A. Down syndrome

    B. Patau syndrome

    C. Turner syndrome

    D. Prune belly syndrome

    E. Beckwith-Wiedemann syndrome

112. With which of the following conditions has caudal regression syndrome been associated?

A. Diabetes mellitus

B. Hyperemesis gravidarum

C. Rh isoimmunization

D. Pregnancy-induced hypertension (PIH)

E. Sickle cell anemia

113. Which statement about bilateral renal agenesis is incorrect?

A. It is accompanied by an increase in the volume of amniotic fluid.

B. Adrenal glands may enlarge and mimic fetal kidneys.

C. It is accompanied by a decrease in amniotic fluid volume.

D. The fetal urinary bladder will not be identified.

E. The condition is terminal.

114. The following is *not* true of the iliac vessels:

A. In the pelvis, the iliac arteries lie anterior to the veins and the ovaries lie medial to both vessels.

B. The ovary can be localized by reference to the external iliac artery.

C. Another name for the internal iliac artery is the hypogastric artery.

D. The branches of the iliac arteries are followed by the pelvic lymph nodes.

E. The internal iliac artery delivers oxygenated blood to the organs of the pelvis.

115. Which sign is associated with thanatophoric dwarfism?

A. Banana head

B. Strawberry head

C. Lemon head

D. Acrania

E. Cloverleaf head

116. All the following conditions exhibit echogenic bowel *except*:

A. Bowel obstruction

B. Down syndrome

C. Cytomegalovirus

D. Cystic fibrosis

E. All of the above

117. In pregnant women, which condition is associated with HELLP syndrome?

A. Rh isoimmunization

B. Pregnancy-induced hypertension

C. Gestational diabetes

D. Maternal gallbladder disease

E. Fetal anemia

118. Which of the following could cause a fetal chest to be smaller than the fetal abdomen?

A. Pulmonary hypoplasia

B. Dwarfism

C. Macrosomia

D. All of the above

E. None of the above

119. Which statement is true?

A. Sonography is an excellent method for imaging the bowel.

B. Contrast agents must be used to image soft tissues.

C. Diagnostic ultrasound can differentiate benign from malignant tissue.

D. Ultrasound imaging can determine organ function and size.

E. A cystic mass can be readily identified with sonography.

120. The part of the heart closest to the anterior chest wall is the:

A. Left atrium

B. Right ventricle

C. Left ventricle

D. Right atrium

E. Aortic arch

121. Which type of physician typically oversees a targeted scan?
    A. Pediatrician
    B. Radiologist
    C. Pathologist
    D. Perinatologist
    E. Obstetrician

122. In the case of a pregnancy with twins, which of the following would require a cesarean section?
    A. Diamniotic twins
    B. Monozygotic twins
    C. A twin that presents breech
    D. Growth discordancy
    E. Monochorionic twins

123. Which ovarian tumor is androgenic?
    A. Fibroma
    B. Arrhenoblastoma
    C. Granulosa cell
    D. Krukenberg tumor
    E. Brenner tumor

124. The landmark for locating the atria of the lateral ventricles is:
    A. The periventricular vasculature
    B. The cisterna magna
    C. The cavum septum pellucidum
    D. The corpus callosum
    E. The choroid plexus

125. If you cannot visualize the fetal gallbladder in the third trimester, the following condition might be affecting the fetus:
    A. Bowel atresia
    B. Cystic fibrosis
    C. Sickle cell anemia
    D. Choledochal cyst
    E. Down syndrome

126. Hematocolpos is most often caused by:
    A. Cervical cancer
    B. Bladder-vaginal fistula
    C. Vaginal agenesis
    D. Imperforate hymen
    E. Acquired gynatresia

127. Chorionic villus sampling is appropriate for all but which of the following objectives?
    A. Performing a karyotype
    B. Examining chromosomes
    C. Ruling out spina bifida
    D. Identifying an inherited disorder
    E. Ruling out Down syndrome

128. In patients with diabetes, which is *not* true of color Doppler and waveform analysis?
    A. The technique assists in diagnosing heart defects.
    B. It provides conclusive evidence of an "at risk" pregnancy.
    C. It assists in physiologic evaluation of placental circulation.
    D. It assists in evaluation of fetal well-being.
    E. It can play a valuable role in evaluating high-risk pregnancies.

129. Which term refers to the space between the anterior uterus and the posterior bladder?
    A. Posterior cul-de-sac
    B. Space of Retzius
    C. Pouch of Douglas
    D. Fornix
    E. Anterior cul-de-sac

130. A limb missing below the elbow or knee is called:
    A. Micromelia
    B. Mesomelia
    C. Phocomelia
    D. Rhizomelia
    E. Hemimelia

131. Polyhydramnios is associated with all but which of the following?

    A. Prematurity

    B. Anomalies

    C. Placental abruption

    D. Fetal demise

    E. Premature rupture of membranes

132. A pregnancy is evaluated by a targeted scan in order to assess:

    A. Placental location

    B. Fetal anomalies

    C. Fetal gender

    D. Multiple gestations

    E. All of the above

133. A profile view of the fetal face will fail to reveal which anomaly?

    A. Micrognathia

    B. Hypotelorism

    C. Prominent occiput

    D. Cleft lip

    E. Frontal bossing

134. Spectral Doppler waveforms from arteries that supply trophoblastic tissue demonstrate:

    A. High-amplitude, low-resistance flow

    B. Low-amplitude, monophasic flow

    C. High-amplitude, high-resistance flow

    D. High-amplitude, triphasic flow

135. A compromised pregnancy is *not* associated with which of these Doppler ultrasound findings?

    A. Increasing resistance on serial surveillance

    B. Decreasing resistance on serial surveillance

    C. Diastolic notching

    D. Diastolic flow reversal

136. Which sonographic mode best displays the soft tissues of the fetal face?

    A. Multiplanar

    B. Brightness

    C. Maximum-intensity

    D. Surface rendering

137. Holoprosencephaly is characteristically accompanied by:

    A. Acrania

    B. Cystic hygroma

    C. Cleft defects

    D. Bowed limbs

    E. Encephalocele

138. The growth of twins is termed *discordant* if:

    A. One of the amniotic sacs has polyhydramnios

    B. The twins' abdominal circumferences differ by 5 mm

    C. Their cephalic indices are different

    D. Their weights differ by more than 500 grams

    E. Their biparietal diameters differ by 2 mm

139. Singleton charts for gestational age can be used for twin and other multiple gestations until which gestational age?

    A. 30 weeks

    B. 35 weeks

    C. 40 weeks

    D. 13 weeks

    E. 25 weeks

140. Adhesions in the endometrial cavity are called:

    A. Adenomyosis

    B. Synechiae

    C. Fibroids

    D. Polyps

    E. Mucosa

141. You should always be able to detect a fetal pole with cardiac motion by the time the gestational sac diameter measures:

    A. 3.5 mm

    B. 2.5 cm

    C. 2 mm

    D. 2 cm

    E. 3 cm

142. What is the term for twins joined at the pelvic region?

A. Craniopagus

B. Xiphopagus

C. Omphalopagus

D. Thoracopagus

E. Pygopagus

143. A ruptured amniotic band can cause which of the following abnormalities?

A. Renal agenesis

B. Situs inversus

C. Facial clefts

D. Alobar holoprosencephaly

E. Duodenal atresia

144. By which gestational age is ossification of the lumbosacral region of the fetal spine sufficient to rule out spina bifida?

A. 12 weeks

B. 16 weeks

C. 10 weeks

D. 18 weeks

E. 14 weeks

145. The most common ovarian condition associated with molar pregnancy is:

A. Polycystic ovaries

B. Theca-lutein cysts

C. Multicystic ovary

D. Hemorrhagic follicular cyst

E. Corpus luteum cyst

146. The cephalic index is performed to identify:

A. Head shape

B. Brain volume

C. Growth restriction

D. Gestational age

E. Hydrocephalus

147. The normal gestational sac should grow at the following daily rate for up to 10 weeks:

A. 1–2 mm

B. 2–3 mm

C. 4–5 mm

D. 3–4 mm

E. 5–6 mm

148. Immune hydrops is caused by:

A. Pregnancy-induced hypertension

B. Diabetes

C. TORCH infections

D. Rh incompatibility

E. Twin-to-twin transfusion syndrome

149. Which condition is *not* associated with gastroschisis?

A. Preterm delivery

B. Elevated alpha-fetoprotein

C. Growth restriction

D. Bowel obstructions

E. Chromosomal abnormalities

150. Which of the following is *not* true regarding grief?

A. Children and adults grieve differently.

B. Young children should be protected from death and grief.

C. Grief should be shared.

D. Almost any feeling associated with grief is normal.

E. Grief can cause physical symptoms.

Answers to Self-Assessment Exercises

CHAPTER 1

1. B is correct: *Linear.* Linear transducers produce a rectangular format. All of the others produce a triangular or wedge-shaped image.

2. D is correct: *A cystic mass can be readily identified with sonography.* Diagnostic ultrasound is of limited value in evaluating the lungs and bowel because air reflects sound, and because it is not sensitive for evaluating function since the outline of the organ will be demonstrated, if present, whether it functions or not. One of the major advantages of diagnostic ultrasound is that it images soft tissue structures without contrast introduction, and cysts can be readily differentiated from solid structures.

3. C is correct: *Poor through-transmission.* The major characteristics for a cyst include posterior enhancement or "through-transmission," which indicates the fluid component, good outline, no internal echoes, and edge shadows. Poor sound transmission through a structure indicates that something is solid or contains something that is highly reflective.

4. E is correct: *A and C.* Abscesses and hematomas can look very similar and vary greatly in echogenicities depending on the stage of the process. However, pus will transmit sound better unless it contains gas-forming organisms.

5. C is correct: *Complex cystic.* Complex masses include those that are predominantly cystic with only some solid parts, those that are predominantly solid with only a small portion of fluid component, and those that contain thick fluid. This is typical of a cyst containing some debris. It has all the characteristics of a cyst, except that it contains echoes.

6. B is correct: *Posterior enhancement.* Posterior enhancement or "through-transmission" is demonstrated by exaggerated echoes (brighter than surrounding echoes) behind a fluid-containing structure.

7. C is correct: *The right side of the image.* See the section headed "Image Orientation" in the section headed "Introduction to Transvaginal Technique."

8. A is correct: *The top of the image.* See the section headed "Introduction to Transvaginal Technique."

9. A is correct: *Solid.* The mass is isoechoic with the uterine myometrium and most likely represents a fibroid, a benign tumor composed of muscle and connective tissues.

10. B is correct: *Retroflexed.* One demonstrates the levo-posed and dextroposed positions from a transverse orientation. Sonography is not a good technique for demonstrating prolapse. If the uterus is anteflexed, transvaginally, the endometrium should point toward the left lower corner of the image.

11. C is correct: *Fluid in the posterior cul-de-sac.* Because the uterus is retroflexed, this fluid would be in the posterior cul-de-sac. The bladder, if seen, would be at the left upper corner of the image, as would the anterior cul-de-sac. The endometrial stripe is clearly imaged and thin.

12. D is correct: *Left lower corner.* See the section headed "Image Orientation." in the section headed "Introduction to Transvaginal Technique."

13. C is correct: *Right side of the image.*

14. E is correct: *It is used to punish the patient.* The split image is produced by scanning through the abdominal wall musculature. Only a change in transducer position will eliminate the problem.

15. A is correct: *Scanning from a different projection.*

CHAPTER 2

1. B is correct: *Cystic teratoma.* The dysgerminoma is a solid malignant tumor seen in the 20–30-year age group and is rare. The other tumors are mostly seen in peri- and postmenopausal women.

2. A is correct: *Normal ovary.* Multicystic and hyper-stimulated ovaries usually are enlarged and would show cysts abutting each other with little visible ovarian parenchyma. Polycystic ovaries show tiny peripheral follicles with ovarian tissue centrally compressed. The postmenopausal ovary should not show follicles at all.

3. D is correct: *Cervix.* Broad ligament cysts are located separate from the ovary. The others listed usually are ovarian in origin and often show complex or mixed components.

4. E is correct: *Pelvic inflammatory disease.* This syndrome causes perihepatitis from pelvic inflammation migrating into the abdomen. A fibroma might be associated with Meigs syndrome, and carcinoid syndrome might be associated with ovarian cancer.

5. D is correct: *Levator ani.* The obturator internus muscles form the lateral pelvic sidewall. The ilio-psoas are anterior to the iliac wing of the pelvis.

The coccygeus muscles are more anterior than the piriformis.

6. B is correct: *Endometrioma.* Cystadenomas and dermoids are often asymptomatic. Fibroids usually cause lumbar pain. Hemorrhagic cysts are usually not regularly cyclic.

7. A is correct: *Anterior cul-de-sac.* The posterior cul-de-sac and pouch of Douglas are located between the uterus and rectum. The fornix is around the cervix. The space of Retzius is between the pubic bone and anterior bladder.

8. E is correct: *Arrhenoblastoma.* All of the other tumors listed are usually estrogenic.

9. A is correct: *Hirsutism.* All of the other symptoms would arise from estrogenic sources.

10. B is correct: *Shadowing from a myomatous uterus.* Normal bowel would not cause these symptoms, which are classic for fibroids. Adenomyosis would cause streaky shadows to emanate from the uterine body. The cystic teratoma would also show some cystic component and be adnexal in location. Poor time gain compensation would affect the whole image in that section.

11. B is correct: *Anteflexed.* When the bladder is fully distended, the uterus is anteverted, but most of us do not maintain a fully distended bladder. Retroverted/retroflexed is an abnormal backward tilt, and a levo-posed uterus deviates to the left of midline as a result of congenital anomaly or pathology.

12. C is correct: *Imperforate hymen.* Cervical cancer is usually diagnosed before it causes such an obstruction. The other choices are rather uncommon.

13. D is correct: *Ovarian hyperstimulation.* Intrauterine contraceptive devices (IUCDs) do not produce hormones that stimulate the ovaries. By irritating the uterine lining IUCDs can cause heavier menses, and there may be a higher incidence of infection. The effectiveness of IUCDs is approximately 98%, and the incidence of ectopic pregnancy is increased.

14. E is correct: *Paraovarian cyst.* Paraovarian cysts are usually simple, unilocular, and large. The other masses listed are usually complex in appearance.

15. A is correct: *Early proliferative.* Late proliferative, peri-ovulatory, and preovulatory phases show a multilayered endometrium. The secretory phase is thick and echogenic.

16. B is correct: *Anteflexed.* Transvaginal images are performed with the bladder empty. A normal uterus is anteverted when the bladder is well distended. With the retroflexed/retroverted uterus, the endometrium points toward the right lower corner of the image. Dextroposition cannot be determined from a longitudinal scan.

17. C is correct: *Ovary.* Muscles are striated and more elongated. Pelvic lymph nodes are not well imaged and, if enlarged, would be multiple and clustered, creating a lobulated appearance. A simple cyst would show some posterior enhancement, and fibroids are usually uterine in origin. Ligamentous fibroids are not common.

18. B is correct: *Most are benign.* The most common ovarian neoplasm in teenage women is the dermoid, which is complex. The most common neoplasm in reproductive and menopausal women is the cystadenoma. Solid, malignant, and androgenic tumors, in general, are not common.

19. E is correct: *They are usually malignant* is *not* true. Only about 2% of dermoids/teratomas are malignant.

20. C is correct: *The external iliac artery can be used to localize the ovary* is the statement that is *not* true. The external iliac artery lies along the top of the iliopsoas muscle anterior to the iliac wing of the pelvis.

CHAPTER 3

1. D is correct: *Ampulla.* Normal fertilization occurs in the lateral one-third or ampullary portion of the fallopian tube. Fertilization in the other areas listed could result in an ectopic pregnancy.

2. B is correct: *Secondary yolk* sac. The primary yolk sac is too small to resolve sonongraphically and develops before all the other structures listed. Identification of the secondary yolk sac is an indication of how many amniotic sacs will be present. The amnion, embryonic disc, and vitelline duct are all seen after visualization of the secondary yolk sac.

3. A is correct: *Decidua basalis. Decidual reaction* refers to the effect of hormone stimulation of the endometrium whether the patient is pregnant or not. During early pregnancy, the *decidua capsularis* is the part of the endometrium covering over the blastocyst. The *decidua vera* and *decidua parietalis* both refer to the rest of the endometrium covering the cavity.

4. E is correct: *Asymptomatic.* A missed abortion refers to demise of the products of conception with failure to expel; it is missed clinically. All the other choices would be clinical indications for a possible problem.

5. E is correct: *12.* Prior to 12 weeks, herniation of the intestines into the base of the umbilical cord is normal because of rapid organ growth.

6. B is correct: *Ampullary.* All of the other choices are considered rare.

7. A is correct: *Theca-lutein cysts.* Excess placental tissue from a mole secretes progesterone and estrogen, which results in bilateral hyperstimulation of the ovaries. Polycystic ovaries are usually associated with infertility, while the other choices are not necessarily related to pregnancy.

8. A is correct: *2 mm.* Normal ranges for the secondary yolk sac are not less than 2 mm and not greater than 6 mm prior to 10 weeks.

9. D is correct: *Morula. Ovum* is the egg, *zygote* is a fertilized egg, *blastomere* is one cell produced by cleavage, and *blastocyst* is the conceptus after the morula stage.

10. C is correct: *8.* All major organ systems have developed by 8 weeks, when an embryo becomes a fetus.

11. B is correct: *2000.* The Second International Standard is always half of the First International Reference Preparation.

12. C is correct: *Embryo with calcified yolk sac.* Secondary yolk sacs should be round and well defined. Those that are flat, irregular in shape, calcified, absent, or solid in appearance would be an indication for an abnormal pregnancy with the possibility of impending abortion.

13. A is correct: *Ectopic pregnancy.* The image shows the uterus to be empty, which rules out threatened abortion and trophoblastic disease. With an hCG level of 5730, one should be able to see an intrauterine gestational sac. There is a mass in the right adnexa that could be a hemorrhagic corpus luteum, but this patient has the classic triad for ectopic pregnancy. Round ligament pain would not be something identified on a sonographic image.

14. C is correct: *Incomplete abortion.* The uterus contains tissue but shows nothing that represents a normal pregnancy. An ectopic pregnancy or pseudocyesis would present with an empty uterus. Molar tissue

usually shows multiple cystic areas representative of hydropic changes within the placenta.

15. B is correct: *Molar pregnancy.* The patient's symptoms and evidence in this image present a classic history for a molar pregnancy.

16. C is correct: *Vitelline duct.* This is the structure connected to the round, cystic yolk sac. The amnion is a thin membrane closely related to and surrounding the embryo. Only limb buds are seen at this stage, and it is too early to see a well-defined umbilical cord.

17. D is correct: *Rhombencephalon.* This is in the fetal head and is a normal structure. One cannot diagnose an enlarged ventricle at this stage. The heart and stomach would be below, while the yolk sac is outside the fetus.

18. E is correct: *Abnormal yolk sac.* The gestational sac and embryo appear normal for the stage of pregnancy; however, the yolk sac should not be so large in comparison with the embryonic pole.

19. D is correct: *12.* Fusion of the amnion and chorion in some cases may be delayed until 16 weeks but should not be seen separately after that. Most will fuse by 12 weeks.

20. A is correct: *1–2 mm/day.*

CHAPTER 4

1. E is correct: *To provide nourishment.* The fetus is nourished by the placenta through the umbilical cord.

2. B is correct: *Choroid plexus.* This structure is located between the medial and lateral walls of the ventricles of the brain and serves as a landmark after 18 weeks.

3. C is correct: *Cisterna magna.*

4. D is correct: *Transversely, one can see one posterior and two anterior ossification centers.*

5. E is correct: *Mitral.*

6. C is correct: *Transposition of the great vessels.*

7. D is correct: *Right ventricle.*

8. E is correct: *Fetal hands and feet.*

9. A is correct: *Head shape.*

10. B is correct: *Fetal demise.* Polyhydramnios is associated with gastrointestinal, central nervous system, and chromosomal anomalies but not demise; oligohydramnios is associated with fetal demise.

11. B is correct: *Anomalies.* A targeted scan will be ordered to enhance detection of abnormalities in high-risk pregnancy; indications include (among many others) substance abuse, maternal compromise because of infection or conditions such as diabetes, and advanced maternal age.

12. E is correct: *1.0 to 2.5 mm.* From gestational weeks 11 to 14, normal nuchal translucency is 1.0 to 2.5 mm, and measurements exceeding 3.0 mm are considered abnormal.

13. B is correct: *Hypotelorism.* Hypotelorism would be seen on the binocular or frontal view of the face.

14. D is correct: *A and B.*

15. B is correct: *Situs transversus. Situs solitus* refers to the normal position of anatomy, *levocardia* refers to the normal angle of the heart toward the left side of the body, and *organomegaly* means enlarged organs.

16. D is correct: *Bowel obstruction.*

17. A is correct: *Clinodactyly.* The lack of or hypoplasia of the middle phalanx of the fifth digit causes the fifth digit to curve toward the fourth digit. *Syndactyly* is fusion of digits, *Down syndrome* is associated with (not caused by) hypoplasia if the middle phalanx of the fifth digit, and *adactyly* is absence of digits.

18. E is correct: *Perinatologist.*

19. B is correct: *15 and 20 weeks.*

20. D is correct: *5 mm.* Formerly the threshold was 6 mm, but the current consensus is that 5 mm is a more sensitive threshold.

21. E is correct: *Cerebellum.*

22. C is correct: *Right ventricular outflow tract.*

23. A is correct: *Aortic arch.*

24. E is correct: *All of the above.*

25. C is correct: *Cystic fibrosis.*

CHAPTER 5

1. D is correct: *4–5 cm.* At 20 weeks, the placenta measure 2–3 cm and at term should measure no more than 4–5 cm. Small placentas put the fetus at risk for intrauterine growth restriction (IUGR). Thick placentas may indicate edema.

2. B is correct: *Intrauterine growth restriction.* Intrauterine growth restriction is associated with a placenta that is small and reaches grade III prior to 35 weeks.

3. A is correct: *Endometrium. Myometrium* is the muscle layer of the uterus. *Perimetrium* is the thin, serous outer layer.

4. C is correct: *Chorioangioma.*

5. B is correct: *Deoxygenated blood leaves the fetus by way of the umbilical vein.*

6. C is correct: *Grade III.* As shown in Figure 5-11A, Grannum's grade III placenta displays large calcifications and indentations of the basal plate.

7. D is correct: *Retroplacental vessels.* The venous channels behind the placenta may be mistaken for an abruption on an image, but the patient would not have the classic symptoms associated with abruptio placentae.

8. B is correct: *Posterior.*

9. C is correct: *Retroplacental space.* The key word here is *asymptomatic,* which rules out abruption and subchorionic hematoma. Contractions will ultimately relax.

10. A is correct: *Bipartite placenta.*

11. B is correct: *Placenta previa.* Symptoms are classic for placenta previa. Except for marginal placenta, all other choices would present with pain.

12. D is correct: *Placenta percreta.* Abruption tears away preterm, previa is where the placenta is presenting, accreta adheres to myometrium, and increta invades myometrium.

13. E is correct: *Facial clefts.* All other choices are anomalies that occur within the fetus developmentally.

14. D is correct: *2.0 cm.*

15. C is correct: *Protects the fetus from infection.* Infection can actually be transmitted to the fetus across the placenta.

CHAPTER 6

1. C is correct: *3 cm.* The cervix can be quite long during pregnancy but rarely exceeds 6 cm. Cervical length should not be less than 3 cm; otherwise dilation would be suspected.

2. D is correct: *Transvaginal sonography.* Transabdominal imaging can falsely elongate measurements of the cervix depending on the degree to which the maternal bladder is distended. Overlying bowel gas in the rectum makes it difficult to image the external os using transperineal or translabial techniques.

3. B is correct: *Gets shorter.* As the cervix dilates, one loses the ability to see the cervical tissue, a condition known as effacement.

4. A is correct: *Funneling.* If the membranes have ruptured (PROM), the endocervical canal cannot be seen. Preterm labor does not necessarily have to be associated with a visibly dilated cervix.

5. E is correct: *Effacement.* Atrophy and degeneration suggest a pathologic event. Engorgement usually denotes enlargement of ducts or vessels, while funneling refers to the bulging of intact membranes within the endocervical canal.

6. B is correct: *Shirodkar cerclage.* Although a *McDonald's procedure* is a type of cerclage suture, it does not require a c-section delivery. A *Valsalva maneuver* is a bearing down on abdominal muscles as if one were trying to have a bowel movement. *Effacement* refers to cervical shortening due to dilation. A *digital examination* is performed by a clinician to palpate the cervix.

7. E is correct: *Placenta previa.* A transvaginal ultrasound of the cervix might be performed in the second or third trimester to rule out placenta previa but is not performed or required as a prophylactic measure.

8. D is correct: *Internal iliac arteries.*

9. B is correct: *Funnel with a shortened cervical length.*

10. A is correct: *Posterior placenta that completely covers the internal cervical os.*

CHAPTER 7

1. C is correct: *Anencephaly.*

2. A is correct: *Chromosomal abnormalities.*

3. A is correct: *Esophageal atresia.*

4. D is correct: *Cleft defects.* Alobar holoprosencephaly is associated with trisomy 13, and severe cleft defects are common. They may also show a proboscis. Cystic hygromas are associated with Turner syndrome, while bowed limbs are associated with dwarfism.

5. B is correct: *Cystic fibrosis.*

6. B is correct: *Holoprosencephaly.*

7. E is correct: *Transposition of the great vessels.* Anomalies that are difficult to identify with the four-chamber view also include truncus arteriosus, coarctation of the aorta, and very small ventricular septal defects.

8. C is correct: *Microcystic adenomatoid malformation.* Both pulmonary sequestration and microcystic adenomatoid malformations appear as hyperechoic masses adjacent to or within the lung and cause displacement of the heart. Although a right-sided diaphragmatic hernia may appear as a solid mass in the chest, the liver is less echogenic than lung tissue.

9. E is correct: *18 weeks' gestation.*

10. E is correct: *Sacrococcygeal region.* Sacrococcygeal teratomas are the most common tumor seen in newborns.

11. B is correct: *Porencephaly.*

12. A is correct: *Arthrogryposis.*

13. A is correct: *Cloverleaf-shaped head.* The strawberry shape is associated with trisomy 18 and the lemon shape is associated with the Arnold-Chiari malformation type II. Acrania is a brain without skull. There is no banana head.

14. D is correct: *Proximal segment of a limb.* A and B refer to acromelia, C to mesomelia, and E to micromelia.

15. B is correct: *Rachischisis.* Also referred to as *myeloschisis. Scoliosis* is lateral curvature of spine, *kyphosis* is a hump back, *lordosis* is a swayback, and *platyspondylisis* (also called platyspondyly) is a flattening or widening of the vertebral bodies.

16. E is correct: *Hemimelia.*

17. C is correct: *Achondroplasia.*

18. B is correct: *Duodenal atresia.* Massive polyhydramnios is also evident.

19. A is correct: *Holoprosencephaly.* Holoprosencephaly is often associated with severe cleft defects of the face, severe hypotelorism, and proboscis. These findings usually indicate trisomy 13.

20. C is correct: *Duodenal atresia.* The classic double-bubble finding is associated with duodenal atresia. This can be an isolated finding, which is more common in males, or it can be associated with Down syndrome.

21. C is correct: *Spina bifida with myelomeningocele.* Spina bifida occulta would not present with a mass and is usually difficult to see sonographically. A meningocele would be cystic. A teratoma would not show a spinal defect, and in rachischisis the spine is open throughout its length and the spinal cord is exposed.

22. E is correct: *Extracorporeal liver.* With gastroschisis, the herniated bowel is free-floating, and extralobar sequestration involves an accessory lung lobe. A simple umbilical hernia would not be this severe. The prune belly syndrome involves severe distention of the urinary bladder.

23. B is correct: *Sacrococcygeal teratoma.*

24. B is correct: *Lemon.*

25. A is correct: *Arnold-Chiari malformation.*

26. D is correct: *Spina bifida.*

27. E is correct: *Hydrocephaly.*

CHAPTER 8

1. C is correct: *Helps regulate fetal blood flow.* Fetal blood flow can be affected by a number of conditions, including those that cause IUGR, placental abnormalities, cord anomalies, and others. Lack of blood flow to the fetal kidneys will cause decreased renal function, resulting in oligohydramnios, but has nothing to do with regulation of the fetal blood flow.

2. B is correct: *It is a quantitative means of calculating amniotic fluid.* "Eyeballing" fluid levels is a qualitative means of evaluating amniotic fluid used by experienced practitioners. The amniotic fluid index (AFI) is an accepted practice and considered reliable. Although an adequate fluid pocket is necessary for amniocentesis, the AFI is not a method for performing the procedure.

3. A is correct: *Lack of cardiac activity demonstrated during real-time examination is the most accurate means of diagnosing fetal demise.* Although *Spalding's sign* is specific for fetal demise, it refers to the collapse and overlapping of fetal cranial bones. *Anasarca* refers to scalp edema and can be associated with demise but also with hydrops and chromosomal abnormalities. Once cardiac motion can be detected sonographically (5–6 weeks transvaginally and 7–8 weeks transabdominally), embryonic as well as fetal demise can be verified.

4. B is correct: *2.5 cm.* With a normal pregnancy, when the gestational sac measures 2.5 cm, one should be able to identify a fetal pole with a heartbeat.

5. B is correct: *Increased fundal height.* With fetal demise, the uterus usually stops growing. Therefore, in most cases the patient presents small for gestational

age. Lack of uterine growth with no detectable fetal movement or heart tones is highly suspicious for demise. An enlarging uterus suggests continued growth of the pregnancy.

6. A is correct: *There is an increase in amniotic fluid volume.* Since the fetal kidneys are responsible for the production of amniotic fluid, no kidneys would mean no fluid in the fetal bladder or amniotic sac. If the kidneys are absent, the large fetal adrenal glands will fill the renal fossae and may look like elongated, flat kidneys.

7. B is correct: *Hyperechoic appearance.* With infantile polycystic kidneys, the cysts are very small and often difficult to appreciate sonographically. The process causes bilateral enlargement of the kidneys, and they have a bright spongy appearance. Usually they maintain their reniform shape.

8. D is correct: *Unilateral and nonfunctional.* Although the multicystic kidney does not function well if at all, the condition is usually unilateral; therefore the opposite kidney compensates for the loss of function on the multicystic side. When multicystic dysplasia is bilateral, usually one kidney is affected more than the other, with some function present.

9. B is correct: *There is an obstruction at the urethral outflow tract.* When the entire urinary tract is obstructed, the source is usually PUV. UPJ obstructions affect the kidneys only, not the ureters and bladder. The prognosis for bilateral obstruction depends on when the process develops and whether intervention can be performed to salvage at least one kidney and allow for enough amniotic fluid production so that the lungs can develop properly.

10. A is correct: *The ratio of the renal pelvis AP diameter to the kidney diameter should be less than 50%.*

11. A is correct: *Obstruction at the ureteropelvic junction (UPJ).* A UVJ and mid-ureteral junction would show hydronephrosis and dilated ureter, usually unilateral. PUV would show dilation of the entire urinary tract including both kidneys, the ureters, and the bladder.

12. C is correct: *It causes unilateral hydronephrosis.* PUV is the result of obstruction at the level of the proximal urethra and results in dilation of the entire urinary tract. Prognosis depends on when the process develops, whether or not the kidneys can be salvaged, and whether or not the fetal lungs have developed. If the

fetus can be delivered and the obstruction relieved, prognosis can be good.

13. D is correct: *Anomalies.* Asymmetric IUGR is caused by an insult late in the pregnancy, and fetuses that can be delivered can experience "catch-up" growth after delivery. When there is an insult to a pregnancy early on, during developmental stages, anomalies are often the result, as seen with symmetric IUGR.

14. A is correct: *Incorrect dates.* Genetic indications should also be considered when evaluating patients for SGA. Parents usually have babies similar to the parents' own size at birth, and smaller people often have smaller babies.

15. C is correct: *Polycystic kidneys.* Normal kidneys show a hyperechoic center and hypoechoic cortex while multicystic and hydronephrotic kidneys are more cystic in appearance.

16. A is correct: *Normal kidneys.* The normal fetal kidney should occupy one-third of the AP or transverse diameter of the fetal abdomen. The fetal kidneys are rounded structures on either side of the spine with a "bull's-eye" appearance, the calyces being central and echogenic and the cortex hypoechoic.

17. C is correct: *Autosomal recessive.* Recessive disorders are usually more serious than dominant disorders, and most cases of infantile polycystic kidney disease are not compatible with life. Autosomal dominant and recessive disorders are hereditary and can be passed on to offspring.

18. D is correct: *10–14 days.* Although the process of maceration begins immediately, it does so in a sterile environment and usually does not become sonographically apparent for 10 to 14 days following fetal demise.

19. B is correct: *Robert's sign. Spalding's sign* refers to collapse and overlapping of cranial bones, *Murphy's sign* refers to gallbladder pain when pressure is applied across the GB region, *Deuel's sign* (the halo sign) is the halo effect that subcutaneous scalp edema produces on radiography of the fetal head in cases of demise, and *Haley's sign* (in reference to the comet) is an irrelevant distractor.

20. A is correct: *Rupture of membranes after 37 weeks' gestation but before onset of labor.*

CHAPTER 9

1. B is correct: *Sacs. Chorionicity* refers to numbers of placentas, and *zygosity* refers to number of eggs fertilized.

2. A is correct: *Trophoblastic disease.* Although trophoblastic disease could occur with a multiple gestation, it usually results from a single gestation where the embryo dies early on and the placenta continues to grow and becomes hydropic. Trophoblastic disease associated with a live fetus is rare.

3. E is correct: *Twin-to-twin transfusion syndrome (TTTS).* Conjoined twins share the same amniotic sac. *TRAP* refers to the acardiac twin malformation, and the *vanishing twin* to when one twin dies in the first trimester and is reabsorbed, resulting in a single gestation at birth. *Twin peak* is a phenomenon in which trophoblastic tissue grows between the amniotic layers, indicating a dichorionic pregnancy.

4. A is correct: *Diamniotic/dichorionic. Diamniotic/ monochorionic* would indicate two sacs and one placenta, *monoamniotic/dichorionic* would indicate one sac and two placentas, *monoamniotic/monochorionic* would indicate one sac and one placenta, and *amniotic band syndrome* occurs when the amniotic membrane separates from the chorion and becomes attached to the fetus.

5. C is correct: *Twin embolization syndrome (TES). Acardiac parabiotic twinning* and *TRAP* refer to the same abnormality, where one twin develops without a heart and is supported by the surviving twin through the sharing of one large circulatory system. *TTTS* results in IUGR of one twin and hydrops in the other as a result of artery-to-vein anastomosis within the common placenta. Dizygotic twins are not at risk for any of these conditions.

6. D is correct: *Thoracopagus. Craniopagus* refers to joined heads, *pygo-* to the anus, *ischio-* to the pelvis, and *omphalo-* to the abdomen.

7. C is correct: *30.* For multiples of three and more the growth diminishes after 20 weeks.

8. C is correct: *Diamniotic.* The root zygote refers to eggs, *amnion* to sacs, and *chorion* to placentas.

9. A is correct: *Zygosity.* The only way zygosity can be determined sonographically is by identifying different sexes between fetuses.

10. D is correct: *They are considered identical twins.* Identical twins are monozygotic, i.e., formed from the fertilization of a single egg that splits into what will become two chromosomally identical individuals.

11. C is correct: *Pygopagus. Cranio-* refers to the head, *thoraco-* to the thorax, *omphalo-* to the abdomen, and *xipho-* to the xiphoid.

12. E is correct: *Their weights differ by more than 500 grams.* A difference of a few millimeters between measurements is not clinically significant. The cephalic index will indicate an abnormal head shape, which is often due to crowding, and affect the BPD measurement, but it should not affect the head circumference for dating and size. Amniotic sacs can have different fluid levels for different reasons and may not always indicate a growth discrepancy.

13. C is correct: *The presenting twin is breech.* This is particularly true if the presenting fetus is a footling or incomplete breech.

14. E is correct: *Twin reversed arterial perfusion (TRAP) sequence.* TTTS and stuck twin syndrome are associated with severe IUGR of one twin and hydrops of the other. Conjoined twins are the result of late splitting (two weeks after fertilization) of a single egg. TES may occur when one twin dies and thromboplastic debris is thrown to the surviving twin through a common placenta, causing obstructions and/or destruction of major organs.

15. D is correct: *Twin-to-twin transfusion syndrome (TTTS).* Simple IUGR can be seen with dichorionic or monochorionic gestations and shows differences in fetal measurements with no other structural abnormalities. TES may cause ischemia, infarction, or even death in the surviving twin. Severe abnormalities of the central nervous, gastrointestinal, and genitourinary systems are not uncommon.

16. B is correct: *Paternal family history.* The female determines the number of fetuses because the number depends on how many eggs are fertilized and on whether or not the fertilized egg splits postfertilization. The male (XY) determines the fetal sex since he contributes either an X or a Y chromosome to the female (XX) chromosome contribution.

17. A is correct: *<2 mm.* Greater than 2 mm would indicate a dichorionic gestation.

18. E is correct: *The twins are diamniotic/dichorionic.* The answer cannot be "identical" because the only way

that can be determined is to identify same sexes with a single placenta. It cannot be "diamniotic/monochorionic" because there is clearly a placenta anterior and one posterior. The twins cannot be conjoined because we see a separating membrane, and discordant growth is determined by fetal measurements.

19. B is correct: *Most complications relate to chorionicity.* Sixty percent of monozygotic twins are diamniotic/monochorionic, 30% are diamniotic/dichorionic, and 10% are monoamniotic/monochorionic. TTTS occurs only when there is a vascular communication between twins in a common placenta. Zygosity refers to the number of eggs fertilized. TES is a complication occurring with monochorionic gestations, but it is not common.

20. C is correct: *Conjoined twins are usually dizygotic.* Conjoined twins are always monozygotic. Several complications are specifically associated with monozygotic twins, including conjoined twins, acardia, and TTTS.

CHAPTER 10

1. C is correct: *Carbohydrates.* Bilirubin is not metabolized but excreted by the liver as a by-product of broken-down red blood cells.

2. D is correct: *28–32 weeks.*

3. C is correct: *4–5 cm.* Maximum dimension at 20 weeks is 2–3 cm.

4. A is correct: *Monozygotic multiple gestations.* Maternal diabetes is associated with a number of malformations but not with multiple births.

5. D is correct: *HgBA1C.* Beta-hCG and MSAFP will determine pregnancy. CEA is a cancer-screening test, and SMA-12 is a blood test that evaluates multiple organ systems for abnormalities.

6. C is correct: *24 and 28 weeks.*

7. B is correct: *Caudal regression syndrome.* Also more common among twin gestations, caudal regression syndrome is 200–600 times more common among diabetics.

8. B is correct: *Type 1 diabetic.* Although the fetuses of all diabetic mothers are at risk for anomalies, the offspring of insulin-dependent diabetics are at significant risk because this type develops earlier in life and carries more significant complications, including circulatory complications, which affect fetal growth.

9. D is correct: *Hyperemesis gravidarum.*

10. B is correct: *It can provide conclusive evidence of the "at risk" pregnancy.* Doppler is used as an adjunct procedure to help confirm suspicious findings and assist with monitoring fetal well-being but should not be considered conclusive.

11. E is correct: *Rh isoimmunization.* The Rh factor is considered an immune cause for hydrops.

12. D is correct: *A and B.* The female estrogenic factors are associated with gallstone formation. Testosterone is the androgenic male hormone.

13. A is correct: *Ectopic pregnancies.* The condition is the result of excess production of estrogens/progesterone. These levels, although present with an ectopic pregnancy, are usually lower than normal.

14. D is correct: *Roll her into a left lateral decubitus position.* This condition is simply the result of the fetus/uterus placing pressure on the maternal IVC and causing a decrease in circulation. A change in maternal position will allow normal blood flow and the symptoms will subside.

15. A is correct: *Pregnancy-induced hypertension.*

16. B is correct: *Progesterone.* Obstruction is the result of hormonal stimulation (progesterone) and mechanical compression of the ureters by the enlarged uterus. Progesterone has a relaxing effect on the smooth muscle of the ureters, which allows for dilation.

17. C is correct: *Cystadenoma.* Although cystadenomas can become quite large, they usually simply displace anatomy painlessly, similar to the way an enlarging pregnant uterus does pain.

18. B is correct: *Rhesus (Rh) incompatibility.* All other choices are causes for nonimmune hydrops.

19. A is correct: *Alpha thalassemia.*

20. E is correct: *Over 140/90 mmHg.*

CHAPTER 11

1. B is correct: *Fetal liver.* Fetal kidneys produce amniotic fluid. The placenta and maternal ovaries produce estrogenic hormones.

2. E is correct: *Congenital nephrosis.* Although demise can be associated with a decrease or increase in AFP (mostly a decrease), the most correct answer would be fetal nephrosis as it causes an elevation in AFP.

3. B is correct: *10–12 weeks.* It is too early for cells to grow out of the specimen at 4–6 weeks. Performing CVS after 12 weeks would require a second trimester abortion if results indicated a serious malformation or syndrome and the patient opted for termination.

4. D is correct: *Down syndrome.* Patau is trisomy 13, Edwards is trisomy 18, and Potter and Meckel syndromes involve the urinary tract.

5. A is correct: *Diabetes mellitus.* Sickle cell anemia and Rh isoimmunization can be associated with hydrops, PIH is associated with IUGR, and hyperemesis can be associated with moles and multiple gestations.

6. E is correct: *Meckel syndrome.* Eagle-Barrett is prune belly syndrome, classic Potter syndrome is bilateral renal agenesis, Potter type I affects infantile kidneys, and Potter type II is multicystic dysplasia.

7. B is correct: *25%.* Dominant disorders carry a 50% chance of being passed on to offspring.

8. A is correct: *Cystic hygromas.* Hydrops may also develop in fetuses with Turner syndrome, but they do not usually show other anomalies.

9. C is correct: *Neural tube defects.* CVS is used to identify chromosomal information.

10. E is correct: *Patau syndrome.* Most infants still viable at birth usually die within a few months.

11. A is correct: *Choroid plexus cysts.*

12. C is correct: *Trisomy 18.*

13. A is correct: *Trisomy 13.*

14. D is correct: *Hypotelorism.*

15. E is correct: *Clubfoot.*

CHAPTER 12

1. B is correct: *Internal iliac arteries. Pelvic organs* is a general term referring to all anatomic structures in the pelvic cavity. The internal iliac arteries are the trunk arteries that direct blood to all of the pelvic organs, and therefore B is the correct answer. The gonadal and spermatic arteries are branches of the internal iliac arteries and supply blood to specific structures. The external iliac artery supplies blood to the lower extremity.

2. A is correct: *Ovarian hyperemia.* Ovarian torsion, which is the twisting of the ovary along its pedicle, results in a diminution or cessation of blood flow into the parenchyma. Hyperemia is a state characterized by an increase in blood flow to an organ. The other choices are, in fact, sonographic findings associated with ovarian torsion.

3. D is correct: *Internal iliac artery Doppler.* Umbilical, fetal cerebral, and uterine artery Doppler studies are all established methods useful in predicting fetal IUGR. Internal iliac artery Doppler has no such use in obstetrics or in any other medical specialty.

4. A is correct: *Pressure of flow.* Ultrasound modalities that present real-time hemodynamic information about a vessel rely on variables included in the Doppler equation. First and foremost, Doppler modalities determine whether flow is present or not (B). Flow direction (C) is displayed based on a positive or a negative Doppler shift, and pulsatility of flow (D) is a real-time display of presence, velocity, and direction of flow over time. Pressure of flow in the blood vessel, while an important hemodynamic factor, cannot be determined using Doppler methods. Sphygmomanometers (blood pressure cuffs) can be used externally to obtain pressures; pressure catheters can be used for internal monitoring of either arterial or venous pressures.

5. D is correct: *Pulsatility index.* Diastolic runoff is a measurement of how much blood continues to flow into a vascular bed after the primary push of systole has subsided. The pulsatility index, which indexes the difference of peak systolic and end-diastolic flow velocities to the average velocity across the cardiac cycle, provides such an indicator. High PI values are associated with little diastolic runoff; low values are consistent with a more robust forward flow during diastole.

6. C is correct: *Early diastolic flow reduction.* The *diastolic notch*—distinct from the *dicrotic notch* referenced in peripheral vascular Doppler studies—is a brief deflection of a spectral waveform obtained from the uterine artery during early diastole. While the hemodynamic mechanism for creation of a diastolic notch is unclear, its appearance early in gestation suggests compromise of placental circulation.

7. A is correct: *High-amplitude, low-resistance flow.* Trophoblastic tissue is metabolically very active. Spectral waveforms obtained from arteries feeding trophoblastic tissue display low-resistance flow, i.e., high-amplitude forward flow throughout the cardiac

cycle, just as they do for arteries feeding other vascular beds that require a constant supply of oxygen and nutrients to meet their very active metabolic needs.

8. A is correct: *The resistance decreases.* Decreasing resistance indicates an increase in demand for the oxygen and metabolites carried by blood. As the uterus prepares for the implantation of a conceptus, the endometrium proliferates under the influence of estrogen.

9. C is correct: *Decreasing resistance on serial surveillance.* Decreasing resistance is a normal finding as a pregnancy progresses. The other choices are all associated with the compromise of a pregnancy.

10. C is correct: *Near the cervix.* All of the protocols employing uterine artery Doppler as an indicator of gestational integrity obtain spectral waveforms from a site near the cervix. Samples should be obtained from uterine arteries on both sides.

CHAPTER 13

1. C is correct: *Varicoceles.* All the choices can be causes of male infertility, but the varicocele is the most common and is correctable.

2. E is correct: *Infertility.* If the FSH is high, the brain has to work harder to stimulate the ovaries.

3. C is correct: *Day 3.*

4. E is correct: *Endometriosis.* Although endometriosis can affect the uterus (adenomyosis), it mostly affects the adnexa. (This question requires the use of deductive reasoning to choose the best answer among several plausible answers—common on the registry examinations.)

5. C is correct: *Hysterogram.* A sonohysterogram is the ultrasound version of imaging the uterine cavity by introducing fluid into the cavity and capturing images with ultrasound. A hysteroscope is a small camera at the end of a tube that is placed inside the uterus through a small incision. Laparoscopy uses a small camera at the end of a tube that is placed through a small incision in the abdomen. The endoscope is placed in the rectum or esophagus for viewing.

6. A is correct: *Ectopic pregnancy.* When more than one embryo is placed in the uterus or fallopian tube, some may migrate and implant in places outside the uterine cavity. With ART methods such as in vitro

fertilization, usually 3–4 are introduced, increasing the risks for abnormal implantation.

7. D is correct: *ZIFT.* Although both GIFT and ZIFT involve placing the egg into the fallopian tube, only in ZIFT is the egg first fertilized in the Petri dish. ZIFT stands for zygote intrafallopian tube transfer. ART stands for assisted reproductive technology, GIFT for gamete intrafallopian tube, IVF for in vitro fertilization, and BBT for basal body temperature.

8. B is correct: *Synechiae.*

9. A is correct: *Ovulation has occurred.* The core body temperature rises about 0.5 degree Fahrenheit upon ovulation.

10. E is correct: *Estradiol.* FSH stimulates follicular growth, LH induces ovulation, progesterone causes symptoms of pregnancy, and clomiphene is a drug used to stimulate follicle growth and maturation. H is a meaningless answer.

CHAPTER 14

1. D is correct: *Dedicated mechanized volume probes.* The dedicated mechanized probes, commonly referred to as volume probes, provide a volume of data that is more spatially and temporally accurate, which allows for more accurate linear and volume measurements.

2. B is correct: *Maximum-intensity projections.* Surface rendering and minimum-intensity projections demonstrate soft tissues and organs, while the multiplanar images show longitudinal, transverse, and coronal planes separately.

3. D is correct: *Volume sonography is mostly used in the cardiology and obstetric specialties.*

4. A is correct: *Voxels.*

5. C is correct: *Surface rendering.* Brightness or B-mode displays images utilizing dots, and the dots create the various multiplanar images. The maximum-intensity projections best demonstrate high-intensity structures such as bone.

6. C is correct: *A and B.* Once a volume scan has been obtained, multiple planes can be reconstructed, allowing all angles of the structure of interest to be viewed.

7. A is correct: *Decreased image quality.* STIC is utilized to increase image quality.

8. B is correct: *Use the lowest frame rate possible.* One should use the highest possible frame rate.

9. A is correct: *Polyhydramnios.* Polyhydramnios would enhance the ability to see fetal structures, while oligohydramnios would be a limiting factor. All other factors limit 2D imaging as well as 3D.

10. D is correct: *Motion.* Motion artifact is the most common artifact and the one over which the sonographer has the least control.

CHAPTER 15

1. D is correct: *To rule out spina bifida.*
2. A is correct: *Pre-eclampsia.*
3. B is correct: *Fetal hydrops due to Rh sensitization.*
4. E is correct: *All of the above.*
5. C is correct: *Twin-to-twin transfusion syndrome.*
6. A is correct: *18 weeks.*
7. A is correct: *1%.*
8. C is correct: *When fetal bradycardia is noted.*
9. C is correct: *To facilitate an amniocentesis.*
10. B is correct: *Pleural effusion.*
11. E is correct: *Spina bifida.*
12. B is correct: *The elevation of the amnion by a needle when the membranes have not fused.*
13. C is correct: *20 gauge.*

CHAPTER 16

1. D is correct: *Social.* Social death is the loss of regular social activities in which one was once able to participate. Casual acquaintances with whom one enjoyed engaging in these activities are often lost, and being confined to the home narrows the opportunities for interacting with others.

2. B is correct: *Biologic.* Biologic death is different from physiologic death because machines will allow the organs to continue their physiologic functions. However, without mechanical assistance, the organs cannot function.

3. A is correct: *Loss.* Loss can be defined in terms of time, physical/emotional relationships, a sense of belonging, a situation, space, or a body part.

4. B is correct: *Bereavement.* Grief is how one feels and psychological death comprises the associated personality changes.

5. C is correct: *Mourning.* Searching and yearning is a phase of the bereavement process; mourning, grief, and depression are all indications of how one may feel after experiencing a loss.

6. A is correct: *Loss is associated only with a death of someone or something loved.* A loss refers to any event that changes the way things have been.

7. E is correct: *24.* Although no one can assign a time frame for mourning, most individuals will begin to feel some renewed energy and show better coping skills after 24 months.

8. C is correct: *Try to be upbeat and always cheerful and encourage the griever to be the same.* It is important to be natural and genuine when offering support, and that does not always mean you have to put on a happy face. You will come across as insincere if you try to mask your own feelings by overcompensating.

9. E is correct: *Mourning and bereavement are synonymous.* Mourning is the actual process of working through and dealing with the conflicts associated with loss. Bereavement describes the signs and symptoms associated with loss.

10. B is correct: *Young children should be protected from death and grief.* Children are people and will vary in how they grieve but they should not be protected from grief. Death is a part of life, and more harm can come from suppressing grief than dealing with it outright. Age-appropriate exchanges with children will help them move through the grieving process in a healthy way.

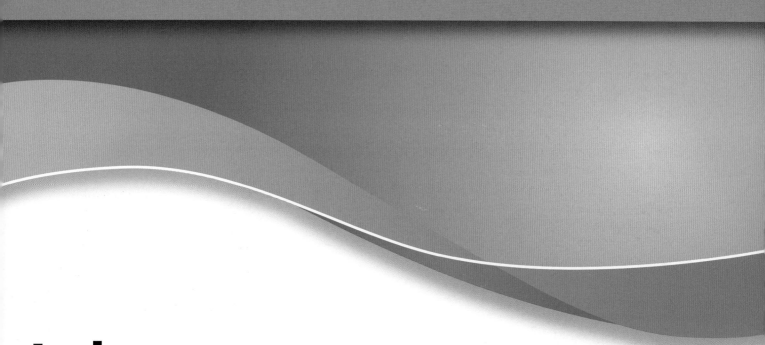

Index